ABroadening the Base of Treatment for Alcohol Problems

Report of a Study by a Committee of the

INSTITUTE OF MEDICINE

Division of Mental Health and Behavioral Medicine

National Academy Press
Washington, D.C. 1990

National Academy Press • **2101 Constitution Avenue, NW** • **Washington, DC 20418**

NOTICE: The project that is the subject of this report was approved by the Governing Board of the National Research Council, whose members are drawn from the councils of the National Academy of Sciences, the National Academy of Engineering, and the Institute of Medicine. The members of the committee responsible for the report were chosen for their special competencies and with regard for appropriate balance.

This report has been reviewed by a group other than the authors according to procedures approved by a Report Review Committee consisting of members of the National Academy of Sciences, the National Academy of Engineering, and the Institute of Medicine.

The Institute of Medicine was chartered in 1970 by the National Academy of Sciences to enlist distinguished members of the appropriate professions in the examination of policy matters pertaining to the health of the public. In this, the Institute acts under both the Academy's 1863 congressional charter responsibility to be an adviser to the federal government and its own initiative in identifying issues of medical care, research, and education.

The work on which this publication is based was performed pursuant to Contract No. ADM-281-87-003 with the National Institute on Alcohol Abuse and Alcoholism of the Department of Health and Human Services.

Library of Congress Cataloging-in-Publication Data

Institute of Medicine (U.S.)
    Broadening the base of treatment for alcohol problems : report of
a study by a committee of the Institute of Medicine, Division of
Mental Health and Behavioral Medicine.
        p.   cm.
    "Committee for the Study of Treatment and Rehabilitation Services
for Alcoholism and Alcohol Abuse"--P. following table of contents.
    "Contract no. ADM-281-87-003 with the National Institute on
Alcohol Abuse and Alcoholism of the Department of Health and Human
Services"--T.p. verso.
    Includes bibliographical references.
    ISBN 0-309-04038-8
    1. Alcoholism--Treatment--Congresses. 2. Alcoholics-
-Rehabilitation--Congress. I. Institute of Medicine (U.S.).
Committee for the Study of Treatment and Rehabilitation Services for
Alcoholism and Alcohol Abuse. II. National Institute on Alcohol
Abuse and Alcoholism (U.S.) III. Title.
    [DNLM: 1. alcoholism--therapy. WM 274 I585bc]
RC565.I4893 1990
362.29'2--dc20
DNLM/DLC
for Library of Congress   90-5702
                                                    CIP

Printed in the United States of America

This book is dedicated to the memory of

E. MANSELL PATTISON, M.D.

1933-1989

in recognition of his many contributions to
the treatment of alcohol problems;

and to the memory of

SARAH CAITLIN GLASER

1987-1988

Committee for the Study of Treatment and Rehabilitation Services for Alcoholism and Alcohol Abuse

ROBERT D. SPARKS, M.D.,* *Chair,* President Emeritus and Senior Consultant, W.K. Kellogg Foundation, Battle Creek, Michigan

THOMAS F. BABOR, PH.D., + Professor of Psychology, Department of Psychiatry, University of Connecticut Health Center, Farmington, Connecticut

ROBERT W. BLUM, M.D., PH.D., Associate Professor of Pediatrics and Maternal and Child Health, University of Minnesota, Minneapolis, Minnesota

CHAD D. EMRICK, PH.D., Assistant Clinical Professor of Clinical Psychology in Psychiatry, University of Colorado Health Sciences Center, Denver, Colorado

JIM FRANCEK, M.S.W., C.E.A.P., President, Jim Francek and Associates, Inc., Norwalk, Connecticut

EDWARD GOTTHEIL, M.D., PH.D., Professor of Psychiatry, Jefferson Medical College, Philadelphia, Pennsylvania

MERWYN R. GREENLICK, PH.D.,* + Vice President (Research), Kaiser Foundation Hospitals, and Director, Center for Health Research, Kaiser Permanente, Portland, Oregon

DAVID C. LEWIS, M.D., Professor of Medicine and Community Health, Donald G. Millar Professor of Alcohol and Addiction Studies, and Director, Center for Alcohol and Addiction Studies, Brown University Medical School, Providence, Rhode Island

G. ALAN MARLATT, PH.D., Professor of Psychology, University of Washington, Seattle, Washington

THOMAS F. MCGOVERN, ED.D., C.A.D.A.C., Associate Professor of Psychiatry, Department of Psychiatry, Southwest Institute for Addictive Diseases, Texas Tech University Health Sciences Center, Lubbock, Texas

MARK V. PAULY, PH.D.,* # Robert D. Eilers Professor of Health Care Management and Economics, Professor of Public Management and Economics, and Executive Director, Leonard Davis Institute of Health Economics, University of Pennsylvania, Philadelphia, Pennsylvania

BARBARA ROSS-LEE, D.O., Professor and Chairman, Department of Family Medicine, College of Osteopathic Medicine, Michigan State University, East Lansing, Michigan.

HARVEY A. SKINNER, PH.D., Professor and Chairman, Department of Behavioural Science, Faculty of Medicine, University of Toronto, and Senior Scientist Addiction Research Foundation, Toronto, Ontario, Canada

CYNTHIA P. TURNURE, PH.D., Executive Director, Chemical Dependency Program Division, Minnesota Department of Human Services, Saint Paul, Minnesota

ROGER DALE WALKER, M.D., Professor of Psychiatry and Behavioral Sciences, University of Washington School of Medicine, and Chief, Addictions Treatment Center, Veterans Affairs Medical Center, Seattle, Washington

CONSTANCE M. WEISNER, M.S.W., DR. P.H., Senior Scientist, Alcohol Research Group, Institute of Epidemiology and Behavioral Medicine, Medical Research Institute of San Francisco Pacific Medical Center, and Lecturer, School of Public Health, University of California at Berkeley, California

STUDY STAFF

FREDERICK B. GLASER, M.D., F.R.C.P.(C), Study Director

HERMAN I. DIESENHAUS, PH.D., Associate Study Director

LEAH MAZADE, Editor

BARBARA A. KELLEY, Project Secretary

FREDRIC SOLOMON, M.D., Director, Division of Mental Health and Behavioral Medicine

ELAINE LAWSON, Administrative Secretary, Division of Mental Health and Behavioral Medicine

*Member, Institute of Medicine
+Liaison, Committee to Identify Research Opportunities for the Prevention and Treatment of Alcohol-Related Problems
#Liaison, Committee for the Substance Abuse Coverage Study

Contents

Broadening the Base of Treatment for

Alcohol Problems

Introduction and Summary

As an aspect of its general responsibility for the health of the American people, the U.S. Congress has been concerned about the treatment of persons with alcohol problems. From time to time Congress has sought information on such treatment to guide its legislative activities. In 1983, for example, the congressional Office of Technology Assessment (OTA) responded to a request from the Senate Finance Committee with a report entitled *The Effectiveness and Costs of Alcoholism Treatment* (Saxe et al., 1983).

During the course of its deliberations in 1986 on the extension of the expiring authorization of appropriations for alcohol and drug research programs, Congress noted (in the words of the report of the House Committee on Energy and Commerce) that the availability of these treatment services "is becoming increasingly important to the nation's health care system." Accordingly, it authorized the present study on the treatment of alcohol problems in Section 4022 of Public Law 99-570, the Alcohol, Drug Abuse, and Mental Health Amendments of 1986, enacted on October 17 of that year. Section 4022 required the secretary of health and human services, acting through the director of the National Institute on Alcohol Abuse and Alcoholism (NIAAA), to arrange for a study to carry out the following charge:

(a) critically review available research knowledge and experience in the United States and other countries regarding alternative approaches and mechanisms (including statutory and voluntary mechanisms) for the provision of alcoholism and alcohol abuse treatment and rehabilitative services;

(b) assess available evidence concerning comparative costs, quality, effectiveness, and appropriateness of alcoholism and alcohol abuse treatment and rehabilitation services;

(c) review the state of financing alternatives available to the public, including an analysis of policies and experiences of third-party insurers and state and municipal governments; and

(d) consider and make recommendations for policies and programs of research, planning, administration, and reimbursement for the treatment of individuals suffering from alcoholism and alcohol abuse.

Congress further specified that the study be carried out by the National Academy of Sciences. In transmitting the congressional request to the Academy, the director of NIAAA, Dr. Enoch Gordis, summarized those topics that might be viewed as having especial importance for potential inclusion in the forthcoming study:

(1) the validity of outcome measures; (2) the role of minimal intervention as a treatment modality; (3) better definition of patient types and treatment modalities; (4) determining feasibility and potential benefits of matching patients with treatments; (5) defining for whom an inpatient setting is appropriate; (6) the controlled drinking issue; (7) getting better data on the costs of alcoholism and on who pays and benefits; (8) choosing among the better of existing studies for more rigorously designed replication.

In 1987, the National Academy of Sciences accepted responsibility for conducting the study. The Academy is a private, nonprofit corporation chartered by Abraham Lincoln in 1863 to provide independent advice to the government on matters of science and technology. Over the years, components of the Academy have developed an interest in dealing with issues relating to alcohol and drug problems. For example, in 1981 the Academy's Assembly of Social and Behavioral Sciences published a report entitled *Alcohol and Public Policy: Beyond the Shadow of Prohibition* (Moore and Gerstein, 1981). Although concerned with prevention rather than treatment, the report detailed a number of concepts that are germane to the development of this study, including the use of alcohol problems as an inclusive framework for consideration of the subject and the importance of attending to those individuals with less severe alcohol problems as well as to those with more severe difficulties.

As the component of the Academy devoted to the improvement of health care, the Institute of Medicine (IOM) was assigned responsibility for conducting the study mandated by Congress. IOM has a history of interest in this field and in the treatment of alcohol and drug problems. At the request of a prior director of NIAAA, for example, IOM produced the 1980 report entitled *Alcoholism, Alcohol Abuse and Related Problems: Opportunities for Research* (IOM, 1980), which outlined a possible research agenda for the next few years. Subsequently, the administrator of the Alcohol, Drug Abuse, and Mental Health Administration (ADAMHA) asked IOM to review research opportunities in its tripartite portfolio (which includes alcohol problems); the resulting document, entitled "Research on Mental Illness and Addictive Disorders: Progress and Prospects," was published in 1985 in the *American Journal of Psychiatry* (Board on Mental Health and Behavioral Medicine, Institute of Medicine, 1985).

More recently, NIAAA requested an update of the 1980 report. The initial portion of the update, which deals with basic research, was published in May 1987 as *Causes and Consequences of Alcohol Problems: An Agenda for Research* (IOM, 1987). The final portion of this study (IOM, 1989), which covers research opportunities in the treatment and prevention of alcohol problems, was conducted at the same time as the present study on the treatment of alcohol problems. To ensure coordination of the two efforts, a liaison member serving on both committees was appointed. That coordination did in fact occur is indicated by the appearance of a chapter of the research opportunities study as an appendix to this report (Appendix B).

In addition, during the same period, IOM conducted a third relevant study (also mandated by Public Law 99-570) on substance abuse coverage. Its overall purpose was to assess the extent and adequacy of financial coverage for the treatment of drug abuse. Again, to ensure coordination of the two studies, a liaison member belonging to both committees was appointed. Although each of the three simultaneous studies was an independent effort, a productive cross-fertilization occurred among them. Several outside experts, for example, served as consultants for more than one study. IOM staff interacted to ensure coordination of activities and the exchange of information.

Yet the three studies have had rather different emphases. The research opportunities study and this study on the treatment of alcohol problems shared a common general interest in treatment. The interest of the former, however, lay more in the area of treatment research opportunities for the future; this study concerned itself with what might be done to improve treatment in the near term and is based largely on current knowledge. In addition, the research opportunities study dealt equally with prevention and treatment. The financial aspects of treatment proved a common interest in the substance abuse coverage study and this study; nevertheless, the interest of the former focused on drugs other than alcohol and on mechanisms of insurance coverage, whereas the treatment study committee concerned itself with more general aspects of the financing of treatment and the issue of cost-effectiveness. These congruities and disparities reflect the differing questions posed to each committee.

The Study Process

IOM studies are carried out by steering committees appointed by the institute's president. Because of the many contributions of the behavioral and social sciences in the area of alcohol problems, in this instance, concurrence of the Commission on Behavioral and Social Sciences and Education (CBASSE), a component of the National Academy of Sciences, was also required for appointments. The membership of the steering committee reflected the wide range of disciplines active in prevention, treatment, and research activities in the field of alcohol problems and was required to be responsive to the questions raised.

Each member of the committee was understood to have not one but two special roles to fulfill in the work of the group. First, each was to bring the benefit of his or her professional experience in dealing with alcohol problems. Second, every member also had a duty to function as an informed and responsible citizen in carrying out the committee's work. It was hoped that such an emphasis would encourage committee members to rise above special interests, current controversies, and loyalties to particular constituencies. The reader must judge whether the committee as a whole enacted this dual role successfully but may rest assured that such duality was diligently pursued.

Staff for the study were drawn from IOM's Division of Mental Health and Behavioral Medicine. The role of staff was technical and supportive; the content of the report is the responsibility of the committee. In addition, a project officer from NIAAA subserved important liaison functions and provided invaluable information throughout but did not participate in executive sessions of the committee when recommendations were formulated. A list of committee members and staff follows the title page of this report.

Studies conducted by the IOM are not experimental in nature, and no primary data are collected. Frequently, however, secondary analyses of existing data are made, and the present study contains a number of examples of this sort of analysis (e.g., the material on the availability of treatment in Chapter 7). Fundamentally, IOM studies consist of the assiduous assembly of available data relevant to the charge of the committee, followed by the consideration and interpretation of the data by the committee as it formulates its recommendations.

In keeping with its legislative charge, this report focuses exclusively on alcohol problems. There is value in retaining such a focus; without it, the magnitude of these problems in our society and the difficulties that arise in dealing with them might be obscured. The committee recognizes that the interest of Congress in directing its attention to alcohol alone reflects the public interest in distinguishing between illegal drugs and all other drugs. Other manifestations of this interest are the existence of separate constituencies, and of separate structures within the executive branch of the federal government, for alcohol and drug problems.

The committee is aware of the widespread impression among clinicians that many persons who are currently seeking treatment for alcohol problems, and especially younger persons, have problems with other drugs; the opinion is also held, conversely, that many persons seeking treatment for drug problems have problems with multiple drugs including alcohol. Longitudinal data are lacking to document a trend toward polydrug problems in populations that are presumptively at risk for them, but this lack may reflect more accurately the paucity of longitudinal data rather than the reality of the phenomenon. Should the trend prove to be widespread and persistent, a reevaluation of the inclination to deal separately with alcohol and drug problems might be in order. However, although the committee appreciates the potential importance of these issues, their consideration is beyond the scope of this report.

Also in keeping with its legislative charge, this report focuses largely on treatment rather than on prevention. The committee recognizes that prevention and treatment are closely related and that primary prevention practices, which are directed at populations that have not yet developed problems, may nevertheless have a significant effect on individuals who have developed problems. The research opportunities study (IOM, 1989), conducted at the same time as the present study (see above) has dealt extensively with primary prevention, which accordingly is not discussed further here. Secondary prevention is considered in both the research opportunities report (Chapter 10) and in the present report (Chapters 3 and 9).

The work of the committee was conducted primarily in a series of six general meetings that were held over the course of the study in various locations. Four task forces were constituted to elaborate critical concepts in particular areas; these groups included but were not limited to members of the committee and held separate meetings. Each task force developed a written report, on which much of the material in the final report is based. Some of the task forces, such as the Task Force on Assessment and Treatment Assignment, developed literally volumes of original written resource materials, some of which are cited as references at appropriate places in the report text. Membership lists of the various task forces appear in Appendix A. In addition to their work on the task forces, committee members also carried out functions for the committee as a whole (e.g., report review and agenda specification).

To expand the range of information available for its deliberations, the committee commissioned three papers on specific areas of interest. Staff and consultants of the World Health Organization in Geneva, Switzerland, prepared an international review of treatment practices, which appears as Appendix C of the report. Kaye M. Fillmore of San Francisco, California, and her colleagues were commissioned to prepare a report on improvement in alcohol problems outside of formal treatment (so-called "spontaneous remission"). This report is a significant source for the text of the report, especially in Chapter 6. (Its authors have revised and extended the paper and are seeking publication elsewhere.) Henrick Harwood, at the time a staff member of the Research Triangle Institute, was commissioned to explore aspects of the financing of treatment. His analyses revealed that a number of these avenues of exploration were unfruitful; other aspects of his work have been incorporated into Section V of the report.

Another source for Section V was a draft paper prepared by members of the Task Forces on Financing and on Treatment Outcome Evaluation working together under the direction of Harold D. Holder. The draft attempted to deal with the specific cost-effectiveness of particular kinds of treatment. At the conclusion of the study it was incomplete; its authors plan to continue their work and will seek publication of the paper elsewhere.

The appendices also contain two additional reports that were felt by the committee to be highly relevant to the study. As noted earlier, Appendix B is Chapter 9, "Treatment Modalities: Process and Outcome," from the research opportunities study. It reviews critically and summarizes the literature on the outcome of treatment for alcohol problems. Although the committee for the research opportunities study took the lead in developing this material, it was considered to be of central importance to both studies. Consequently, rather than duplicate efforts, a joint project was undertaken, with many committee members, task force members, and staff from the Study on the Treatment of Alcohol Problems participating actively in the development of Chapter 9. Appendix B is a significant source for Chapter 5 of this report, although it is generally relevant to the report as a whole. Appendix D is a paper entitled "Coercion in Alcohol Treatment," which was authored by committee member Constance M. Weisner. The paper principally reflects her understanding of this complex area, although other committee members and staff contributed to its development as well. It is a significant source for Chapter 6 of the report.

Widespread solicitation of viewpoints on all issues was made by mail, telephone, and personal interview. A day-long public meeting was held to hear testimony from many of the groups with particular interests in the field. Numerous site visits were carried out by committee members and staff. Relevant congressional hearings as well as meetings of professional societies were scrupulously attended. Current and past literature was reviewed. If despite these efforts every relevant viewpoint failed to receive its due, the failure stems not from lack of effort but from the complexity of the subject matter.

In preparing its report, the committee attempted to keep several potential audiences in mind. Because the report was prepared at the behest of Congress, a primary goal was to respond to the congressional mandate and to provide information that would be useful in developing a legislative agenda at both the federal and state levels. Many other federal, state, and local governmental agencies are significantly involved in the support of treatment efforts for alcohol problems, and it is hoped the report will also be useful to these organizations. Another very important audience for the report is what those who are in it often refer to as "the field"—those indispensable persons and organizations whose work focuses on the understanding and treatment of alcohol problems.

Finally, because the use of alcohol and the domain of alcohol problems and their consequences touch all members of our society, we have tried to prepare a report that will be understandable and useful to all. In attempting to serve many masters, we may have succeeded in serving none as well as they individually might wish. We can only hope that these few words about the committee's intentions, although not an excuse for its shortcomings, will nevertheless explain their origin.

The report discusses those issues pertinent to the charge of the committee that were thoroughly reviewed by the committee as a whole; it presents the consensus of the group. As such, it constitutes an achievement rather than an initial "given." In a group as diverse as the committee, working in an area as complex and difficult as the treatment of alcohol problems, disagreement was expected and, indeed, materialized. Points of contention were put forward and discussed in professional and agreeable exchanges. Where such disagreements proved to be significant, the chairman played an active role in working out a satisfactory resolution. Compromise was usually effected through this process. In the few instances in which disagreements persisted, they are noted in the text.

The following section is a summary of the contents of the report. A common practice is to accompany each portion of such a summary with succinct, discrete recommendations for action, often set off by typographical "bullets." The committee gave this approach due consideration and ultimately rejected it, not only for the report as a whole but for various sections of the report. For example, the committee actively considered including a fully specified assessment battery in Chapter 10 but decided this degree of specification would prove counterproductive; the committee believes such batteries might most appropriately emerge from a consensus process that draws on a much wider base of opinion and interests than could be found in the committee. It did, however, provide guidelines for the construction of an assessment battery, as well as a general outline of what such a battery might look like.

As another example, much effort was expended to provide careful financial estimates of the cost of implementing the approach advocated by the committee, the cost benefits that were likely to ensue in comparison with alternative methods of procedure, and the mechanisms whereby the costs might be met. Ultimately, however, such specification seemed more illusory than real, because the data on which to base reasonable estimates of costs and benefits are simply not available (see Chapters 8, 19, and 20). There are many potential funding mechanisms, and preferences for their differential use vary widely. The committee considered it appropriate to confine its contribution in the area of financing to a more general discussion, expressing its opinion, for example, that there seemed likely to be a rough parity between the costs of the changes it advocated and the cost benefits that were likely to arise. The available data do not allow the committee to go beyond a general discussion.

In sum, the committee made a deliberate and conscious choice in many instances not to be prescriptive. It did not believe that it *could* be prescriptive because many of the relevant data were not available. Neither did it believe, however, that it *ought* to be prescriptive; evolution toward the treatment systems it sees as desirable is best accomplished through a broadly based process of consensus involving the field as a whole and all of its diverse elements—indeed, a process involving society as a whole. In the balance of this report the committee presents what it has called its vision of the direction in which it believes and hopes treatment will evolve, as well as a number of guidelines on how to negotiate the terrain of the future. What the committee has presented is not a finely detailed map: it considers the drawing of such a map to be the future task of the many rather than the present task of a few.

A Summary of the Text

To summarize the large volume of information it received and the conclusions it reached, the committee has proceeded by (1) describing its vision of the endpoint toward which it believes treatment is evolving and toward which it ought to evolve; (2) providing its answers to a series of fundamental questions about treatment; (3) discussing in detail particular aspects of the treatment process that it believes require special attention; (4) reviewing the issue of special populations in treatment; (5) examining the financing of treatment; and (6) evaluating the opportunities for leadership in the treatment area for the future. The numbers of the points in this paragraph correspond to the six sections of the report. A brief summary of their contents follows; full details are contained in the text.

Our Vision

During its deliberations the committee was guided by its vision of the probable structure toward which treatment for alcohol problems seems to be evolving. That structure is a treatment system in which a broad community-wide treatment effort is coupled closely with a comprehensive specialized treatment effort. The role of community agencies in treatment would include the identification of individuals with alcohol problems, the provision of brief interventions to a portion of those identified, and the referral of others to specialized treatment. Specialized treatment would emphasize comprehensive pretreatment assessment, the matching of particular individuals to specific treatment interventions, and the regular determination of the outcome of treatment. Assuring the continuity of care and providing for the feedback of outcome results in the reformulation of matching guidelines are also viewed as important functional elements of the emerging treatment system. *The most fundamental recommendation of the committee is that this vision be shared, tested, refined, and implemented.*

Some Fundamental Questions

What Is Being Treated? The committee has elected to refer to the target of treatment throughout the report as alcohol problems. This terminology is intentionally broad and reflects the committee's view that the focus of treatment needs to be expanded. While maintaining and, indeed, increasing its present concern for individuals with severe problems, treatment must also address the vast and heterogeneous spectrum of problems that are of less than maximum severity. The committee defines alcohol problems as those problems that may arise in individuals around their use of beverage alcohol and that may require an appropriate treatment response for their optimum management. "Alcohol problems" is felt to be a more inclusive definition of the object of treatment than such current alternatives as "alcoholism" or "alcohol dependence syndrome," but it is nevertheless compatible with these widely used conceptual frameworks.

What Is Treatment? In keeping with its broadened definition of the focus of treatment, the committee believes that the definition of treatment itself needs to be broadened. Treatment is herein defined as those activities that must be undertaken to deal with an alcohol problem and with the individual manifesting such a problem. A comprehensive continuum of interventions is required to cope with the expanded focus of treatment the committee is proposing. In specifying the elements of this continuum, the committee uses a framework that includes the treatment philosophies of providers, the settings in which treatment takes place, and the specific modalities used in each of the stages of treatment—acute intervention, rehabilitation, and maintenance.

Who Provides Treatment? Recent years have seen a broadening of the programmatic contexts of treatment and of the kinds of experience and training that are considered appropriate for treatment personnel. A variety of disciplines is now involved, including physicians, social workers, counselors, and psychologists. Alcoholism counselors, many of them "recovering persons" who have experienced difficulties with alcohol themselves, have become the major providers of treatment in all organized settings. Of particular note has been the growth in nontraditional treatment settings and in the provision of care through private funding sources. Alcoholics Anonymous continues to be the best-known source of care, and its approach is embodied in programs beyond its own, including professional programs. However, the evolving network of service providers, both individual and programmatic, has not been adequately described and studied. The committee sees a need for expanded efforts to obtain more detailed, timely information regarding the provision of treatment.

Does Treatment Work? The committee has expanded this frequently asked question to the following: Which kinds of individuals, with what kinds of alcohol problems, are likely to respond to what kinds of treatments by achieving what kinds of goals when delivered by which kinds of practitioners? Although the answer to this reframed question is still being developed, the committee feels that its general outlines are clear. There is no one uniformly effective treatment approach for all persons with alcohol problems. Providing appropriate specific treatments, however, can substantially improve outcome.

Is Treatment Necessary? The committee considers the answer to this question to be a qualified "yes." The complexities of treatment necessitate that such activities be approached cautiously and on an individualized basis; thus, treatment is usually but not invariably necessary for alcohol problems. The committee's response is constrained by several considerations. First, improvement in alcohol problems can occur without formal treatment. Second, although treatment is often helpful, it can sometimes be harmful. Third, the growing use of coercion in bringing people into treatment for alcohol problems is of concern to the committee. Although some positive outcomes may be achieved, the results of coerced treatment are by no means uniformly positive. The committee believes that additional study is required to determine who does not need treatment, who will be harmed by treatment (especially when coerced into undertaking it), and who will benefit from treatment only under coercion.

Is Treatment Available?   Treatment for alcohol problems is not equally available throughout the United States.   There is wide variability among jurisdictions in total available treatment capacity, and there are major differences in the availability of each of the types of care and in per capita expenditure of funds.   The cause or causes of this variability are unknown (and largely unstudied), but it does not seem to reflect differences in the prevalence of alcohol problems.   Careful study of the reasons for differences in treatment availability is a necessary prelude to effective action to bring about a more equitable distribution of the broad spectrum of required treatment resources.

Who Pays for Treatment?   Private health insurance is now the largest single source of funding for the treatment of alcohol problems across jurisdictions.   State and local government contributions are next in aggregate size; federal funding for treatment, now provided through the alcohol, drug abuse, and mental health services block grant, represents a substantial component of state funding.   Direct patient payments and federal insurance programs (primarily Medicare and Medicaid) provide a lower proportion of funding; an expected growth in coverage by Medicare and Medicaid has not occurred.   Overall, there has been a steady increase in the number of public and private sources of financing.   Yet although there have been some improvements in coverage, it does not appear that the goal of obtaining nondiscriminatory coverage equivalent to that provided for other illnesses has been reached.   Consistent, precise reporting is required from providers and the states on their expenditures for treatment services to persons with alcohol problems in order to understand the financing of treatment fully, both at present and in the future.

Aspects of Treatment

The Community Role   Although some persons have many alcohol problems and are suitable candidates for specialized treatment, most persons with alcohol problems have a small number of such difficulties.   Because there are many more persons with fewer problems, the burden that alcohol problems constitute for society arises principally from this group. There is a need for a comprehensive effort to identify persons having few but significant alcohol problems and to deal with them effectively and efficiently outside of the context of specialized treatment and within the community itself.   Fortunately, suitable methods of identification and readily learned brief intervention techniques with good evidence of efficacy are now available.   The committee recommends that consideration be given to the broad deploying, in a wide variety of community settings, of identification and brief intervention capabilities, coupled with the referral of appropriate individuals to the specialized treatment system for alcohol problems.

Assessment   Specialized treatment for alcohol problems should begin with a comprehensive assessment.   The assessment should be carried out prior to the selection of a particular treatment intervention, and it should be designed to provide the information necessary to determine which kind of treatment is likely to be most appropriate for each individual. Multiple dimensions of both the problem and the individual manifesting the problem should be assessed in an efficient process that proceeds in a series of logical stages.   Care needs to be taken to ensure that the assessment process is a positive experience and that its objectivity is maximized.   In addition to its benefits for the individual entering treatment, the gathering of compatible assessment data across treatment settings would contribute greatly to our understanding of many aspects of the treatment process.

Matching Because no treatment is universally effective but some treatments are effective for some persons, it is necessary to match individuals to particular treatments. Less is known about how this should be done than is desirable; however, potentially appropriate matching guidelines can be developed in a number of ways. If guidelines are made explicit and are tested by determining the outcome of treatment, they can be appropriately modified to produce increasingly positive outcomes. Effective matching will also require increased specification of treatment interventions (to complement the specification of individuals and problems through assessment) and the specification of treatment outcomes. Because it views the process of matching as central to the treatment of alcohol problems, the committee recommends that conferences of clinicians and researchers be regularly convened to explore what is currently known and to identify promising directions for the future.

Outcome Determination For a variety of reasons it is rapidly becoming untenable to provide treatment in the absence of knowledge of its outcome. There is a tendency to rely on randomized controlled trials (RCTs) to evaluate treatment outcome. Although the RCT is a powerful tool with many advantages and its more widespread use is to be commended, its application in many clinical settings is problematic. As an alternative, outcome monitoring is more readily applicable and importantly complements information gained from RCTs. Yet although outcome monitoring data may be *consistent* with treatment efficacy, positive results following treatment may be due to factors other than treatment. The external examination of treatment outcome (by those not connected with the provision of treatment) provides protection against bias and is in general to be preferred; however, internal examination of treatment outcome can provide important guidance for program decision making.

Implementing the Vision Implementing separately each of the aspects of treatment discussed above (the community role, assessment, matching, and outcome determination) is of value to the treatment enterprise. But the committee's preference is for the simultaneous implementation of all of these aspects of treatment, together with the addition of mechanisms to assure continuity of care and the feedback of outcome data into the treatment process in a meaningful manner. Some treatment programs have accomplished this implementation to varying degrees, but a much more determined effort to implement and evaluate comprehensive treatment systems embodying all of these functions is now indicated. The committee recommends that four or five model comprehensive treatment systems be implemented as demonstration projects in the immediate future, with provision for full, objective evaluation of all aspects of their functioning and of their treatment outcomes.

Special Populations in Treatment

Overview and Definitions Special population groups are defined in legislation, research, and practice not only in terms of their unique biological and sociocultural characteristics but also in terms of extant concerns regarding access to services. The committee has concentrated on those subgroups that have been seen as needing specifically tailored, "culturally sensitive" treatment programs. Since the early 1970s women and youth have received the most attention, but interest in each of the identified special populations has waxed and waned. There have been no systematic evaluations to determine whether access is improved and treatment outcome positively affected when special population treatment programs are implemented.

Populations Defined by Structural Characteristics Some special population groups tend to be defined primarily in terms of relatively fixed characteristics—principally gender, race, ethnicity, and age. Yet the members of populations so defined vary on other important dimensions that have implications for treatment outcome (e.g., socioeconomic status, employment status); hence, the cogency of such a classification is problematic. Structural characteristics are widely believed to have an important effect on access to treatment. Although there is some evidence for this belief, it is confounded by financial considerations; minority group members, for example, are less likely to be able to pay for treatment themselves or to have insurance coverage. In addition, biomedical and psychosocial approaches to treatment across ethnic and cultural groups in the United States seem to be essentially similar, even in the hands of treatment personnel of differing characteristics. Because most persons will continue to be treated in mainstream programs, taking structural characteristics into account in assessment, matching, and outcome determination is important for determining how effectively these subgroups are being served. For racial and ethnic minorities, the degree of acculturation to the majority culture may be a crucial variable to examine.

Populations Defined by Functional Characteristics Other special population groups are defined by less fixed characteristics, such as their common social, clinical, or legal status. For some of these functionally defined special populations (e.g., the drinking driver, the public inebriate), specifically targeted treatment programs have been developed. The conclusions that emerge from the committee's consideration of populations defined by functional characteristics are not very different from those reached in looking at the groups defined by structural characteristics. Members of functionally defined special populations also vary on other important dimensions that have implications for treatment outcome—including those structural characteristics discussed earlier. Again, the cogency of the classification is problematic. The same lack of evidence favoring the application of specific treatment approaches for populations defined by structural characteristics holds for those special populations defined by functional characteristics.

Conclusions and Recommendations Regarding Special Populations The committee recommends a dual approach to the issue of culturally relevant treatment for special populations. One aspect of this approach is to look more closely at those programs that provide such treatment. The lack of evidence as to their particular efficacy may be due in large measure to a lack of testing. The committee has concluded that there is evidence that access has been improved by these programs. It recommends that funding for them be continued, together with funding for discrete evaluations of treatment for each of the major special populations. These evaluations should compare culturally specific and mainstream programs for the special population in terms of treatment processes and outcomes. At the same time, because many members of special populations will continue to be treated in majority-staffed, mainstream programs, a major effort is recommended to train staff working in mainstream programs in the skills required to deal most effectively with members of special populations. The committee has concluded that special populations, as commonly defined, are actually heterogeneous. It can foresee the possibility that a variety of both "culturally sensitive" and mainstream programs may be required to deal successfully with members of these populations, as well as with people in the "general" population who manifest alcohol problems.

Aspects of Financing

The Evolution of Financing Policy Over the past 20 years, there has been a partially successful effort to develop adequate funding mechanisms and structures for financing treatment for alcohol problems. Such financing is now accepted, albeit not without reservations, as the conjoint responsibility of state and local governments, of the federal government acting on behalf of selected poor, elderly, and chronically disabled individuals, and of private insurers acting on behalf of employers and individuals who purchase health insurance. Inconsistencies in financing policy remain; funding varies considerably among jurisdictions and between the public and private treatment efforts within jurisdictions. In the light of current concerns over rapidly rising health care costs, the major question now being raised is whether current financing and reimbursement policies promote access to the most cost-effective treatments. The committee recommends the development of a common framework of criteria for matching individuals to the most appropriate treatment as a significant contribution to this effort. Better data on expenditures, expanded research on the impact of financing policies on treatment, and a detailed understanding of the cost-effectiveness of alternative treatments are also required if a truly nondiscriminatory financing policy is to be realized.

Cost-Effectiveness The justification of increased insurance coverage for the treatment of alcohol problems has often been based on studies of cost offset (i.e, the decline in health care expenditures to be expected if alcohol problems are successfully treated). Review of the recent literature suggests that, although studies demonstrating cost offset have been methodologically flawed, there is some indication, although not conclusive evidence, that spending money on treatment for alcohol problems today does lower medical costs tomorrow. The question that must be answered now is the cost-effectiveness of alternative forms of treatment. We do not know whether more costly treatments provide additional benefits sufficient to offset their greater cost. Accordingly, the committee recommends an intensive program of research to compare the costs of alternative treatments relative to their benefits. In addition, studies of matching and of treatment effectiveness should include the consideration of cost-effectiveness questions.

Paying for the Treatment System The committee considered the changes that would be required in the methods used to pay for treatment for two scenarios: first, to improve the current system and second, to pay for the ideal comprehensive treatment system.

Given the lack of adequate cost-effectiveness studies comparing alternative treatments, it is not possible to say definitively to what degree particular treatments should or should not be covered. Although committee members held different opinions regarding the criteria that should be used for admission to intensive treatment, as a whole the committee considered a significant redistribution of resource utilization from more intensive to less intensive treatments to be desirable. The committee anticipates that such a redistribution would take place if alternative programs, guidelines for their use, and outcome monitoring were available. To facilitate this redistribution, public and private insurance coverage should be available for a broad variety of treatment options. Given the current state of knowledge, medical supervision should not necessarily be required for the provision of insurance benefits. At the same time, however, medical consultation should be readily available when required for the diagnosis and treatment of medical and psychiatric disorders in all treatment programs.

Implementing the new treatment system proposed by the committee will require comprehensive and flexible benefit plans offered by all payer sources. Underlying the development of all such plans is the principle that public and private insurance financing should cover effective care that is worth the cost. The committee is aware of the fears its recommendations may evoke that, in suggesting the development and implementation of treatment systems, it is at the same time recommending vast increases in funding. There is not an adequate data base on which to develop projections of any additional costs that may arise. Nevertheless, the committee believes that, to a significant extent, the additional costs incurred by recruiting more people into treatment through the establishment of a widespread community role will be offset by future savings in medical costs and by more efficient and effective treatment through the use of assessment, matching, outcome determination, feedback, and continuity assurance. Should a net increase in the cost of treatment ensue, the committee is confident that it would not be excessive and that the total costs of treatment would continue to represent only a small fraction of the social costs of alcohol problems.

Guiding the Ongoing Effort

Although it is tempting to charge a single designated leader—an individual, a federal agency, an advocacy group, a profession, Congress—with ongoing stewardship of the treatment of alcohol problems, realistically the base of leadership must be broad. The committee believes that, to ensure progress, community and voluntary organizations, government agencies, treatment providers, professional organizations, employers, insurance companies, consumers of treatment services, and other interested parties will need to evaluate its recommendations and take appropriate and concerted action. The committee has offered suggestions on how each of these groups can provide leadership. Alcohol problems are sufficiently pervasive, sufficiently complex, and sufficiently massive in the aggregate that dealing with them effectively requires multifocal leadership representing society as a whole.

REFERENCES

Board on Mental Health and Behavioral Medicine, Institute of Medicine. 1985. Research on mental illness and addictive disorders: Progress and prospects. American Journal of Psychiatry 142(Suppl.):1-41.

Institute of Medicine. 1980. Alcoholism, Alcohol Abuse, and Related Problems: Opportunities for Research. Washington, D.C.: National Academy Press.

Institute of Medicine. 1987. Causes and Consequences of Alcohol Problems: An Agenda for Research. Washington, D.C.: National Academy Press.

Institute of Medicine. 1989. Prevention and Treatment of Alcohol Problems: Research Opportunities. Washington, D.C.: National Academy Press.

Moore, M. H., and D. R. Gerstein, eds. 1981. Alcohol and Public Policy: Beyond the Shadow of Prohibition. Washington, D.C.: National Academy Press.

Saxe, L., D. Dougherty, K. Esty, and M. Fine. 1983. The Effectiveness and Costs of Alcoholism Treatment. Washington, D.C.: U.S. Congress, Office of Technolgy Assessment

1 Our Vision

Where there is no vision, the people perish.
—Proverbs 29:18

In the introduction to and summary of this study, the steering committee detailed the process by which it responded to its mandate. During this process much information was brought forward and is presented in considerable detail in the multiple chapters of this report, together with the recommendations that arose from it. As is the custom in such presentations, the material is divided into chapters, each of which covers an important aspect of the whole.

Yet the whole itself also requires consideration. During the committee's prolonged and detailed examination of information on multiple aspects of the subject matter, an overarching view of the probable evolution of treatment for people with alcohol problems emerged with considerable clarity. Once this had happened, the overarching view guided the development of the report. Because it is difficult to understand the parts of the report without reference to the whole, the committee has decided to begin its exposition with a brief description of this view, which it has chosen to call its vision.

From several possible definitions of "vision," the committee has selected one that dates from 1592 to convey its meaning—"a mental concept of a distinct or vivid kind; a highly imaginative scheme or anticipation" (Oxford English Dictionary). In choosing both the term and this definition of it, the committee deliberately underscores the subjectivity of its viewpoint. It recognizes that other groups of individuals considering the same material may develop alternative visions. The committee welcomes these alternatives as compatible with its belief that future progress can only benefit from the availability of differing viewpoints.

Briefly put, the committee's vision is that the treatment of people with alcohol problems has undergone an historical evolution. From an originally and perhaps necessarily circumscribed focus, the base of the treatment enterprise has begun to broaden in a number of important ways, a development the committee believes should be encouraged. Yet together with, and largely because of, the development of a broader base, there is a concomitant need for a more structured approach to treatment. That structure takes the form of treatment systems, each of which may combine many important properties and functions of treatment into a coherent whole.

In the balance of this chapter, which concludes Section I of the report, the committee will further describe its vision. The report then attempts in Section II to address questions that are often put to those involved in the treatment enterprise; they are not necessarily the most appropriate questions, but they are the ones most frequently asked (e.g., "Does treatment work?"). In Section III, several critical aspects of treatment, such as assessment, are addressed, as well as the advantages of joining these aspects together into a carefully articulated whole.

The needs of special populations, as defined by various structural and functional descriptors, are considered in some detail in Section IV. Financing, the crucial "bottom line" that has more frequently determined rather than facilitated the provision of treatment, is discussed in Section V. Finally, in Section VI, the committee discusses the multiple leadership initiatives needed for a fuller realization of its vision.

A Brief History of Treatment

As noted above, the committee's vision rests in part on a view of the development of treatment as an evolving historical process. The history of treatment for alcohol problems in the United States can be traced back to the beginning of national history and, like that history, is in broad perspective quite brief. Dr. Benjamin Rush of Philadelphia (1746-1813), a signer of the Declaration of Independence and surgeon general of the Continental Army, is clearly the starting point.

Rush's classic work, *An Inquiry into the Effects of Ardent Spirits upon the Human Body and Mind, with an Account of the Means of Preventing and of the Remedies for Curing Them*, first appeared in 1785 (Jellinek, 1943). Although it contained novel ideas about therapeutics, they were largely ignored; his colonial American contemporaries viewed alcohol problems as a moral rather than a medical matter (Levine, 1978). More proximately, Rush's work was cited by the founders of the American temperance movement as the source of their activity (Kobler, 1973), which was, however, preventive rather than therapeutic in orientation. Justin Edwards, a principal leader of the temperance movement, proclaimed in 1822: "Keep the temperate people temperate; the drunkards will soon die, and the land be free" (Maxwell, 1950).

Nevertheless, some interest in therapeutics did persist. The Washingtonian Movement, which flourished between 1840 and 1860, was initiated by and directed at heavy drinkers (Maxwell, 1950). By the 1870s sanitaria for "inebriates" had begun to appear. In the words of one such establishment, they "afforded [inebriates] time to come to themselves, and allow their better nature to assert itself, with the hope that during the lucid interval thus secured, they might be re-assurred of their manhood, and add the force of a moral purpose, to the physical means employed for their benefit" (Parrish et al., 1871).

With the coming of Prohibition (the Eighteenth Amendment to the U.S. constitution became law on January 6, 1919), any other approach to alcohol problems appeared unnecessary. Probably as a joint result of Prohibition and of wartime restrictions, there was a sharp decline in alcohol consumption and the related index of death from liver cirrhosis (Jellinek, 1947; Terris, 1967). Alcohol became an issue for law enforcement, and treatment fell into disuse.

Repeal, however, became official on December 5, 1933, and a renewed treatment response followed. Less than two years later, on June 10, 1935, Alcoholics Anonymous was formed (Alcoholics Anonymous World Services, Inc., 1955). During the next few years the impact of E. M. Jellinek (1890-1963), a founder of the scientific study of alcohol problems, was apparent in the publication of the first major review of treatment (Bowman and Jellinek, 1941) and in the establishment in 1942 of the Yale School of Alcohol Studies (which was later relocated to Rutgers). Another significant date was 1948; in that year the drug disulfiram (Antabuse) was introduced into therapeutics (Hald and Jacobsen, 1948).

Yet the present shape of treatment for alcohol problems in the United States has largely been a consequence of the passage of the Comprehensive Alcohol Abuse and Alcoholism Prevention, Treatment, and Rehabilitation Act of 1970 (P.L. 91-616), often called the Hughes Act, after its sponsor, Senator Harold Hughes of Iowa (see Chapter 18). The act created the National Institute on Alcohol Abuse and Alcoholism and initiated large-scale federal funding for the treatment of alcohol problems. Today, federal funding continues to play an important role in treatment financing, although federal monies since 1982 have been provided through a block grant mechanism to the individual states for administration. The growth of the private sector in treatment has been a feature of recent years (Yahr, 1988).

Thus, the treatment of alcohol problems in the United States can be traced back for about 200 years—a brief span by historical standards—but it is, in many significant respects, a much more recent phenomenon. On account of the hiatus introduced by

Prohibition and the "Great War," treatment had in some respects to start from scratch following repeal in 1933. Alcoholics Anonymous, the oldest significant feature of the current scene, is but 50 years old, and the changes introduced by the Hughes Act and by private initiatives are even more recent.

During the course of this study, the committee had an opportunity to examine much of the current treatment effort, and it was deeply and positively impressed. It is convinced that people seeking help with alcohol problems at present often receive effective and even invaluable assistance. Much, indeed, has been accomplished.

But the historical record is as yet brief, and significant changes continue to occur. The evolution of treatment has not ceased but is ongoing. The committee would fix our current position with respect to the evolution of treatment by echoing Churchill: "Now, this is not the end. It is not even the beginning of the end. But it is, perhaps, the end of the beginning."

Broadening the Base

The historical record also suggests that treatment for any problem tends to originate as a result of attention being drawn to severe cases. Initially, treatment consists of applying to these cases the existing remedies that are available when the problem is first recognized. As time passes, however, it becomes increasingly clear that (a) cases other than severe cases exist and (b) other methods can be used to deal with them. The history of the treatment of most problems follows this progression; diabetes, tuberculosis, and cancers offer illustrations. Thus, it is not surprising to find the same progression in the treatment of persons with alcohol problems.

The committee has elected to refer to the principal target of therapeutic activities as *alcohol problems*, including, as necessary, appropriate modifiers for time course and severity (e.g., acute mild alcohol problems; chronic severe alcohol problems). This broadened frame of reference is discussed in Chapter 2; Chapter 10, which deals with assessment, discusses the multiple dimensions along which alcohol problems should be specified.

It is now accepted that *individuals experience many different kinds of problems around their consumption of beverage alcohol.* Such problems range from the hyperacute to the severely chronic and from the mild to the extremely severe. They are manifest at different levels and in different patterns of alcohol consumption that in turn are associated with differing symptoms and with consequences in differing life areas. *Alcohol problems are heterogeneous.* There is not one problem but rather many problems. The committee believes that this broad range of problems requires the attention of a knowledgeable individual who can gather the appropriate information and make a reasonable decision about what to do (or what not to do). As will be further discussed in Chapter 9, these activities constitute an important aspect of treatment.

It is also accepted that *the individuals who manifest the problems are themselves diverse.* These individual differences are important for many reasons; for example, they affect the selection of treatment. Different individuals prefer and may benefit from different kinds of treatment. Chapters 2, 10, and 11 discuss these differences, how they may be taken into account in the treatment process, and the improvements in treatment outcome that may result. The whole of Section IV of the report, "Special Populations in Treatment," also deals with this issue.

As the field has developed over time, new treatment methods have been proposed and tested, with the result that *there are now many different methods of treatment* for people with alcohol problems. These methods are described in some detail in Chapter 3, and the evidence for their efficacy is discussed in Chapter 5 and the related Appendix B. Moreover additional personnel have entered the field over time—the development of the counselor's role is but one example—with the result that *there are now many persons with differing backgrounds who are providing treatment in a variety of settings.* Chapter 4 discusses these providers.

Treatment that is provided must be paid for. Originally, it was either paid for directly by the individual who received it or provided as a charity by the treater. With the growth of a complex society, the payment issue has become much more complex, and *there are now many different ways in which treatment is paid for.* Payment methods are detailed in Chapter 8, as well as in the related three chapters of Section V, "Aspects of Financing."

Thus, there has been a fundamental broadening of the base of treatment with the passage of time. Originally, a restricted number of treatment options were applied to a relatively homogeneous group of persons with similarly severe problems by a small number of therapists who were reimbursed for their efforts in a restricted number of ways. Today, treatment involves a large number of very different people with very different problems who are treated in a variety of ways by a diverse group of therapists who are reimbursed for their efforts through multiple mechanisms. There is every reason to suppose that this evolutionary trend will continue, a course of development with which the committee is comfortable.

Yet there is another sense in which the base of treatment has been broadened, and the committee believes this aspect of the evolution of treatment is worthy of special emphasis. Until quite recently, the treatment of alcohol problems was viewed as the exclusive province of a specialized treatment sector. Specialized treatment for alcohol problems is a vital and necessary component of the overall therapeutic approach. There has been increasing recognition, however, that it cannot constitute the whole of the therapeutic approach to alcohol problems.

Particularly from epidemiological studies of the general population, it has become apparent that, although some people have multiple alcohol problems, most people who have alcohol problems have a small number of such problems (the relevant evidence on this point is discussed in Chapter 9). Because they have few problems, they are likely to seek help for the individual consequences of their problems—for example, health consequences. Thus, many individuals will seek help from their physicians for "nerves" or "stomach trouble," or from their welfare worker for "family problems," or from their school guidance counselor for "trouble concentrating," without recognizing the critical role that may be played in such problems by excessive alcohol consumption.

Two considerations become critical under these circumstances. One is that the role of alcohol consumption in the genesis of such problems be identified by the individual to whom these problems are presented. The other is that the individual identifying the alcohol problem be able to deal with it directly through a brief intervention, without necessarily making a referral to specialized treatment. There is now very good evidence (see Chapter 9) that brief interventions may be effective for a large number of people with alcohol problems. Moreover, many such people will not accept a referral to specialized treatment. Without the option of brief intervention, an important opportunity to deal effectively with these individuals will be lost. In addition, because most individuals with alcohol problems are of this kind, an important opportunity will be missed for reducing the total burden of alcohol problems on society.

This brief intervention strategy, which is discussed extensively in Chapter 9, in many ways represents the greatest degree of broadening the base of treatment. It posits that *the effective reduction of the burden of alcohol problems cannot realistically be viewed as the sole responsibility of specialized treatment programs.* Rather, the reduction of alcohol problems must be a much more broadly disseminated responsibility, involving a great many different personnel in a large number of different human services arenas, all of whom must learn to recognize such problems and intervene effectively.

In some quarters this conclusion will be viewed as surprising, but it is really quite straightforward. The burden of alcohol problems is a heavy one; the specialized treatment sector is necessarily limited in size and quite costly. The committee believes that only a shared effort can succeed in lifting this burden to any significant degree. For humanitarian and other reasons it is necessary to focus on those with more serious problems; but for practical reasons it is necessary to focus on those with less serious problems as well.

Toward Treatment Systems

If the base of treatment for alcohol problems needs to be broadened, the apex of treatment needs to be sharpened. In other words, although more needs to be done to deal broadly with people who have less severe problems, it is true at the same time that *more needs to be done to deal effectively with people who have more severe problems.* This conclusion, which the committee feels leads toward the development of treatment systems, is the outgrowth of many of the same considerations that lead toward the broadening of the treatment base.

The committee's reasoning with respect to the specialized treatment of alcohol problems begins with the observation that alcohol problems are diverse and that they are manifested by very different kinds of individuals. This observation is as true of people with substantial to severe alcohol problems as it is of people with mild or moderate alcohol problems. As well, there are many different treatment approaches. A major conclusion from research on the outcome of treatment is that there is no one treatment approach that is effective for all persons with alcohol problems (see Chapter 5 and Appendix B).

Several major consequences arise from these fundamental observations. First, differences in the problems presented and in the individuals who manifest them must be taken into account before a decision is made regarding which kind of treatment is most appropriate; this goal is accomplished through pretreatment assessment (Chapter 10). Second, every possible effort must be made to ensure that each individual receives the kind of treatment most likely to produce a positive outcome for him or her; this goal is accomplished through a process of matching (Chapter 11). Third, because treatment outcome cannot be assumed to be positive, it must be determined in all cases and on a regular basis (Chapter 12).

Logical as these considerations may be, pretreatment assessment, treatment matching, and the regular determination of treatment outcome are not at present being widely implemented. In addition, the multiple treatment options implied by these processes are not now usually available to individuals entering treatment. It is quite true that there is a need for further research into all of these activities, and also for research on the feasibility of implementing them on any scale. The committee believes, however, that implementation should not wait upon the final completion of an extensive program of research. Relevant research is well under way and, if the reasons for implementing these processes are compelling, as the committee believes they are, ways must be found to make them broadly available. To some extent, these critical processes have already been implemented or are planned to be implemented (see Chapter 13).

No doubt there are many different implementation scenarios. For example, one possible way to achieve the provision of pretreatment assessment leading to careful matching to a variety of treatment methods with regular determination of treatment outcome might be through the coalescence of individual treatment programs. Most programs offer only one kind of treatment. By joining together with other programs they could offer a greater variety of treatments. Their combined resources would also be better able to support the added processes of pretreatment assessment, matching, and outcome determination and would offer a more commanding position from which to garner the new resources that are likely to be needed. Some larger treatment programs might be able to restructure themselves internally to achieve the same end. The committee has formulated some suggestions for initiating these changes (see Chapter 12).

Almost by definition, and irrespective of the scenario that is followed, such a restructuring will result in the formation of a treatment *system*, that is "a set or assemblage of things connected, associated, or interdependent, so as to form a complex unity; a whole composed of parts in orderly arrangement according to some scheme or plan" (Oxford English Dictionary). What this structure might look like is outlined in greater detail in Chapter 13 but will be briefly presented here. Figure 1-1 shows the committee's vision of the system toward which the treatment of alcohol problems is evolving.

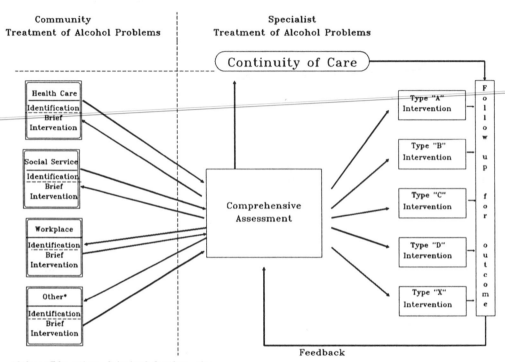

*Other=Education, Criminal Justice, etc.

FIGURE 1-1 The committee's view of the evolving treatment system. All persons seeking services from community agencies are screened for alcohol problems. A brief intervention is provided by agency personnel for persons with mild or moderate problems. Persons with substantial or severe problems are referred for a specialized comprehensive assessment. Where treatment is indicated they are matched to the most appropriate specialized type of intervention. The outcome of treatment is determined, and feedback of outcome information is used to improve the matching guidelines. Continuity of care is provided as required to guide individuals through the treatment system.

On the left of the diagram appears that portion of the treatment system that is optimally located within various agencies and organizations in the community that provide services and subserve other functions. The task of the community treatment sector (see Chapter 9) is to (a) identify those individuals within it who have alcohol problems; (b) provide a brief intervention for persons who have mild or moderate alcohol problems; and (c) refer to specialized treatment those persons with substantial or severe alcohol problems, or those for whom a brief intervention has proven insufficient. The operational location of the community role in treatment is diverse; it is partly in the health care sector, partly in the social services sector, and partly in the workplace, in educational settings, and in the criminal justice arena. Implementation of this aspect of the system greatly broadens its base and is more related to the training of personnel in relevant techniques than to the coalescence of treatment programs described earlier.

Although the available evidence suggests that direct and relatively straightforward treatment within community settings can deal effectively with a substantial proportion of the population of individuals with alcohol problems, others will need specialized treatment. Specialized treatment is shown on the right side of the diagram and is concerned with persons who have substantial or severe alcohol problems, as well as other persons for whom a brief intervention has not proven sufficient. As the diagram indicates, all persons who are referred are first provided with a comprehensive assessment and on that basis are matched to one or more of a variety of available programs.

After treatment, follow-up interviews are conducted to determine the outcome of treatment. If individuals have achieved a positive outcome, no further therapeutic attention may be necessary. If the outcome has not been satisfactory, further treatment may be indicated, perhaps of a different kind. As the arrows indicate, outcome determination and redirection of the individual are the result of a process of reassessment.

It is worthwhile stressing that *the determination of outcome provides a crucial feedback function of the treatment system.* Feedback allows the system to correct for any lack of treatment success, perhaps its most obvious function. But it also provides, even in instances in which treatment is successful, an ongoing check on the matching guidelines used to select treatment so that the guidelines can be continually reexamined and confirmed or modified in the light of known outcomes. In addition, the feedback of outcome results provides an accumulating record of experience with particular individuals and particular problems in particular treatments. This record ultimately can be used to guide the future matching efforts of the treatment system.

One further function that becomes increasingly important when a relatively more complex system is approached by individuals with substantial to severe problems is *continuity of care* (see Chapters 13 and 20.) Although some individuals may be quite capable of negotiating the system on their own, others will be unable to do so. This determination can be made as part of the pretreatment assessment, and appropriate steps can be taken to provide for continuity, either through the use of special personnel (expediters, ombudsmen, patient advocates, etc.) or by other methods. There is also a need to assure continuity of care between the specialized treatment system and treatment in the community; for the most part this task can be undertaken by community providers. The contribution to continuity of care rendered by Alcoholics Anonymous and other elements of the mutual help network is noteworthy.

Advice to the Reader

Such is the vision of this committee regarding the treatment of persons with alcohol problems. It seemed to arise naturally from the premises that the committee developed, to offer a reasonable promise of improved care, and to provide pathways for guidance into the future. A vision has to do with the future; the definition chosen by the committee includes the phrase "a highly imaginative scheme or anticipation." Because our vision for the future differs from the reality of the present, change will be required.

To change to a new perspective, even when that change involves a broadening rather than a replacement of the current perspective, is often very difficult. There is a natural and even laudable allegiance to concepts that have served well and faithfully over a long period of time. Although the current perspective is rich and does not lend itself well to a simple summary, it may be said with some justice that at present alcohol problems are largely viewed as arising more or less directly from the relatively predictable and uniform actions of the drug, alcohol, on the human organism.

Alcohol is a drug, and its direct, relatively predictable, and uniform actions on the human organism have been well documented (cf. Michaelis and Michaelis, 1983; Popham et al., 1984; Palmer et al., 1986; Institute of Medicine, 1987; Koob and Bloom, 1988.) Yet alcohol problems are experienced by specific individuals, who live and move and have their being within very different social, psychological, and cultural environments. The committee's view is that, although the interaction of the drug, alcohol, and the human organism may be a consistent part of alcohol problems, the alcohol problems are deeply and profoundly modified by a multiplicity of other factors that are highly relevant for treatment. The focus in this report, therefore, is on an expanded perspective that includes the actions of the drug alcohol, as well as the totality of the context in which those actions occur (see Chapters 2 and 3).

A change in perspective similar to that called for by the committee in dealing with alcohol problems has been advocated for medicine. In his forward to Kerr White's *The Task of Medicine* (White, 1988), Alvin R. Tarlov has written that the "prevailing paradigm" in medicine

> envisages disease as the end result of disordered molecular and biochemical processes. Such processes lead to cellular, tissue, organ and system disturbance or destruction, resulting in disease, a characteristic constellation of specific biochemical, physiological, and pathological anomalies. These anomalies are responsible for the specific loss of physical and other functions experienced by the patient and observed by the physician.
>
> Dissatisfaction with the prevailing paradigm as a complete explanation of disease and illness has arisen in the past couple of decades. Coming largely from behaviorists, a broadened paradigm of medicine has emerged out of the certain knowledge that one disease may be manifest among a group of patients in widely divergent ways and that illness as experienced by patients may be as highly individualized as fingerprints. The modern paradigm, not by any means intended by its protagonists to replace but rather to broaden prevailing thought, interacts disease with personal, social, and psychological factors to explain individual differences in illness. Despite face and experiential validity, the broadened paradigm has not achieved wide acceptance. (Tarlov, 1988:ix)

In an appendix to the same book (White, 1988), a "patient-centered clinical method" (rather than one centered on disease) is viewed as responsive to such a change in perspective (McWhinney, 1988.) The reader will find that a similar approach to treatment is outlined in this report, particularly in Section III. It is an approach that is to some extent already under way (see Chapter 13). Nevertheless, *the committee would like to see a more direct, intentional, and multifocal approach to the testing, refinement, and implementation of its vision. That is the fundamental recommendation of this report.*

A *caveat* should, however, be posted. Despite its commitment to its vision, the committee believes that further progress should be gradual rather than abrupt. Because what is proposed is an extension of, rather than a replacement for, what exists, the intent of the present report would be violated if it were used as an excuse for dismantling what is currently being done. Rather, the committee feels its vision should be used as a catalyst to inform and accelerate a process that has already begun. Its intention is to extend and increase—not reduce—services to persons with alcohol problems, although with the extension and increase of services it sees the necessity of a redistribution of emphasis.

The committee anticipates that reactions to its vision may be mixed. Some reactions will be positive and will lead smoothly to a close inspection of the much more detailed text that follows. Other reactions, however, may not be positive. The committee urges those who have an unfavorable response to this initial summary to read on. We suspect that in some instances you will be reassured. If you are not, you will at least have more substantial grounds for your objections. Although our vision emerged with some sense of inevitability from the deliberations of the group, we recognize that it is not the only possible vision. To the extent that our efforts serve to sharpen a different vision that contributes to the future of treatment, we will also consider that our work has been worthwhile.

REFERENCES

Alcoholics Anonymous World Services, Inc. 1955. Alcoholics Anonymous. New York: Alcoholics Anonymous World Services, Inc.

Bowman, K., and E. M. Jellinek. 1941. Alcohol addiction and its treatment. Quarterly Journal of Studies on Alcohol 2:98-176.

Hald, J., and E. Jacobsen. 1948. A drug sensitizing the organism to ethyl alcohol. Lancet 2:1001-1004.

Institute of Medicine. 1987. Causes and Consequences of Alcohol Problems: An Agenda for Research. Washington, D.C.: National Academy Press.

Jellinek, E. M. 1943. Benjamin Rush's "An Inquiry into the Effects of Ardent Spirits upon the Human Body and Mind, with an Account of the Means of Preventing and of the Remedies for Curing Them." Quarterly Journal of Studies on Alcohol 4:321-341.

Jellinek, E. M. 1947. Recent trends in alcoholism and in alcohol consumption. Quarterly Journal of Studies on Alcohol 8:1-42.

Kobler, J. 1973. Ardent Spirits: The Rise and Fall of Prohibition. New York: G. P. Putnam's Sons.

Koob, G. F., and F. E. Bloom. 1988. Cellular and molecular mechanisms of drug dependence. Science 242:715-723.

Levine, H. G. 1978. The discovery of addiction: Changing conceptions of habitual drunkenness in America. Journal of Studies on Alcohol 39:143-174.

Maxwell, M. A. 1950. The Washingtonian Movement. Quarterly Journal of Studies on Alcohol 11:410-451.

McWhinney, I. R. 1988. Through clinical method to a more humane medicine. Pp. 218-231 in The Task of Medicine: Dialogue at Wickenburg, K. L. White. Menlo Park, Calif.: The Henry J. Kaiser Family Foundation.

Michaelis, E. K., and M. L. Michaelis. 1983. Physico-chemical interactions between alcohol and biological membranes. Pp. 127-173 in Research Advances in Alcohol and Drug Problems, vol. 7, R. G. Smart, F. B. Glaser, Y. Israel, H. Kalant, R. E. Popham, and W. Schmidt, eds. New York: Plenum Press.

Palmer, M. R., T. V. Dunwiddie, and B. J. Hoffer. 1986. Cellular mechanisms underlying differences in acute ethanol sensitivity: Effects of tolerance and genetic factors upon neuronal sensitivity to alcohol. Pp. 157-178 in Research Advances in Alcohol and Drug Problems, vol. 9, H. D. Cappell, F. B. Glaser, Y. Israel, H. Kalant, W. Schmidt, E. M. Sellers, and R. G. Smart, eds. New York: Plenum Press.

Parrish, J., H. Lewis, M. Baird, G. Milliken, et al. 1871. Address to the People by the Directors, Pennsylvania Sanitarium. Philadelphia: Henry B. Ashmead.

Popham, R. E., W. Schmidt, and S. Israelstam. 1984. Heavy alcohol consumption and physical health problems: A review of the epidemiologic evidence. Pp. 148-182 in Research Advances in Alcohol and Drug Problems, vol. 8, R. G., Smart, H. D. Cappell, F. B. Glaser, Y. Israel, H. Kalant, R. E. Popham, W. Schmidt, and E. M. Sellers, eds. New York: Plenum Press.

Tarlov, A. R. 1988. Forward. Pp. ix-x in The Task of Medicine: Dialogue at Wickenburg, K. L. White. Menlo Park, Calif.: The Henry J. Kaiser Family Foundation.

Terris, M. 1967. Epidemiology of cirrhosis of the liver: National mortality data. American Journal of Public Health 57:2076-2088.

White, K. L. 1988. The Task of Medicine: Dialogue at Wickenburg. Menlo Park, Calif.: The Henry J. Kaiser Family Foundation.

Yahr, H. T. 1988. A national comparison of public- and private-sector alcoholism treatment delivery system characteristics. Journal of Studies on Alcohol 49:233-239.

2   What Is Being Treated?

George, aged 19, is a college freshman from a comfortable middle-class home in which his parents drink on occasion. He was forbidden to do so, and has continued to drink very little while in college. However, he recently pledged the local chapter of his father's fraternity, where heavy weekend drinking is common. Wanting to "fit in," he has learned to enjoy beer, although ordinarily he does not consume large amounts. But last weekend he became intoxicated and, while pursuing a dare, crashed his car and fractured his pelvis.

Sally has had a speech impediment from childhood. Despite considerable attention from speech therapists, her ability to speak clearly has been only intermittent. In her adolescence she developed the notion that she was able to speak much more clearly while under the influence of alcohol; she did not like its taste, however, and so used it only sparingly. Recently she accepted a position as an assistant receptionist. When her coworker is absent, she is called upon to be the interface between the office and the outside world, something she has found difficult because of her impediment. Accordingly, she has turned increasingly to the use of alcohol, taking vodka in the mornings before work and at lunchtime. As yet her drinking has gone undetected in the workplace, but she has recognized that what was initially self-medication has become a practice that she is beginning to find gratifying in itself.

Patrick, a foundry worker, is one of a pair of fraternal twins. His father was a foundry worker as well, and had a small local reputation as "a man who could hold his liquor." Peter, his twin, has reacted strongly to his father's drinking (which was not as well controlled within the home as outside it) and has become an abstainer. Patrick, however, enjoys the conviviality of before-dinner drinks at the local bar with his workmates. A small group of them has taken to attending the races on weekends and skipping work on Monday if they make money on the horses, in part to recover from "being under the weather." On two occasions in the past half-year, Patrick's foreman has spoken sharply to him regarding his absenteeism.

David is the star salesman for a small company that specializes in corporate liability insurance. Because of the pressures of his clients' work, and because of his own view that an important factor in his success is his personal relationship with them, much of his business is transacted at luncheons or dinners. In part because they are underwritten as legitimate business expenses, these occasions tend to be lavish both in terms of food and drink. On weekends, feeling "let down" from "the excitement of the working week," David has taken to having two to four drinks per day, preferring to remain at home. Increasing tension has developed with his wife and children for this as well as other reasons. Both his wife and his private physician have cautioned him about the level of his alcohol consumption, his weight, and his gradually rising blood pressure. In dismissing their objections, he points out that they have never seen him in an intoxicated state.

Ordinarily, William is a sober and well-mannered man. A loner, he lives in a rented room and rarely goes out except to work. However, from time to time, and increasingly in recent years, he will suddenly start drinking enormous quantities of alcohol in the form of cheap fortified wine. Except to purchase his gallon jugs he does not leave his room at these times, but he can be heard at all hours, pacing up and down and talking loudly to himself. After a week or two (or three, in recent months) his room becomes quiet, and some time later, looking much the worse for wear, William emerges to seek a new temporary job. When asked by his sympathetic landlady what causes him to behave in this way, he says, simply, "I don't know."

23

Elizabeth and her family have lived in the California wine country ever since their ancestor migrated to North America several generations ago. For as long as anyone can remember, both in the Old World and the New, most family members have been involved in the production of wine. Plentiful and inexpensive, it is always in evidence, and not only at mealtimes. For most of her adult life Elizabeth has accounted for between one and three bottles daily, depending in part on whether there was something to celebrate. Aside from a tendency toward stoutness, she has been in good general health and of a pleasant disposition. Last week, however, she suddenly began to vomit bright red blood and then passed out. Although she is now out of immediate danger, the doctors have told the family that her "condition" is "serious."

Gregory does not drink. Yesterday, however, he took two drinks of whiskey; they proved to be two too many. He and his close circle of friends had been celebrating, and (primarily to deflect their insistent teasing) he participated in their good cheer. After doing so, he developed what his friends recall as a "glazed" appearance and briefly left the group. He returned with a shotgun that he promptly discharged at point blank range into the chest of his closest friend, killing him instantly. Returning home, he immediately fell into a deep sleep, from which he awakened with a professed amnesia for what had happened. Informed of the death of his friend, he reacted with an outpouring of grief. As he waits in his detention cell to be evaluated by a forensic psychiatrist, he maintains that he could not possibly have killed his friend deliberately but must have been temporarily insane at the time.

Jimmy did not drink a great deal until he entered the military, where a combination of boredom, the ready availability of alcohol, and boon companions led to excesses that occasionally resulted in disciplinary action. Nevertheless, he compiled an impressive service record and was considered a war hero in his neighborhood at the time of discharge. Initially successful as a junior executive, he soon found that coping with the adjustment to civilian life, a sharply competitive business environment, a joyless marriage, advancing age, and the sudden death of his father from cirrhosis of the liver was a burden that was bearable only with the daily consumption of alcohol and frequent extramarital affairs. He has had a long series of admissions to inpatient medical care for gastritis and pancreatitis; during the course of one of these hospitalizations he developed delirium tremens. On three separate occasions in the last five years he attended well-known 28-day residential treatment programs and briefly affiliated afterwards with Alcoholics Anonymous; subsequently he did reasonably well for several weeks to several months. On this occasion he is accompanied to the emergency room of the local hospital by a police officer; he was found wandering about the streets intoxicated and bleeding profusely from both wrists, which he had slashed with his army sheath knife after an especially bitter encounter with his estranged wife.

* * *

The foregoing vignettes are based upon actual individuals encountered by clinicians in the course of providing services to persons seeking assistance for alcohol problems. In light of the limited number of instances that are portrayed, the vignettes cannot be considered fully representative of the great variety of individuals who develop alcohol problems, or of the problems themselves. Yet those who have worked in treatment settings will recognize all or most of these people and their problems—and many more besides. They are the focus of the treatment enterprise.

In the sense that they possess a number of common characteristics, these individuals form an identifiable group. For example, all are experiencing problems around their consumption of beverage alcohol. All may need to be dealt with effectively in some manner by someone with special knowledge of alcohol problems ("treated," in the older sense of the term, which survives when one speaks of a literary or other artistic treatment of a person or subject).

Yet within even this small group there are marked differences. Some of the problems experienced by these individuals are relatively mild (e.g., George, Sally), others are quite severe (e.g., Gregory, Jimmy), and the remainder occupy intermediate positions. Some problems are relatively acute or intermittent (e.g., Patrick, William, Gregory) while others are relatively chronic (e.g., Sally, David, Elizabeth). Some problems have occurred in the context of heavy consumption and some in the context of comparatively light consumption. Some problems are clearly secondary to specific, preexisting conditions; others are not. Some individuals have developed various signs and symptoms or have experienced specific consequences associated with the use of alcohol; others have not. The individuals described here differ widely in terms of age, sex, cultural background, occupation, education, and other factors.

That both important commonalities and important diversities exist in such a group of persons presents a major challenge to those who deal with them. To what degree should each be emphasized, and for what purposes? Some frameworks which are currently employed in dealing with these phenomena, such as those for which the key terms are *alcoholism* and the *alcohol dependence syndrome,* tend to emphasize the diversity of the group as a whole, and at the same time the commonalities between individual members of the group, especially at the more serious end of the spectrum.

An alternative approach is to emphasize the commonalities of the group as a whole and at the same time the diversities between individual members of the group, even at the more serious end of the spectrum. This approach has been taken in the present study, as will be discussed in the balance of this chapter. These two approaches are alternative perspectives upon the same phenomena. Both represent attempts to cope with the combination of commonalities and diversities that are intertwined in this complex and perplexing human problem.

The Alcohol Problems Perspective

Alcohol problems are defined for the purposes of this report as those problems that may arise in individuals around their use of beverage alcohol and that may require an appropriate treatment response for their optimum management. Alcohol problems can be conveniently described in terms of their duration (acute, intermittent, chronic) and severity (mild, moderate, substantial, severe). Yet such abbreviated descriptions should not be permitted to conceal the fact that alcohol problems are extremely diverse; they vary continuously along many dimensions. For example, the manifestations of these problems will sometimes be primarily physical, sometimes social, sometimes psychological; most often they will be variable combinations of all of these. Alcohol problems also vary greatly in terms of the kinds of treatment responses that may be appropriate, responses ranging from simple advice to elaborate combinations and/or sequences of biological, social, and psychological interventions. Access to a comprehensive and coherent system of care that is capable of identifying and implementing the appropriate responses is desirable for all persons with alcohol problems.

The term *alcohol problems* was first used as an organizing concept in a 1967 report of the Cooperative Commission on the Study of Alcoholism (Plaut, 1967). In that context it referred "both to any controversy or disagreement about beverage alcohol use or nonuse, and to any drinking behavior that is defined or experienced as a problem" (p. 4). The first part of this definition has been seen as problematic (cf. Levine, 1984). As used herein the term is consistent with, as well as an extension of, only the second part of the 1967 definition.

If the vignettes of the opening section of this chapter are examined in the light of the foregoing definition, each individual can be viewed as manifesting an alcohol problem. As already noted these problems can be usefully described (though not, to be sure, fully characterized) by duration and severity; for example, George exhibits an acute mild alcohol problem and Jimmy a chronic severe alcohol problem. A measured therapeutic response may be advisable in all instances. The need for treatment is more apparent at Jimmy's end of the spectrum. But George might benefit considerably from some well-chosen words of advice from the physicians attending to his injury, as well as assistance to help him modify at least aspects of his conformity to his present social environment.

From the committee's perspective, the principal advantage of the alcohol problems approach is that it identifies the population of individuals toward which the treatment activities it sees as necessary can be directed. It provides a succinct answer to the question posed in the title of this chapter: what is being treated are alcohol problems. People with alcohol problems are the group that should be dealt with in a variety of ways relevant to the charge to the committee. Treatment should be provided for this group in all its diverse manifestations, which means that policy should be formulated around this group and—as a crucial enabling development—financing mechanisms should be developed to cover the entire spectrum of possible therapeutic responses.

At the same time that the alcohol problems perspective provides a broad, overall approach useful in terms of policy and planning, it also emphasizes the diversity of the problems which are presented and of the individual who present them. The committee feels that this perspective of diversity in individual instances, of what in this report will often be referred to as heterogeneity, is essential to the development of an informed therapeutic response. Such a response involves the systematic identification of salient individual differences and the tailoring of treatment in the light of those differences. It is related to, though not identical with, the classic medical paradigm of differential diagnosis followed by specific treatment

A final possible advantage is that, in employing a relatively limited and deliberately neutral set of terms, the alcohol problems perspective is not freighted with a large body of theory. Accordingly, it does not constrain thinking about many issues that continue to be actively debated. The use of some alternative terminologies (see below) implies the acceptance of particular positions on certain issues. As will be seen, the alcohol problems perspective does not contradict the validity of these alternative perspectives but sees them as appropriately addressed to parts of the overall picture, rather than to the overall picture itself.

Other Perspectives

Alcoholism

The term *alcoholism* was first used by the Swedish physician and temperance advocate Magnus Huss in 1849 to refer "only to those disease manifestations which, without any direct connection with organic changes of the nervous system, take on a chronic form in persons who, over long periods, have partaken of large quantities of brandy" (Jellinek, 1943:86). It enjoys widespread use, though there been no consensus as to its meaning (Babor and Kadden, 1985; IOM, 1987). A recent definition, derived through a Delphi process that surveyed persons felt to possess appropriate expertise nominated by 23 professional organizations, is "a chronic, progressive, and potentially fatal biogenetic and psychosocial disease characterized by tolerance and physical dependence manifested by a loss of control, as well as diverse personality changes and social consequences" (Rinaldi et al., 1988:556).

Most persons with clinical experience will immediately recognize this description as applicable to individuals they have seen in practice. This applicability is attested to by the high levels of interrater agreement achieved for the similarly defined diagnosis "alcohol use disorder" in the field trials (Spitzer et al., 1979) of the third edition of the *Diagnostic and Statistical Manual of the American Psychiatric Association* (DSM-III) (American Psychiatric Association, 1980). Indeed, persons without clinical experience will nevertheless recognize that the definition applies to some people they have encountered during the course of their everyday lives, as well as to current popular notions of the nature and course of heavy drinking (Mulford and Miller, 1964; Rodin, 1981; Caetano, 1987).

The question, however, is not whether the formulation or formulations embodied in the term alcoholism represents with a high degree of validity *some* persons with problems around the consumption of beverage alcohol. It does. The question, rather, is whether the formulation or formulations validly represent *all* those whom the committee would wish to include within the scope of planning, policy development, and treatment. The committee's view is that the answer is negative—some persons, but not all persons, whom it would wish to include are encompassed by the term *alcoholism.* The term may with substantial accuracy describe a subset of the target population but does not describe the target population as a whole.

If one consults the vignettes presented at the outset of this chapter, the problem posed for the committee in the use of the term *alcoholism* can be illustrated. Jimmy is the only one of the eight individuals who would unequivocally meet the definition. Others, such as David and William, might or might not qualify. Elizabeth represents a particular problem; while she has been brought to clinical attention by an acute medical emergency most commonly seen only in individuals who would meet the definition of *alcoholism,* and while she is certainly tolerant and almost certainly physically dependent (although given the consistency of her consumption, this has not been tested), "loss of control," whether subjective or objective, is not clear. Moreover, in many respects the course of her life does not feature the diverse personality changes and social consequences of the definition. Gregory, although in some respects the person with the most serious problem of all, would clearly not meet the definition. Nor, for other reasons, would George, Sally, or Patrick.

A possible qualification might be introduced: some at least of the individuals in the vignettes and elsewhere who do not qualify as "alcoholics" in terms of the full definition might instead be considered to exhibit the early stages of alcoholism. For example, a 72 year-old widow who was a total abstainer from alcohol for the 52 years of her marriage was prescribed sherry as a sedative-hypnotic by an attending physician. Although she "never drank more than three cordial glasses of sherry in any twenty-four hour period" she is described as "fully alcoholic" because "she would make anyone around her miserable until she got her sherry" (Talbott and Cooney, 1982:15). This behavior is viewed as consistent with the fundamental symptom of alcoholism, defined as "inappropriate, irresponsible, illogical, compulsive lack of control of the drinking" (Talbott and Cooney, 1982:27). Although it does not preclude the possibility that some form of assistance might be useful in this case, the committee feels that the extension of the definition of alcoholism in such instances is not realistic.

Widespread acceptance of the term *alcoholism* may be due in part to the remarkable saga of Alcoholics Anonymous (AA), a fellowship devoted to helping those who wish to stop drinking. From its original two members in 1935—Bill W., a stockbroker, and Dr. Bob, a surgeon—it has become an international organization consisting of more than 73,000 groups worldwide, with a current active membership in the United States and Canada of approximately 800,000 (Jackson, 1988). E. M. Jellinek (1890-1963), considered the founding father of scientific studies in this area, did most of his early research on AA members, and his book, *The Disease Concept of Alcoholism* (Jellinek, 1960), is considered a classic. The National Council on Alcoholism (NCA), the principal citizen's group involved in the field, was an outgrowth of both AA and the Yale (later Rutgers) Center of Alcohol Studies.

Yet the key individuals involved in these significant developments did not see *alcoholism* as a useful synonym for the totality of problems. Bill W., for example, spoke in "The Big Book" of "moderate drinkers" and of "a certain type of hard drinker" who could experience serious consequences but who were not "real alcoholics" (Alcoholics Anonymous World Services, Inc., 1955:20-21). In like manner Marty Mann, the first woman to come through Alcoholics Anonymous and the founder of the National Council on Alcoholism, identified "two groups . . . whose drinking is not so easy to distinguish from alcoholic drinking," which she labeled "heavy drinkers" and "occasional drunks." She placed many of her New York friends, with whom she lost contact during her sojourn abroad and her own successful struggle with alcohol problems, in the former category. When she eventually returned to New York,

> I met once again many of my own acquaintances of the Twenties. Some of them were still drinking exactly as they had when I had first known them, with no visible harmful effects. The majority, however, today drink comparatively little—at most, social drinking in the strictest sense of the term. None that I have met again has stopped drinking entirely—and none has become an alcoholic. (Mann, 1981:82)

In *The Disease Concept of Alcoholism,* E. M. Jellinek (1960) identified what he called different "species" of alcoholism. He was particularly concerned with five such species, to which he assigned as identifiers the first five letters of the Greek alphabet—alpha, beta, gamma, delta, and epsilon. Jellinek felt that only the gamma and delta species could be viewed as diseases. He noted that "obviously there are species of alcoholism . . . which cannot be regarded as illnesses" (p. 35), and added that "all the remaining 19 letters of the Greek and if necessary other alphabets are available for labelling them" (p. 39).

Jellinek also mentioned "other species of alcoholism" such as "explosive drinking" and "fiesta drinking," with the admonition that "the student of the problems of alcohol cannot afford to overlook these behaviors, whether or not he is inclined to designate them as species of alcoholism" (p. 39). Finally, he observed that "By adhering strictly to our American ideas about `alcoholism´ (created by Alcoholics Anonymous in their own image) and restricting the term to these ideas, we have been continuing to overlook many other problems of alcohol which need urgent attention" (Jellinek, 1960:35). Jellinek's view of alcoholism as a diverse phenomenon, and of the need to look beyond it in a broad perspective, is consistent with the view of the committee.

Alcohol Dependence Syndrome

In 1976 Edwards and Gross first described the alcohol dependence syndrome. Their stated aim was "to help further to delineate the clinical picture," and even the brief "provisional" description contained in the original article includes memorable descriptions of clinical phenomena. The authors proposed that the "essential elements" of the syndrome might include "a narrowing in the repertoire of drinking behavior; salience of drink-seeking behavior; increased tolerance to alcohol; repeated withdrawal symptoms; repeated relief or avoidance of withdrawal symptoms by further drinking; subjective awareness of a compulsion to drink; reinstatement of the syndrome after abstinence" (Edwards and Gross, 1976:1058).

Edwards and Gross further stated that "all these elements exist in degree, thus giving the syndrome a range of severity." They also proposed a category of "drink-related disabilities" (subsequently "alcohol-related disabilities"). It consisted of various problems (in the original paper the examples given were the development of cirrhosis, the loss of a job, the breakup of a marriage, and the crashing of a car) that could occur as a result of drinking but "without suffering from the dependence syndrome." Although the authors suggested that the syndrome "should therefore not monopolize medical and social concern," they emphasized that such disabilities would "often accumulate for the person who is dependent and are more likely to occur the greater his dependence."

In the more than a dozen years since its enunciation, the concept of the alcohol dependence syndrome has undergone much examination and testing, as well as amplification and some modification. (For summaries see Edwards [1977, 1986]; the most detailed explication of the alcohol dependence syndrome is in Edwards and coworkers [1977]). The concept has received its share of criticism (e.g. Shaw, 1979; Caetano, 1985; Skinner, 1988). Overall, however, it has gained currency, having been adopted by both of the major diagnostic classification systems that are now in use for mental disorders. With respect to the *International Classification of Diseases,* it replaced the term *alcoholism* as a designation in the 9th edition (ICD-9), implemented in 1979 (World Health Organization, 1979), and operationalized criteria are now being tested for inclusion in the forthcoming tenth edition. With respect to the *Diagnostic and Statistical Manual of the American Psychiatric Association,* the alcohol dependence syndrome has become the conceptual basis for the diagnosis of "psychoactive substance use disorders" in the revised version of the 3rd edition of the manual, or DSM-III-R, implemented in 1987 (American Psychiatric Association, 1987).

In the United States, DSM-III-R is more widely used than ICD-9; the DSM-III-R version of the alcohol dependence framework thus requires some additional comment. In keeping with the high degree of specificity introduced into the prior edition (DSM-III), this version of the alcohol dependence framework is quite detailed. It enumerates nine specific "criteria" (similar to but not identical with the symptoms enumerated in the original paper by Edwards and Gross) and specifies that three or more of these must be met to make a diagnosis. An important consequence is that neither physical dependence nor tolerance need be present to diagnose the dependence syndrome. DSM-III-R also specifies an "abuse" category that is similar to but not identical with Edwards and Gross's category of "alcohol-related disabilities."

Finally, in DSM-III-R the criteria and the diagnostic category itself are to be applied not only to alcohol but to all drugs; hence the category is labeled "psychoactive substance use disorders." A more extensive detailing of the criteria for this version of the alcohol dependence framework, its rationale, and the results of field trials carried out in the United States is available in the literature (Rounsaville et al., 1986, 1987). Efforts are under way currently to attempt to resolve some of the differences between the DSM-III-R and the forthcoming ICD-10 versions of this framework.

There can be little doubt that the concept of the alcohol dependence syndrome has presented a significant and highly sophisticated challenge to researchers and clinicians, requiring them to rethink many fundamental concepts and definitions. The ensuing dialogue has enriched the field. Nevertheless, for the purposes of this report, the same question must be posed regarding the alcohol dependence framework as was articulated for the alcoholism framework: does it encompass all of the individuals the committee feels must be included within the scope of planning, policy formulation, and treatment?

Once again, the committee feels that the answer is in the negative. Many such persons are included within the concept of "alcohol-related disabilities." In terms of the vignettes presented at the outset of this chapter, George's fractured pelvis, Patrick's absenteeism, and even Gregory's homicide would be classified in this category rather than as instances of the alcohol dependence syndrome. Nor would George, Sally, or Gregory meet DSM-III-R criteria for *either* alcohol abuse or alcohol dependence. From planning, policy, and treatment perspectives, the potential hazard is that individuals failing to be classified as alcohol dependent might readily come to be assigned a lower priority, while those manifesting the genuine syndrome might be accorded a higher priority.

A Terminological "Map"

The committee feels that the alcohol problems perspective, as defined above, most readily encompasses the target population of the present report. Nevertheless, it does not feel that this perspective is contradictory to, or even precludes the use of, other perspectives such as that of alcoholism or the alcohol dependence syndrome. In many ways the perspectives are compatible, at least over portions of the range of problems. For the sake of simplicity and uniformity, the committee has used the alcohol problems perspective and its associated terminology throughout the balance of this report. As an aid to understanding, however, Figure 2-1 shows in an organized manner the interrelationships between these various perspectives.

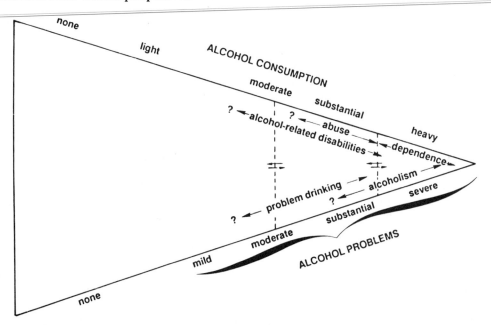

FIGURE 2-1 A terminological map. The triangle represents the population of the United States. The alcohol consumption of the population ranges from none to heavy (along the upper side of the triangle) and the problems experienced in association with alcohol consumption range from none to severe (along the lower side of the triangle). The two-way arrows and the dotted lines indicate that, both from an individual and a population perspective, consumption levels and the degree of problems vary from time to time. The scope of terms that are often used to refer to individuals and groups according to their consumption levels and the degree of their problems are illustrated; question marks indicate that the lower boundary for many of the terms is uncertain.

The triangle in the figure represents the population of the United States, partitioned into drinking categories according to level of alcohol consumption, which is indicated along the upper arm of the triangle. In the United States there is a substantial population that does not consume alcoholic beverages, and most individuals' consumption would be classified as light or moderate; such categories account for approximately three-quarters of the population. Approximately one-fifth consumes substantial amounts of alcohol, and approximately 5 per cent drink heavily. Too much should not be made of these figures, however, as they tend to change over time and are extremely variable depending on location, degree of urbanization, and other factors.

As suggested in the figure, there is a generally positive and direct relationship between the level of alcohol consumption in a population and the nature and severity of the problems experienced by that population (Hilton, 1987; Babor et al., 1988). This relationship is less consistent at the individual level, where discrepancies between consumption levels and problems are often observed. These discrepancies are the basis for the committee's recommendation of a routine assessment of both consumption levels and problems in evaluating individuals for treatment (see Chapter 10). In aggregate data, however, these individual differences tend to balance out, and a relatively direct relationship between consumption and alcohol problems emerges.

By drawing dotted rather than solid lines, and by placing two-way arrows in the figure, the committee intends to indicate that both alcohol consumption and alcohol problems lie along a continuum and that categories, such as moderate or severe, are conveniences for communication rather than fixed entities. In addition, the relative size of the categories, as well as the positioning of a single individual within the confines of the diagram, are not static but vary substantially over time. The principal purpose of the diagram is not to apportion drinkers in the United States into categories but to indicate graphically the committee's view of the scope of the alcohol problems framework and alternative conceptual frameworks.

Thus, the committee sees alcohol dependence and alcoholism as occupying primarily the apex of the triangle, together with heavy alcohol consumption. Their analogue in the alcohol problems framework would be severe, chronic alcohol problems (the figure does not show a temporal dimension). Alcohol-related disabilities, alcohol abuse, and problem drinking occupy portions of the less severe area of the diagram. (Problem drinking was not discussed as an alternative framework because, as the concept is currently used, it would exclude the apex of the triangle; for a different viewpoint, however, see Cahalan [1970].) The question marks indicate that the placement of various terms within this context is hardly precise, particularly at the lower end.

What emerges principally from the diagram is that the alcohol problems perspective encompasses within a single category a larger portion of the relevant spectrum than other perspectives but at the same time is not incompatible with them. This property makes it particularly useful for the committee's purposes and influenced its choice as the frame of reference for the present report. Those who are more comfortable with or more accustomed to an alternative frame of reference can use the figure to place what is said in a more familiar perspective.

The Heterogeneity of Alcohol Problems

Having selected a broad, overarching framework within which all problems requiring treatment in a broad sense are viewed as similar in important ways for policy, planning, and treatment purposes, the committee proposes to explore the marked diversity within this unitary framework, principally for treatment purposes. On its surface, this seems contradictory. Yet the seeming paradox is readily resolved. The committee wishes to assure the availability of treatment for the broad spectrum of individuals with alcohol problems but at the same time recognizes that different individuals will manifest different problems and will require different treatment or treatments.

Toward the end of the 18th century Dr. Thomas Trotter, an English physician, anticipated a major conclusion of the present report when he wrote with regard to alcohol problems that "in treating these various descriptions of persons and characters, it will readily appear, to a discerning physician, that very different remedies will be required" (Jellinek, 1941). The differential treatment of alcohol problems is not a new idea. To an important degree, however, it seems to have been disregarded until comparatively recently, and the committee believes it requires re-emphasis.

Perhaps the reasons for its relative neglect are historical. Following the long hiatus in treatment efforts occasioned by Prohibition in the United States and elsewhere (see Chapter 1) a new beginning was required. Under such circumstances it is the more chronic and more severe cases that come immediately to attention, and it is perhaps not surprising that they should have become the major focus of clinical efforts. Only in the last two decades, through large-scale epidemiological studies of general populations, has the existence of a large population of persons with less than maximally severe alcohol problems become apparent, and only subsequent to that discovery have treatment approaches been developed that may be particularly suitable for such problems.

An emerging perspective on the diversity or heterogeneity of alcohol problems can be traced in the contemporary literature. By law, the secretary of Health and Human Services is required to report to Congress periodically on the health consequences of alcohol consumption and on research findings regarding alcoholism and alcohol abuse. The Secretary's *Fifth Special Report to Congress on Alcohol and Health* states:

> The traditional concept of alcoholism as a unitary disease has been challenged. Over the past decade, researchers and clinicians have come to realize that multiple patterns of alcohol use may result in multiple forms of disability. Accordingly, a new emerging model of treatment stresses the heterogeneous nature of the client population, the need for more specific and efficient treatments, and the importance of maintaining gains after treatment. This model differentiates among alcoholics . . . and attempts to match each type with the most appropriate combination and configuration of treatments. (USDHHS, 1983:116)

By the time the next special report appeared in January 1987, what had been a "new emerging model of treatment" only three years before was now itself described as "traditional" (USDHHS, 1987:121). Four months later the Institute of Medicine (1987) published *Causes and Consequences of Alcohol Problems.* It stressed that one of the two "developments of particular note" during 1980-1985 was that "increasing numbers of examples have been found to support the concept of heterogeneity among individuals in the impact of heredity and environment on both the social and biological aspects of drinking" (p.1). The other development noted was the contribution made by genetic studies in humans and animals, which stressed the heterogeneity of the contribution of genetics to alcohol problems (cf. Cloninger, 1987).

The disease concept of alcoholism has sometimes been viewed (see above) as retarding an acceptance of the heterogeneity of alcohol problems. Yet Jellinek's concept of alcoholism, as discussed earlier, included at least two types that he considered diseases and that differed from each other, as well as other types that he did not consider diseases. This report will not deal extensively with the disease concept debate, which is well detailed elsewhere (cf. Keller, 1976; Fingarette, 1977; Kissin, 1983; Room, 1983; Fingarette, 1988). However, many diseases are heterogeneous—for example diabetes, hypertension, asthma, cancer, schizophrenia, end-stage renal disease, syphilis, and tuberculosis. Dealing with severe and institutionalized cases of post-encephalitic Parkinson's disease, a gifted observer noted:

What excited me . . . was the spectacle of a disease that was never the same in two patients, a disease that could take any possible form . . . [P]ost-encephalitic illness could by no means be considered a simple disease, but needed to be seen as an individual creation of the greatest complexity, determined not simply by a primary disease-process, but by a vast host of personal traits and social circumstances . . . a coming-to-terms of the sensitized individual with his total environment. (Sacks, 1987:21)

Some time ago, Griffith Edwards observed that "the decision as to alcoholism being a disease will still rest very much on the definition of alcoholism on the one hand and of `disease´ on the other" (Edwards, 1970:161). Within the perspective of alcohol problems it would not be surprising if particular individuals were most effectively and realistically viewed as suffering from a disease, whereas others should not be so viewed. *It is part of this perspective that all individuals with alcohol problems should have broad access to appropriate and effective treatment*; it follows that access should not be contingent on whether a disease is present. As diseases themselves can be heterogeneous, differential treatment is required even if a disease *is* present. There may be reasons for continuing the debate over the disease concept, but progress in treatment need not await its resolution.

Heterogeneity of Presentation

There are a number of ways in which alcohol problems are heterogeneous. One is the manner in which they initially present. They are protean; they can imitate the presentation of any other disorder, but even if they present as alcohol problems they are extraordinarily diverse (as demonstrated in the vignettes at the outset of this chapter). Based on longitudinal research on several different populations, George Vaillant has eloquently stated the case:

Alcoholism is a syndrome defined by the redundancy and variety of individual symptoms. Efforts to fit all alcohol users who are problems to themselves or others into a single, rigid definition will prove procrustean. It is the variety of alcohol-related problems, not a unique criterion, that captures what clinicians really mean when they label a person alcoholic (Vaillant et al., 1982:229).

This summary statement is concretely embodied in the lengthy lists of medical history items and clinical signs that may alert a physician to the presence of an alcohol problem (cf. Tables 1 and 2 in Skinner et al., 1986).

In an earlier era Sir William Osler remarked that "to know syphilis is to know medicine." Some medical educators feel that this is now true of alcohol problems precisely because of their seemingly infinite variety of clinical presentations. At Johns Hopkins Medical School, alcohol problems have become the central focus of teaching: "the purpose of the program is to get every medical student and every clinician at the institution acquainted with the early signs of alcoholism and competent to detect and recommend appropriate treatment for the disorder" (Holden, 1985). As part of this approach researchers carried out a study of all new admissions to adult inpatient services at Johns Hopkins Hospital. They confirmed that approximately 20% of all admissions had significant alcohol problems and that these problems frequently went unrecognized by the hospital staff (Moore et al., 1989).

Heterogeneity of Course

As noted earlier, a progressive course in which a problem becomes increasingly severe as time passes is a part of at least some definitions of alcoholism. Although it is understandable that individuals pursuing such a course should make a strong impression on clinicians who are trying to help them, further experience has documented that a progressive course is by no means the only direction pursued by individuals manifesting alcohol problems. The observations of Marty Mann (see above) are an example that has been confirmed by more systematic research many times over.

Vaillant's longitudinal studies, for example, delineated a group of "atypical alcoholics," individuals "who spend a lifetime abusing alcohol but never progress." He commented that "the atypical alcohol abusers by no means were individuals who were not *really alcoholic*" and illustrated this point by a statistical comparison with his clinic sample (Vaillant, 1983:144-45). He labeled as an "illusion" the notion that "alcoholism is a progressive disease that ends in abstinence or death" (p.160) and indicated that the assumption of universal progression may be an artifact produced by a focus upon skewed clinic samples: ". . . if one looks at those individuals whose alcoholism *has* been progressive (that is, relapsing alcohol-dependent individuals seen in alcohol clinics and emergency rooms) then alcoholism certainly appears to be progressive" (p.309).

There is ample evidence that, even in clinic samples of individuals with severe problems, the progression of these problems is by no means a universal course. This statement is even true for some groups of patients who continue to consume alcohol—not an ideal treatment goal for persons with severe problems but certainly a critical test of the universal progression notion. For example, in a recent study that followed a large sample for three years after treatment, in excess of 18 per cent of the sample had continued to drink at different levels without experiencing any further problems (Helzer et al., 1985; see also Miller, 1985). Similar findings indicating a lack of progression for some persons even in the face of continuing alcohol consumption have been reported in the post-treatment period by others (Armor et al., 1978; Gottheil et al., 1979; Paredes et al., 1979.)

Studies in nontreatment populations find a similarly variable mixture of progression and other patterns (Cahalan, 1970; Clark and Cahalan, 1976; Fillmore and Midanik, 1984; Temple and Fillmore, 1985; Fillmore, 1987). In the largest study yet mounted of nontreatment populations, the so-called Epidemiologic Catchment Area (ECA) study, fully 84 per cent of those who met DSM-III lifetime criteria for alcoholism and had reported especially heavy consumption at some time (7 or more drinks daily for two or more weeks) reported no periods of such drinking during the past year. Rates of remission (defined as the proportion of lifetime cases that had no alcohol problems in the past year) were found to be high, ranging from 45 to 55 per cent across the different sites of the study and averaging 51 per cent for the study overall. Most remitted cases dated their first and last symptoms at less than 5 years apart; more than three-quarters of the entire sample provided an estimated duration of less than 11 years (Helzer and Burnham, in press).

Thus, some persons with alcohol problems run a progressive course, and some do not. Systematic examination of the courses actually traversed in any reasonably sized population, whether of persons who have been treated or persons who have not, regularly finds a multiplicity of courses. A number of factors that may affect the course of alcohol problems have been identified, but no determinative factors, either biological or otherwise, that invariably result in a particular course have come to light (Babor and Kadden, 1985; IOM, 1987).

Heterogeneity of Etiology

What is the cause of alcohol problems? Although this question has been repeatedly and insistently asked over the years, no ready answer, in terms of the identification of a single cause, has emerged, and the committee believes none is likely. As noted in the 1987 IOM report, "these are complex phenomena, occurring at the junction of biologic, behavioral, and social forces" (IOM, 1987).

In light of this conclusion, the committee's response to the commonly-asked question about the cause of alcohol problems is fourfold:

1. *There is no likelihood that a single cause will be identified for all instances of alcohol problems.*

2. *There is every likelihood that the range of causes that interact to produce alcohol problems in the population can be identified.*

3. *Alcohol problems will prove to be the result of different interactions of different etiological factors in different individuals.*

4. *While effective treatment will be served by a more precise knowledge of etiology, effective treatment is possible in the absence of such knowledge.*

This viewpoint on etiology is similar to that of the biopsychosocial model of etiology in medicine (Engel, 1977; Engel, 1980; Engel, 1988) and to the multifactorial model of etiology in human behavior (cf. Babor and Kadden, 1985). A representative statement of this perspective for alcohol problems is the following:

> This way of thinking views every drinker as being at some stage of a dynamic, lifelong process influenced by a multitude of weak, interacting social, psychological, and physical forces with no single factor, except alcohol, being necessary, and none at all being sufficient to cause advancement in the process to the point of being labelled "alcoholic" or "problem drinker." From this viewpoint, the alcohologist's task of identifying the forces influencing the alcoholic process and untangling their complex interrelationships is much like that of the meteorologist's attempts to understand the process called "the weather." (Mulford, 1982:451)

This type of multidimensional approach has been taken by investigators in the area of genetics. That genetic factors play a role in the etiology of alcohol problems, as in most aspects of human behavior, has been thought likely for some time. Recently, however, it has been felt that the available data are more understandable if that role is viewed as diverse rather than identical in all instances, and an attempt has been made to delineate those instances in which genetic influences are likely to be of greater or of lesser importance (Murray and Gurling, 1982; Murray et al., 1983; Cloninger, 1987). "An important general principle in genetic epidemiology," writes a group of involved investigators, "is that disorders as prevalent as alcoholism have complex patterns of development involving the interaction of many genetic and environmental influences. Accordingly, such common disorders are expected to be heterogeneous both clinically and etiologically (Cloninger et al., 1988:500).

It has long been recognized that treatment can be effective in the absence of detailed knowledge of etiology. Mortality from many of the common infectious diseases declined steadily long before the bacteriologic identification of the offending organisms and the development of specific antibiotics as a result of general measures of public hygiene and the provision of adequate nutrition (McKeown, 1976). The etiology of essential hypertension is unknown, but its effective treatment is commonplace. Schizophrenia is a devastating problem of unknown etiology, but the appropriate deployment of pharmacotherapy, psychotherapy, and social restructuring can be effective in dealing with it. Many other examples are available. It is also the case, regrettably, that precise knowledge of etiology does not in all instances lead to effective treatment (cf. Luzzatto and Goodfellow, 1989).

This is not to deny that the elucidation of etiological factors for alcohol problems is a pressing need; it is, and it should be attended to. But the development of an effective treatment response need not and, indeed, cannot be viewed as contingent upon such an elucidation. Much can be done—must be done—even as that knowledge unfolds. Knowledge of etiology will unfold slowly, and its applicability will be limited by the diversity and complexity of the problems and of the human condition. Nevertheless, effective assistance is now available, and further delays in deploying it would be both unnecessary and unfortunate.

Implications of Heterogeneity for Treatment

In closing, it seems desirable to address again and to refine the implications of the foregoing discussion for treatment, the principal subject of this report. If persons with alcohol problems are viewed as heterogeneous in significant ways, there are potentially important implications for treatment. One is that *no one form of treatment is likely to be effective for all persons with alcohol problems.* A related implication is that *each treatment may be effective for some persons with alcohol problems* (see Chapter 5). It follows that *a principal task in providing treatment is to identify the kind of treatment that is most likely to prove effective for a given person with a given problem* (see Chapter 11).

Some of those who have acknowledged the wide differences among alcohol problems and among the individuals who manifest them have nevertheless questioned the significance of these differences. Keller's law holds that "the investigation of any trait in alcoholics will show that they have either more or less of it." Keller's overall conclusion, however, is that "alcoholics are different in so many ways that it makes no difference" (Keller, 1972:1147). A similar conclusion has sometimes been applied to treatment:

> Practically, differences that do not make any difference are not differences.
> It does not seem warranted at our present level of therapeutic knowledge
> to develop separate programs for different categories of alcoholics . . . .
> Within a single treatment approach it is possible to acknowledge and deal
> with individual differences thereby treating both the common problem of
> alcoholism-chemical dependency and the problems unique to individual
> patients. (Laundergan, 1982:36)

The committee favors a combined approach. Not *all* differences between problems or between individuals manifesting them will necessarily require different treatments all of the time. For example, experience suggests that it is not always necessary to provide different treatments for men and women with alcohol problems. However, *some* differences among problems or individuals will require different treatments some of the time. Thus experience, as well as a substantial body of experimental evidence (Annis, 1988), also suggests that at times it *may* be necessary to provide different treatments for men and women with alcohol problems to achieve the best possible outcomes for each (see Chapters 15 and 18).

Much of the remainder of this report is devoted to spelling out the implications of this view for treatment. To summarize briefly, however, the committee believes that, for persons with problems that do not appear to require specialized treatment or for those who are unwilling to undertake such treatment, it is reasonable, as well as practical at present, for nonspecialists to offer a generalized brief intervention (see Chapter 9). In addition, although the committee considers as potentially important differences those characteristics which distinguish what have been called special populations, it believes that, at present, such differences should be dealt with in the context of standard treatment programs (see Section IV).

On the other hand, the committee feels that some differences will at some times require differential treatment. Hence, in each instance of an individual seeking specialized treatment, individual differences must be carefully assessed (see Chapter 10) and, where indicated, taken into account by selecting the most appropriate treatment (see Chapter 11). Fortunately, there is a considerable variety of treatment programs that have already been developed (see Chapter 3), although the availability of different programs may still be a problem (see Chapter 7).

Treatment so conceived is not a simple matter. There is no standard formula; instead, the constant exercise of judgment is required in deciding when individual differences are likely to be crucial to the choice of treatment. It is a heavy responsibility. The committee recommends that steps be taken to inform that judgment to a much greater extent than is now usually the case—for example, through the development of knowledge regarding outcome (see Chapter 12) and the development of treatment systems (see Chapter 13). Even if these recommendations are implemented, however, the committee recognizes that the treatment of people with alcohol problems will remain a complex, arduous task for both the treaters and the treated.

Summary and Conclusions

To focus concretely on its response to the question, "What is being treated?", the committee has presented a series of vignettes of individuals in whom problems have arisen around their use of beverage alcohol and who may require an appropriate treatment response for their optimum management. The committee's preference is to refer to these problems simply and directly as "alcohol problems," and it has used this terminology consistently throughout the report. It recognizes, however, that other frames of reference (e.g. "alcoholism," "alcohol dependence syndrome") may be more familiar or preferred by some and, viewing these as compatible if ultimately less satisfactory frameworks, provides a terminological "map" to facilitate understanding.

Although it is convenient to use a single term to designate the focus of treatment efforts, the committee places strong emphasis on the heterogeneity of the target population. In many crucial respects alcohol problems, as well as the individuals who manifest them, are quite different from one another. Present knowledge suggests that the causes of alcohol problems are multiple and diverse, and long experience indicates that alcohol problems present for treatment in many different forms and guises and follow a variety of courses.

The implications of this impressive diversity for treatment are discussed in the next sections of the report. The differences among alcohol problems and among individuals are viewed as potentially relevant to treatment. Hence, they must be comprehensively assessed on an individual basis prior to treatment and taken into account in selecting that treatment or treatments that are most likely to be associated with a favorable outcome. Treatment so conceived is a more complex matter than is sometimes recognized. Nevertheless, considering the complexity of the problems themselves and of the individuals who manifest them, the committee believes that effective approaches to treatment for alcohol problems must be able to cope with these complexities.

REFERENCES

Alcoholics Anonymous World Services, Inc. 1955. Alcoholics Anonymous. Second edition, revised. New York: Alcoholics Anonymous World Services, Inc.

American Psychiatric Association (APA). 1980. DSM III: Diagnostic and Statistical Manual of Mental Disorders, 3rd edition. Washington, D.C.: APA.

American Psychiatric Association (APA). 1987. DSM III-R: Diagnostic and Statistical Manual of Mental Disorders, 3rd edition revised. Washington, D.C.: APA.

Annis, H. M. 1988. Patient-treatment matching in the management of alcoholism. Presented to the 50th Annual Scientific Meeting of the Committee on Problems of Drug Dependence, Incorporated, North Falmouth, Mass., June 28.

Armor, D. J., J. M. Polich, and H. B. Stambuhl. 1978. Alcoholism and Treatment. New York: John Wiley and Sons.

Babor, T. F., and R. Kadden. 1985. Screening for alcohol problems: conceptual issues and practical considerations. Pp. 1-30 in Early Identification of Alcohol Abuse, N.C. Chang and H. M. Chao, eds. Washington, D.C.: U.S. Government Printing Office.

Babor, T. F., Z. Dolinsky, B. Rounsaville, and J. Jaffe. 1988. Unitary versus multi- dimensional models of alcoholism treatment outcome: An empirical study. Journal of Studies on Alcohol 49:167-77.

Caetano, R. 1985. Alcohol dependence and the need to drink: A compulsion? Psychological Medicine 15:463-69.

Caetano, R. 1987. Public opinions about alcoholism and its treatment. Journal of Studies on Alcohol 48:153-60.

Cahalan, D. 1970. Problem Drinkers: A National Survey. San Francisco: Jossey-Bass.

Clark, W. B., and D. Cahalan. 1976. Changes in problem drinking over a four-year span. Addictive Behavior 1:251-59.

Cloninger, C. R., S. Sigvardsson, A.-L. von Knorring. 1988. The Swedish studies of the adopted children of alcoholics: A reply to Littrell. Journal of Studies on Alcohol 49:500-509.

Cloninger, C. R. 1987. Neurogenetic adaptive mechanisms in alcoholism. Science 236:410-16.

Edwards, G. 1970. The status of alcoholism as a disease. Pp. 140-63 in Modern Trends in Drug Dependence and Alcoholism, R. V. Phillipson ed. New York: AppletonCentury-Crofts.

Edwards, G. 1977. The alcohol dependence syndrome: Usefulness of an idea. Pp. 136-56 in Alcoholism: New Knowledge and New Responses, G. Edwards and M. Grant, eds. Baltimore: University Park Press.

Edwards, G. 1986. The alcohol dependence syndrome: A concept as stimulus to enquiry. British Journal of Addiction 81:171-83.

Edwards, G., and M. M. Gross. 1976. Alcohol dependence: provisional description of a clinical syndrome. British Medical Journal 1:1058-61.

Edwards, G., M. M. Gross, and M. Keller. 1977. Alcohol Related Disabilities. Geneva: World Health Organization.

Engel, G. L. 1977. The need for a new medical model: a challenge for biomedicine. Science 196:129-36.

Engel, G. L. 1980. The clinical application of the biopsychosocial model. American Journal of Psychiatry 137:535-44.

Engel, G. L. 1988. How much longer must medicine's science be bounded by a seventeenth-century world view? Pp. 113-36 in The Task of Medicine: Dialogue at Wickenburg, K. L. White. Menlo Park, Calif.: Kaiser Family Foundation.

Fillmore, K. M. 1987. Women's drinking across the life course as compared to men's. British Journal of Addiction 82:801-11.

Fillmore, K. M., and L. Midanik. 1984. Chronicity of drinking problems among men: A longitudinal study. Journal of Studies on Alcohol 45:228-36.

Fingarette, H. 1983. Philosophical and legal aspects of the disease concept of alcoholism. Pp. 1-45 in Research Advances in Alcohol and Drug Problems, vol. 7, R. G. Smart, F. B. Glaser, Y. Israel, H. Kalant, R. E. Popham, and W. Schmidt, eds. New York: Plenum Press.

Fingarette, H. 1988. Heavy Drinking: The Myth of Alcoholism as a Disease. Berkeley: University of California Press.

Gottheil, E., C. C. Thornton, and T. E. Skoloda. 1979. Follow-up study of alcoholics at 6, 12, and 24 months. Currents in Alcoholism 6:91-109.

Gottheil, E., C. C. Thornton, and T. E. Skoloda, 1982. Follow-up of abstinent and non-abstinent alcoholics. American Journal of Psychiatry 139:560-65.

Helzer, J. E., L. N. Robins, J. R. Taylor, 1985. The extent of long-term moderate drinking among alcoholics discharged from medical and psychiatric treatment facilities. New England Journal of Medicine 312:1678-82.

Helzer, J. E., and A. Burnham. In press. Alcohol abuse and dependence. In Psychiatric Disorders in America, L. N. Robins and D. A. Regier, eds. New York:The Free Press.

Hilton, M. E. 1987. Demographic characteristics and the frequency of heavy drinking as predictors of self-reported drinking problems. British Journal of Addiction 82:913-25.

Holden, C. 1985. The neglected disease in medical education. Science 229:741-42.

Institute of Medicine. 1987. Causes and Consequences of Alcohol Problems: An Agenda for Research. Washington, D.C.: National Academy Press.

Jackson, J. K. 1988. Testimony presented before the U.S. Senate Governmental Affairs Committee hearing regarding the causes of and governmental responses to alcohol abuse and alcoholism, Washington, D.C., June 16.

Jellinek, E. M. 1941. An early medical view of alcohol addiction and its treatment: Dr. Thomas Trotter's Essay, Medical, Philosophical, and Chemical, on Drunkenness. Quarterly Journal of Studies on Alcohol 2:584-91.

Jellinek, E. M. 1943. Magnus Huss' Alcoholismus Chronicus. Quarterly Journal of Studies on Alcohol 4:85-92.

Jellinek, E. M. 1960. The Disease Concept of Alcoholism. Highland Park, N.J.: Hillhouse Press.

Keller, M. 1976. The disease concept of alcoholism revisited. Journal of Studies on Alcohol 37:1694-1717.

Keller, M. 1972. The oddities of alcoholics. Quarterly Journal of Studies on Alcohol 33:1147.

Kissin, B. 1983. The disease concept of alcoholism. Pp. 93-126 in Research Advances in Alcohol and Drug Problems, Vol. 7. R. G. Smart, F. B. Glaser, Y. Israel, H. Kalant, R. E. Popham, and W. Schmidt, eds. New York: Plenum Press.

Laundergan, J. C. 1982. Easy Does It: Alcoholism Treatment Outcomes, Hazelden, and the Minnesota Model. Center City, Minn.: The Hazelden Foundation.

Levine, H. G. 1984. What is an alcohol-related problem? (or, what are people talking about when they refer to alcohol problems)? Journal of Drug Issues 14:45-60.

Luzzatto, L., and P. Goodfellow. 1989. A simple disease with no cure. Nature 337:17-18.

Mann, M. 1981. Marty Mann's New Primer on Alcoholism: How People Drink, How to Recognize Alcoholics, and What to Do About Them. New York: Henry Holt and Company.

McKeown, T. 1976. The Modern Rise of Population. London: Edward Arnold.

Miller, W. R. 1985. Letter to the editor. New England Journal of Medicine 313:1661-62.

Moore, R. D., L. R. Bone, and G. Geller. 1989. Prevalence, detection, and treatment of alcoholism in hospitalized patients. Journal of the American Medical Association 261:403-07.

Mulford, H. A., and D. E. Miller. 1964. Measuring public acceptance of the alcoholic as a sick person. Quarterly Journal of Studies on Alcohol 25:314-24.

Mulford, H. A. 1982. The epidemiology of alcoholism and its implications. Pp. 441-457 in Encyclopedic Handbook of Alcoholism, E. M. Pattison, and E. Kaufman, eds. New York: Gardner Press.

Murray, R. M., C. A. Clifford, and H. M. D. Gurling. 1983. Twin and adoption studies: how good is the evidence for a genetic role? Pp. 25-48 in Recent Developments in Alcoholism,. vol. 1, M. Galanter, ed. New York: Academic Press.

Murray, R. M., and H. M. D. Gurling. 1982. Alcoholism: polygenic influence on a multifactorial disorder. British Journal Hospital Medicine 27:328-34.

Paredes, A., D. Gregory, O. H. Rundell. 1979. Drinking behavior, remission, and relapse: the RAND report revisited. Alcoholism: Theory, Research, and Practice 3:3-10.

Plaut, T. F. A., ed. 1967. Alcohol Problems: A Report to the Nation by the Cooperative Commission on the Study of Alcoholism. New York: Oxford University Press.

Rinaldi, R. C., E. M. Steindler, and B. B. Wilford, 1988. Clarification and standardization of substance abuse terminology. Journal of the American Medical Association 259:555-57.

Rodin, M. B. 1981. Alcoholism as a folk disease: the paradox of beliefs and choices of therapy in an urban american community. Journal of Studies on Alcohol 42:822-35.

Room, R. 1983. Sociological aspects of the disease concept of alcoholism. Pp. 47-91 in Research Advances in Alcohol and Drug Problems, vol 7, R. G. Smart, F. B. Glaser, Y. Israel, H. Kalant, R. E. Popham, and W. Schmidt, eds. New York: Plenum Press.

Rounsaville, B. J., T. R. Kosten, and J. B. W. Williams. 1987. A field trial of DSM-III-R psychoactive substance dependence disorders. American Journal of Psychiatry 144:351-55.

Rounsaville, B. J., R. L. Spitzer, and J. B. W. Williams. 1986. Proposed changes in DSM-III substance use disorders: Description and rationale. American Journal of Psychiatry 143:463-68.

Sacks, O. 1987. Awakenings. New York: Summit Books.

Shaw, S. 1979. A critique of the concept of the alcohol dependence syndrome. British Journal of Addiction 74:339-48.

Skinner, H. A. 1988. Validation of the dependence syndrome: have we crossed the half-life of this concept? Manuscript prepared for the meeting on "The Nature of Dependence," sponsored by the Society for the Study of Addiction, at Cumberland Lodge, Windsor Great Park, England, April 27-29.

Skinner, H. A., S. Holt, W.-J. Sheu, and Y. Israel. 1986. Clinical versus laboratory detection of alcohol abuse: The Alcohol Clinical Index. British Medical Journal 292:1703-1708.

Spitzer, R. L., J. B. W. Forman, and J. Nee. 1979. DSM-III field trials: I. Initial interrater diagnostic reliability. American Journal of Psychiatry 136:815-17.

Talbott, G. D., and M. Cooney. 1982. Today's Disease: Alcohol and Drug Dependence. Springfield, Ill.: Charles C. Thomas.

Temple, M. T., and K. M. Fillmore. 1985. The variability of drinking patterns and problems among young men, ages 16-31: a longitudinal study. International Journal of the Addictions 20:1595-1620.

U.S. Department of Health and Human Services (USDHHS). 1983. Fifth Special Report to the U.S. Congress on Alcohol and Health. Rockville, Md.: National Institute on Alcohol Abuse and Alcoholism.

United States Department of Health and Human Services (USDHHS). 1987. Sixth Special Report to the U.S. Congress on Alcohol and Health. Rockville, Md.: National Institute on Alcohol Abuse and Alcoholism.

Vaillant, G. E. 1983. The Natural History of Alcoholism: Causes, Patterns, and Paths to Recovery. Cambridge: Harvard University Press.

Vaillant, G. E., L. Gale, and E. S. Milofsky. 1982. Natural history of male alcoholism. II. The relationship between different diagnostic dimensions. Journal of Studies on Alcohol 43:216-32.

World Health Organization (WHO). 1979. International Classification of Diseases, 9th ed. Geneva: WHO.

3   What Is Treatment?

Just as it is necessary to clarify what is being treated in the realm of alcohol problems, it is also important to review and crystallize what is meant by treatment because there are many differing definitions. In most research studies, no single definition is offered; instead, one often finds a series of procedures or a specific program and setting being described and "evaluated." At other times, a rather complex and all-embracing definition is presented. As a result, there are arguments and controversy about what constitutes treatment for alcohol problems and who needs such treatment.

Is Alcoholics Anonymous a form of treatment? Are minor tranquilizers, when prescribed for anxiety reduction after detoxification is completed, treatment or symptom substitution? Are social model recovery centers and halfway houses treatment for alcohol problems? Is providing a supportive, alcohol-free living environment for homeless persons with alcohol problems treatment? Is family therapy a required element of the treatment of alcohol problems? Is education and counseling for incipient problem drinkers who have been arrested for a drinking-and-driving offense treatment?

Sometimes treatment is defined by what is reimbursable under a third-party payment plan. This definition, however, does not so much answer the question as raise alternative questions. Are biofeedback and stress management training for college students who are drinking excessively at weekend fraternity parties reimbursable treatment procedures under private health insurance? Is individual psychotherapy conducted by a certified alcoholism counselor in a private-practice setting a reimbursable service? Is chemical aversion therapy a safe and effective treatment for alcohol problems that should be reimbursed under Medicare and private health insurance? Is Antabuse monitoring by a certified alcoholism counselor working in a state-licensed outpatient clinic a treatment for which private health insurance or the state alcoholism authority, or both, should provide reimbursement? Is social model detoxification in a freestanding facility a form of treatment for which Medicare should provide reimbursement?

Much of the argument surrounding this issue appears to reflect a failure to agree on the definition of treatment for alcohol problems and on the active ingredients of the treatment process (Moos and Finney, 1987/1988; Filstead, 1988a,b; IOM, 1989). Consider the following definitions, which have been offered in federal government reports over the years:

> "Treatment" means the broad range of emergency, outpatient, intermediate, and inpatient services and care, including diagnostic evaluation, medical, psychiatric, psychological, and social service care, vocational rehabilitation and career counseling, which may be extended to alcoholic and intoxicated persons. (U.S. Department of Health, Education, and Welfare [USDHEW], 1971:106)

> Treatment/Treatment Services—The broad range of planned and continuing services, including diagnostic assessment, counseling, medical, psychiatric, psychological, and social service care for alcohol-related dysfunction, that may be extended to program patients and influence the behavior of such individuals toward identified goals and objectives. (Bast, 1984:11)

> Alcohol treatment refers to the broad range of services, including diagnostic assessment, counseling, medical, psychiatric, psychological, and

42

social services care for clients or patients with alcohol-related problems. Treatment activities involve intervention after the development and manifestation of alcohol abuse and alcoholism in order to arrest or reverse their progress, or to prevent illness or death from associated medical conditions . . . Treatment is essentially composed of two elements, (1) the therapeutic procedure, i.e., a specific set of protocols and activities, and (2) the therapeutic process, i.e., the milieu, setting, and interpersonal context in which a procedure can be implemented for optimal success. Treatment is a complex, interpersonal admixture of procedures and processes. (U.S. Department of Health and Human Services [USDHHS], 1986:42)

The first definition given above was included in the Uniform Alcoholism and Intoxication Treatment Act and as such became the basis for the definitions adopted by state licensure and national accreditation bodies, thus setting the broad parameters that underlie existing treatment and financing efforts. The Uniform Act had as its focus decriminalization of public drunkenness and destigmatization of all persons with alcohol problems (Plaut, 1967; Grad et al., 1971; Finn, 1985). Its definition was to a large extent based on the image of the typical alcoholic as the indigent, socially deteriorated public inebriate who required extensive psychological and social support services along with treatment of physical disabilities and direct treatment of the alcohol problem. This image was embodied in the original legislation and in resource development carried out by the federal government and the states.

The breadth of the various "official" definitions of treatment for alcohol problems reflects the importance that has been placed on including within the treatment process additional supportive activities (e.g., vocational counseling, family therapy). Thus, the definitions reflect the professional judgment that the treatment of alcohol problems cannot be limited only to those direct activities that are designed to reduce alcohol consumption. Supportive activities are seen as required if relapse is to be avoided and continued sobriety and recovery are to be maintained by individuals who have few personal and social resources and who are experiencing very severe physical, vocational, family, legal, or emotional problems around their use of alcohol (e.g., Boche, 1975; Kissin, 1977b; Costello, 1982; McClellan et al., 1980; Pattison, 1985; Moos and Finney, 1986/1987).

Socially deteriorated public inebriates or homeless alcoholics do require many additional supportive services if they are not to relapse and return to destructive alcohol consumption (Blumberg et al., 1973; Costello et al., 1977; Costello, 1980, 1982; Pattison et al., 1977; Shandler and Shipley, 1987; IOM, 1989). The extent of the person's dysfunction in other key life areas (e.g., employment, physical health, emotional health, marital and family relations) determines the breadth of the treatment response required (Pattison et al., 1977; Costello, 1980, 1982; Longabaugh and Beattie, 1985; Kissin and Hansen, 1985; Sanchez-Craig, 1988; see also Kissin, 1977a,b; Armor et al., 1978; Brown University Center for Alcohol Studies, 1985; Pattison, 1985).

The second and third definitions given earlier (Bast, 1984; USDHHS, 1986) are derivative of the Uniform Act definition and reflect the variety of treatment services that have been supported by federal and state categorical funding in the early years of the struggle to establish the treatment of alcohol problems as a distinct, legitimate activity (Chafetz, 1976; Booz-Allen and Hamilton, Inc., 1978; Anderson, 1981; J. Lewis, 1982; Weisman, 1988). To a certain extent, federal and state governments have supported this wide array of approaches to treatment because of differing theories about the causes of alcohol problems. As Saxe and colleagues (1983:4) note: "[t]he treatments for alcoholism are diverse, in part because experts have different views about the causes of alcoholism. At least three major views of the etiology of alcoholism can be identified: medical, psychological, and sociocultural. Treatments are generally based on one or a combination of these views."

There has been a continuing effort not only to define the treatment of alcohol problems as a primary condition (i.e., not a symptom of underlying psychopathology) but also to develop a separate, nonpsychiatric specialist system of treatment resources. The specialty programs directly treat the primary condition (Anderson, 1981; Weisman, 1988; see Chapters 4 and 7). The emphasis has been on creating a specialized continuum of care that can assist individuals in dealing with the complex set of biological, psychological, and sociocultural forces that create and maintain problem drinking behavior. As Glasscote and colleagues (1967:13) have stated:

> [I]t is abundantly clear that no single treatment approach or method has been demonstrated to be superior to all others. Although numerous kinds of therapy and intervention appear to have been effective with various kinds of problem drinkers, the process of matching patient and treatment method is not yet highly developed. There is an urgent need for continued experimentation for modifying and improving existing treatment methods, for developing new ones and for careful and well designed evaluative studies. Most of the facilities that provide services to alcoholics have made little if any attempt to determine the effectiveness of the total program or its components.

These observations remain appropriate today. Treatment for alcohol problems, as described in many of the studies and practice settings that have been reviewed for this report, has been found to be just such an unspecified admixture of medical, psychological, and sociocultural approaches. Research that organizes and evaluates the components of treatment in a systematic fashion is only now beginning to be carried out (Saxe et al., 1983; Walsh et al, 1986; Moos and Finney, 1987/1988; Filstead, 1988a,b; Holder et al., 1988; IOM, 1989; T. McLellan, Philadelphia VA Medical Center, personal communication, May 25, 1989). This committee's emphases on heterogeneity in etiology, presentation, and course and on the need for individualized comprehensive treatment are not new developments. Rather, they represent an approach that, although long advocated, has not been systematically applied in the design of funding policies and effective treatment programs.

Refining the Definition of Treatment for Alcohol Problems

Treatment for alcohol problems has come to include a very broad range of activities that vary in content, duration, intensity, goal, setting, provider, and target population.   Research data are available on the effectiveness of "treatments" or "interventions" that cover a broad spectrum: from brief, one-session outpatient treatment episodes for married, socially stable adult males in which the intervention is information about the hazards of continuing to drink excessively and advice on how to control drinking given by a physician or nurse (e.g., Edwards et al., 1977; Edwards, 1987) to months-long hospital and residential stays that remove the affected person from the stresses and seductions of an environment in which alcohol is easily available (e.g., Wallerstein, 1956, 1957; Blumberg et al., 1973). Given this range, it has become customary to distinguish between intervention and treatment when reviewing research and discussing available services. Intervention is generally discussed in connection with primary prevention; a prominent example of this approach is the most recent report on alcohol and health submitted to Congress by the secretary of health and human services (USDHHS, 1987b).

However, the term intervention has come to have two distinct meanings in the treatment of alcohol problems in addition to its usual meaning in medicine and education (i.e., an activity designed to modify a condition). First, intervention is used to describe a specific technique for confronting persons who are thought to have problems around their use of alcohol and to motivate them to enter treatment (Johnson, 1980, 1986; Beyer and Trice, 1982; Trice and Beyer, 1984; see Appendix D). As a technique used to bring people into treatment, intervention involves nonjudgemental confrontation by family, friends, or coworkers to break down an individual's rationalization and denial of the problems related to excessive drinking (Blume, 1982).

Second, intervention may be used to describe case finding and treatment of "early-stage" problem drinkers, as noted by Cohen (1982:127):

> Early intervention consists of the identification of persons or groups whose drinking behavior places them at risk and of persons in the early stages of destructive drinking practices. It includes their involvement in corrective learning and emotional experiences designed to help them develop abstinence or more benign drinking patterns.

In this use of the term, early intervention is identified with secondary prevention, and treatment is identified with tertiary prevention. The distinction is made primarily on the basis of the target population, and secondarily on the goal chosen (abstinence or controlled drinking), rather than on the basis of the activity that is actually performed. Thus, intervention is described as being aimed at the "early-stage drinker" or less impaired youthful drinker; treatment and rehabilitation are described as being directed toward "those with established disabling, psychosocial disorders":

> Early intervention is conceptualized as the equivalent of secondary prevention, the attempted reversal of the early stages of dysfunctional drinking by individuals or homogeneous groups at risk. Secondary prevention contrasts with primary prevention, i.e., the educational approaches that attempt to reinforce healthful drinking attitudes especially, but not exclusively among youths. Tertiary prevention consists of the formal treatment and rehabilitation measures for those with established disabling, psychosocial disorders. (Cohen, 1982:128)

> Intervention activities are those that seek to detect alcohol-related problems in their early stages and to intervene in such problems in such a way as to arrest their progression . . . . Treatment activities involve intervention after the development and manifestation of alcohol abuse and alcoholism in order to arrest or reverse their progress, and/or to prevent progressive illness or death from associated medical conditions. (USDHHS, 1986:69)

It is important to distinguish between intervention activities and primary prevention activities, which are aimed at those persons, whether abstainers or social drinkers, for whom no alcohol-related problems have as yet been identified by themselves or by others. Although sometimes labeled as early intervention, primary prevention more accurately describes those specific activities that are aimed at persons who are not engaged in risky or problematic drinking but who are designated as high risk because of such factors as a family history of alcohol problems or childhood behavior problems. Secondary prevention activities—activities that could more accurately be labeled "early intervention"—involve the identification of individuals who are drinking in a risky fashion and are beginning to experience problems and symptoms. Actually, however, in view of the heterogeneity of course discussed in the previous chapter, the designation "early" is inappropriate. Many persons so identified will not progress to more serious problems although some will (see Chapter 6). Examples of "early intervention" (secondary prevention activities) are counseling heavy drinkers among college students (Marlatt, 1988a) or counseling patients who are receiving medical treatment for alcohol-related physical illnesses or injuries (D. C. Lewis and Gordon, 1983; Williams et al., 1985).

There are many organizational entities in this country that sponsor and conduct early intervention programs—social service agencies, drinking-driver programs, student assistance programs, employee assistance programs, to name a few. It has been customary, however, to view these locales and activities as intervention programs rather than treatment; they are considered to be separate from the overall treatment system and engaged in performing only referral and case monitoring (e.g., Saxe et al., 1983; USDHHS, 1987b), even though many also provide counseling and education. *The committee considers it an error to continue to omit these resources from consideration as elements of the continuum of treatment services that should be available in each community to all persons who need them.* Therefore, intervention programs which offer referral, education, and short term counseling as well as continuity of care assurance and follow-up monitoring (e.g., employee assistance programs, student assistance programs) are included in the committee's definition of the treatment system, along with more traditional locales (e.g., hospital and freestanding detoxification and rehabilitation units, outpatient clinics, halfway houses) (see Chapter 9).

The most direct and simple definition of intervention and treatment for alcohol problems is "any activity that is directed toward changing a person's drinking behavior and reducing their alcohol consumption." Treatment and intervention are both aimed at changing the person's drinking behavior after a problem has been identified. Moreover, both intervention and treatment generally involve additional activities that are designed to alleviate other physical, psychological, and social problems as well as the conditions that are assumed to cause or maintain the hazardous level of drinking.

Thus, activities that previously were classified separately as either intervention or as treatment are included in the definition of treatment used in this report. The committee clearly identifies and distinguishes any use of the term *intervention* to describe the confrontational technique for motivating persons to seek treatment. At all other times, *intervention* is used synonymously with treatment.

To guide its deliberations and recommendations, the committee has adopted the following definition of treatment, which builds on the definitions reviewed earlier in the report and incorporates both intervention and treatment:

> *Treatment refers to the broad range of services, including identification, brief intervention, assessment, diagnosis, counseling, medical services, psychiatric services, psychological services, social services, and follow-up, for persons with alcohol problems. The overall goal of treatment is to reduce or eliminate the use of alcohol as a contributing factor to physical, psychological, and social dysfunction and to arrest, retard, or reverse the progress of any associated problems.*

The committee has formulated this expanded definition of treatment because it agrees with those who have suggested that efforts to treat alcohol problems in this country have been too narrowly focused on those persons with the most severe problems (see Chapter 9). The guiding principle it has espoused is that all of those individuals who are identified as having a problem around their use of alcohol should receive some assistance with their problems. The traditional approach to the management of alcohol problems has often been the so-called Minnesota model of treatment (discussed later in this chapter), which focuses on the smaller number of individuals who show major symptoms of alcohol dependence, physical disability, and psychosocial dysfunction. The committee favors a broader approach that also deals with the much larger group of individuals who have engaged in excessive drinking and experienced some negative consequences (e.g., Skinner, 1985, 1988; Babor et al., 1986; Skinner and Holt, 1987; IOM, 1989). This approach will include the use of sites that provide brief interventions and brief therapy for persons with low or moderate levels of alcohol problems. The successful utilization of brief interventions will require changes in our conceptualization of the treatment system as well as additional training in the conduct of brief interventions for workers in the specialty alcohol problems treatment sector as well as in the general medical and social services sectors (see Section III).

Other countries have developed similar strategies, some of which are described in Appendix C. The effort to expand treatment availability in France is described by Babor and coworkers (1983). During the 1970s, the French developed a national network of outpatient clinics to provide secondary prevention, in the form of early intervention services to "habitual excessive drinkers" who were to be identified through screening in various industrial, legal, and health care settings. Generally staffed by a physician, a nurse, and a social worker, these specialty clinics provide a combination of clinical diagnosis of alcohol problems, medical treatment and counseling about the effects of continued excessive alcohol use, dietary counseling, health education, family counseling, and assistance in resolving social and legal problems. The focus of the clinics' education and counseling is that excessive alcohol consumption is the primary source of the patient's physical health, work, and family problems; sobriety or temperance, rather than abstinence only, are stressed as the means of eliminating these problems. Thus, a person is told to reduce drinking to the amount he or she can tolerate without risk.

Another example of the development of an expanded network of services is the methodology used by drinking-driver programs (see Chapter 16). This approach identifies persons arrested for a driving-while-impaired (DWI) offense and assigns them to an education (intervention) or treatment experience on the basis of a screening that categorizes individuals as social drinkers, incipient problem drinkers, or problem drinkers. The military, which initially modeled its approach on that used by drinking-driver programs, uses a similar methodology to assign individuals to education, outpatient counseling, or inpatient treatment, (Borthwick, 1977; Armor et al., 1978; Zuska, 1978; Orvis et al., 1981). The approaches of all these programs are based on the view that alcohol problems must be broadly addressed within an expanded treatment context.

Defining the Expanded Continuum of Care

Given the complexities of dealing with the wide range of medical, psychological, and social difficulties presented by persons with alcohol problems, it has become customary to speak of the need for a comprehensive continuum of available treatment services. This continuum has become the operationalized definition of treatment for alcohol problems:

> It is important that any funding mechanism for alcohol and drug services cover a broad enough spectrum of services and service providers to insure that the individual patients or clients are provided with a continuum of care which is adequate and appropriate to their needs. Such care may include a combination of inpatient hospital services, direct medical care, residential care in various sheltered environments, counseling, job training and placement assistance and aid in dealing with various life problems. (Boche, 1975:3)

Similarly, Sections 1, 8, and 10(5) of the Uniform Alcoholism and Intoxication Treatment Act explicitly called on the states to ensure that a continuum of coordinated treatment services with reasonable geographic access was established within each state (USDHEW, 1971). The act emphasized a coordinated network of services within each community to ensure that individuals would receive all the care appropriate to their needs and not be denied access to services because of agency boundaries. The Uniform Act was a major source for the treatment definitions presented earlier in this chapter; it is also the major source for contemporary definitions of the components of the continuum of care and the practices that currently represent the operational definition of treatment for alcohol problems.

The continuum of care called for in the Uniform Act had four major elements: (1) emergency treatment provided by a facility affiliated with or part of the medical service of a general hospital; (2) inpatient treatment; (3) intermediate treatment; and (4) outpatient and follow-up treatment. The description of the continuum was based on observed practices and on contemporary efforts by several states to redefine what treatment should be, based on research (Plaut, 1967) and surveys of existing programs (Glasscote, 1967; Grad et al., 1971).

As the first element of the continuum, the Uniform Act used the concept of emergency treatment in a hospital-related facility rather than the more popular "detoxification center" (the latter was seen as stigmatizing persons with alcohol problems by setting them apart from people with other illnesses or difficulties). These specialized emergency services were to be readily available 24 hours a day to anyone who needed them; they comprised medical services, social services, and appropriate diagnostic and referral services. Inpatient treatment, the second element called for in the act, was to provide 24-hour care in a short-stay community hospital for that limited percentage of persons who were thought to need to begin treatment in a restricted environment. Long-term hospital inpatient services were considered to be inappropriate for persons with alcohol problems; the short-term units were to be designed to facilitate the individual's return to his family and the community or to other appropriate care services as rapidly as possible.

Intermediate treatment was the term used to refer to residential treatment that was less than full time and that could be provided in a variety of community facilities (e.g., halfway houses, day or night hospitals, foster homes). Intermediate treatment settings, the third element in the continuum of care, were seen as alternatives to hospital inpatient settings and as extensions of initial inpatient services. The Uniform Act's final element, outpatient and follow-up treatment, was to include the same wide range of treatment services and modalities offered in the inpatient or intermediate service settings. The difference was that these services would be offered in a wide variety of settings in the community: for example, clinics, social centers, and even in the patient's own home (USDHEW, 1971).

In its 1986 report to Congress setting forth a comprehensive national plan to combat alcohol abuse and alcoholism, the Department of Health and Human Services (USDHHS) continued to discuss the need to provide and fully finance a "comprehensive continuum of care approach" to the treatment of alcohol abuse and alcoholism. The approach it described was derived primarily from the continuum of care that had been developed over the years in Minnesota (Anderson, 1981; Research Triangle Institute, 1985):

> A comprehensive alcohol treatment program provides care that recognizes the physical, social, psychological, and other needs of the patient. The major components of a comprehensive continuum of care approach are recognition, diagnosis and referral, detoxification, primary residential treatment, extended care, outpatient care or day care, aftercare, and a family program. (USDHHS, 1986:42)

More recently, the continuum of care needed for the treatment of alcohol problems has been described in another USDHHS report:

> Although necessarily limited by cost effectiveness considerations, alcoholism treatment has become increasingly multimodal and multidisciplinary. As is generally recognized, a comprehensive system of services includes at least the following: detoxification; inpatient rehabilitation; outpatient services including clinic, day hospital, and partial hospital services; family treatment; aftercare; residential or supervised living services; and sobering up services. These categories of services are not mutually exclusive. (USDHHS, 1987b:124)

These slightly different descriptions show that the continuum has not been clearly and consistently defined—neither in terms of the elements that constitute it, the combinations of elements required for particular groups within the population of persons with alcohol problems (see, for example, Section IV), nor the sequence in which the elements are required. The original Uniform Act description of the continuum focused on the settings in which treatment took place, whereas the later descriptions called for additional elements. Yet even in these key reports, many of the terms used to describe the components are not defined. There is no clear statement in either the 1986 national plan or the more recent report to Congress about how the continuum should be organized or the desired relationship among the listed elements.

For example, in the most recent description of the continuum (USDHHS, 1987b), the "sobering up services" element is introduced but without definition or discussion. Both detoxification and sobering-up services are included as necessary elements, but no distinction is made between them. Both are emergency treatment in terms of the original Uniform Act definitions. The context of the report suggests that the inclusion of sobering-up services as an essential element is to reflect the distinction that is now commonly made among the two or more levels of detoxification care included by many of the state alcoholism authorities in their planning and funding efforts.

In fact, the reference in the DHHS report is most likely drawn from a particular element (now, no longer used) of the New York state continuum, the sobering-up station. The sobering-up station was a particular form of the non-hospital-based, subacute, inpatient detoxification unit and was initially introduced as a lower cost alternative to jail or to expensive hospital-based detoxification for public inebriates (Zimberg, 1983). Recently, the New York state alcoholism authority developed a new model to describe its view of the ideal continuum of care. The new plan introduced a more comprehensive emergency treatment element, the alcohol crisis center, which replaces the sobering-up station; the plan also maintains a reduced hospital detoxification element (New York Division of Alcoholism and Alcohol Abuse, 1986). This new model recognizes, as has been shown in the research literature, that only a limited percentage of all persons who require detoxification—and not just public inebriates—need hospital-based services. Withdrawal for the majority can be safely managed in a subacute, nonhospital social setting or in an ambulatory medical model setting (O'Briant et al., 1973; Feldman et al., 1975; Whitfield et al., 1978; DenHartog, 1982; Diesenhaus, 1982; Alterman et al., 1988; Hayashida et al., 1989; Klerman, 1989).

Another example of the lack of agreement on definitions among the various continua are the descriptions of a "family program" or "family treatment." Again, it is not clear what is meant. In the alcohol problems field, family therapy, in common with other treatment modalities, is considered appropriate for some but not necessarily all persons in treatment (McCrady, 1988). In addition, family therapy may constitute different activities in different programs or settings. The importance of the family in supporting recovery (i.e., changing drinking behavior) is recognized; yet there is little research on the effectiveness of the various techniques or structured programs with particular kinds of persons with alcohol problems the various subgroups (McCrady, 1988). Looking beyond settings in defining the desired elements of the continuum of care is of value, but there is not enough evidence available to single out specific treatment modalities as appropriate for inclusion.

Yet this is exactly what has occurred in a number of definitions of the ideal continuum of care. In addition, these descriptions tend to condense and confuse the settings in which treatment takes place, the procedures or modalities that are used, the stages or phases of treatment that are offered, and the philosophical model that underlies a given treatment approach. The descriptions also do not sufficiently recognize that different subgroups will require different elements in combination to sufficiently address their alcohol problems. This imprecision is one of the factors that creates tensions between providers, regulators, funders, and policymakers regarding the resources that are needed and the proportions of treatment costs that should be financed either through public or private third-party payment.

That the federal government continues to view the concept of a continuum of care as important, however, can be seen in several of the recommendations made in the 1986 national plan proposed by the Department of Health and Human Services:

> States and the private sector should develop a continuum of care based on an assessment of need which accurately reflects age, ethnicity, sex, service needs and other significant variables based on appropriate State and local level data. (USDHHS, 1986:47)

> Third party payers should selectively expand financing throughout the continuum of care, thereby increasing the availability of treatment in a variety of settings. (p. 46)

> Public and private treatment programs should improve the match between client and treatment by evaluating diagnostic techniques and the continuum of care that is provided. (p. 50)

In keeping with this view, each state has defined its own continuum of care, some (e.g., New York, Colorado, Indiana) very consciously tying the elements together to reflect the stages or functions of treatment (in part to serve planning, funding, and evaluation purposes). Others (e.g., California, Minnesota) continue to view the components more as distinct entities. Some states include identification and intervention services in their treatment continuum; others do not. The federal government has implicitly defined its existing continua of care through the policies of the various federal agencies that fund and/or operate treatment programs (e.g., the Veterans Administration, the Department of Defense, the Health Care Financing Administration, the Alcohol, Drug Abuse, and Mental Health Administration) and through the definitions used in its national surveys. Yet consistency is lacking even in the federal arena; thus the definitions are not consistent from state to state, agency to agency or from survey to survey (Kusserow, 1989; Lewin/ICF, 1989a), a limitation that prevents the development of a comprehensive national approach.

If progress is to be made in defining treatment for alcohol problems, the elements of the continuum of care that constitutes such treatment must be specified. In addition, agreement must be reached on how those elements are defined and sequenced and how they can best be used in matching various subgroups of persons with alcohol problems to an appropriate series of interventions. Because there are still no widely accepted models for describing either the course of treatment and recovery for persons with alcohol problems or the settings in which each stage of that course can be most reasonably and least expensively accomplished, the committee has provided a preliminary framework for a taxonomy of treatment elements as a starting point for defining the expanded continuum of care.

Defining the Elements of Treatment in the Continuum of Care

In the attempts that have been made to describe the continuum of care needed for the treatment of alcohol problems, there appears to have been some confusion among its various elements: the philosophy or orientation of treatment, the stages of treatment, the settings in which treatment takes place, the levels of care required by persons of varying clinical statuses, the modalities to be used to decrease or eliminate alcohol consumption, and the supportive services that are required by some individuals with extensive physical, psychological, or social problems. To organize systematically the elements that should make up the continuum of care, the committee proposes to employ a multidimensional framework that distinguishes among treatment philosophy and orientation, treatment stage, and treatment setting and level of care. This approach separates the specific treatment modalities and supportive services that are used from the environmental context in which they are applied (USDHHS, 1981, 1987b). In addition, the framework can serve multiple purposes. Among them is its potential for organizing the studies that are necessary to determine how best to match an individual with appropriate treatment. The framework also provides a structure for analyzing the variety of placement methods that have recently been introduced (Weedman, 1987; Hoffmann et al., 1987a).

Treatment Philosophy or Orientation

A model for treatment consists of a certain perspective on or orientation toward the etiology of alcohol problems that in turn specifies the preferred methods of intervention and suggests expected outcomes (Armor et al., 1978). A variety of models have been identified as guiding the development of treatment for alcohol problems—for example, the disease model endorsed by the majority of treatment programs, the social learning model developed by behavioral psychologists (Nathan, 1984; Donovan and Chaney, 1985), and the social-community model of recovery that is now widely used in California (Borkman, 1986, 1988). Three major orientations have been identified as providing the rationale for the differing approaches to the treatment of alcohol problems: the physiological, the psychological, and the sociocultural (Armor et al., 1978; Saxe et al., 1983).

Before proceeding with a discussion of these orientations, the committee would emphasize that any description of these models constitutes an abstraction that does not necessarily describe current practice. Nevertheless, the models have historical value in that they inform us about the development of contemporary approaches—for example, the evolving biopsychosocial model that is now endorsed by many practitioners.

The physiological or biological perspective, which underpins what is generally known as the medical model of treatment, often considers "alcoholism" to be a progressive disease that is caused by physiological malfunctioning and that requires treatment by or under the direct supervision of a physician. Genetic risk factors are seen as important in the etiology of the disease. Physiological treatment strategies focus on the person with severe alcohol problems as the unit of treatment and may incorporate the use of pharmacotherapy to produce change in the individual's drinking behavior. Medical treatments include drugs to diminish anxiety and depression and such alcohol-sensitizing agents as disulfiram (Antabuse).

The psychological perspective views alcohol problems as arising from motivational, learning, or emotional dysfunctions in the person. Like the physiological approach, psychological treatment strategies also focus on the individual and use psychotherapy or behavior therapy to produce changes in drinking behavior. The psychological model can also be further differentiated into variants that reflect differing theories about the etiology of problem drinking behavior—for example, whether alcohol problems are symptoms of underlying psychopathology (intrapsychic conflicts) or are the results of social learning (the behavioral model). Treatment based on psychoanalytically oriented dynamic theory is another such variant. In this approach the individual psychotherapeutic relationship is seen as the key element; adjunctive psychotherapies (e.g., group therapy, psychodrama, occupational therapy) and supportive social rehabilitative services (Alcoholics Anonymous, vocational counseling) help the individual to consolidate the gains he or she has made (e.g., Khantzian, 1981, 1985; Zimberg et al., 1985; Khantzian and Mack, 1989; Nace, 1987).

The characteristic structure of a psychological model treatment regimen is a course of intensive psychotherapy sessions (either individual or group, or a combination of both) over an extended period of time in either a private practice or clinic setting. The primary therapist is usually a mental health professional (psychiatrist, clinical psychologist, psychiatric social worker, psychiatric nurse, or clergyman). An antianxiety, antidepressant, or antipsychotic medication is often used as an adjunctive therapy. Disulfiram is sometimes used to provide external controls on drinking until the individual can develop internal controls. However, the stress here is on the adjunctive or secondary nature of these psychopharmacological approaches. Family therapy may also be used. Other strategies include blood-alcohol-level discrimination training, biofeedback, and desensitization training.

One development of the past few years relating to the psychological treatment model has been the increasing use of behavior therapy techniques, primarily by psychologists (Poley et al., 1979; Lazarus, 1981; Marlatt and Gordon, 1985; Abrams and Niaura, 1987; Marlatt et al., 1988). The predominant approach is the social learning model, which proposes that what a person believes about the effects of alcohol use on his or her ability to cope with the demands of everyday life is a crucial determinant of how involved with alcohol he or she will become. The social learning approach stresses the important contribution of cultural norms, role models, and learned expectations about the effects of alcohol in a given situation in determining drinking patterns. Social learning theory views persons with deficits in general coping skills, such as the inability to manage everyday stress, as vulnerable to the use of alcohol as an artificial method to modulate their everyday functioning. Biological factors are seen to interact with these psychosocial determinants, resulting in harmful drinking patterns (Abrams and Niaura, 1987).

The sociocultural perspective, the third major treatment orientation, considers alcohol problems to be the result of a lifelong socialization process in a particular social and cultural milieu. Sociocultural treatment strategies focus on both the person and his or her social and physical environment as the units of treatment; they use a variety of techniques, including environmental restructuring, to change the individual's drinking behavior by creating new social relationships. Sociocultural interventions include changing the social environment by providing an alcohol-free living arrangement such as a halfway house; active involvement in Alcoholics Anonymous (AA) or other mutual help groups; social setting (as opposed to hospital-based) detoxification; and a social model of rehabilitation. The sociocultural perspective emphasizes the importance of social groups (e.g., church, family) in influencing not only the person's drinking behavior but also the response to treatment and the potential for relapse. The most prominent example of the use of the sociocultural model in formal treatment is the California social model of recovery (see the discussion later in this chapter).

In recent years there have been a number of attempts to develop an integrative model that could bring together these diverse orientations and perspectives. Such a model has evolved, the biopsychosocial orientation, which has its roots directly in work with persons with alcohol problems (Kissin 1977a,b; Kissin and Hansen, 1985) as well as in behavioral medicine (Engel, 1977; Donovan, 1988; see Chapter 2). Generally, the biopsychosocial model provides a framework within which the biological, psychological, and sociocultural approaches to health can be integrated (Engel, 1977; Zucker and Gomberg, 1986; Marlatt et al., 1988).

More specifically, the model offers a way to bring together varying orientations or philosophies for treating the individual with alcohol problems. This approach implies that the problems are determined by multiple factors and recognizes the heterogeneity of causes and courses that are involved. Problem etiology and the maintenance of the excessive, harmful pattern of drinking behavior are seen as a complex interaction among the biological, psychological, and sociocultural risk factors. Physiological factors include, for example, the genetic predispositions that are presumed to reflect differences in the metabolism of alcohol owing to the absence or presence of certain neurochemicals as well as the physiological changes (e.g., tolerance, dependence, and withdrawal) that follow repeated consumption. Psychological factors may include an individual's personality and character structure as well as variations in mood states and expectations. Sociocultural factors may include variations in drinking norms and expectations, in work environments, and in family structure. The biopsychosocial model recognizes that, for each individual, all three sets of factors are potentially involved but that in different individuals one or the other sets of causes may predominate. Similarly, the major consequences of excessive alcohol use for an individual may be biological (e.g., physical dependence, neuropsychological deficits, physical illnesses such as pancreatitis and cirrhosis), psychological (e.g., depression, anxiety, cognitive dysfunction), or social (e.g., marital dysfunction, job difficulties, legal problems).

Recently, a new approach, the transtheoretical "stages of change" model, has shown promise for studying and organizing the treatment of alcohol problems within the biopsychosocial framework (Prochaska and DiClemente, 1982, 1983, 1986; Marlatt et al., 1988; IOM, 1989). This model emerged from a comparative analysis of 18 theories about psychotherapy and behavioral change, including theories that serve as the basis for the physiological, psychological, and sociocultural models described above. Several researchers have begun to use the model as a framework for studying the treatment process. Such researchers are generally those who utilize the integrative biopsychosocial model to understand the etiology and maintenance of excessive, harmful drinking and other addictions (e.g., smoking and drug use) (Marlatt et al., 1988; IOM, 1989).

The stages of change model posits that there is a common sequence of changes that individuals experience in developing a problem behavior, in ending that behavior, and in either maintaining the cessation of the behavior or relapsing. The behavior change sequence is divided into four stages: (1) precontemplation, in which the individual is not considering change because the drinking behavior is not seen as a problem; (2) contemplation, in which the individual begins to think seriously about changing his or her drinking behavior because of the perception that it is causing increasing difficulties in a variety of life function areas; (3) action, in which the individual takes positive steps to change drinking behavior, either on his or her own or with the assistance of formal treatment; and (4) maintenance, in which the individual engages in active efforts to avoid drinking, again, either alone or with assistance. Preparation for maintenance requires an explicit assessment of the conditions under which an individual is likely to relapse. A person who relapses goes through the same stages where maintenance represents active efforts to continue drinking.

In practice there appear to be programs and practitioners that offer either a single treatment type or modality (e.g., traditional individual psychotherapy in the private practice setting; disulfiram in the primary care physician's office) or a wide range of modalities that can be selectively pursued (e.g., multidisciplinary, multimodality milieu therapy in the freestanding or hospital-based alcohol rehabilitation unit). Often, treatments are combined, with psychologically oriented treatment programs using medications as adjuncts and drug treatments being offered together with psychological and sociocultural strategies (Saxe et al., 1983; Kissin and Hansen, 1985). Although research is lacking to confirm the perception, multicomponent programs have been seen as more successful than single-component programs because they can address the wide variety of difficulties generally presented by persons with chronic alcohol problems (Costello et al., 1977; Costello, 1980; Paredes et al., 1981). Nevertheless, in most of those programs that do offer a range of modalities, it is usually (although not always) possible to discern which of the various treatment philosophies is the dominant orientation.

To understand the intense feeling that underlies the ongoing controversy about treatment in the alcohol problems field, it is helpful to view these differing treatment philosophies as professional ideologies that guide the development of both particular programs and of movements within the field (Strauss et al., 1964; Klerman, 1984; Weisner and Room, 1984; Borkman, 1988). A professional ideology not only includes beliefs and theories about etiology but also provides prescriptive norms for what should be applied in clinical practice, teaching, and research. Strauss and colleagues (1964) used the concept of professional ideologies to explain the variations in psychiatric treatment that could be observed in hospital settings. They demonstrated how the treatment philosophies held by those who worked at a given institution shaped the ways in which services were organized and delivered, the definition of "proper" treatment, and the appropriate divisions of labor. Other aspects of the effects of professional ideologies are that adherents of a particular approach seek each other out, participate in both informal social networks and formal associations, and seek legitimization and institutionalization of their viewpoint. Strong emotions become attached to adherents' beliefs about etiology and practice and sometimes lead to conflicts over the proper way to provide treatment.

One of the potential benefits of such strongly held beliefs may involve matching. It has been suggested that dominant treatment orientation can be an important variable for matching persons with alcohol problems to the most effective form of treatment (Kissin, 1977a; Kissin and Hansen, 1985; Pattison, 1985; Annis, 1988). For example, Welte and colleagues (1978) studied the relationship of the orientation of treatment units to outcome (see also Lyons et al., 1982). Scales were developed to measure each orientation. Medical orientation was measured by the frequency of the use of drug therapies, the number of beds used for detoxification, the number of medical and nursing staff, and the degree of importance placed on staff academic training. Rehabilitation orientation was measured by the frequency of use of relationship therapy, family therapy, occupational therapy, and vocational counseling, and by the number of staff who were psychologists, social workers, rehabilitation counselors, and occupational or recreational counselors. The unit's peer group or sociocultural orientation was determined by measuring the frequency of the use of alcohol education, Alcoholics Anonymous, and Al-Anon; the level of self-government activity; and the type of grievance activity. These three orientations roughly correspond to the treatment models described earlier (i.e., the biological, psychological, and sociocultural).

In the Welte team's study, individuals in treatment were classified according to whether they exhibited either behavioral signs and symptoms of alcohol dependence, physical signs and symptoms, or both behavioral and physical signs and symptoms. The expectation that strongly medically oriented rehabilitation units would be more successful in treating those who exhibited physical signs and symptoms was not borne out; rather, those individuals who exhibited physical signs and symptoms were more successfully treated in the high peer group orientation units. Units with a high medical orientation appeared to be more effective in treating persons who showed signs of little physiological impairment. However, treatment units were not "pure" types and treatment orientation was not as strong a predictor of treatment outcome as were patient characteristics and length of stay.

The work of Brickman and colleagues (1982) also suggests that treatment orientation is an important variable for matching persons to the most effective form of treatment. These investigators developed a social psychological framework to investigate how beliefs about etiology and the treatment of alcohol problems—on both the part of the treatment provider and on the part of the person seeking treatment—influence treatment outcome. Their approach, which has been continued by Marlatt and his colleagues, suggests that there are four models that underlie contemporary efforts to help people to change their drinking behavior. They have labeled these the moral model, the medical model, the enlightenment model, and the compensatory model (Brickman et al., 1982; Marlatt et al., 1988). These models are differentiated by the extent to which the individual is considered responsible for the development of the problem and the extent to which the individual is considered responsible for resolving it.

As interpreted by Brickman and his colleagues, the moral model's position is that individuals are held responsible for both the etiology of the alcohol problem and for creating the solution. Drinking in this model is seen as a weakness in character, and people are expected to change their drinking behavior through personal effort, by an exercise of will power. Examples of this orientation are the temperance movement and Prohibition. The moral model has little support in contemporary literature on treatment and is often dismissed as "old fashioned." Yet because there is an inescapable moral element in all behavior, such a dismissal may be premature. In the enlightenment model, a person is considered to be responsible for developing the alcohol problem but requires external help in changing his and her behavior. Alcoholics Anonymous is given by the Brickman team as an example of the enlightenment model because of its emphasis on requiring the help of a "higher power" in maintaining sobriety.

In the medical model, as described by Brickman and his coworkers (1982), neither the development of the problem nor the responsibility for its resolution is seen as the person's responsibility. The disease model of alcohol problems, with its emphasis on a progressive disease process that arises from an underlying genetic predisposition and is exemplified by increasing physical dependence, is given as an example of this approach: alcohol problems are the result of uncontrollable biological and genetic factors, and treatment is administered by experts who apply biomedical treatments that arrest the underlying condition (Marlatt et al., 1988). The disease model was explicitly developed as an alternative to the moral model and is the dominant approach in U.S. treatment programs. The characteristic structure of the medical model is most evident in those hospital and nonhospital inpatient units in which the physician is either the primary therapist or is influential in determining the treatment plan to be carried out by an alcoholism counselor who acts as the primary therapist. In these units pharmacologically assisted detoxification is the standard regimen, and antianxiety, antidepressant, and sensitizing medications are used as a major component of long-term treatment (e.g., Gallant, 1987). The program milieu and any psychotherapies that are offered are seen as supporting these physiological treatments.

The characteristic structure of the medical model is also seen in those inpatient units that offer a blend of the sociocultural and medical models. In these programs, the physician is not the primary therapist but retains medicolegal responsibility for the overall regimen (Bast, 1984); the primary therapist is very often a counselor who is a recovering alcoholic. Here, the physician most often diagnoses and treats the physical consequences and complications of prolonged excessive alcohol use, prescribes and monitors medications if needed, and serves as a consultant and backup while participating with the multidisciplinary team in planning and evaluating the person's long-term treatment.

The orientation expressed in the compensatory model, the fourth model in the Brickman team's scheme, does not hold the individual responsible for the etiology of his or her alcohol problems; however, the person is responsible for the changes required to resolve them. This approach views the cause of alcohol problems as a combination of biological, psychological, and social factors. In treatment, individuals are taught how to avoid alcohol problems and are then expected to monitor and control their own performance. The compensatory model is reflected in treatment that uses the biopsychosocial model and social learning theory (Marlatt et al., 1988).

Because therapists and persons seeking help may each subscribe to a different model of treatment (i.e., to a different view of the cause of problems and the source of their solution), Brickman and his coworkers (1982) have hypothesized that matching by orientation would improve the chance of a successful outcome. Yet such matching is not easy to effect. All practitioners and researchers neither endorse the Brickman taxonomy nor agree with the classification of specific treatment approaches. Other interpretations of the medical model, for example, would say that the person is not responsible for the development of the problem, but that the person is responsible for its resolution. Many in the medical profession and in Alcoholics Anonymous would see the compensatory model as more nearly approximating their orientation. More research is needed to determine how best to describe the orientation of a given program and whether orientation is a critical matching variable (Annis, 1988).

The orientation that over the recent past has probably evoked the most controversy is the social model of recovery. In the late 1960s and early 1970s, a shift occurred in the orientation of many treatment providers as they began to consider and take into account environmental and social influences on drinking behavior (Beigel and Ghertner, 1977). The dramatic impact of Alcoholics Anonymous as well as the development of the therapeutic community approach for psychiatric patients and drug abusers contributed to and were themselves strengthened by this shift. These approaches shared a critique of the medical and psychological models' use of diagnosis, professional domination by physicians, reliance on somatic forms of treatment, and the passivity of the patient role (Borkman, 1982, 1986; Klerman, 1984). The formalized approach that developed out of this change in orientation, the so-called social model or social setting model, was applied both to detoxification and to long-term treatment (O'Briant et al., 1973 Armor et al., 1978).

The social treatment or social setting model advocated by O'Briant and colleagues (1973) was also a reaction against what was seen as treatment taking place only within the short time frames of the structured program in the hospital or residential treatment center; in the social model, emphasis was placed on continued active involvement in the "social living space" of the alcoholic after discharge from the structured inpatient treatment program. The deemphasis on inpatient rehabilitation extended to detoxification; in addition, proponents of the social setting model of detoxification argued that pharmacologically assisted detoxification in the acute hospital setting, in which the alcoholic assumed the passive role of patient, actually interfered with the process of recovery, the process of learning to live without relying on alcohol. They pointed to the success achieved by the Addiction Research Foundation of Ontario in developing nonhospital detoxification centers in which staff support and encouragement, good food, and pleasant surroundings, rather than physiological treatments, were emphasized. In 1969, the model received a boost of support from the National Institute on Alcohol Abuse and Alcoholism's (NIAAA) sponsorship of a demonstration of the safety of social model detoxification (O'Briant et al., 1973; DenHartog, 1982). The basic methods and goals of the social model approach were soon appropriated by many state alcoholism authorities when they adopted the Uniform Act provisions for decriminalizing public intoxication and qualified for federal incentive grants to provide alternatives to jail for public inebriates (USDHHS, 1981; DenHartog, 1982; Finn, 1985; Sadd and Young, 1986). Nevertheless, there were critics who questioned the degree to which medical procedures were being rejected (Pittman, 1974, Pisani, 1977).

There was a similar effort to shift the philosophical orientation underlying long-term treatment (O'Briant et al., 1973; Beigel and Ghertner, 1977; Kissin, 1977a,b; Borkman, 1982, 1983). The social rehabilitation model was quickly incorporated into the design of many freestanding and hospital-based programs, surviving in its purest form primarily in California (Borkman, 1988; Reynolds and Ryan, 1988). The parallel development in other areas of psychiatric care of the psychosocial rehabilitation and social model concepts has been described by Noshpitz and coworkers (1984) and Gottlieb and colleagues (1984), among others.

Current California social model programs are seen as third-generation mutual-help or self-help organizations that have evolved from the original first-generation efforts of Alcoholics Anonymous and the second-generation social setting detoxification centers, "Twelve Step" houses, halfway houses, and recovery homes that were founded by recovering alcoholics in the 1950s and 1960s (Rubington, 1974; Borkman, 1982, 1983; Orford and Velleman, 1982). In a later report Borkman (1986a) described the nine elements of the community-social model prevalent in the California programs:

1. The experiential knowledge of successfully recovering alcoholics is the basis of authority.
2. The primary foundation of recovery is the 12-step mutual aid process (AA or Al-Anon).
3. Recovery is viewed as a lifelong learning process, which is experiential in nature.
4. In recovery, staff manage the recovery environment, not the individuals; there is an absence of superordinate-subordinate, therapist-client roles or accompanying paraphernalia, such as case files with progress notes on each individual.
5. Participants who embrace recovery become "prosumers," persons who simultaneously give aid to others and receive services from others.
6. Participants feel they own their program and contribute to its upkeep voluntarily.
7. Participants, alumni, volunteers, and staff enjoy a relationship analogous to an extended family network.
8. Participants, alumni, and volunteers (and not just selected staff in specialized roles) represent the recovery process and program to the community.
9. The alcohol problem is viewed as occurring at the level of collectivities (e.g., family, community), rather than solely at the level of the individual; activities to change policies, norms, and practices of collectivities regarding alcohol use are carried out as part of the recovery process.

The current emphasis on social model recovery services in California represents the efforts of an evolving ideology that is actively seeking to confront and change the current system for organizing, accrediting, evaluating, and financing alcohol treatment services (Wright, 1985; Holden, 1987; Borkman, 1988; Reynolds, 1988a,b; Reynolds, and Ryan, 1988). In California, social model concepts have become institutionalized in the public sector, and many of the major counties (e.g., San Diego, Los Angeles, Alameda) have adopted the social model philosophy as the basis for funding treatment programs. Medical and psychological model programs are favored in the private sector.

One of the major points of contention regarding the California social model programs is that they eschew the involvement of professional staff (i.e., medical practitioners, psychotherapists, case managers) (Dodd, 1974, 1986; Borkman, 1986; DeMiranda, 1986; Reynolds and Ryan, 1988). They see themselves as differentiated from second-generation social setting detoxification and rehabilitation programs in California and in other states by their rejection of the "professional/clinical model" that is embodied in the data-gathering, licensing, and accreditation requirements of the majority of third-party payers--for example, staffing by degreed professionals, elaborate recordkeeping and documentation, the case management form of monitoring, and funding tied to individual patients and individual units of service. Second-generation social setting programs subscribe to these requirements to retain their funding. California's social model programs, on the other hand, are funded mainly through specific jurisdictional mechanisms; because they do not have to meet traditional health insurance requirements, they are presented as cost-effective alternatives to standard treatment programs (Reynolds, 1988a,b; Reynolds and Ryan, 1988). Evaluations of these claims are currently in progress.

Although treatment programs continue to vary along ideological lines, the field has seen in recent years the evolution and emergence of hybrid programs that claim to reflect the biopsychosocial model. The major hybrid is the Minnesota Model of Chemical Dependence Intervention and Treatment (Laundergan, 1982), a treatment strategy that blends AA and professional concepts and practices. It is widely believed that today the vast majority of U.S. treatment programs, both in the public and private sectors, subscribes to the philosophy and organization of treatment services that has become known simply as the Minnesota model (Anderson, 1981; Laundergan, 1982; Hoffmann et al., 1987b). For example, the continuum of care proposed by the Funding Task Force of the North American Congress on Alcohol and Drug Problems (Boche, 1975), which is discussed later in this chapter under "Treatment Stages," was to a large extent based on the Minnesota system in place at that time. Any attempt to understand treatment for alcohol problems in this country must include a review of the Minnesota model as well as an understanding of the role played by Alcoholics Anonymous in promoting particular concepts about the nature of alcohol problems and their treatment.

Although one could trace a number of early precursors of the Minnesota approach (e.g., Zimberg, 1983, Weisman, 1988), the model had its origins in the 1950s in work carried out at three institutions in the state: Willmar State Hospital, the Hazelden Foundation, and the Johnson Institute. The approach blends professional diagnostic and treatment activities with the 12-step recovery program developed by Alcoholics Anonymous (see Chapter 4). The standardized treatment program, which is typically delivered to all individuals in the course of a four-week inpatient stay, either in a hospital or in a freestanding facility, consists of detoxification, education (based on the disease concept) about the harmful medical and psychosocial effects of excessive alcohol consumption, confrontation, attendance at AA meetings and use of AA materials in developing a recovery plan ("stepwork"), and disulfiram therapy (Weisner and Room, 1984; Babor, 1986). The approach places strong emphasis on the use of recovering alcoholics as primary counselors, who guide the person through a multidisciplinary program that attempts to merge the medical, psychological, and sociocultural models. Laundergan (1982:2) describes it as follows:

> The alternative treatment program that became seminal to the Minnesota Model was a blend of professional behavioral science and AA principles. . . .Their program involved unlocking the treatment wards and using as counselors recovering alcoholics with five years or more of sobriety and at least a high school education. They also used lectures and group and individual therapy integrated with a working knowledge of Alcoholics Anonymous principles.

This new active (rather than custodial) treatment program that developed and evolved throughout the 1950s at Willmar introduced the distinction between detoxification and rehabilitation (Anderson, 1981). The Minnesota model also included a definition of a continuum of care with specialized service components integrated into a network (Anderson, 1981). These elements included a diagnostic and referral center, a detoxification center, a primary residential rehabilitation program, an extended care program, residential intermediate care (e.g., halfway houses), outpatient care (diagnostic, primary, and extended), aftercare, and a family program.

The new model that had been developed at Willmar was soon adopted by the Hazelden Foundation; following further development, it was refined into what became known as the Hazelden variant of the model. With this approach, after detoxification, which lasted from 2 to 7 days, patients were transferred to a "primary care program." In the original version of the Hazelden variant, this stage of treatment lasted 60 days.) The primary care program was an intensive, highly structured inpatient treatment regimen that included a psychological evaluation and two treatment "tracks," a general program track and an individualized prescriptive track. The components of the general program track were small, task-oriented group meetings (two to three times a week) and lectures (five mornings a week). The components of the individualized prescriptive track were meetings with the assigned "focal counselor" (twice a week, or more, if necessary), a work assignment, and referral to a professional staff member if additional medical, psychiatric, or social services were needed.

Another major variant of the Minnesota model developed at Minnesota's Johnson Institute. Like the Hazelden version, the Johnson model stressed the need to view alcohol problems as a primary disorder that required treatment in its own right and not simply the symptomatic expression of an underlying psychiatric disorder. Johnson (1980:2) described it as follows: "Very simply, the treatment involves a therapy designed to bring the patient back to reality. The course of treatment consists of an average of four weeks of intensive inpatient care of the acute symptoms in the (general) hospital, and up to two years of aftercare as an outpatient." The recommended setting for intensive treatment of the disorder's acute symptoms was the general hospital; the inpatient stay was divided into two phases, observation and detoxification followed by initiation of rehabilitation. Although the Johnson model saw treatment as a multidisciplinary endeavor involving physicians, nurses, psychiatrists, psychologists, counselors, and administrators, it considered rehabilitation to be a nonmedical process that was best carried out under the direction of the counselor. The third phase, outpatient treatment, was described as weekly contact with the nonmedical program for up to two years after inpatient discharge. This nonmedical outpatient program included weekly group therapy sessions, consultation and counseling as needed, weekly AA meetings, and spouse and family weekly participation in Al-Anon and Alateen. Participation in the entire two year period was seen as necessary for all individuals, with extensions of the length of formal treatment required for some.

The Johnson variant of the Minnesota model eventually spread throughout the country through consultations by Johnson Institute personnel with newly developing treatment programs and through the influential writings of Vernon Johnson. The first of these units was opened in 1968 at St. Mary's Hospital in Minneapolis; other units based on the same philosophy were subsequently opened in Nebraska, Louisiana, Ohio, and California. Another important development in the evolution and dissemination of the Minnesota model was the movement of several key staff from the Willmar State Hospital program to Park Ridge, Illinois, where they helped to found the Lutheran General Hospital program. This inpatient treatment center was the forerunner of Parkside Medical Services, which is now the largest single nongovernment provider of alcohol and drug abuse treatment services in the country, operating a nationwide network of hospital and freestanding facilities and units that subscribe to the Minnesota model philosophy.

Proprietary firms also served to diffuse the Minnesota model throughout the nation by the development of management contracts to initiate and operate hospital-based, fixed-length of stay "alcohol rehabilitation units" (Saxe et al., 1983; Weisner and Room, 1984; Cahalan, 1987). All of these organizations engaged in outreach and educational efforts to employers and professionals, stressing that "alcoholism" was treatable and that treatment in the end was cost-effective. All of these organizations produced education and training materials and conducted seminars, influencing potential reformer and also shaping the ideologies of those entering the field. All stressed the involvement of recovering counselors, who came into their new roles strongly imbued with the philosophical orientation of and belief in the Minnesota model of treatment for "alcoholism": inpatient rehabilitation followed by outpatient aftercare for a condition defined as a physical disease and characterized by progressive deterioration if abstinence were not the goal of treatment.

These principles were also finding voice in many of the treatment programs that were being developed in other parts of the country simultaneously with the Minnesota model. These programs tended to follow a similar course, growing out of the union of recovering persons and professionals working in specialized programs in acute care or psychiatric hospitals. Stuckey and Harrision described the type of program that often developed in the eastern states:

> A typical rehabilitation center is a residential therapeutic community of recovering alcoholics sharing experiences and feelings in a chemical-free environment. The average stay is approximately 28 days utilizing the following key ingredients:
>
> 1. Strong AA orientation
> 2. Skilled alcoholism counselors as primary therapists
> 3. Psychological testing and psychosocial evaluations
> 4. Medical and psychiatric support for coexisting problems
> 5. Therapists trained in systematized methods of treatment including Gestalt, psychodrama, reality therapy, transactional analysis, behavior therapy, activity therapy, and stress management
> 6. Use of therapeutic community and crisis intervention
> 7. Systems therapy, especially with employers and later including a strong family component
> 8. Family- and peer-oriented aftercare. (Stuckey and Harrison, 1982:865-867)

Today, the modal pattern of treatment has become the fixed-length inpatient rehabilitation program, with disagreement about the amount of aftercare required. Current inpatient primary care programs that follow this orientation usually involve a three- to six-week length of stay. Aftercare following the completion of the inpatient phase of treatment varies greatly in both format and duration (Vannicelli, 1978; Harrison and Hoffmann, 1986). Aftercare may consist of diverse activities ranging from monthly telephone contact or attendance at alumni meetings to continuing treatment in weekly counseling sessions for patients and significant others provided at the programs. Alternatively, aftercare can be referral to a halfway house or referral to another agency for continuing outpatient treatment. Most commonly aftercare is referral to Alcoholics Anonymous.

Treatment Stages

Programs for treating alcohol problems have long used a stage or phase model.

For some programs this model has been explicit; for others it has been implicit (Diesenhaus, 1982). Nevertheless, it has become customary to break down episodes of treatment for alcohol problems into stages or phases that mirror current practices and the natural process of recovery (e.g., Mulford, 1979, 1988; Pattison, 1985; Anderson, 1981; Costello and Hodde, 1981; Blume, 1983; Vaillant, 1983). The simplest and most commonly used division is the distinction between detoxification, rehabilitation, and aftercare or relapse prevention (e.g., Glatt, 1974; IOM, 1989). This sequence of components of a treatment episode now appears not only in the model benefit design developed by the Blue Cross/Blue Shield Association (Berman and Klein, 1977) but also in the accreditation standards of the Joint Commission for Accreditation of Health Care Organizations and the Commission on the Accreditation of Rehabilitation Facilities. The sequence also appears in state licensure standards and insurance mandates, in state resource allocation models, in the U.S. military's CHAMPUS benefit design, and most recently in the Medicare prospective payment system using diagnosis-related groups. Such a sequence provides a framework for what was referred to earlier in this chapter as a continuum of care for persons with alcohol problems.

The efforts of the Blue Cross/Blue Shield Association in developing its model benefit plan are one of the first instances in which the phases of treatment were made explicit. In 1977 NIAAA funded Blue Cross/Blue Shield to determine the feasibility of providing private health insurance benefits for alcoholism treatment. To estimate the costs of specific benefit designs more precisely, this effort clearly differentiated between those procedures that addressed acute physical problems arising out of excessive alcohol consumption and those procedures that focused on alleviating the chronic problems that arise out of the compulsive use of alcohol. Thus, the association's design for a model benefit package differentiated between "acute phase services" (e.g., emergency medical treatment, withdrawal management) and "chronic phase activities" (Berman and Klein, 1977). Making such distinctions among the phases or stages of treatment had two important advantages: (1) it allowed the differentiation of the specific costs associated with treating the varied consequences of alcohol misuse and (2) it emphasized that one activity cannot substitute for the other; that is, neither the treatment of intoxication and withdrawal nor the treatment of the medical consequences of excessive alcohol use are substitutes for comprehensive treatment for alcohol problems (although they may need to precede such treatment).

A number of models of sequenced or phased treatment have been developed by researchers, practitioners, and planners. A review of several such models can be helpful in two ways: in understanding the variation that exists in practice and as a first step in designing a framework for an expanded continuum of care. Pattison (1974, 1985) has attempted the most ambitious description of the existing and required continua, seeking to link agencies, facilities, programs, settings, target populations, and phases of treatment into an organized whole or "system" of treatment. His model has seven phases:

Phase A, *Identification*—the determination of whether an individual has an alcohol use problem of any degree (mild, moderate, or severe) that requires treatment.

Phase B, *Triage Referral*—active referral of the individual to the "appropriate" treatment facility, "appropriateness" being determined through mutual exploration with individuals of their perceptions, needs, and desires regarding acceptable types of facilities and treatment.

Phase C, *Program Entry*—the response of an agency to the individual's immediate needs and its involvement of the person in an emotionally receptive "social climate" oriented to his or her personal needs. At program entry the individual's immediate needs for acute medical care or psychiatric care are established. Motivation is to be enhanced and program dropout avoided.

Phase D, *Initial Treatment Processes* (acute care)—the implementation of specific procedures to guard against the person's dropping out of treatment and to provide a preparatory treatment experience that is supportive, symptom relieving, and nonthreatening, as well as reality oriented and option oriented. The goal of this phase is positive involvement of the individual with the program's social environment (i.e., staff, other persons in recovery) so as to instill a shared motivation to continue in the ongoing process of rehabilitation.

Phase E, *Selection of Goals and Methods* (rehabilitation)—cooperatively working with the now stabilized alcoholic to develop and carry out a long-range individualized plan, specifying which of the wide variety of treatment methods and goals are appropriate and desirable, based on a comprehensive differential assessment of drinking behavior, personality, degree of socialization, extent of disability in each area of life (e.g., work, physical health, emotional health), and social status.

Phase F, *Treatment Maintenance and Monitoring*—regular review of progress toward the individual's goals, including determinations of whether specific treatment methods are being adequately carried out and redefinition of the methods and goals when necessary.

Phase G, *Termination and Follow-up*—similarly, the assessment of gains achieved and maintained, with termination of formal treatment when treatment goals are reached.

The Funding Task Force of the North American Congress on Alcohol and Drug Problems also defined a continuum of care that included the following components (roughly corresponding to stages in a treatment episode): (1) outreach, assessment, and referral; (2) crisis management/detoxification; (3) primary treatment and rehabilitation; (4) transitional/aftercare/ extended care; and (5) supportive services (Boche, 1975). The task force defined its three active treatment components much as they were defined in the original Minnesota model of care:

Crisis management is defined as activities associated with addressing an emergent or immediate situation perceived by a client as being threatening to himself or others. This category includes activities generally identified as protective services, subacute detoxification, and acute detoxification.

Primary treatment and rehabilitation is defined as a set of intensive activities, of limited duration, designed to provide the person in treatment with a positive substitute or alternative to addiction, dependency and associated behavioral activities.

Transitional/aftercare is defined as a set of ongoing supportive activities, including professional and self-help programs, designed to maintain behavioral change. (Boche, 1975:5)

In keeping with the perspective of the Uniform Act, the task force asserted that the continuum of care must include supportive services to reduce the patient's personal and social impairments as well as primary treatment activities that focus on changing drinking behavior: "Supportive services are services provided to the client as part of ongoing care, either as a direct part of a program or as "ancillary" services arranged for by the program, such as vocational rehabilitation, income maintenance and family counseling (Boche, 1975:5)." The task force saw such services as essential to the effectiveness of treatment offered by specialty programs and to the avoidance of relapse. It therefore sought multiple-source funding for all primary and supportive treatment services (e.g., health insurance for medical care, social services funding for supportive services, categorical grants for noncovered activities).

Glaser and colleagues (1978) developed what they called a "practical taxonomy" of treatment programs as a means of organizing their findings from a survey of 80 Pennsylvania alcoholism treatment programs. This taxonomy uses as its major organizing principle the "function" of the principal means of intervention provided by a given treatment program. These investigators defined six unitary functions that alone or in combination were seen to characterize all 80 of the programs surveyed: (1) acute intervention—the immediate resolution of an acute physical, social, or psychological emergency; (2) evaluation—the development of an individualized treatment strategy by thorough assessment of the person's clinical and social status; (3) intensive intervention—the application of therapeutic activities to bring the individual to a better level of functioning; (4) stabilization—the consolidation of gains through continued participation in supportive activities in a sheltered living environment; (5) maintenance—the continued provision of some therapeutic input to maintain the gains in functioning achieved through intensive intervention or stabilization (or both); and (6) domiciliary care—the provision of an ongoing supportive, protected living environment for those too disabled by alcohol use to return to independent community living.

The analysis of the Pennsylvania programs by the Glaser team (1978) also involved an attempt to describe and classify the existing service delivery system. The analysis pointed out that the separate functions were usually embedded in characteristic organizational structures and that the functions represented the possible sequence of movement through a comprehensive treatment system. Each function with its characteristic structure was a component of the system. These six components, which are listed in table 3-1, can be viewed as another way to describe the stages and settings that make up the continuum of care.

Blume (1982, 1983, 1985) used a similar model of the treatment episode to organize her recommendations on how to perform and evaluate treatment. She divided the alcoholism treatment episode into four phases (identification/intervention, detoxification,

TABLE 3-1 Stages and Settings of the Contimuum of Care

Component	Function	Structure
I	Acute intervention	Medical or nonmedical detoxification unit
II	Evaluation	Centralized diagnostic center
III	Intensive intervention	Residential facility; Day program
IV	Stabilization	Halfway house
V	Maintenance	Outpatient clinic; AA
VI	Domiciliary Care	State hospital; Rescue mission

rehabilitation, and long-term follow-up) and indicated that the phases must be applied in the appropriate sequence for each individual. She also identified private practice and organized program settings in which each phase could take place, as well as the treatment modalities appropriate to each phase. Blume noted that one of the reasons for negative perceptions in the past regarding the effectiveness of treatment for persons with alcohol problems has been the inappropriate use of selected modalities in a particular phase of treatment.

Blume saw these combinations of treatment phase, setting, and modality as useful both for designing an overall treatment delivery system and for treating the individual:

> Therefore, as an overall treatment system we try to provide appropriate services for different types and stages of alcohol problems in a coordinated continuum. As individual practitioners, we try to motivate patients and their families to use these services, to stick with them, and to return immediately to the appropriate form of treatment in case of relapse (Blume, 1983:174).

In a paper prepared for this committee, Holder and colleagues (1988) reviewed various studies of the effectiveness of individual modalities, placing the modalities within the context of the stage and setting of treatment and considering the cost of each combination. They defined three treatment functions or stages: (1) entry and assessment—to determine the next steps in the system; (2) acute care—to stabilize the patient and deal with life threatening conditions; and (3) rehabilitative care—to return the person to a life unhampered by the adverse consequences of alcohol use. These functions are further explained as follows:

> While the routes used by people to enter treatment are varied there are, in general, common steps. The first function is entry and assessment illustrated by triage. The function could be undertaken in an actual emergency room triage or by admission desk at an alcoholism treatment facility or in a private provider's office. It is possible to consider the triage function undertaken by a case manager or treatment broker who makes decisions on the basis of patient need. Such a case manager could select treatment types and interventions based on patient need, not on a particular program.
>
> If the client is neither intoxicated nor has an acute medical problem then he is able to skip detoxification and acute care and move directly into rehabilitative care if desired.
>
> If a physical health problem (other than the need to address detoxification exists) than medical care usually in an emergency room or trauma setting is required. Detoxification can occur concurrently with attention to trauma. If detoxification only is required, then except for the stabilization of the patient with medication (for example with librium), detoxification (removal of ethanol from the body) is metabolic and thus a natural process. It can occur in a variety of settings from an acute care hospital to a social model detoxification center.
>
> If the patient is not intoxicated then rehabilitative care can begin. (Holder et al., 1988:9-10)

Despite the varying language these different proposals use to describe the stages or phases of treatment, they are nevertheless responding to common features of the recovery process, as well as to both research and clinical evidence for inducing and maintaining behavior change. The committee's review of the various programs indicated that treatment programs varied in the emphasis they placed on each stage and in the delineation of substages; however, the review also showed more similarity than dissimilarity, suggesting that it is possible to develop a general model that can be used not only for planning and resource allocation and development but also for matching persons to the appropriate treatment.

A taxonomy of treatment stages must address both the acute and the chronic care needs of persons with alcohol problems. The stage models developed by Blume (1985) and Glaser and coworkers (1978) appear to come closest to actual practice as manifest in the planning and resource allocation models used by various states. They describe both the active treatment of acute states (detoxification and primary rehabilitation) and the supportive treatment of chronic states (aftercare, long-term follow-up) that are needed when dealing with persons whose psychosocial resources and level of impairments range so widely. Both models also recognize the need for careful assessment to plan the treatment course. In defining the continuum of care and its elements, it is critical to distinguish between those elements that are designed to provide detoxification, rehabilitation, and aftercare or relapse prevention and to acknowledge that in each of these stages the person's clinical status and physical, psychological, and social resources will determine which setting, level of care, and combination of treatment modalities are required.

Drawing on the various proposals that have attempted to depict the course of treatment, the committee has used three major stages (acute intervention, rehabilitation, and maintenance) to organize its review of the current status of treatment services and research. The stages incorporate the commonly used activities, stages, and phases that have been identified by other researchers and practitioners:

Stage 1: Acute Intervention

Emergency treatment—the immediate resolution of an acute physical, social, or psychological emergency caused by excessive alcohol use.

Detoxification—the management of acute alcohol intoxication and withdrawal while in either independent living or in a sheltered living environment; the medical process of taking the affected person safely through the predictable sequence of symptoms that occur when blood alcohol levels drop during withdrawal.

Screening—the identification, by the person seeking treatment or another individual (whether a family member, supervisor, or law enforcement or medical professional), of the existence of a problem with alcohol, followed by a referral for treatment.

Stage 2: Rehabilitation

Evaluation and assessment—the development of an individualized treatment strategy aimed at eliminating or reducing alcohol consumption by a thorough assessment of the person's physical, psychological, and social status and a determination of the environmental forces that contribute to the drinking behavior.

Primary care—the application of therapeutic activities to help the individual reduce alcohol consumption and attain a higher level of physical, psychological, and social functioning while in either independent living or in a sheltered living environment. (Primary care includes both brief intervention and intensive intervention.)

Extended care (stabilization)—the consolidation of gains achieved in primary care through continued participation in treatment and supportive activities while in either independent living or in a transitional supportive, sheltered living environment.

Stage 3: Maintenance

Aftercare—the continued provision of some therapeutic input to maintain the gains in functioning achieved through intensive intervention and stabilization while in either independent living or in a transitional or long-term supportive, sheltered living environment.

Relapse prevention—the continued provision of therapeutic activities to avoid the return to prior patterns of drinking and to maintain the gains in functioning achieved through brief intervention or intensive intervention and stabilization while in either independent living or in a transitional or long-term supportive, sheltered living environment.

Domiciliary care—the provision of an ongoing supportive, protected living environment for those too disabled by prior alcohol use to return to independent community living.

Follow-up (monitoring and reassessment)—the maintenance of ongoing contact with the individual during and after each stage of treatment to determine how effective the treatment has been and to provide the opportunity to revise the treatment plan as necessary (e.g., to change treatment settings or modalities)—is not included as a distinct stage or activity. Follow-up has traditionally been linked with aftercare, but it is a distinct activity, not tied to any of the stages. Because different settings and modalities may be appropriate during the various stages, the committee wishes to stress the importance of including initial assessment at the beginning of each stage and reassessment at the end of each stage (i.e., follow-up). Follow-up will be discussed in more detail in Section III under the rubric "continuity assurance."

In the past, when providers and policymakers have spoken about treatment for "alcoholism," they focused on the totality of efforts required to end ongoing misuse and excessive consumption. "Treatment," however, was considered to be only the short-term activities involved in detoxification, in emergency treatment of alcohol-related physical and psychiatric problems, and in rehabilitation in fixed-length programs; everything else was "aftercare." This report focuses on the entire treatment episode and attempts to distinguish among the three major stages (acute intervention, rehabilitation, and maintenance) that are necessary to achieve and maintain sustained recovery.

The acute intervention stage includes emergency treatment and detoxification, which are likely to be needed by persons with severe alcohol problems. It also includes the screening of individuals in various community settings to detect the presence of alcohol problems. Screening is intended mainly to detect persons with mild or moderate problems, but it will also detect persons with more severe problems who may have escaped notice. Not all individuals with severe alcohol problems will require detoxification as the first phase of the treatment episode; all will require acute intervention, even if it only screening.

Rehabilitation describes the efforts involved in helping an individual change his or her drinking behavior. Rehabilitation comprises all activities designed to change directly the pattern of excessive consumption of beverage alcohol and prevent a return to the pattern. The rehabilitation stage may require that an individual learn new coping skills and develop new patterns of living and thinking (Johnson, 1980; Abrams and Niaura, 1987). It can be further divided into two substages: primary care and extended care or stabilization. Primary care is a period in which the treatment is undertaken to initiate change in an individual's alcohol consumption, to uncover the root causes of the excessive drinking behavior, and to provide positive substitute behaviors. The extent of primary care will vary with the severity of impairment and can be categorized as a brief intervention or an intensive intervention. Extended care in the committee's scheme is defined as a period in which the person is involved in supportive activities to strengthen and consolidate the changes that were initiated during primary care. The primary care period tends to be of limited duration, whereas the extended care or stabilization period can be prolonged. Individuals will vary in the length of time they require for primary care or extended care, in part as a function of the degree of severity of their problem and their level of social competence.

Each model of the treatment course that was reviewed earlier has attempted to provide for such substages using a variety of terms and descriptions for the settings in which primary care and extended care take place. Often, the setting and stage of treatment have been combined. Most frequently, there has been confusion between the stage of treatment and the setting for extended care (e.g., halfway house, domiciliary, nursing home). This confusion has resulted in a continuing problem in matching the needs of individuals for extended care with appropriate sources of funding because of the difficulty in specifying which funding source bears the responsibility for providing formal treatment and which is responsible for providing a supportive alcohol-free living environment while in each stage of treatment. This separation of responsibilities appears to have originated in the development of Twelve Step houses and early halfway houses (Booz-Allen and Hamilton, Inc., 1978). A key element of the committee's proposed taxonomy is to separate the concept of extended care from the concept of residence or living situation and to recognize that, for some persons, extended care on an ambulatory (outpatient) basis is both necessary and possible (Edwards, 1987).

Another goal of the committee's taxonomy is to make a clear distinction between extended care and aftercare. In the committee's proposed scheme, extended care is part of the rehabilitation stage, and aftercare is part of the maintenance stage. Extended care or stabilization differs from what has been called aftercare in that formal contact with the treatment program is maintained while the intensity and frequency of the contacts are gradually reduced as part of an ongoing treatment plan. "Aftercare," on the other hand, has been used to describe the long-term efforts that help the individual maintain the changes made during formal treatment. Exactly what efforts fall under this rubric, however, is sometimes difficult to determine, in part because programs vary in their use of the term and because its meaning has shifted over the years.

For example, in an early set of accreditation standards, aftercare was defined as "postdischarge services designed to help a patient maintain and improve on the gains made during treatment" (Joint Commission on the Accreditation of Hospitals, 1983). Thus, initially, the term was applied to all of the services provided to individuals following discharge from inpatient treatment. Its general intent was to ease the transition between hospital and home and provide continuity of care beyond the inpatient phase of treatment. Such a transition was needed because, in the early days of development of the Minnesota model and of other similar approaches, persons in the majority of inpatient programs experienced an abrupt leap from total immersion in a highly structured, 24-hour alcohol-free milieu to an aftercare plan that often called only for once-a-month alumni meetings and referral to Alcoholics Anonymous. As with many of the terms used in the alcohol field, however, there was little consensus on what aftercare really was; as a result there has been some confusion among aftercare, the continued formal treatment which is required by many persons (what the committee refers to an extended care), and the ongoing support for avoiding relapse required by most, if not all, persons with alcohol problems. This confusion has been engendered by the idea that "treatment" is limited to a 28-day inpatient stay, the primary care treatment duration often found in programs subscribing to the Minnesota model.

Aftercare thus came to mean arrangements made for the person discharged from formal treatment for continued informal support from self-help groups, a program alumni group, or informal, nonscheduled contact with the treatment program. Today, however, given the high rate of relapse that was seen following the limited treatment offered by the

28-day inpatient stay, the term aftercare has also come to mean continued formal treatment in a nonhospital setting following an initial hospital stay as an inpatient (in the committee's taxonomy, this is "extended care"). For example, Stuckey and Harrison offered the following descriptions:

> Formal aftercare should be a commitment and extend a minimum of 8 weeks after discharge. Many rehabilitation centers have extensive aftercare up to 2 years after discharge and others have patients return for week-long refresher periods during early sobriety. The debate over the length of formal aftercare revolves around developing an overreliance of the patient on the treatment center. (1982:871)

> The backbone of true aftercare support, however, is AA. There was no epidemic of treatment centers until the AA support network was in place and effective throughout the country. Rehabilitation centers using AA aftercare uniformly report that better than 80% of their clients are not drinking at a point 2 years after treatment. (1982:873)

And Filstead (1988a:182) noted, "[as] a practical matter, employee assistance programs are concerned not only with the intensive phase of treatment, be it outpatient, residential, or hospital based, but also with the aftercare or continuing-care phase that provides the supportive environment following residential intervention." Yet despite the efforts of many in the field, there is still no agreement on what constitutes appropriate aftercare or on the appropriate duration of such services (Vannicelli, 1978; Costello, 1980; Gilbert, 1988). In addition, there has been a general shift away from viewing the specialized unit in the general hospital or psychiatric hospital as the most appropriate and most cost-effective setting for the long-term effort required to facilitate the significant behavioral changes required. For all psychiatric illnesses as well as for alcohol and drug problems, hospitals and residential treatment centers now tend to be viewed as the appropriate setting for short-term crisis intervention, problem resolution, and stabilization ("primary care"); continuing treatment is seen as being more appropriate to less expensive residential or outpatient settings ("extended care").

In the face of continuing ambiguity surrounding the make-up of "aftercare," many in the field of alcohol problems have begun to use the concepts of continuing care, follow-up, and relapse prevention have begun to replace the concept of aftercare. The committee prefers these concepts to that of aftercare, which implies that treatment has ended with discharge from the primary rehabilitation stage in the inpatient setting. In particular, relapse prevention is an area of continuing treatment that is becoming more defined. Relapse prevention is the term now used to describe the more formal activities that are designed to prevent "slips," or "lapses," from leading to full-blown relapses—that is, a return to the individual's pattern of drinking before treatment (Marlatt, 1985; Gorski, 1986; IOM, 1989). In developing the rationale for his self-managed relapse prevention program, Marlatt (1985) makes a distinction between the methods used to initiate abstinence or moderate use and the methods used to maintain abstinence or moderate use: "Once an alcoholic has stopped drinking, for example, RP [relapse prevention] methods can be applied toward the effective maintenance of abstinence regardless of the methods used to initiate abstinence (e.g., attending AA meetings, aversion therapy, voluntary cessation, or some other means)" (p. 4).

In its taxonomy of treatment, the committee has combined the activities known as relapse prevention, continuing care, and aftercare under the rubric "maintenance" as a more acceptable description of the third major stage of treatment. *All persons who receive treatment for alcohol problems should be involved in maintenance activities following the treatment for alcohol problems should be involved in maintenance activities following the completion of the formal treatment activities of the rehabilitation stage.* The specific form, content, and duration of the maintenance stage should be determined by the ongoing follow-up reassessment that has been incorporated into the treatment process (see the discussion of outcome monitoring in Chapter 12). By including an option for continued support in the maintenance stage, the committee's proposed framework recognizes the heterogeneity of alcohol problems and the differing needs of the individuals who experience them. For example, for some severely impaired individuals (e.g., the chronic public inebriate), domiciliary care in a long-term sheltered living environment is required whereas for only mildly impaired individuals, periodic follow-up visits with their physician may be all that is required.

There have been relatively few studies of the treatment and recovery process that use such a continuum of stages, despite earlier calls for such research (Vannicelli, 1978; Costello, 1980; IOM, 1980; Costello and Hodde, 1981; Moberg et al., 1982; Moos et al., 1982). As described in Section III, the committee considers the need for such an organizing scheme and the conduct of studies on the treatment process, through follow-up and reassessment, to be critical for future research and practice.

Treatment Settings

The term *treatment setting* is used in several different ways in the literature on the treatment of alcohol problems. Sometimes it is used to describe the organizational location in which treatment is provided (e.g., a health care facility, mental health center, private practitioner's office). Sometimes it is used to describe the underlying treatment philosophy (e.g., social setting detoxification, medical setting detoxification). At still other times it is used to describe a person's living arrangement while in treatment (e.g., inpatient, outpatient; hospital, prison, residential facility, group home, nursing home, day treatment center, halfway house). As noted by the Department of Health and Human Services (DHHS), the most common use of the term in research and program planning for the treatment of alcohol problems has been to describe the environment within which treatment takes place:

> Treatment can be delivered in two basic types of settings—inpatient and outpatient—although some settings represent a combination of the two. The major distinction is whether care involves overnight care in a residential facility. Inpatient care involves the provision of medical, social, and other supporting services for patients who require 24-hour supervision. Outpatient care is the provision of nonresidential evaluative and alcohol treatment services on both a scheduled and nonscheduled basis. The choice of treatment setting is related to a variety of factors, including the ability to pay, the severity of alcohol abuse and attendant problems, the ability to leave the home environment to be treated in inpatient settings, and the client's orientation toward help-seeking. The varied inpatient and outpatient settings thus often serve a distinctive client population. (USDHHS, 1986:72)

DHHS's recent categorization of two basic treatment settings (inpatient and outpatient) is not fully consistent with prior usage or with the differentiation among settings used by the states in their planning and funding. It is also not fully consistent with the differentiation used by payers in their determination of the level of care that is appropriate for a given procedure (treatment modality) and for an individual's clinical status. For example, inpatient care has generally been further divided into 24-hour treatment and supervision in a hospital and in a freestanding facility such as a halfway house or recovery home (Armor et al., 1978; Research Triangle Institute, 1985).

In contrast to the DHHS structure, the first major national study of treatment for alcohol problems identified three types of settings: inpatient, intermediate, and outpatient (Armor et al., 1978). These settings were used by NIAAA in its original monitoring system for federally funded alcohol treatment centers, which provided the data for the Armor study. The inpatient care or hospital setting included all facilities that were licensed as general or specialty hospitals. Common features of the hospital setting were the use of the medical model, removal from the environment that supported the excessive drinking, and a highly structured program offering a range of treatment modalities.

The intermediate care setting grouped together all residential facilities (primarily halfway houses) that provided transitional living arrangements for severely impaired individuals who were moving from hospital inpatient care to independent living. The common feature of intermediate care facilities included staffing by nonprofessionals whose responsibility was to provide a supportive, alcohol-free communal living milieu; any continuing professional treatment was carried out elsewhere. The Armor team's study also acknowledged the existence of a graded series of nonhospital residential settings (i.e., residential care facilities, quarterway houses, halfway houses) that offered varying intensities of treatment and support.

The introduction by NIAAA of the quarterway house concept, however, shifted the definition of the intermediate care setting from a supportive transitional living facility to an active treatment facility that provided primary care similar to that provided in hospital settings (Diesenhaus and Booth, 1977; Armor et al., 1978). Once this shift occurred, intermediate care settings, many of which were still identified as halfway houses, were seen to be occupying three positions on the treatment continuum: (1) less expensive, social model primary rehabilitation settings (quarterway houses); (2) extended care or transitional living settings (halfway houses) for persons who did not need the level of nursing and medical care associated with hospitals or nursing homes but who required removal from a stressful environment during rehabilitation; and (3) extended care or transitional living settings (residential care) for persons who had completed primary treatment but who were not yet seen as ready to return to their original life situation or for persons who needed to reconstruct a new social reality (O'Briant et al., 1973; Armor et al., 1978). These new functions were similar to those called for in the Uniform Act's definition of intermediate care.

The outpatient care setting delineated by the Armor team included all facilities in which the person did not reside and received one to several hours of treatment per week. These facilities ranged from private practitioners' offices to community social services agencies to hospital outpatient clinics. Like intermediate care settings, outpatient care settings subserved three functions: primary treatment, extended care, and follow-up or aftercare.

The definitional difficulties that plague other aspects of the alcohol problems field extend to treatment settings in that the definitions used in national planning and policymaking efforts have not been consistent. This problem is seen in the 1987 National Drug and Alcoholism Treatment Unit Survey (NDATUS) conducted by NIAAA. In the 1987 survey the agency uses a different classification scheme to obtain data on treatment settings than that used in earlier surveys. For capturing data on individuals in treatment in its 1987 survey, NIAAA used the categories "Facility Location" and "Type of Care" to describe the treatment setting in which active clients were enrolled (USDDHS, 1987a). The two facility locations on the survey were (1) hospital inpatient and (2) nonhospital. The five types of care listed are (1) inpatient/residential social detoxification, (2) inpatient/residential medical detoxification, (3) inpatient/residential custodial/domiciliary care, (4) inpatient/residential rehabilitation/ recovery care, and (5) outpatient/nonresidential rehabilitation/recovery care. In contrast, the 1982 NDATUS used hospital, quarterway house, halfway house, recovery home, other residential facility, outpatient facility, and correctional facility for its facility location classifications.

Various states have tried to deal with these inconsistencies by developing their own definitions of treatment setting. For example, in 1978 the Colorado Alcohol and Drug Abuse Division introduced its Treatment Needs Model, which distinguished among four different settings in which the major treatment activity was to take place: (1) outpatient, (2) partial (day) care, (3) residential, and (4) hospital inpatient. Settings were primarily differentiated by (a) the amount of time per day that the individual was to spend in either treatment activities or under observation and control (restriction) by clinical staff (i.e., part time, which was indicated for outpatient and day-care settings, or full time, which was indicated for residential and inpatient facilities and (b) the relationship of the setting to a hospital. Hospital-based programs were to be used for patients whose conditions required a greater amount of nursing and medical care; they were differentiated from residential programs in terms of licensing requirements for physical structure, patient safety, staffing composition and ratios, and nature of medical control and supervision (Colorado Alcohol and Drug Abuse Division, 1978).

In medical care the term *treatment setting* has been most often used to describe the individual's status in treatment or enrollment in a particular level of care: hospital (inpatient care), nursing home (intermediate care), or outpatient clinic (ambulatory care). Both the halfway house and nursing home designations imply a convalescent as opposed to an active treatment role; however, in the treatment of alcohol problems, as in the treatment of psychiatric disabilities, persons who require noncomplicated detoxification or rehabilitation are ambulatory and do not need the full services of a hospital. Consequently, in recent years the field has seen the development and acceptance of the nonhospital, freestanding facility for providing residential detoxification and rehabilitation services as well as convalescent, supportive, and custodial services.

The issue of medical control and supervision of the treatment process and of the setting in which the treatment takes place has been a critical factor in attempting to reconcile the dilemmas posed by the different requirements of the funding available for patients (Holden, 1987; Reynolds, 1988a,b). Health insurance mechanisms, whether public or private, require medical control; community services funds do not (Booz-Allen and Hamilton, Inc., 1978). To broaden the extent and range of reimbursement for treatment, a number of states have introduced new licensing standards to allow for reimbursement of detoxification and rehabilitation services provided to ambulatory patients in nonhospital settings (DenHartog, 1982; Diesenhaus, 1982; Lawrence Johnson and Associates, Inc., 1983). For example, Colorado developed its nonhospital community intensive residential treatment program licensure category for public- and private-sector programs (mixed medical-social setting models) as well as program standards for alcohol detoxification and rehabilitation units in licensed hospitals (medical model). Oregon adopted a similar program licensure category. Similar concerns about capturing third-party payer funds led California to develop its chemical dependency rehabilitation hospital licensure category for private-sector programs (modified medical model) and recovery home standards for public-sector programs (social model).

In an attempt to develop a single national framework, NIAAA sponsored a project to develop guidelines for the classification of the essential characteristics of treatment settings in which services were provided (Chatham, 1984). A major impetus for this effort was the desire to provide legitimization of reimbursement for treatment of alcohol problems by private and public health insurers in both the expanded traditional and the new nontraditional settings that had developed as a result of NIAAA's categorical grant programs (see Chapter 18). There were also other reasons for developing such a classification: (1) to provide a common definition of treatment settings for information and evaluation reporting systems; (2) to provide guidelines for state alcoholism authorities to use in their licensure activities; (3) to familiarize the general health planning community with the type and character of settings in which alcoholism services were provided; and (4) to acquaint the general public with the types of resources that might be available in their communities (Bast, 1984). The classification system was modeled after the American Hospital Association's Classification of Health Care Institutions (American Hospital Association, 1974). There has not been widespread adoption or use of the framework, however; thus, it does not appear to be serving the purposes for which it was intended.

Nevertheless, in the review of treatment cost-effectiveness prepared for the committee by Holder and colleagues (1988:10), this framework was used as part of the basis for definitions of the general types of settings in which rehabilitative care can take place. These definitions are summarized below.

> *Inpatient* The provision of medical services and supportive services including board, laundry, and housekeeping for patients who require 24-hour supervision in a hospital or other suitably equipped and licensed medical facility for the treatment of alcohol problems and other problems related to alcohol use.

> *Residential* The provision of 24-hour care or support, or both, for individuals who live on the premises of the program.

> *Intermediate* The provision of care or support, or both, in a partial (less than 24-hour) treatment or recovery setting for individuals who need more intensive care, treatment, and support than are available through outpatient settings or who can benefit from supportive social arrangements during the day.

> *Outpatient* The provision of nonresidential evaluative and treatment services on both a scheduled and nonscheduled basis.

These definitions for rehabilitative care are quite similar to those used by several of the states. The definitions include the differentiation between the requirements of treatment in a hospital and in a freestanding facility. They also include, as the intermediate care setting, the partial care or day-care option that has become increasingly important in obtaining appropriate level of care placement.

Although Holder and his colleagues note that acute care (detoxification) can also take place in a variety of settings, they do not attempt a similar differentiation of the settings in which rehabilitation can take place. *The committee considers it possible to carry out any of the stages of treatment for alcohol problems in any of the settings, should the individual's clinical status merit that placement.* There was similar recognition of the independence of the setting in which treatment took place and the treatment process itself in all the other models that were reviewed earlier (Glaser et al., 1978; Blume, 1983; Pattison, 1985). In addition, the Funding Task Force of the North American Congress of Alcohol and Drug Problems clearly stated that all three stages or active treatment elements could take place in either a hospital, nonhospital, or nonresidential setting (Boche, 1975).

The various proposals suggest important commonalities that must be considered in developing a general framework for classifying treatment settings. The committee has chosen to use the same four categories proposed by Holder and colleagues (1988), with slightly modified definitions. These categories in turn define the levels of care, which the committee employs as its framework for describing the continuum of care:

> *Inpatient* The provision of treatment for alcohol problems, comprising, as needed, medical services, nursing services, counseling, supportive services, board, laundry,

and housekeeping for persons who require 24-hour supervision in a hospital or other suitably equipped and licensed medical setting.

Residential The provision of treatment for alcohol problems, comprising, as needed, medical services, nursing services, counseling, supportive services, board, laundry, and housekeeping for persons who require 24-hour supervision in a freestanding residential facility or other suitably equipped and licensed specialty setting.

Intermediate The provision of treatment for alcohol problems, comprising, as needed, medical services, nursing services, counseling, supportive services, board, laundry, and housekeeping for persons who require care or support, or both, in a partial (less than 24-hour) treatment or recovery setting. Such persons generally will be those who need more intensive care, treatment, and support than are available through outpatient settings or who can benefit from supportive social arrangements during the day in a suitably equipped and licensed specialty setting.

Outpatient The provision of treatment for alcohol problems, comprising, as needed, medical services, nursing services, counseling, and supportive services for persons who can benefit from treatment available through ambulatory care settings while maintaining themselves in their usual living arrangements.

Treatment Modalities

The content of treatment is usually referred to as the technique, method, procedure, or modality. The specific activities that are used to relieve symptoms or to induce behavior change are referred to as modalities. Treatment modalities are additional elements of the continuum of care that are implemented within each of the philosophies, stages, and settings that have already been described. Many treatment modalities have been used to address alcohol problems, alone or in combination, including advice, psychotherapy, self-help groups, aversive counterconditioning, antianxiety medication, self-control training, stress management, massage therapy, antidipsotropic medication, physical exercise, vocational counseling, marital and family therapy, hypnosis, education about the effects of alcohol, milieu management, and social skills training. The committee has used three general categories—(1) pharmacological, (2) psychological, and (3) behavioral—in the paragraphs below to organize its description of the variety of treatment modalities. More critical review of the effectiveness of the modalities appears in Appendix B.

Pharmacological Treatment Modalities There have been a number of attempts to classify the different drugs used in the treatment of alcohol problems. The major distinctions have been in terms of (a) drugs used to counter or antagonize the acute effects of alcohol intoxication, (b) drugs used in the management of withdrawal (detoxification), and (c) drugs used in long-term treatment (rehabilitation and relapse prevention).

Drugs used to manage intoxication At present there is no known compound that can counteract or antagonize the acute effects of alcohol intoxication. Such a drug would be useful in a variety of situations frequently encountered in hospital emergency rooms, ranging from the treatment of serious, life-threatening overdoses in comatose admissions to the calming of combative public inebriates (Noble, 1984; Jaffe and Ciraulo, 1985). Previously, research has focused on finding a single all-purpose drug that could reverse alcohol-induced respiratory depression, reduce alcohol-induced cognitive and motor impairments, and lessen the subjective state of intoxication (Liskow and Goodwin, 1987). There has been little success to date, but some agents appear promising, notably, zimelidine, ibuprofen, lithium, and the narcotic antagonist nalaxone.

Drugs used to manage withdrawal Most persons who become intoxicated experience a mild form of withdrawal, which is usually self-limited. In mild withdrawal a person may experience irritability, anxiety, tremor of the hands, sweating, rapid heart beat, nausea, vomiting, diarrhea, and sleep disturbance. The onset of these withdrawal symptoms is within hours of the last drink. The peak experience of these symptoms comes one or two days after the cessation of drinking; most symptoms gradually disappear after three to seven days.

A small percentage of persons will experience more severe withdrawal symptoms, with an estimated 1 to 3 percent experiencing seizures or delirium tremens (DTs), or both. DTs are characterized by profound confusion and disorientation, hyperactivity, and hallucinations. The onset of DTs typically occurs on the second or third day after drinking has stopped; DTs typically peak on the fourth day and gradually subside over another three to five days (Femino and Lewis, 1982; Jaffe and Ciraulo, 1985). Seizures generally occur within the first 24 hours. The severity of the withdrawal syndrome varies greatly among individuals and is generally proportional to the duration of the preceding period of alcohol consumption, although other factors are involved in determining severity. Persons who have experienced withdrawal symptoms in the past are more likely to experience severe withdrawal than are persons who have not experienced such symptoms; in general, severity increases each time withdrawal occurs (Jaffe and Ciraulo, 1985). In addition, other concurrent physical illnesses (e.g., trauma, pneumonia, gastritis) can increase the severity of withdrawal.

Benzodiazepines, the most commonly prescribed antianxiety drugs, are considered the drugs of choice in the pharmacological management of alcohol withdrawal (Noble, 1984; Jaffe and Ciraulo, 1985; Liskow and Goodwin, 1987; Cushman, 1988). These drugs are chosen in part because of the cross-tolerance between alcohol and the benzodiazepines (e.g., chloridiazepoxide, diazepam, fluorazepam, and orazepam).

Two distinct approaches to detoxification have developed, which reflect different treatment orientations rather than the selective placement of individuals based on their clinical status and a knowledge of the effectiveness of various treatment modalities. The first approach, pharmacologically assisted detoxification, is identified with the medical model and is referred to as medical detoxification. The second approach is identified with the sociocultural model and is referred to either as nonmedical detoxification or social model detoxification. Currently, these are seen as rival rather than as complementary approaches (Klerman, 1989).

Although it has long been recognized that careful nursing, counseling, and supportive care alone can reduce the severity of withdrawal, advocates of the medical model continue to urge the use of drugs and other physical procedures to help control the withdrawal process (Whitfield et al., 1978; Jaffe and Ciraulo, 1985). Their concern has been to have qualified medical care in an inpatient setting available to ensure the safety and comfort of the person should severe withdrawal develop. However, recent studies have used random assignment to demonstrate that pharmacologically assisted withdrawal can be safely carried out in an ambulatory setting (Alterman et al., 1988; Hayashida et al., 1989).

Medical detoxification also involves the use of other "physical procedures" in the treatment of withdrawal. Standard practice is to prescribe thiamine on admission and the use of multivitamins, given daily either orally or by injection (Jaffe and Ciraulo, 1985). Social setting detoxification uses behavioral and environmental techniques (e.g., reassurance and reality orientation) to achieve the same ends.

Although there is no single instrument in general use to predict the severity of withdrawal, there are several scales that have been employed in order to determine which orientation and which setting or level of care is necessary for a given individual. For example, the Selective Severity Assessment Scale has been suggested as promising (DenHartog, 1982). The Clinical Institute Withdrawal Assessment for Alcohol is another scale which has been used to measure symptoms of withdrawal and to monitor the severity of the withdrawal syndrome (e.g., Sellers and Naranjo, 1985). Such scales could be helpful in placement decisions if all levels of care and both types of treatment orientation (medical and sociocultural) were available in each community.

Drugs used during rehabilitation and maintenance A wide variety of drugs has been used in the long-term treatment of alcohol problems. Although there are limited clinical data to demonstrate that any of the drug therapies are effective in preventing a return to drinking, drugs continue to be used for certain persons in certain situations, and research continues to pursue pharmacological agents that can be used to decrease the appetite to drink. Several categories of such drugs are discussed in the following paragraphs.

Disulfiram (Antabuse) is described as the most commonly prescribed drug for the treatment of alcohol problems (Saxe et al., 1983; Schuckit, 1985). The agent is identified as an *alcohol-sensitizing drug*, which is a medication that precipitates unpleasant symptoms if the person drinks. Disulfiram is the only such drug in regular use in the United States, although calcium carbide is used in Canada and Europe. Calcium carbide is a shorter acting drug of this kind and could be used as a complement to disulfiram in certain cases; however, it has not been approved for use in the United States. Another alcohol-sensitizing drug, metronidazole, has also been tried and discarded, primarily because of its side effects.

Disulfiram was introduced as a pharmacological treatment for chronic alcoholism in 1948 with much enthusiasm, following the serendipitous discovery of its action by two researchers who became ill at a cocktail party. The disulfiram-ethanol reaction (DER) results from the blocking of the complete oxidation of alcohol to acetate, producing an accumulation of acetaldehyde. Disulfiram inhibits the enzyme aldehyde dehydrogenase, thereby causing a toxic reaction that consists of marked vasodilation and hypotension. The DER involves an initial sensation of heat and a bright red flushing; there is coughing and labored breathing. Nausea is common, and vomiting may occur if a large amount of alcohol has been consumed. There is also a painful feeling of apprehension.

Initially, when the drug was introduced, the person was given a demonstration of the DER, but this practice was dropped in favor of an explanation and description of the results if the person were to drink while taking disulfiram. A DER can be experienced two to three days after discontinuation of the medication. In certain cases, a DER can occur up to two weeks after discontinuation. Standard practice is a starting dose of 500 mg daily for one to two weeks, and a maintenance dose of 250 mg daily. The medication is usually taken in the morning but may sometimes be taken at night if a sedative effect is present. Disulfiram is usually continued until the person has shown substantial personal, social, and vocational improvement; maintenance or relapse prevention may be required for years.

When it was first introduced, disulfiram was routinely prescribed in many treatment programs to all persons who were admitted as part of the standard rehabilitation protocol. Because of its side effects and the potential of dangerous DERs in some individuals, questions about its relative effectiveness and safety have led to recommendations for its more selective use as an adjunct to other treatment modalities (Kwentus and Major, 1979; Noble, 1984; Schuckit, 1985; Forrest, 1985; Jaffe and Ciraulo, 1985; Liskow and Goodwin, 1987; Sellers, 1988).

The effective use of disulfiram requires a cooperative individual who will comply with the treatment regimen, taking the prescribed dose consistently. Because of this requirement, there has been research to determine whether an implant can be used; thus far, such efforts have not been successful, and compliance is achieved through monitoring (the ingestion of the medication observed by treatment personnel or a family member, checked by self-report in a weekly follow-up session, or investigated through urine testing).

Various theories have been advanced for the action of disulfiram in preventing relapse, but a general consensus has not yet developed. The use of disulfiram appears to be most successful for those individuals who have decided to abstain and who need an external aid in carrying out this decision. Fuller and colleagues (1986) recently reported the results of a controlled, blinded multicenter study of the effectiveness of disulfiram treatment as it is used in clinical practice: in combination with counseling and given to patients to take at home (rather than ingested daily in the presence of a monitor). Male subjects were randomly assigned to one of three conditions: (1) counseling plus a daily 250 mg dose of disulfiram (the standard regimen in which the subject is exposed to both pharmacological action of disulfiram and the pharmacological threat of DER); (2) counseling plus a daily 1 mg dose of disulfiram (a placebo regimen to control for the pharmacological action of disulfiram while the subject is exposed to the psychological threat of DER); and (3) counseling plus a daily 50 mg dose of riboflavin (a regimen in which the subject is exposed to counseling while controlling for the psychological threat of DER as well as the pharmacological action of disulfiram). Fuller and coworkers (1986) did not find that disulfiram as it is customarily used with outpatients was any more effective than counseling alone in achieving continuous abstinence. Their results, as those of previous studies, did suggest that disulfiram may be useful for older, more socially stable men who have a history of relapses. The results also highlight the need to investigate in more detail the factors associated with compliance: these researchers found that those men who did comply with the prescribed treatment regimen in all three conditions were more likely to remain abstinent than those who did not comply.

Another class of drugs, *psychotropic medications*, are also used in rehabilitation and relapse prevention and can be said to decrease drinking by improving associated psychopathology (i.e., anxiety, depression) (Noble, 1984; Jaffe and Ciraulo, 1985; Meyer, 1986; Liskow and Goodwin, 1987). The current use of psychoactive medications to decrease anxiety or depression in persons with alcohol problems recognizes the heterogeneity that exists. Clinicians seek to identify those persons for whom excessive drinking is clearly associated with anxiety or depression and to find an appropriate drug that will decrease the target symptom (Jaffe and Ciraulo, 1985).

For example, *antidepressant drugs* have been extensively prescribed for persons with alcohol problems because depression is so often seen in the immediate postwithdrawal phase. The original justification for prescribing antidepressant drugs was based on clinical studies that showed that persons with severe alcohol problems were frequently depressed and that their depressions were similar to those seen in persons with primary affective disorders. The assumption was that the depression caused the excessive drinking and that eliminating the depression would eliminate the drinking. Critics contended that the depression was the consequence and not the cause of the excessive drinking and that when the drinking ended, the depression would lift. In many individuals, such depression clears without pharmacological intervention (Liskow and Goodwin, 1987). Current practice is to recommend the use of antidepressant drugs only if a major depression is found to coexist with the chronic alcohol problem after a reasonable evaluation period of at least three weeks following detoxification (Gallant, 1987; Nace, 1987).

Tricyclic antidepressants (TCAs) are a family of drugs that show a high level of effectiveness in relieving symptoms of depression. Studies are continuing on three of the TCAs that have been used to treat persons with alcohol problems (amitrytyline, imipramine, and doxepin). These medications are sometimes recommended as treatments for persons who are assessed as having a severe depression that preceded their alcohol problems or who manifest persistent depression after the postdetoxification clearance period (Jaffe and Ciraulo, 1985; Liskow and Goodwin, 1987). A critical factor in the use of TCAs is to ensure that an adequate dose has been prescribed and that there is compliance with the regimen. Earlier studies have been criticized for using therapeutically inadequate doses; Liskow and Goodwin (1987) suggest that, to be effective, TCAs should be given in higher doses than those used for depressed persons without alcohol problems.

Monoamine oxidase inhibitors (MAOIs) constitute the second group of antidepressant drugs that have been used with some success to treat persons with both depressive and anxiety symptoms. There is less evidence regarding their effectiveness in persons with alcohol problems (Jaffe and Ciraulo, 1985). Another drug, lithium, is the third major antidepressant that has been employed. Its original use was based on clinical experience and the etiologic theory that the underlying problem in difficulties with alcohol was a lack of impulse control similar to that found in hypomanic states. It has been used both experimentally and clinically to treat depression in persons with alcohol problems. Lithium is used to treat bipolar conditions (where there are mood swings between manic and depressed states) rather than unipolar depression (Gallant, 1987); however, its effectiveness has not yet been demonstrated in controlled trials. A recent clinical trial (Dorus et al., 1989) found no difference in outcome for males with alcohol problems, with or without depression, who received lithium or an inactive placebo.

As with the antidepressant drugs, experienced clinicians now recommend that *antianxiety drugs* (anxiolytic agents) be administered to that subgroup of persons with alcohol problems who have a comorbid diagnosable anxiety disorder (Meyer, 1986). The judicious prescription of antianxiety agents, primarily the benzodiazepines, is also recommended for persons who continue to experience anxiety symptoms (e.g., insomnia, nightmares, palpitations) in the immediate postwithdrawal phase, which can last for three weeks to six months (Jaffe and Ciraulo, 1985; Meyer, 1986; Gallant, 1987; Liskow and Goodwin, 1987). One of the rationales for the use of antianxiety drugs is that they improve retention in ongoing treatment and relapse prevention efforts. Yet there has been a great deal of controversy regarding their use in long-term rehabilitation and relapse prevention because of their own dependence-producing properties (Jaffe and Ciraulo, 1985; Meyer, 1986; Gallant, 1987). Newer anxiolytic agents that apparently do not produce dependence are currently under investigation; these agents include beta blockers, propranalol, and buspirone. In the search for a tranquilizing drug to be used in rehabilitation, the criteria have been (a) low abuse potential; (b) effectiveness in maintaining individuals in treatment; and (c) lack of potentiation (augmentation) of the effects of alcohol. Buspirone is one of a new class of anxiolytic agents that do not have sedative effects; it does not appear to create physical dependence or to potentiate the effects of alcohol. More studies are required to determine whether it can fulfill its early promise and whether it is truly nonaddictive.

Drugs used to attenuate drinking behavior   Much of the current research on pharmacological agents is focused on finding a drug that will directly reduce the desire or craving for alcohol. The physiological model, understandably, considers craving to be primarily physiological, although environmental and social cues are also seen as contributors to the inability of an individual to abstain from drinking and his or her vulnerability to relapse in given situations (Meyer, 1986; Liskow and Goodwin, 1987). Each of the psychotropic medications, which are now reserved for treatment of so-called "dual-diagnosis patients"—those individuals with alcohol problems and a concomitant psychiatric condition—has been used and studied as much for its effectiveness in decreasing the desire to drink as for its effectiveness in reducing the associated anxiety or depressive symptoms (see Chapter 16). Lithium in particular is regarded with interest because several studies have shown that lithium may block the euphoria felt when drinking and reduce the desire to drink (Judd et al., 1977; Noble, 1984; Liskow and Goodwin, 1987; Sellers, 1988).

More recently, interest has focused on those drugs—dopamine, serotonin, and gamma aminobutyric acid (GABA)—that affect the neurotransmitters that are assumed to play a role in the effects of alcohol on the central nervous system. The antidepressant serotonin uptake inhibitors (e.g., femeldine, fluoxetine, fluovramine) have been shown in preliminary studies to decrease alcohol consumption. The relevance of such drugs to treatment, however, remains uncertain until more extensive clinical trials are carried out (Liskow and Goodwin, 1987; Sellers, 1988).   Similarly, positive results of preliminary studies with bromocriptine and apomorphine (dopamine antagonists) and homotaurine (a GABA receptor antagonist) require follow-up (Liskow and Goodwin, 1987).

Psychological Treatment Modalities   There is, as noted at the beginning of this section, a wide variety of psychological treatments, both behavioral and psychodynamic, that have been used in the treatment of alcohol problems.   Sometimes it is difficult to determine whether a specific approach is primarily behavioral or psychodynamic.   Group therapy and marital and family therapy, for example, cannot truly be classified as either psychodynamic or behavioral because they are used by practitioners from each orientation.   In fact, current practice is to combine different modalities and orientations to fashion multimodal treatment approaches.   There are, however, certain specific modalities that for descriptive purposes are identified with one or the other model because of the rationale for their use and effect.

Behavioral treatment modalities   The first clinical use of techniques derived from learning theory to reduce alcohol consumption was by the Soviet physician Kantorovich more than 50 years ago.   Kantorovich used electrical aversion, but the method was shown to be ineffective, and its use as a clinical procedure discontinued (Wilson et al., 1975; Nathan, 1984).   The major continuing use of behavioral methods over the intervening years was as chemical aversion, a technique initiated at the Shadel Sanatorium in Seattle (Lemere and Vogetlin, 1950).   The more widespread application of behavioral methods to a range of psychopathological disorders began in the early 1960s (Nathan, 1984).   These initial efforts reflected a comparatively simple view of the etiology of problem drinking as an attempt to reduce conditioned anxiety.   The first, unidimensional learning theories about the cause of excessive drinking were primarily derived from animal laboratory studies (e.g., Conger, 1951, 1956) and clinical observations that alcohol eased high levels of anxiety in persons under treatment for alcohol problems.   However, behavioral research with humans challenged the view that conditioned anxiety was the sole cause of excessive drinking (e.g., Nathan and O'Brien, 1971; Mello, 1972; Okulitch and Marlatt, 1972) and suggested that cognitive elements must also be considered.   Indeed, contemporary behavioral theories see learning as occurring within a context that comprises sociocultural, genetic, and physiological etiologic factors.   The newer conceptualizations of etiology that have been derived from social learning theory view problem drinking as multiply determined; equal attention must be paid to the determinants of drinking behavior and to the consequences of drinking because these consequences maintain the behavior (Marlatt and Donovan, 1982).

Behavior therapy for persons with alcohol problems starts with a detailed, comprehensive behavioral assessment that includes five critical elements (Nathan, 1984):

1.   the target behavior itself—its frequency, intensity, and pattern;
2.   the antecedent events—the "setting" events for the individual's maladaptive behavior;
3.   the maintaining stimuli—the environmental factors that reinforce the target behaviors;
4.   the reinforcement hierarchy—the range of factors in the environment that reinforce both target and nontarget behaviors; and
5.   the potential for remediation in the environment.

Behavior therapies have sometimes been controversial because they have been associated with challenges to the premise that total abstinence should be the goal of treatment (e.g., Miller and Caddy, 1977; Sobell and Sobell, 1973, 1986/1987; Pendery et al., 1982).   The current expression of this position is that for some moderately impaired persons, a goal of reduced consumption can be useful, whereas for more severely impaired persons a goal of abstinence is required (Nathan and McCrady, 1986; Sanchez-Craig and Wilkinson, 1986/1987; Skinner, 1985, 1988). At present, this conclusion is based more on ideology than on scientific evidence.

Nathan (1984) has classified behavioral treatments as (a) those using a single procedure that focuses on abusive drinking, (b) those focusing on antecedents and consequences, and (c) those using a broad spectrum approach, that is, a combination of specific procedures either simultaneously or sequentially. Some examples of specific procedures are presented below, although this discussion is by no means comprehensive or exhaustive.

Chemical aversion remains the best-known behavioral treatment procedure that focuses on drinking behavior (Wilson, 1987). In chemical aversion as currently practiced, a noxious stimulus (nausea induced by oral ingestion or intramuscular injection, or both, of an emetic drug) is paired with a drink of the person's favorite alcoholic beverage. Vomiting is induced to condition the individual to react adversely to the sight, smell, or taste of alcohol. Five aversion treatments are generally administered on alternate days during a 10- to 15-day hospitalization. Some persons develop adequate aversion in fewer than five treatments; others require additional treatments. Because aversion does not generalize to all alcoholic beverages, the individual receives a number of different beverages at some time during the treatment.

Covert sensitization is a verbal aversion therapy (Cautela, 1977) that uses the person's imagination to repeatedly pair unpleasant, often nausea provoking events with the anticipated acts involved in drinking. The person visualizes the drinking sequence—ordering of a drink, touching the glass to the lips, drinking itself—all in his or her usual drinking environments. At the moment the person brings the glass to his lips, he is instructed to imagine an aversive stimulus, usually vomiting. He is asked to imagine that relief occurs when he turns away from the drink. Treatment involves repeated sessions (20 presentations per session over 6 to 12 months) with the person practicing twice a day and using the procedure whenever he or she feels the urge to drink.

Stress management training has also been found to help persons with alcohol problems in staying sober, particularly when anxiety is a significant concomitant problem (Miller and Hester, 1986). Biofeedback is one such technique. It uses an electronic apparatus to monitor physiological responses and to display them to the individual through visual or auditory feedback. The individual is trained to produce the feedback by practicing the desired response (usually the relaxation of muscle groups or meditation). The person learns to recognize the subjective states that indicate heightened muscle tension as measured in electromyographic (EMG) biofeedback or alpha waves as measured by the electroencephalograph (EEG). Subjects practice producing the desired response, using the visual or auditory feedback as cues and reinforcers. Biofeedback training has been found to contribute to reductions in drinking but only for individuals with high levels of anxiety. Other forms of stress management training that have been used in the treatment of alcohol problems have been progressive relaxation training, meditation, systematic desensitization, and exercise.

A variety of behavioral social skills training procedures has been developed by those who believe that excessive drinking is caused by the inability to perform to one's own satisfaction in interpersonal situations (Oei and Jackson, 1980, 1982). Individuals are taught in either group or social settings how to respond in typical social encounters; sessions focus on such specific skills as how to express and receive positive and negative feelings, how to initiate contact, and how to reply to criticism. The modeling of skills, role playing, and videotapes of role-playing situations are all techniques that have been used in this type of behavioral approach.

Contingency management, another behavioral technique, attempts to formalize, through contracts, the naturally occurring contingencies, both positive and negative, reinforcing and punishing, that result from excessive drinking. This approach involves identifying the target behavior to be changed (i.e., drinking), identifying an appropriate reward or punishment to be administered for continued performance of the behavior to be changed, and dispensing rewarding or punishing events or activities contingent on a predetermined level of performance of the target behavior. The keys to developing effective contingency management are to (a) identify, through assessment, consequences that are meaningful to the person; (b) develop mutual agreement about the contingency, and (c) carefully and consistently carry out the contingency with all parties to the agreement (e.g., spouse, employer) performing their designated roles.

Community reinforcement counseling is a contingency management approach that is designed to provide focused behavioral training to persons with chronic alcohol problems. The goal of the counseling is to improve longstanding vocational, interpersonal, and familial problems (Hunt and Azrin, 1973; Azrin et al., 1982; Nathan and Niaura, 1985; IOM 1989). The reinforcers used in these studies were access to family, to jobs, and to friends, which were contingent on sobriety. Community reinforcement counseling is a broad-spectrum treatment strategy that includes the use of disulfiram; a regular reporting system to provide counselors with feedback from friends, family, and employers on the individual's drinking behavior or other problems; a source of continuing social support through a neighborhood "buddy," or peer advisor; and ongoing group counseling.

In the 1980s new treatment procedures have been introduced that may be broadly described as relapse prevention strategies. These include Marlatt's cognitive-behavioral strategies (Marlatt and Gordon, 1985), Annis's (1986) self-efficacy approach, and Littman's (1986) "survival" model. The three models overlap, all relying heavily on cognitive therapy techniques to avert posttreatment relapse. In recent years, relapse prevention strategies have been widely publicized, and training has been offered to practitioners (Gorski and Miller, 1982; Gorski, 1986). The addition of relapse prevention procedures to a treatment program is intended to reduce the probability and rapidity of relapse, although the techniques can be used for primary rehabilitation as well as relapse prevention. Annis's self-efficacy approach, a behavioral treatment strategy derived from Bandura's (1982, 1985) social learning theory of self-efficacy, is described below as an example of these techniques.

The self-efficacy treatment strategy uses careful assessment of the situations in which the person drank heavily during the past year to determine which contexts present a high risk of return to excessive drinking. The approach also involves careful assessment of the person's confidence in his or her ability to handle conflictual or stressful situations without resorting to heavy drinking. The key assumption underlying this strategy is that it is not the drinking alone that leads to a return to chronic, excessive drinking; also of importance are the meaning of the act of drinking for the person, the alternative behaviors that the person has available for coping with the stressful drinking situation, and the strength of the individual's belief in his or her ability to handle the situation effectively without resorting to drinking. Treatment consists of developing a hierarchical series of performance-based homework assignments that the person can perform successfully, thereby experiencing a sense of mastery in what were formerly seen as problematic drinking situations. The therapist monitors the person's feelings of self-efficacy as each assignment is completed. A variety of techniques can be used, including rehearsal of the activity during the therapy sessions and joint performance of the task with a responsible friend or the therapist. During the treatment process, the person may also use an alcohol-sensitizing drug as additional protection (Annis and Davis, 1988).

Behavioral self-control training is another relapse prevention strategy that uses a set of self-management procedures designed to help individuals stop or reduce alcohol consumption (Sanchez-Craig and Wilkinson, 1986/1987; Sanchez-Craig et al., 1987;

Sanchez-Craig, 1988). Treatment using this modality involves self-observation of drinking behavior through self-monitoring and the setting of specific behavioral objectives based on an analysis of the functions served by drinking (roughly categorized as drinking to cope and drinking for pleasure). The self-monitoring of drinking behavior through the use of structured record keeping provides information both about the functions of drinking and situations of high risk. Self-monitoring also provides feedback about progress. For persons who use drinking for coping, treatment involves the establishment of alternative cognitive and behavioral responses. For persons who use drinking for pleasure, treatment involves the establishment of self-control skills to avoid intoxication and the development of alternative recreational skills.

Reactivity to alcohol stimuli has been found to be predictive of relapse. A plausible but still experimental relapse prevention strategy is cue exposure, in which the goal is to diminish a drinker's responsivity to cues that may precipitate the desire to drink or relapse. Empirical support for the cue exposure approach is currently limited to case reports (Blakey and Baker, 1980) and evidence that cue exposure decreases the subjective desire to drink and reduces the individual's perceived difficulty of resisting relapse (Rankin et al., 1983).

Cue therapy consists of a series of treatment sessions in which the person is presented with the sight and smell of alcohol but consumption is strictly forbidden after the person has imagined himself in a high risk situation for drinking (e.g., having a fight with their spouse or attending a fraternity party). The person and therapist then review the feelings aroused by the alcohol and may practice responses that can lead to refusing a drink. Cue therapy is based on extinction theory: the cues lose their arousal value through repeated exposure without reinforcement.

Psychodynamic modalities A simple yet helpful definition of psychotherapy is that it is "an interpersonal process designed to bring about modifications of feelings, [thoughts], attitudes, and behaviors which have proven troublesome to the person seeking help from a trained professional" (Strupp, 1978:3). Contemporary psychotherapy is characterized by a variety of theoretical orientations (e.g., psychoanalytic, Gestalt, cognitive, rational-emotive). Very often the psychotherapy offered to a person with alcohol problems reflects the orientation and training of the therapist; there have been no real comparisons of the effectiveness of the different theoretical varieties of psychotherapy in treating persons with alcohol problems. What has emerged, however, is a set of principles or techniques that are recommended for use with persons experiencing alcohol problems (Zimberg et al., 1985; Nace, 1987). As with the other modalities described, current practice is to include psychotherapy as a component in a multimodality approach. Psychotherapeutic principles are often embodied in the overall design of these multicomponent programs.

Psychotherapy also varies in the format through which it is delivered: it can be offered in individual sessions, in groups of unrelated persons, and in groups of family members. In addition, types of psychotherapy vary in duration—the number of sessions and the period of time over which those sessions are spaced. Durations have ranged from short term (12 or fewer sessions) to long-term (up to 7 years) (Saxe et al., 1983). There does not appear to be substantial evidence supporting the greater effectiveness of longer periods of time in the few studies that have considered this variable (IOM, 1989). The various formats are discussed in the paragraphs below.

In recent years *individual dynamic psychotherapy* has not been seen as a major contributor to the treatment of persons with alcohol problems. The lack of support for use of this approach comes from a history of failure in the use of psychoanalytically oriented methods, which viewed problem drinking as a symptom of underlying pathology and sought to resolve the underlying conflict through the use of interpretations and development of insight (Zimberg, 1985; Nace, 1987). There are those, however, who feel that individual psychotherapy or counseling continues to play an important role in the treatment of alcohol problems (Zimberg et al., 1985; Johnson, 1986). Most psychotherapists and counselors focus on contemporary life problems and the drinking behavior rather than on historical, developmental issues. Supportive rather than uncovering therapy is the primary mode.

Specific variations of the approach have developed based on clinical experience (Blume, 1983; Nace, 1987) in which the therapist is advised to take a more active role, to be both supportive and confrontative, and to be aware of the characteristic defense structure and ego disturbances of persons with alcohol problems. Individual psychotherapy generally is recommended only as part of a more comprehensive rehabilitation effort that can include alcohol education, referral to Alcoholics Anonymous, family intervention with referral to Al-Anon and Alateen, the prescription of disulfiram, and specific efforts (e.g., vocational training) to remove life problems that contribute to continued problem drinking.

Unlike individual psychotherapy, *group psychotherapy* is among the most commonly used psychotherapeutic techniques for the treatment of alcohol problems (Blume, 1985). Group therapy is used in most primary and extended care rehabilitation programs—indeed, has been required by some licensing authorities—in keeping with the belief that it is the most effective and economical treatment modality available for alcohol problems. This belief, however, is based primarily on clinical experience and earlier studies, which did not involve sophisticated controls (Kansas, 1982; Brandsma and Pattison, 1985).

Group therapy as a distinct singular treatment is rare. As with individual psychotherapy, group therapy is offered in concert with alcohol education, referral to Alcoholics Anonymous, and additional supportive activities. Similarly to individual psychotherapy, groups tend to vary according to the orientation and training of the therapists or the ideology of the overall program of which they are a component. Consequently, variety is a prominent feature of group therapy for alcohol problems, and there is no standardization as to length of participation in the group, frequency of group meetings, length of group sessions, number of therapists, and style of group interaction.

The advantages that are often cited for the use of group psychotherapy focus on the technique in which persons with alcohol problems share experiences surrounding alcohol use with others who have had similar experiences. In this approach, group members provide both support for the difficulties to be encountered in staying sober while confronting the behaviors that are assumed to be characteristic of such persons: denial, manipulativeness, and grandiosity.

As a primary rehabilitation modality in either an inpatient or outpatient setting, group psychotherapy generally involves a daily (or three to five times a week) 1- to 1-1/2 hour session led by a staff member. When group therapy is used as an extended care or aftercare modality, groups may meet as frequently as three times a week and as infrequently as once a month. The optimal size for a group is generally considered to be 8 to 12 persons, although in practice groups vary from 4 to more than 20 persons. As with other kinds of group psychotherapy, the use of male and female cotherapists is seen as optimal for facilitating the group process.

In addition to group psychotherapy, organized programs often use the principles of group dynamics in conducting other components of the overall treatment program. These components may include educational groups that present factual material about the physiological action of alcohol, the physical consequences of prolonged excessive drinking, the potential familial, social, legal, and vocational consequences, and the characteristics of this problem state. Educational groups vary in size and style. The most common format is large-group presentations of material through lectures, films, and videotapes, followed by a discussion period in which the goal is both to clarify and amplify the factual material and to correct misconceptions and emotional reactions. Such educational groups are the main component of many drinking driver programs in which format, content, number and length of sessions, and instructor qualifications are prescribed by state government regulations.

Activity groups are another type of group psychotherapy organized around a specific recreational event and used widely in organized programs. The objectives of activity group participation are to relearn social skills by interacting with other people in a sober context, to learn and practice alternative recreational activities that will eventually replace drinking, and to become familiar with community resources. Many organized programs also use community meetings or ward management meetings as group therapy vehicles.

Over the past 25 years there has been an increase in the development of family-oriented theories about the causes and treatment of alcohol problems (Ablon, 1976, 1984; Kaufman, 1985). To a certain extent these efforts to develop techniques specifically directed at families with alcohol problems arose out of the failure to achieve successful outcomes using psychoanalytically oriented individual psychotherapy (Baekeland et al., 1975; Edwards et al., 1977). *Marital and family treatments* focus on both the drinking behavior of the identified individual with alcohol problems and the patterns of family interaction and communication. There is no one family therapy approach; rather, there is a variety of theories and interventions being used in clinical practice. Different schools of family therapy (e.g., structural, behavioral, interactional, psychodynamic) use different languages, strategies, and techniques. Some of the family intervention methods that have been utilized in the alcohol problems field include joint hospitalization of marital couples (although only one spouse has alcohol problems) (Steinglass, 1979a); group therapy for married couples in which one or both spouses has alcohol problems; intensive three- to seven-day family intervention programs as part of fixed-length Minnesota model primary rehabilitation programs (Laundergan and Williams, 1979); day treatment for marital couples (McCrady et al., 1986); Al-Anon; family education; and the involvement of the multigeneration family in a series of therapy sessions. A number of fixed-length inpatient rehabilitation programs have introduced a one week residential stay for family members who attend a highly structured program of lectures, films, discussion meetings, milieu therapy sessions, group therapy or counseling sessions, and family counseling sessions. Similar outpatient family programs have been introduced as part of fixed-length outpatient rehabilitation programs, although it is more common for these programs to spread family participation out over the full course of the primary care period (e.g., involving family members in two sessions per week over a four-week course). There have been no comprehensive studies of the comparative effectiveness of these varied approaches (Kaufman, 1985; McCrady, 1988; IOM, 1989).

One of the reasons difficulties arise in describing and studying family treatment approaches is that there is such a wide variety of family types (McCrady, 1988). Some examples are married couples without children; nuclear families consisting of two parents and children living in the same household; remarried families consisting of two married adults with children from the current marriage or from the previous marriage, or both, who may or may not be living in the same household; multigenerational families living in the same household; single-parent families; cohabiting heterosexual couples; cohabiting same-sex couples; engaged or involved couples who do not live together; long-term roommates without sexual involvement; and adult offspring, either married or unmarried, who do not live in the family household but who are available and involved with the parents. Alcohol problems may be identified in any adult or child member of the family, and more than one family member may be experiencing problems with alcohol.

Goals for family treatment also vary considerably. They may comprise facilitating a better outcome in terms of reduced consumption by the identified problem drinker(s); enhancing the personal adjustment and functioning of all family members; enhancing family functioning, communication, and relationships; or all of these objectives. The goals that are chosen vary with the type of treatment provided and with the stage of treatment (McCrady, 1988).

Another area of variability is the specific timing and nature of the family involvement in treatment. Family involvement can occur prior to treatment in attempts to "intervene" and persuade the drinker to enter treatment; it can also occur during treatment primarily to keep the drinker participating in treatment efforts and complying with specific requirements (e.g., taking prescribed medication) and to work on "family issues." Family members can also be involved in treatment when the drinker is not to help them cope with the situation and their own reactions and behaviors.

There has been some question about the appropriate setting for the initiation of family involvement (McCrady, 1988). For example, there are no data that suggest that family treatment is more effectively initiated on an inpatient basis, as is common practice. Indeed, two studies find little support for the effectiveness of family treatment on an inpatient basis (Steinglass, 1979a; McCrady et al., 1982). Reviews of the limited research that has been done do support the belief that family involvement may increase the likelihood that a person with alcohol problems will enter and remain in treatment; the review also suggests that family involvement may increase the likelihood that the problem drinker will successfully reduce the quantity or frequency of drinking or remain abstinent after treatment (Steinglass, 1979b; McCrady, 1988). McCrady (1988) concludes her review of the status of family treatment by suggesting that research data support superior outcomes for family-involved treatment, enough so that the modal approach should involve family members in carefully planned interventions. She suggests that the questions that now need to be addressed to guide future research and practice are the following: What family members should be involved at what stages in treatment, and what kinds of family treatment methods should be used? She also recommends that in planning treatment, "family" should be defined broadly to comprise all those members of the person's immediate social environment who have a substantial emotional commitment to the individual, whether or not they are biological or legal relatives.

Summary and Conclusions

As a way to clarify the dimensions of treatment for alcohol problems, the committee has reviewed the many different definitions offered in previous studies, reviews, and planning documents. It has developed a definition of treatment that can encompass all efforts to reduce alcohol consumption by persons who experience problems surrounding such consumption, as well as the additional supportive services required to prevent relapse and a return to destructive alcohol use. The committee's definition incorporates those activities that are currently labeled intervention as well as those labeled treatment and rehabilitation:

> *Treatment refers to the broad range of services, including identification, brief intervention, assessment, diagnosis, counseling, medical services, psychiatric services, psychological services, social services, and follow-up, for persons with alcohol problems. The overall goal of treatment is to reduce or eliminate the use of alcohol as a contributing factor to physical, psychological, and social dysfunction and to arrest, retard, or reverse the progress of associated problems.*

This expanded definition reflects the committee's conclusion that efforts to treat alcohol problems in this country have in the recent past been too narrowly focused on those persons with the most severe problems. Its review of prior efforts has suggested a preliminary framework for identifying the elements of an expanded continuum of care that incorporates intervention (secondary prevention) activities as well as treatment and rehabilitation (tertiary prevention) efforts and that can address the treatment needs of persons at each level of severity of alcohol problems.

The committee's definition also reflects the professional judgment that the treatment of alcohol problems cannot be limited only to those direct activities designed to reduce alcohol consumption. Supportive services are required if relapse is to be avoided and continued sobriety and recovery is to be maintained by individuals who may have few personal and social resources and who are experiencing very severe physical, vocational, family, legal, or emotional problems surrounding their use of alcohol. The extent of the person's dysfunction in other key life areas (e.g., employment, physical health, emotional health, marital and family relations) should determine the breadth of the treatment response needed.

Treatments for alcohol problems are diverse, in part because experts have different views about the causes of such problems. Three major views or models of the etiology of alcohol problems have been guiding treatment provision in recent years; these are the medical, psychological, and sociocultural models. Treatment regimens generally have been based on one or a combination of these views. The committee is encouraged that these differing approaches are now evolving toward a comprehensive approach, the biopsychosocial model, which recognizes the contribution of genetic, physiological, psychological, and sociocultural factors to the etiology and treatment of alcohol problems.

The committee reviewed the development of the current network of services in this country, with particular attention to the origin and spread of the so-called Minnesota model of treatment and the California social model of recovery, their relationship to Alcoholics Anonymous, and the shift in underlying ideologies. To understand the current status of treatment in this country, it is important to understand the evolution of Minnesota model inpatient treatment programs, a standardized specialist treatment system that has been criticized as emphasizing an overly expensive, inpatient-focused medical model (e.g., Miller and Hester, 1987; Yahr, 1988). The standardized treatment program typically delivered to persons in treatment in the course of a four week inpatient stay, either in a hospital or in a freestanding facility, consists of detoxification, education (based on the disease concept) about the harmful medical and psychosocial effects of excessive alcohol consumption, confrontation, attendance at AA meetings and use of AA materials in developing a recovery plan ("stepwork"), and disulfiram therapy. Although one could trace a number of early precursors of this approach, the efforts begun in Minnesota at the Willmar State Hospital, the Hazelden Foundation, and the Johnson Foundation were particularly influential in the development and spread of this program model and in its adoption as the standard treatment regimen. The Minnesota model is the orientation for both public- and private-sector programs across the nation (e.g., Kelso and Fillmore, 1984; Yahr, 1988; see Chapter 4). Programs are generally based on the disease model, and the primary goal of treatment is abstinence. Arising from the same tradition, California's social model recovery programs share an ideology based on mutual aid and self-help principles. These programs stress the value of peer support—reliance on the experiential knowledge base of other recovering alcoholics to help the person with alcohol problems take responsibility for maintaining lifelong abstinence, rather than professionalized treatment.

The committee's review of earlier efforts to describe the treatment system and the variety of therapies that have been employed has suggested a preliminary framework that can be used to describe the resources in the continuum of care. Four orientations can be identified, although in reality the major distinction is now whether the orientation of a given program is a mixed medical-social model or a social model. Three major stages (acute intervention, rehabilitation, and maintenance) and four settings (hospital, residential, intermediate, and outpatient) have been proposed. Any endeavor to implement this framework as a uniform classification should be preceded by a comprehensive review of how well the framework can incorporate the elements of the original continuum of care, as defined in the Uniform Act, and the modifications that have been introduced in the many state and county jurisdictions that have developed a maturing system of local treatment services.

As a result of its deliberations, the committee found that treatment for alcohol problems includes a broad range of activities that vary in content, duration, intensity, goals, setting, provider, and target population and that no single treatment approach or modality has been demonstrated to be superior to all others. The committee also found that although there is agreement that an organized continuum of care is required, there is no agreement on the definition of that continuum, on the definitions of the service elements, or even on what constitutes a single treatment episode for purposes of evaluating treatment appropriateness and success. The federal government, state and local governments, and other third-party payers, in their planning, funding, and regulatory efforts, use very different labels and definitions for the elements in the continuum of care, often confusing the orientation of the providers, the stage of treatment, the setting of treatment, and the modality or procedure used. It is only recently that research has begun to investigate these elements in a systematic fashion. Additional studies are needed to determine the effectiveness of the different modalities, alone and in combination.

The committee sees a need to develop a consensually accepted system for describing the treatment episode. This system can then serve as the basis for defining the required continuum of care—the orientations, stages, settings, and modalities of treatment—to be used in both research and program development. There have been a number of prior efforts to develop classifications of treatment programs for evaluating and funding treatment from a national perspective. These efforts have used such variables as treatment philosophy, settings, and modalities, but there has been no acceptance of a uniform classification. Consequently, there is no consistent definition of treatment in this country or of the elements of the continuum of care that are necessary to meet national objectives to reduce the prevalence of alcohol problems.

The rich diversity of treatment options reviewed by the committee reflects the dynamic vitality of the field. The committee is encouraged by the evolution that has occurred and wishes to encourage that growth by assisting in the development of a comprehensive framework for evaluation and program development.

REFERENCES

Ablon, J. 1976. Family structure and behavior in alcoholism: A review of the literature. Pp. 205-242 in Social Pathology, Vol. 4 of The Biology of Alcoholism, B. Kissin and H. Begleiter, eds. New York: Plenum Press.

Ablon, J. 1984. Family research and alcoholism. Pp. 383-396 in Recent Developments in Alcoholism, vol. 2, M. Galanter, ed. New York: Plenum Press.

Abrams, D. B., and R. S. Niaura. 1987. Social learning theory. Pp. 131-178 in Psychological Theories of Drinking and Alcoholism, H. T. Blane and K. E. Leonard, eds. New York: Guilford Press.

Alterman, A. I., M. Hayashida, and C. P. O'Brien. 1988. Treatment response and safety of ambulatory medical detoxification. Journal of Studies on Alcohol 49:160-166.

American Hospital Association. 1974. Classification of Health Care Institutions. Chicago: American Hospital Association.

Anderson, D. J. 1981. Perspectives on Treatment: The Minnesota Experience. Center City, Minn.: Hazelden Foundation.

Anderson, J. G., and F. S. Gilbert. 1989. Communication skills training with alcoholics for improving performance of two of the Alcoholics Anonymous recovery steps. Journal of Studies on Alcohol 50:361-367.

Annis, H. M. 1986. A relapse prevention model for treatment of alcoholics. Pp. 407-433 in Treating Addictive Behaviors, W. R. Miller and N. Heather, eds. New York: Plenum Press.

Annis, H. M. 1988. Optimal treatment for alcoholism and drug dependencies. Presented to the Kaiser Permanente Southern California Medical Group, Los Angeles, March 30.

Annis, H. M., and C. S. Davis. 1988. Assessment of expectancies. Pp. 84-111 in Assessment of Addictive Behaviors, D. M. Donovan and G. A. Marlatt, eds. New York: Guilford Press.

Armor, D. J., J. M. Polich, and H. B. Stambul. 1976. Alcoholism and Treatment. Santa Monica, Calif.: RAND Corporation.

Azrin, N. H., R. W. Sisson, R. W. Meyers, and M. Godley. 1982. Alcoholism treatment by disulfiram and community reinforcement therapy. Journal of Behavior Therapy and Experimental Psychiatry 13:105-112.

Babor, T. F. 1986. Management of alcohol use disorders in developing and developed countries: Research evidence as a basis for the rational allocation of treatment services. Presented at the Symposium on Alcohol and Drug Abuse of the National Institute of Mental Health and Neuro-sciences of India and the U.S. Alcohol, Drug Abuse, and Mental Health Administration, Bangalore, India, November 18-21.

Babor, T. F., M. Treffardier, J. Weill, L. Feguer, and J. P. Ferrant. 1983. The early detection and secondary prevention of alcoholism in France. Journal of Studies on Alcohol 44:600-616.

Babor, T. F., E. B. Ritson, and R. J. Hodgson. 1986. Alcohol-related problems in the primary health care setting: a review of early intervention strategies. British Journal of Addiction 81:23-46.

Bandura, A. 1982. Self-efficacy mechanism in human agency. American Psychologist 37:122-147.

Bandura, A. 1985. Social Foundations of Thought and Action. Englewood Cliff, N.J.: Prentice-Hall.

Baekeland, F., L. Lundwall, and B. Kissin. 1975. Methods for the treatment of chronic alcoholism: A critical appraisal. Pp. 247-327 in Research Advances in Alcohol and Drug Problems, vol. 2, R. J. Gibbins, Y. Israel, H. Kalant, R. E. Popham, W. Schmidt, and R. G. Smart, eds. Toronto: John Wiley and Sons.

Bast, R. J. 1984. Classification of Alcoholism Treatment Settings. Rockville, Md.: National Institute on Alcohol Abuse and Alcoholism.

Beigel, A., and S. Ghertner. 1977. Toward a social model: An assessment of social factors which influence social drinking and its treatment. Pp. 197-233 in Treatment and Rehabilitation of the Chronic Alcoholic. Vol. 5 of The Biology of Alcoholism, B. Kissin and H. Begleiter, eds. New York: Plenum Press.

Berman, H., and D. Klein. 1977. Project to Develop a Comprehensive Alcoholism Benefit Through Blue Cross: Final Report of Phase I. Prepared for the National Institute on Alcohol Abuse and Alcoholism. Chicago: Blue Cross Association.

Beyer, J. A., and H. M. Trice. 1982. Design and implementation of job-based alcoholism programs: Constructive confrontation strategies and how they work. Pp. 181-239 in Occupational Alcoholism: A Review of Research Issues. (Proceedings of a workshop held May 24-26, 1980, by the National Institute on Alcohol Abuse and Alcoholism.) Washington, D.C.: U.S. Government Printing Office.

Blakey, R., and R. Baker. 1980. An exposure approach to alcohol abuse. Behavioral Research and Therapy 18:319-325.

Blumberg, L., T. Shepley, and I. W. Shandler. 1973. Skid Row and Its Alternatives. Philadelphia: Temple University Press.

Blume, S. B. 1982. Alcoholism. Pp. 921-925 in Current Therapy, H. Conn, ed. Philadelphia: W. B. Saunders.

Blume, S. B. 1983. Is alcoholism treatment worthwhile? Bulletin of the New York Academy of Medicine 59:171-180.

Blume, S. B. 1985. Group psychotherapy in the treatment of alcoholism. Pp. 7-107 in Practical Approaches to Alcoholism Psychotherapy, S. Zimberg, J. Wallace, and S. B. Blume, eds. New York: Plenum Press.

Boche, H. L., ed. 1975. Funding of Alcohol and Drug Programs: A Report of the Funding Task Force. Washington, D.C.: Alcohol and Drug Problems Association of North America.

Booz-Allen and Hamilton, Inc. 1978. The Alcoholism Funding Study: Evaluations of the Sources of Funds and Barriers to Funding Alcoholism Treatment Programs. Prepared for the U.S. Department of Health Education and Welfare. Washington, D.C.: Booz-Allen and Hamilton, Inc.

Borkman, T. 1982. Third generation mutual self-help organizations: Social model recovery organizations. Presented at the Southern Sociological Society Annual Meeting, Memphis, Tennessee, April 15.

Borkman, T. 1983. A Social-Experiential Model in Programs for Alcoholism Recovery: A Research Report on a New Treatment Design. Rockville, Md.: National Institute on Alcohol Abuse and Alcoholism.

Borkman, T. 1986. The Alcohol Services Reporting System (ASRS) Revision Study. Prepared for the California Department of Alcohol and Drug Programs, Health and Welfare Agency, Sacramento.

Borkman, T. 1988. Executive summary: social model recovery programs. Prepared for the IOM Committee for the Study of Treatment and Rehabilitation Services for Alcoholism and Alcohol Abuse, May.

Borthwick, R. B. 1977. Summary of Cost-Benefit Study Results for Navy Alcohol Rehabilitation Programs. Technical Report No. 346. Washington, D.C.: U.S. Navy Bureau of Naval Personnel.

Brandsma, J. M., and E. M. Pattison. 1985. The outcome of group psychotherapy with alcoholics: An empirical review. American Journal of Drug and Alcohol Abuse 11:151-162.

Brickman, P., V. C. Rabinowitz, J. Karuza, D. Coates, E. Cohn, and L. Kidder. 1982. Models of helping and coping. American Psychologist 37:368-384.

Brown University Center for Alcohol Studies. 1985. Substance Abuse Treatment in Rhode Island: Population Needs and Program Development. Providence, R.I.: Rhode Island Department of Mental Health, Retardation and Hospitals and Department of Health.

Cahalan, D. 1987. Understanding America's Drinking Problem: How to Combat the Hazards of Alcohol. San Francisco: Jossey-Bass.

Cautela, J. R. 1977. The treatment of alcoholism by covert sensitization. Psychotherapy: Theory, Research, and Practice 7:86-90.

Chafetz, M. E. 1976. Alcoholism. Psychiatric Annals 6:107-141.

Chatham, L. R. 1984. Foreword. Pp. iii-v in Classification of Alcoholism Treatment Settings, by R. J. Bast. Rockville, Md.: National Institute on Alcohol Abuse and Alcoholism.

Cohen, S. 1982. Methods of intervention. Pp. 127-143 in Prevention, Intervention, and Treatment: Concerns and Models, J. de Luca, ed. Washington, D.C.: U.S. Government Printing Office.

Colorado Alcohol and Drug Abuse Division. 1978. State Plan for Alcohol and Drug Abuse Treatment, Prevention, and Quality of Care: FY1979. Denver: Colorado Department of Health.

Conger, J. J. 1951. The effects of alcohol on conflict behavior in the albino rat. Quarterly Journal of Studies on Alcohol 12:1-29.

Conger, J. J. 1956. Alcoholism: Theory, problem and challenge. II. Reinforcement theory and the dynamics of alcoholism. Quarterly Journal of Studies on Alcohol 17:291-324.

Costello, R. M. 1980. Alcoholism aftercare and outcome: Cross-legged panel and path analysis. British Journal of Addictions 75:49-53.

Costello, R. M. 1982. Evaluation of alcoholism treatment programs. Pp. 1197-1210 in Encyclopedic Handbook of Alcoholism, E. M. Pattison and E. Kaufman, eds. New York: Gardner Press.

Costello, R. M. and J. E. Hodde. 1981. Costs of comprehensive alcoholism care for 100 patients over 4 years. Journal of Studies on Alcohol 42:87-93.

Costello, R. M., P. Biever, and J. G. Baillargon. 1977. Alcoholism treatment programming: Historical trends and modern approaches. Alcoholism: Clinical and Experimental Research 1:311-318.

Cushman, J. 1988. Alcohol withdrawal: A look at recent research. Presented at the "Treatment" meeting of the National Institute on Alcohol Abuse and Alcoholism Ad Hoc Scientific Advisory Board, Rockville, Md., May 3.

DeMiranda, J. 1986. California's social model of recovery from alcoholism: Report of a conference. Alcohol Health and Research World 10:74-75.

Diesenhaus, H. I. 1982. Current trends in treatment programming for problem drinkers and alcoholics. Pp. 219-90 in Prevention, Intervention, and Treatment: Concerns and Models, J. de Luca, ed. Washington, D.C.: U.S. Government Printing Office.

Diesenhaus, H. I., and R. Booth, eds. 1977. Cost-benefit Study of State Hospital Drug and Alcohol Treatment Programs. Prepared for the Joint Budget Committee, Colorado Legislature. Denver: Alcohol and Drug Abuse Division, Colorado Department of Health.

DenHartog, G. L. 1982. "A Decade of Detox": Development of Non-hospital Approaches to Alcohol Detoxification—A Review of the Literature. Substance Abuse Monograph Series. Jefferson City, Mo.: Division of Alcohol and Drug Abuse.

Dodd, M. H. 1974. The community model of alcoholism. Working paper. Sun Street Centers, Salinas, California.

Dodd, M. H. 1986. What does social model mean? Presented at the Conference on California's Social Model Recovery from Alcoholism. University of California Extension, San Diego, Program on Alcohol Issues, February 23-25.

Donovan, D. M. 1988. Assessment of addictive behaviors: Implications of an emerging biopsychosocial model. Pp. 3-48 in Assessment of Addictive Behaviors, D. M. Donovan and G. A. Marlatt, eds. New York: Guilford Press.

Donovan, D. M., and E. F. Chaney. 1985. Alcoholic relapse prevention and intervention: Models and methods. Pp. 351-416 in Relapse Prevention: Maintenance Strategies in the Treatment of Addictive Behaviors, G. A. Marlatt and J. R. Gordon, eds. New York: Guilford Press.

Dorus, W., D. G. Ostow, R. Anton, P. Cushman, J. F. Collins, M. Schaefer, H. L. Charles, P. Desai, M. Hayashida, U. Malkerneker, M. Willenbring, R. Fiscella, and M. R. Sather. 1989. Lithium treatment of depressed and nondepressed alcoholics. Journal of the American Medical Association 262:1646-1652.

Edwards, G. 1987. The Treatment of Drinking Problems: A Guide for the Helping Professions. Oxford, England: Blackwell Scientific Publications.

Edwards, G., J. Orford, S. Egert, S. Guthrie, A. Hawker, C. Hensman, M. Mitcheson, E. Oppenheimer, and C. Taylor. 1977. Alcoholism: A controlled trial of "treatment" and "advice." Journal of Studies on Alcohol 38:1004-1031.

Engel, G. L. 1977. The need for a new medical model: A challenge for biomedicine. Science 196:129-136.

Feldman, D. J., E. M. Pattison, L. C. Sobell, T. Graham, and M. B. Sobell. 1975. Outpatient alcohol detoxification: Initial findings on 564 patients. American Journal of Psychiatry 132:407-412.

Femino, J., and D. C. Lewis. 1982. Clinical Pharmacology and Therapeutics of the Alcohol Withdrawal Syndrome. Program in Alcoholism and Drug Abuse Medical Monograph No. 1. Providence, R.I.: Brown University Program in Medicine.

Filstead, W. J. 1988a. Monitoring the process of recovery. Pp. 181-191 in Recent Developments in Alcoholism, vol. 6, M. Galanter, ed. New York: Plenum Press.

Filstead, W. J. 1988b. Statement presented at the open meeting of the Committee for the study of Treatment and Rehabilitation Services for Alcoholism and Alcohol Abuse, Institute of Medicine, Washington, D.C., January 25.

Finn, P. 1986. Decriminalization of public drunkenness: Response of the health care system. Journal of Studies on Alcohol 46:7-22.

Finny, J. W., R. H. Moos, and D. A. Chan. 1981. Length of stay and program components in the treatment of alcoholism: A comparison of two techniques for process analyses. Journal of Consulting and Clinical Psychology 49:120-131.

Forrest, G. G. 1985. Antabuse treatment. Pp. 451-460 in Alcoholism and Substance Abuse: Strategies for Clinical Intervention, T. E. Bratter and G. G. Forrest, eds. New York: Free Press.

Fuller, R. K., L. Branchey, D. R. Brightwell, R. M. Derman, C. D. Emrick, F. L. Iber, K. E. James, R. B. Lacoursiere, K. K. Lee, I. Lowenstam, I. Maany, D. Neiderhiser, J. J. Nocks, and S. Shaw. 1986. Disulfiram treatment of alcoholism: A Veterans Administration cooperative study. Journal of the American Medical Association 256:1449-1455.

Gallant, D. M. 1987. Alcoholism: A Guide to Diagnosis, Intervention, and Treatment. New York: Norton and Company.

Gilbert. F. S. 1988. The effect of type of aftercare follow-up on treatment outcome among alcoholics. Journal of Studies on Alcohol 49:149-159.

Glaser, F. B., S. W. Greenberg, and M. Barrett. 1978. A Systems Approach to Alcohol Treatment. Toronto: Addiction Research Foundation.

Glasscote, R. M., T. F. A. Plaut, D. W. Hammersley, F. J. O'Neil, M. E. Chafetz, and E. Cumming. 1967. The Treatment of Alcohol Problems: A Study of Programs and Problems. Washington, D.C.: Joint Information Service of the American Psychiatric Association and the National Association of Mental Health.

Glatt, M. M. 1974. A Guide to Addiction and Its Treatment. New York: John Wiley and Sons.

Gorski, T. T. 1986. Relapse prevention planning: A new recovery tool. Alcohol Health and Research World 10:6-11, 63.

Gorski, T. T., and M. Miller. 1982. Counseling for Relapse Prevention. Independence, Mo.: Herald House.

Gottlieb, F., M. Kirkpatrick, J. Marmor, and M. Galanter. 1984. Self-help groups. Pp. 815-831 in The Psychiatric Therapies, T. B. Karazu, ed. Washington, D.C.: American Psychiatric Association.

Grad, F. P., A. L. Goldberg, and B. A. Shapiro. 1971. Alcoholism and the Law. Dobbs Ferry, N.Y.: Oceana Publications.

Harrison P. A., and N. G. Hoffmann. 1986. Chemical dependency inpatients and outpatients: Intake characteristics and treatment outcome. Prepared for the Chemical Dependency Program Division, Minnesota Department of Human Services. St. Paul-Ramsey Foundation, St. Paul, Minnesota.

Hart, L. A review of treatment and rehabilitation legislation regarding alcohol abusers and alcoholics in the United States: 1920-1971. International Journal of the Addictions 12:667-678.

Hayashida, M., A. I. Alterman, A. T. McLellan, C. P. O'Brien, J. J. Purtill, J. R. Volpicelli, A. H. Raphaelson, and C. P. Hall. 1989. Comparative effectiveness and costs of inpatient and outpatient detoxification of patients with mild-to-moderate alcohol withdrawal syndrome. New England Journal of Medicine 320:358-365.

Hoffmann, N. G., J. A. Halikas, and D. Mee-Lee, 1987a. The Cleveland Admission, Discharge, and Transfer Criteria: Model for Chemical Dependency Treatment Programs. Cleveland, Ohio: The Greater Cleveland Hospital Association.

Hoffmann, N. G., F. Ninonuevo, J. Mozey, and M. G. Luxenberg. 1987b. Comparison of court-referred DWI arrestees with other outpatients in substance abuse treatment. Journal of Studies on Alcohol 48:591-594.

Holden, C. 1987. Alcoholism and the medical cost crunch. Science 235:1132-1133.

Holder, H. D., R. Longabaugh, and W. R. Miller. 1988. Cost and effectiveness of alcoholism treatment using best available information. Prepared for the IOM Committee for the Study of Treatment and Rehabilitation Services for Alcoholism and Alcohol Abuse, July.

Hunt, G. M., and N. H. Azrin. 1973. The community reinforcement approach to alcoholism. Behaviour Research and Therapy 11:91-104.

Institute of Medicine (IOM). 1980. Alcoholism, Alcohol Abuse, and Related Problems: Opportunities for Research. Washington, D.C.: National Academy Press.

Institute of Medicine (IOM). 1989. Research Opportunities in the Prevention and Treatment of Alcohol-Related Problems. Washington, D.C.: National Academy Press.

Jaffe, J. H., and D. A. Ciraulo. 1985. Drugs used in the treatment of alcoholism. Pp. 355-389 in The Diagnosis and Treatment of Alcoholism, 2nd ed., J. H. Mendelson and N. K. Mello, eds. New York: McGraw-Hill.

Johnson, V. E. 1980. I'll Quit Tomorrow. San Francisco: Harper and Row.

Johnson, V. E. 1986. Intervention: How to Help Someone Who Doesn't Want Help. St. Paul, Minn.: Johnson Institute.

Joint Commission on the Accreditation of Hospitals (JCAH). 1983. Consolidated Standards Manual for Child, Adolescent and Adult Psychiatric, Alcoholism, and Drug Abuse Facilities. Chicago: JCAH.

Judd, L., R. B. Hubbard, L. Y. Huey, P. A. Attewell, D. S. Janowsky, and K. I. Takashi. 1977. Lithium carbonate and ethanol induced "highs" in normal subjects. Archives of General Psychiatry 34:463-467.

Kansas, N. 1982. Alcoholism and group psychotherapy. Pp. 1011-1021 in Encyclopedic Handbook of Alcoholism, E. M. Pattison and E. Kaufman, eds. New York: Gardner Press.

Kaufman, E. 1985. Family therapy in the treatment of alcoholism. Pp. 376-397 in Alcoholism and Substance Abuse: Strategies for Clinical Intervention, T. E. Bratter and G. G. Forrest, eds. New York: Free Press.

Kelso, D., and K. M. Fillmore. 1984. Alcoholism Treatment and Client Functioning in Alaska: A Summary of Findings and Implications of a Followup Study of Individuals Receiving Alcoholism Treatment. Report prepared for the Alaska State Office of Alcoholism and Drug Abuse. Anchorage, Alaska: Alam Associates.

Khantzian, E. J. 1981. Some treatment implications of the ego and self-disturbances in alcoholism. Pp. 163-188 in Dynamic Approaches to the Understanding and Treatment of Alcoholism, M. H. Bean and N. E. Zinberg, eds. New York: Free Press.

Khantzian, E. J. 1985. Psychotherapeutic interventions with substance abusers—the clinical context. Journal of Substance Abuse Treatment 2:83-88.

Khantzian, E. J., and J. E. Mack. 1989. A.A. and contemporary psychodynamic theory. Pp. 67-89 in Recent Developments in Alcoholism, vol. 7, M. Galanter, ed. New York: Plenum Press.

Kissin, B. 1977a. Medical management of the alcoholic patient. Pp. 53-103 in Treatment and Rehabilitation of the Chronic Alcoholic. Vol. 5 in The Biology of Alcoholism, B. Kissin and H. Begleiter, eds. New York: Plenum.

Kissin, B. 1977b. Theory and practice in the treatment of alcoholism. Pp. 1-51 in Treatment and Rehabilitation of the Chronic Alcoholic, Vol. 5 in The Biology of Alcoholism, B. Kissin and H. Begleiter, eds. New York: Plenum Press.

Kissin, B., and M. Hansen. 1982. The bio-psychosocial perspective in alcoholism. Pp. 1-19 in Alcoholism and Clinical Psychiatry, J. Solomon, ed. New York: Plenum Press.

Kissin, B., and M. Hansen. 1985. Integration of biological and psychosocial interventions in the treatment of alcoholism. Pp. 63-103 in Future Directions in Alcohol Abuse Treatment Research, B. S. McCrady, N. E. Noel, and T. D. Nirenberg, eds. Washington D.C.: U.S. Government Printing Office.

Klerman, G. L. 1984. Ideological conflicts in combined treatment. Pp. 17-34 in Combining Psychotherapy and Drug Therapy in Clinical Practice, B. D. Beitman and G. L. Klerman, eds. New York: Spectrum Publications.

Klerman, G. L. 1989. Treatment of alcoholism. New England Journal of Medicine 320:394-395.

Kusserow, R. P. 1989. An Assessment of Data Collection for Alcohol, Drug Abuse, and Mental Health Services. Washington, D.C.: Office of the Inspector General, U.S. Department of Health and Human Services.

Kwentus, J., and L. F. Major. 1979. Disulfiram in the treatment of alcoholism: A review. Journal of Studies on Alcohol 40:428-446.

Laundergan, J. C. 1982. Easy Does It: Alcoholism Treatment Outcomes, Hazelden and the Minnesota Model. Minneapolis: Hazelden Foundation.

Laundergan, J. C., and T. Williams. 1979. Hazelden: Evaluation of a residential family program. Alcohol Health and Research World 3(4):13-16.

Lawrence Johnson and Associates, Inc. 1983. Evaluation of the HCFA Alcoholism Services Demonstration: Final Evaluation Design. Prepared for the Office of Research and Demonstrations, Health Care Financing Administration. Washington, D.C., March.

Lazarus, A. 1981. The Practice of Multimodal Therapy. New York: McGraw-Hill.

Lemere, F., and W. L. Vogetlin. 1950. An evaluation of the aversion treatment of alcoholism. Quarterly Journal of Studies on Alcohol 11:199-204.

Lewin/ICF. 1989a. Analysis of State Alcohol and Drug Data Collection Instruments, vols. 1-6. Prepared for the Office of Finance and Coverage Policy, National Institute on Drug Abuse (NIDA). Washington, D.C.: NIDA.

Lewin/ICF. 1989b. Feasibility and Design of a Study of the Delivery and Financing of Drug and Alcohol Services. Prepared for the National Institute on Drug Abuse (NIDA). Washington, D.C.: NIDA.

Lewis, D. C., and A. J. Gordon. 1983. Alcoholism and the general hospital: The Roger Williams intervention program. Bulletin of the New York Academy of Medicine 59:181-197.

Lewis, J. S. 1982. The federal role in alcoholism research, treatment and prevention. Pp. 385-401 in Alcohol, Science and Society Revisited, E. Gomberg, H. White, and J. Carpenter, eds. Ann Arbor, Mich., and New Brunswick, N.J.: University of Michigan Press and Center of Alcohol Studies, Rutgers University.

Liskow, B. I., and D. W. Goodwin. 1987. Pharmacological treatment of alcohol intoxication, withdrawal, and dependence: a critical review. Journal of Studies on Alcohol 48:356-370.

Littman, G. K. 1986. Alcoholism survival: The prevention of relapse. Pp. 294-303 in Treating Addictive Behaviors, W. R. Miller and N. Heather, eds. New York: Plenum Press.

Longabaugh, R., and M. Beattie. 1985. Optimizing the cost effectiveness of treatment for alcohol abusers. Pp. 104-136 in Future Directions in Alcohol Abuse Treatment Research, B. S. McCrady, N. E. Noel, and Ted D. Nirenberg, eds. Washington, D.C.: U.S. Government Printing Office.

Los Angeles County Office of Alcohol Programs. 1987. 1987-1988 Los Angeles County Plan for Alcohol-Related Services. Los Angeles: Department of Health Services.

Lyons, J. P., J. Welte, J. Brown, L. Sokolow, and G. Hynes. 1982. Variation in alcoholism treatment orientation: Differential impact upon specific subpopulations. Alcoholism: Clinical and Experimental Research 6:333-343.

Manov, W. F., and N. N. Beshai. 1986. Alcohol-free living centers: Long term, low cost, alcohol recovery housing. Presented at the 114th Annual Meeting of the American Public Health Association, September 28-October 2.

Marlatt, G. A. 1985. Relapse prevention: Theoretical rationale and overview of the model. Pp. 3-70 in Relapse Prevention: Maintenance Stategies in the Treatment of Addictive Behaviors, G. A. Marlatt and J. R. Gordon, eds. New York: Guilford Press.

Marlatt, G. A. 1988a. Executive summary: Intervention strategies for college students. Prepared for the IOM Committee for the Study of Treatment and Rehabilitation Services for Alcoholism and Alcohol Abuse, February.

Marlatt, G. A. 1988b. Matching clients to treatment: Treatment models and stages of change. Pp. 474-483 in Assessment of Addictive Behaviors, D. M. Donovan and G. A. Marlatt, eds. New York: Guilford Press.

Marlatt, G. A., and D. M. Donovan. 1982. Behavioral psychology approaches to alcoholism. Pp. 560-577 in Encyclopedic Handbook of Alcoholism, E. M. Pattison and E. Kaufman, eds. New York: Gardner Press.

Marlatt, G. A., and J. R. Gordon, eds. 1985. Relapse Prevention: Maintenance Stategies in the Treatment of Addictive Behaviors. New York: Guilford Press.

Marlatt, G. A., J. S. Baer, D. M. Donovan, and D. R. Kivlan. 1988. Addictive behaviors: Etiology and treatment. Annual Review of Psychology 39:223-252.

McClellan, A. T., L. Luborsky, G. E. Woody, and C. P. O'Brien. 1980. An improved diagnostic instrument for substance abuse patients: The Addiction Severity Index. Journal of Nervous and Mental Disorders 168:26-33.

McCrady, B. S. 1988. Executive summary: Criteria and issues to consider when deciding to intervene at the marital/family level, the individual level, or both. Prepared for the IOM Committee to Identify Research Opportunities for the Prevention and Treatment of Alcohol-Related Problems.

McCrady, B.S., J. Moreau, T. J. Paolina, and R. Longabaugh. 1982. Joint hospitalization and couples therapy for alcoholism: A four-year follow-up. Journal of Studies on Alcohol 43:1244-1250.

McCrady, B.S., N. E. Noel, D. B. Abrams, R. L. Stout, H. F. Nelson, and W. M. Hay. 1986. Comparative effectiveness of three types of spouse involvement in outpatient behavioral alcoholism treatment. Journal of Studies on Alcohol 47:459-467.

Mello, N. K. 1972. Behavioral studies of alcoholism. Pp. 219-292 in Physiology and Behavior. Vol. 2 of The Biology of Alcoholism, B. Kissin and H. Begleiter, eds. New York: Plenum Press.

Meyer, R. E. 1986. Anxiolytics and the alcoholic patient. Journal of Studies on Alcohol 47:269-273.

Miller, B., W. F Manov, and A. Wright. 1987. The community model approach: Los Angeles County's application of public health principles to alcohol problems. Presented at the American Public Health Association Meeting, New Orleans, Louisiana, October.

Miller, W. R., and G.R. Caddy. 1977. Abstinence and controlled drinking in the treatment of problem drinkers. Journal of Studies on Alcohol 38:986-1003.

Miller, W. R., and R. K. Hester. 1986. Inpatient alcoholism treatment: Who benefits? American Psychologist 41:794-805.

Moberg, D. P., W. K. Krause, and P. K. Klein. 1982. Posttreatment drinking behavior among inpatients from an industrial alcoholism program. International Journal of Addictions 17:549-567.

Moos, R. H., and J. W. Finney. 1987/1988. Alcoholism program evaluations: The treatment domain. Drugs and Society 2(2):31-51.

Moos, R. H., R. C. Cronkhite, and J. W. Finney. 1982. A conceptual framework for alcoholism treatment evaluation. Pp. 1120-39 in Encyclopedic Handbook of Alcoholism. E.M. Pattison and E. Kaufman, eds. New York: Gardner Press.

Mulford, H. 1979. Treating alcoholism versus accelerating the natural recovery process: A cost-benefit comparison. Journal of Studies on Alcohol 40:505-513.

Mulford, H. 1988. Enhancing the natural control of drinking behavior: Catching up with common sense. Presented at the Conference on Evaluating Treatment Outcomes, University of California, San Diego, Extension Program on Alcohol Issues, February 5.

Nace, E. P. 1987. The Treatment of Alcoholism. New York: Bruner/Mazel.

Nathan, P. E. 1984. Contributions of learning theory to the diagnosis and treatment of alcoholism. Pp. 328-338 in Psychiatry Update. Vol. 3 of the American Psychiatric Association Annual Review, L. Grinspoon, ed. Washington D.C.: American Psychiatric Association.

Nathan, P. E., and B. S. McCrady. 1986/1987. Bases for the use of abstinence as a goal in the treatment of alcohol abusers. Drugs and Society 1(2/3):109-131.

Nathan, P. E., and R. S. Niaura. 1985. Behavioral assessment and treatment of alcoholism. Pp. 391-455 in The Diagnosis and Treatment of Alcoholism, 2d ed., J. H. Mendelson and N. K. Mello, eds. New York: McGraw-Hill.

Nathan, P. E., and J. S. O'Brien. 1971. An experimental analysis of the behavior of alcoholics and nonalcoholics during prolonged problem drinking. Behavior Therapy 2:455-476.

New York Division of Alcoholism and Alcohol Abuse (NYDAAA). 1986. Five Year Comprehensive Plan for Alcoholism Services in New York State 1984-1989: Final 1987 Update. Albany, New York: NYDAAA.

Noble, E. P. 1984. Pharmacotherapy in the detoxification and treatment of alcoholism. Pp. 346-359 in Psychiatry Update. Vol. 3 of the American Psychiatric Association Annual Review, L. Grinspoon, ed. Washington, D.C.: American Psychiatric Association.

Noshpitz, J. D., T. Shapiro, M. Sherman, J. M. Oldham, L. Lazarus, and N. A. Newton. 1984. Milieu therapy. Pp. 619-629 in The Psychiatric Therapies, T. B. Karazu, ed. Washington, D.C.: American Psychiatric Association.

O'Briant, R. G., H. L. Lennard, S. D. Allen, and D. C. Ransom. 1973. Recovery from Alcoholism. Springfield, Ill.: Charles C. Thomas.

Oie, T. P. S., and P. Jackson. 1980. Long-term effects of group and individual social skills training with alcoholics. Addictive Behaviors 5:129-136.

Oie, T. P. S., and P. Jackson. 1982. Social skills and cognitive behavioral approaches to the treatment of problem drinking. Journal of Studies on Alcohol 43:532-547.

Okulitch, P. V., and G. A. Marlatt. 1972. Effects of varied extinction conditions with alcoholics and social drinkers. Journal of Abnormal Psychology 79:205-211.

Orvis, B. R., D. J. Armor, C. E. Williams, A. J. Barras, and D. S. Schwarzbach. 1981. Effectiveness and Cost of Alcohol Rehabilitation in the United States Air Force. Santa Monica, Calif.: RAND Corporation.

Paredes, A., D. Gregory, and O. H. Rundell. 1981. Empirical analysis of the alcoholism services delivery system. Pp. 371-404 in Research Advances in Alcohol and Drug Problems, vol. 6, Y. Israel, F. B. Glaser, H. Kalant, R. E. Popham, W. Schmidt, and R. G. Smart, eds. New York: Plenum Press.

Pattison, E. M. 1974. Rehabilitation of the chronic alcoholic. Pp. 587-658 in Treatment and Rehabilitation of the Chronic Alcoholic. Vol. 3 of The Biology of Alcoholism, B. Kissin and H. Begleiter, eds. New York: Plenum Press.

Pattison, E. M. 1985. The selection of treatment modalities for the alcoholic patient. Pp. 189-294 in J. H. Mendelson and N. K. Mello, eds. The Diagnosis and Treatment of Alcoholism, 2d ed. New York: McGraw-Hill.

Pattison, E. M., M. B. Sobell, and L. C. Sobell. 1977. Emerging Concepts of Alcohol Dependence. New York: Springer Publishing Company.

Pendery, M. L., I. M. Maltzman, and L. J. West. 1982. Controlled drinking by alcoholics? New findings and reevaluation of a major affirmative study. Science 217:169-175.

Pisani, V. 1977. The detoxication of alcoholics—aspects of myth, magic or malpractice. Journal of Studies on Alcohol 38:972-985.

Pittman, D. J. 1974. Role of detoxification centers in alcoholism treatment. Presented at the North American Congress on Alcohol and Drug Problems, San Francisco, December.

Plaut, T. F. A., ed. 1967. Alcohol Problems: A Report to the Nation. New York: Oxford University Press.

Poley, W., G. Lea, and G. Vibe. 1979. Alcoholism: A Treatment Manual. New York: Gardner Press.

Polich, M. J., D. J. Armor, and H. B. Braiker. 1980. The Course of Alcoholism: Four Years After Treatment. Santa Monica, Calif.: The RAND Corporation.

President's Commission on Law Enforcement and Administration of Justice. 1967. The Challenge of Crime in a Free Society, Task Force Report: Drunkenness. Washington, D.C.: U.S. Government Printing Office.

Prochaska, J. O., and C. C. DiClemente. 1982. Transtheoretical therapy: Toward a more integrative model of change. Psychotherapy: Theory and Practice 19:276-278.

Prochaska, J. O., and C. C. DiClemente. 1983. Stages and processes of self-change of smoking: Toward an integrative model of change. Journal of Consulting and Clinical Psychology 51:390-395.

Prochaska, J. O., and C. C. DiClemente. 1986. Toward a comprehensive model of change. Pp. 3-27 in Treating Addictive Behaviors: Processes of Change, W. E. Miller and N. Heather, eds. New York: Plenum Press.

Rankin, H. J., R. Hodgson, and T. Stockwell. 1983. Cue exposure and response prevention with alcoholics: A controlled trial. Behaviour Research and Therapy 21:435-446.

Research Triangle Institute (RTI). 1985. Toward a National Plan to Control Alcohol Abuse and Alcoholism: Draft Report. Prepared for the National Institute on Alcohol Abuse and Alcoholism. Research Triangle Park, N.C.: Research Triangle Institute.

Reynolds, R. I. 1988a. Opening remarks: Evaluating recovery outcomes. Presented at the Conference on Evaluating Recovery Outcome, University of California, San Diego, Extension Program on Alcohol Issues, February 4.

Reynolds, R.I. 1988b. Executive summary: Social model services as an alternative to medical/clinical model services in San Diego county. Prepared for the IOM Committee for the Study of Treatment and Rehabilitation Services for Alcoholism and Alcohol Abuse, February.

Reynolds, R. I., and B. E. Ryan. 1988. Executive summary: Policy implications of social model alcohol recovery services. Prepared for the IOM Committee for the Study of Treatment and Rehabilitation Services for Alcoholism and Alcohol Abuse, July.

Rubington, E.. 1974. The role of the halfway house in the rehabilitation of alcoholics. Pp. 351-383 in Treatment and Rehabilitation of the Chronic Alcoholic. Vol. 5 of The Biology of Alcoholism, B. Kissin and H. Begleiter, eds. New York: Plenum Press.

Sadd, S., and D. W. Young. 1986. A Controlled Study of Detoxification Alternatives for Homeless Alcoholics. New York: Vera Institute of Justice.

Sadd, S., and D. W. Young. 1987. Nonmedical treatment of indigent alcoholics: A review of recent research findings. Alcohol Health and Research World 11:48-49,53.

Sanchez-Craig, M. 1988. Procedures for assessing change after alcoholism treatment. Drugs and Society 2(2):53-67.

Sanchez-Craig, M., and D. A. Wilkinson. 1986/1987. Treating problem drinkers who are not severely dependent on alcohol. Drugs and Society 1(2/3):39-67.

Sanchez-Craig, M., D. A. Wilkinson, and K. Walker. 1987. Theory and methods for secondary prevention of alcohol problems: A cognitively based approach. Pp. 287-331 in Treatment and Prevention of Alcohol Problems: A Resource Manual, W. M. Cox, ed. New York: Academic Press.

Saxe, L., D. Dougherty, K. Esty, and M. Fine. 1983. The Effectiveness and Costs of Alcoholism Treatment. Washington, D.C.: U.S. Congress, Office of Technology Assessment.

Schuckit, M. A. 1985. Treatment of alcoholism in office and outpatient settings. Pp. 295-324 in The Diagnosis and Treatment of Alcoholism, 2d ed., J. H. Mendelson and N. K. Mello, eds. New York: McGraw-Hill.

Sellers, E. M., and C. A. Naranjo. 1985. Strategies for improving the treatment of alcohol withdrawal. Pp. 157-168 in Research Advances in Psychopharmacological Treatments for Alcoholism, C. A. Naranjo and E. M. Sellers, eds. Amsterdam: Excerpta Medica.

Sellers, E. M. 1988. Issues of treatment modalities. Prepared for the "Treatment" meeting of the National Institute on Alcohol Abuse and Alcoholism Ad Hoc Scientific Advisory Board, Rockville, Md., May 3.

Shadle, M., and J. B. Christianson. 1988. The Organization and Delivery of Mental Health, Alcohol, and Other Drug Abuse Services within Health Maintenance Organizations. Final Report. vol. 1. Prepared for the Alcohol, Drug Abuse, and Mental Health Administration. Minneapolis: Interstudy.

Shandler, I. W., and T. E. Shipley. 1987. New focus for an old problem: Philadelphia's response to homelessness. Alcohol Health and Research World 11:54-56.

Skinner, H. A. 1985. Early detection and basic management of alcohol and drug problems. Australian Alcohol/Drug Review 4:243-249.

Skinner, H. A. 1988. Executive summary: Spectrum of drinkers and intervention responses. Prepared for the IOM Committee for the Study of Treatment and Rehabilitation Services for Alcoholism and Alcohol Abuse.

Skinner, H. A., and S. Holt. 1987. The Alcohol Clinical Index: Strategies for Identifying Patients with Alcohol Problems. Toronto: Addiction Research Foundation.

Sobell, M. B., and L. C. Sobell. 1973. Individualized behavior therapy for alcoholics. Behavior Therapy 4:49-72.

Sokolow, L., J. Welte, G. Hynes and J. Lyons. 1980. Treatment-related differences between male and female alcoholics. Journal of Addictions and Health 1.

Steinglass, P. 1979a. An experimental treatment program for alcoholic couples. Journal of Studies on Alcohol 40:159-182.

Steinglass, P. 1979b. Family therapy with alcoholics: A review. Pp. 147-186 in Family Therapy of Drug and Alcohol Abuse, E. Kaufman and P. Kaufman, eds. New York: Gardner Press.

Strauss, A., L. Schatzman, D. Ehrlich, and M. Sabshin. 1964. Psychiatric Ideologies and Institutions. New York: Free Press.

Strupp, H. H. 1978. Psychotherapy research and practice: An overview. Pp. 3-22 in Handbook of Psychotherapy and Behavior Change: An Empirical Analysis. 2d ed., S. Garfield and A. E. Bergin, eds. New York: John Wiley and Sons.

Stuckey, R. F., and J. S. Harrison. 1982. The alcoholism rehabilitation center. Pp. 865-873 in Encyclopedic Handbook of Alcoholism, E. M. Pattison and E. Kaufman, eds. New York: Gardner Press.

Trice, H. M., and J. A. Beyer. 1984. Work related outcomes of the constructive confrontation strategy in a job based alcoholism program. Journal of Studies on Alcohol 45:393-404.

U.S. Department of Health and Human Services (USDHHS). 1981. Fourth Special Report to the U.S. Congress on Alcohol and Health. Rockville, Md.: National Institute on Alcohol Abuse and Alcoholism.

U.S. Department of Health and Human Services (USDHHS). 1986. Toward a National Plan to Combat Alcohol Abuse and Alcoholism. Report submitted to the United States Congress. Rockville, Md.: National Institute on Alcohol Abuse and Alcoholism.

U.S. Department of Health and Human Services (USDHHS). 1987a. 1987 National Drug and Alcoholism Treatment Unit Survey: NDATUS Instruction Manual for States and Reporting Units. Rockville, Md.: National Institute on Drug Abuse and National Institute on Alcohol Abuse and Alcoholism.

U.S. Department of Health and Human Services (USDHHS). 1987. Sixth Special Report to the U.S. Congress on Alcohol and Health. Rockville, Md.: National Institute on Alcohol Abuse and Alcoholism.

U.S. Department of Health, Education, and Welfare (USDHEW). 1971. First Special Report to the U.S. Congress on Alcohol and Health. Rockville, Md.: National Institute on Alcohol Abuse and Alcoholism.

Vaillant, G. E. 1983. The Natural History of Alcoholism: Causes, Patterns, and Paths to Recovery. Cambridge, Mass.: Harvard University Press.

Vannicelli, M. 1978. Impact of aftercare in the treatment of alcoholics: A cross-legged panel analysis. Journal of Studies on Alcohol 39:1875-1886.

Walker, R. D., D. M. Donovan, D. R. Kivlahan, and M. R. O'Leary. 1983. Length of stay, neuropsychological performance, and aftercare: Influences on alcohol treatment outcome. Journal of Consulting and Clinical Psychology 51:900-911.

Wallerstein, R. S. 1956. Comparative study of treatment methods for chronic alcoholism: The alcoholism research project at Winter VA Hospital. American Journal of Psychiatry 113:228-233.

Wallerstein, R. S. 1957. Hospital Treatment of Alcoholism: A Comparative, Experimental Study. New York: Basic Books.

Walsh, D. C., R. W. Hingson, and D. M. Merrigan. 1986. A randomized trial comparing inpatient and outpatient alcoholism treatments in industry—A first report. Presented at the Annual Meeting of the Alcohol Epidemiology Section of the International Council on Alcohol and Addictions, Dubrovnik, Yugoslavia, June.

Weedman, R. D. 1987. Admission, Continued Stay and Discharge Criteria for Alcoholism and Drug Dependence Treatment Services. Irvine, Calif.: National Association of Addiction Treatment Providers.

Weisman, M. N. 1988. Musings on the art of treatment. Alcohol Health and Research World 12:282-287.

Weisner, C., and R. Room. 1984. Financing and ideology in alcohol treatment. Social Problems 32:167-184.

Welte, J., G. Hynes, L. Sokolow, and J. Lyons. 1978. Alcoholism Treatment Effectiveness: An Outcome Study of New York State Operated Rehabilitation Units. Albany N.Y.: Research Institute on Alcoholism.

Whitfield, C. L., G. Thompson, A. Lamb, V. Spencer, M. Pfeifer, and M. Browning-Ferrando. 1978. Detoxification of 1024 patients without psychoactive drugs. Journal of the American Medical Association 239:1409-1410.

Williams, C. N., D. C. Lewis, J. Femino, L. Hall, K. Blackburn-Kilduff, R. Rosen, and C. Samella. 1985. Overcoming barriers to identification and referral of alcoholics in a general hospital setting: one approach. Rhode Island Medical Journal 68:131-138.

Wilson, G. T., R. Leaf, and P. E. Nathan. 1975. The aversive control of excessive drinking by chronic alcoholics in the laboratory. Journal of Applied Behavioral Analysis 8:13-26.

Wilson, G.T. 1987. Chemical aversion conditioning as a treatment for alcoholism: A re-analysis. Behavioral Research and Therapy 25:503-515.

Wright, A. 1985. What is a social model program? Los Angeles County Office of Alcohol Programs, Department of Health Services, Los Angeles, Calif.

Wright, A. 1986. A community model approach to alcohol-related problems. Los Angeles County Office of Alcohol Programs, Department of Health Services, Los Angeles, Calif.

Yahr, H. T. 1988. A national comparison of public- and private-sector alcoholism treatment delivery system characteristics. Journal of Studies on Alcohol 49:233-239.

Zimberg, S. 1974. Evaluation of alcoholism treatment in Harlem. Quarterly Journal of Studies on Alcohol 35:550-557.

Zimberg, S. 1983. Comprehensive model of alcoholism treatment in a general hospital. Bulletin of the New York Academy of Medicine, 59(2):222-229.

Zimberg, S. 1985. Principles of alcoholism psychotherapy. Pp. 3-22 in Practical Approaches to Alcoholism Psychotherapy, S. Zimberg, J. Wallace, and S. B. Blume, eds. New York: Plenum Press.

Zimberg, S., J. Wallace, and S. B. Blume, eds. 1985. Practical Approaches to Alcoholism Psychotherapy. New York: Plenum Press.

Zucker, R. A., and E. S. Lisansky Gomberg. 1986. Etiology of alcoholism reconsidered: The case for a biopsychosocial process. American Psychologist 41:783-793.

Zuska, J. J. 1978. Beginnings of the Navy program. Alcoholism: Clinical and Experimental Research 2:352-357.

4   Who Provides Treatment?

Persons with alcohol problems receive care in a wide variety of health care, social services, educational, corrections, and specialty mental health organizations, as well as in organizations that specialize in treating alcohol and drug problems. Treatment is provided by personnel from a variety of disciplines, including physicians, social workers, counselors, and psychologists. This chapter provides an overview of the various types of providers and personnel that make up the existing treatment services network and reviews the services they provide within the continuum of care.

Describing the System to Treat Persons with Alcohol Problems

In recent years there has been tremendous expansion of both institutional and community-based treatment programs within traditional agencies (e.g., general hospitals, psychiatric hospitals, primary care clinics, family service agencies) and in nontraditional facilities (e.g., social setting detoxification centers, public inebriate shelters, drinking-driver programs, quarterway houses). There has also been a concerted effort to obtain increased acceptance for the treatment of alcohol problems within the mainstream of health care services; yet many of these newer agencies now treating persons with alcohol problems are not located in traditional health care settings. These agencies reflect the historical evolution of the field in this country in that the major impetus for expanded treatment originated with Alcoholics Anonymous and the recovered persons who established pioneering halfway houses (Pattison, 1974, 1977; D. J. Anderson, 1981; Saxe et al., 1983; Weisner and Room, 1984; Weisner, 1986).

There have been a number of efforts to describe the system that has evolved for treating persons with alcohol problems, but the difficulties that surround this task have prevented the formulation of an acceptable, comprehensive classification scheme that fully incorporates the developments of the past 20 years. As discussed in the previous chapter, the states, third-party payers, and key federal agencies use very different labels and definitions for the elements in the continuum of care; one result of this variability is the differing classification schemes used by funders to obtain data from treatment providers to monitor utilization and appropriateness, to evaluate treatment effectiveness, and to develop reimbursement strategies (Bayer, 1980; Wilson and Hartsock, 1981; Bast, 1984; Brown University Center for Alcohol Studies, 1985; Institute for Health and Aging, 1986; McAuliffe et al., 1988).

Confronted with a similar lack of a uniform national and state approach for describing relationships among the various service providers, D. A. Regier and his coworkers (1978) divided what they called the "de facto mental health services system" into three major sectors: general health, other human services, and specialty mental health. Their goal was to provide an initial systematic description of the services provided to persons with behavioral and emotional problems in order to make analysis possible. This framework can also be used to describe the "de facto system" that has developed to treat persons with alcohol problems. Of most interest is Regier's view of the "specialty mental health sector." He and his colleagues defined this sector as including those facilities and practitioners that devoted themselves exclusively to the treatment of psychiatric disorders. The specialty mental health sector included a wide range of facilities that provided inpatient care, outpatient care, or both; these facilities ran the gamut from state and county psychiatric mental hospitals, through halfway houses for the mentally ill, to college campus mental health clinics.

Originally, treatment services for persons with alcohol and other drug problems were considered to be part of the specialty mental health sector. Yet the Regier team in its categorization excluded from the mental health specialty sector all facilities that exclusively treated persons with alcohol problems; they also excluded those other special-purpose facilities that treated drug abusers and the mentally retarded. (However, persons with alcohol problems who were treated in mental health facilities were considered to be part of the specialist sector.) The omission from the specialty mental health services sector of specialty facilities treating only persons with alcohol problems reflected the changes that were taking place in the organization and financing of treatment for mental health, alcohol, and drug problems in the 1970s. In particular, this omission reflects the insistence that alcohol problems were not always a symptom of mental illness but a disease that required "primary treatment" within a specially designed continuum of care (Plaut, 1967; USDHEW, 1971; Grad et al., 1971; D. J. Anderson, 1981; Weisner and Room, 1984). This perspective influenced some of the states (e.g., California) to stop treating persons with alcohol problems in state mental hospitals; however, other states (e.g., New York, Minnesota, Colorado) developed specialty units within their state hospitals (Diesenhaus and Booth, 1977; D. J. Anderson, 1981; Weisner, 1986).

Over the past 20 years, two overlapping yet distinct specialty sectors have emerged: the alcohol problems treatment sector and the drug abuse services system. Each sector appears to have different structural and dynamic qualities that are shaped by ideology and pragmatic survival needs (Weisner and Room, 1984; Cahalan, 1987). If one applies the framework developed by the Regier team (1978), then the specialist alcohol problems treatment sector comprises those facilities and practitioners that treat only persons with alcohol problems. In fact, what has emerged is a distinct network that embraces not only facilities and practitioners but also funding agencies, regulatory agencies, interest and advocacy groups, referral agencies, trade associations, and professional societies linked to the treatment providers in the alcohol problems sector.

In addition to the independent facilities of the specialist alcohol problems sector, provider organizations that belong to each of the other three sectors identified by the Regier team (i.e., general health, other human services, specialty mental health) have also developed specialized programs for treating alcohol problems. Currently, however, more is known about the treatment of alcohol problems in the specialty sector than in these other nonspecialist (i.e., non-alcohol specialty) sectors. *The committee suggests that more accurate descriptions and studies of each of these sectors be developed as a first step toward formulating recommendations for changes in practice and financing.* These sectors are briefly described in the paragraphs below.

Treatment of Alcohol Problems in the Nonspecialist Community Sectors

Following the definitions of Regier and colleagues (1978), the general health care sector comprises all of those facilities and practitioners that offer treatment for alcohol problems within their regular programs or practices. It includes the primary care clinician—whether pediatrician, general practitioner, internist, nurse practitioner, physician's assistant, or family practitioner—who attempts to care for a person who is concerned that she or he may be drinking too much. In this instance, there may be physical problems that bring the person to the attention of the care giver and that become the focus of the treatment, rather than the drinking behavior itself. There is some evidence that the majority of persons seen in this sector are women (Weisner, 1986). The management of the person with alcohol problems may consist of prescribing a minor tranquilizer (e.g., Valium) because the reason given for the excessive drinking is anxiety, brought on by stress at home or at work, or both, and providing supportive counseling. The proportion of patients seen for this type of treatment is unknown.

As discussed in Chapter 9, estimates have been made and studies conducted in various health clinics and other primary health care facilities of the number of persons in treatment who are experiencing alcohol problems. However, these studies vary substantially in the methodologies they use to determine the nature and severity of problems, and they rarely review the treatment that was received. P. D. Cleary and coworkers (1988) reported on a study that evaluated the ability of primary care physicians to identify and address their patients' alcohol problems. Although physicians were aware of the problems in 77 percent of the serious cases and in 36 percent of the less serious cases, they did not routinely address them. The need to improve physician education in identifying and treating alcohol problems is well recognized, and efforts are under way to provide such improvement (see the discussion later in this chapter).

The general health sector also includes the short-term general hospital that has no designated unit for detoxification or rehabilitation. It may be that more persons with alcohol problems may be treated within this sector than are treated in the specialty sector (Harwood et al., 1985; Davis, 1987). Their treatment, however, is likely to be limited to detoxification without rehabilitation or to treatment of the alcohol-related physical problems. The general hospital without a designated detoxification or rehabilitation program nevertheless can develop a screening and intervention program to increase the number of persons with alcohol problems who are identified, counseled, and referred (if necessary) to the appropriate specialist treatment (Lewis and Gordon, 1983; Williams et al., 1985).

The Roger Williams General Hospital in Providence, Rhode Island, initiated such a program, site visited by members of the committee, in which a multidisciplinary consultation team screens all admissions and assesses those that are found to have alcohol or drug problems, or both. The team is able to identify approximately 10 percent of the hospital's admissions as having alcohol or drug problems. The team then intervenes with an assessment of the patient's problems, followed by advice and referral to specialist treatment when indicated. Most of the persons identified by the screening procedures do not have a previous alcohol problem diagnosis but did have a medical or social complication directly related to alcohol intoxication or dependence. More than 80 percent of those referred for further care followed through with their first treatment appointment, usually in an ambulatory clinic (Lewis and Gordon, 1983; Williams et al., 1985). *The committee considers this type of program worthy of replication and rigorous evaluation.* The New York State Division of Alcoholism and Alcohol Abuse is currently providing grants to eleven general hospitals to carry out such screening and interventions (New York State Division of Alcoholism and Alcohol Abuse, 1989a,b). More efforts of this kind are needed.

Investigation of Regier's second sector, "other human services," finds similar activities occurring. This sector embraces social services, correctional facilities and programs, and educational agencies in which efforts are made to work with clients, residents, inmates, students, and others who have problems with alcohol. Many correctional institutions that have no organized program encourage volunteers from Alcoholics Anonymous (AA) to come and work with their inmates, holding AA meetings within the institution and attempting to link those who are released with a formal treatment program or a sponsor, or both. Educational agencies may also provide services. Many school districts have established student assistance programs (SAPs) to work with youth at who are risk for or are already experiencing problems with alcohol and other drugs (G. L. Anderson, 1979; Morehouse, 1984). Some SAPs are linked to a district's health program; others are linked to its school counseling program; still others may be freestanding.

The approaches used by various school districts may vary, but there is a common theme that the treatment of alcohol problems is secondary to the agency's main educational mission. Thus, the focus of most SAPs is identification and referral. The treatment offered is most likely to be a brief intervention (e.g., rap groups, peer helper programs, education) provided by guidance counselors, school psychologists, social workers, and, increasingly, specialist substance abuse counselors (USDHHS, 1987b). Students who experience low or moderate levels of alcohol problems are treated within the educational sector; those who are identified as having more severe problems are referred to the alcohol problems specialist sector, often through the juvenile justice system. The extent of the services offered through SAPs is largely unknown, and for the most part, these programs have not been rigorously evaluated.

The specialty mental health care sector, Regier's third category, includes those mental health practitioners and facilities that offer treatment for alcohol problems within their regular programs or practices. The sector includes the psychiatrist, psychologist, psychiatric social worker, psychiatric nurse, and marriage and family counselor who attempts to treat a person who has been referred either for a drinking problem or for another psychiatric problem. In some instances there may be independent comorbid problems; in others, one difficulty may have contributed to the other. Treatment is likely to consist of prescribing an antidepressant, antianxiety, or antipsychotic drug and providing supportive or insight oriented psychotherapy. As discussed in Chapter 3, the vehicle for providing such psychotherapy (individual, group, or family) may vary with the therapist's discipline and ideology.

This sector also comprises the public or private psychiatric hospital that has no designated unit for withdrawal or rehabilitation but that admits persons with dual psychiatric and alcohol problems or persons with alcohol problems only to a general psychiatry ward. In addition, the specialty mental health care sector includes those community mental health centers, psychiatric outpatient clinics, and sheltered workshops that have no designated units but that do not exclude persons with alcohol problems. The extent of the services provided to persons with alcohol problems in this sector is largely unknown.

Treatment in the Specialist Alcohol Problems Sector

This sector includes those facilities, those units within larger facilities, and those private practitioners that concentrate solely on the treatment of alcohol problems and that provide organized programs of care for persons who require any or all of the treatment stages identified in Chapter 3. The term *facility* is used rather than *hospital* because many treatment services are now offered in settings that are not organized or licensed as general or specialty hospitals or as other health care agencies (e.g., neighborhood health clinics). Some of these facilities are freestanding residential programs, outpatient clinics, and day programs that may be licensed by the state alcoholism authority or by the state social services agency rather than by the state health facilities licensing agency. There is no national standard for making these differentiations, a situation typical in other health care areas as well. Rather, facility and program licensure is seen as a state regulatory function.

The specialist sector can be broken down further according to attributes that affect organization and service delivery. The first grouping is those practitioners and organizations that treat only persons with alcohol problems; the second is those organizations and practitioners that have a specialty unit with a structured program which is embedded within a larger organization or practice. Examples of components that constitute the first grouping are the halfway house that admits only men who have completed a hospital or residential primary rehabilitation program and who are determined to be in need of continued support in a residential setting (i.e., extended care); the outpatient clinic that provides alcohol education and intervention services to persons convicted of a drinking-related traffic offense; and a 58-bed specialty hospital that provides primary rehabilitation to persons who have been detoxified and medically stabilized in a general hospital.   Examples of the second grouping are the 250-bed not-for-profit community hospital that has a discrete 20-bed alcohol rehabilitation unit managed by a national for-profit firm; the 100-bed private psychiatric hospital that has one 30-bed ward offering a rehabilitation program and a second 30-bed unit offering a program dedicated to the treatment of dual-diagnosis patients (i.e., those with coexisting psychiatric syndromes); and the minimum security correctional institution that offers a three-week primary rehabilitation day program for inmates that continue to reside in their cells or dormitories.

Another categorization of the specialist sector that can be made is to group practitioners and programs that treat only persons with alcohol problems and practitioners and programs that treat persons with alcohol or other drug problems. In recent years, the number of such combined programs has been increasing (Reed and Sanchez, 1986; NIDA/NIAAA, 1989). Recent national surveys of treatment facilities have found that most persons are now being seen in combined alcohol and drug units, although this percentage varies by setting and by state.   Many states now have an overwhelming majority of combined units reporting data on service delivery (e.g., Pennsylvania, Louisiana, Michigan). Only a few states have a greater number of alcoholism-only units reporting (e.g., New York, New Jersey, Rhode Island) (Butynski et al., 1987). What is clear is that there has been a definite increase in the number of combined programs and that many units that formerly admitted only persons with alcohol problems now also admit drug abusers. What, if any, impact this change has on treatment availability and accessibility for persons with alcohol rather than drug problems remains to be determined.

The specialist sector can also be subdivided according to the type of population that a given group of providers serves. The populations seen in different facilities may differ on important sociodemographic and clinical variables (e.g., Kissin, 1977b; Kissin and Hansen, 1985; Research Triangle Institute, 1985; Weisner, 1986).   An early study by Pattison and colleagues (1978), which has been replicated a number of times, compared the population characteristics at four different facilities: (1) an aversion conditioning medical model hospital program, (2) a mental health outpatient clinic, (3) a social model halfway house, and (4) a county police work rehabilitation center. The persons served in each of the facilities were found to differ along a continuum of social competence; those treated at the aversion conditioning hospital were the most socially competent and stable and required fewer additional supportive services to achieve and maintain a positive treatment outcome; those served in the police work rehabilitation program were the least socially competent and stable and required many additional supportive services to achieve and maintain a positive outcome. Some of the differences observed among the populations in different facilities appeared to be caused by ideological considerations; others, by funding source policies; and still others, by community pressures. Research on the relationship of treatment ideology and organization to outcome is sorely lacking (e.g., Gilbert and Cervantes, 1986, 1988; National Council on Alcoholism, 1987; Wallen, 1988). *These earlier studies should be expanded and extended; the evolution of the specialist and nonspecialist alcohol problems treatment sectors should be monitored to ensure that the various special populations that might use these services are not excluded from obtaining the resources they require* (see Section IV).

A number of other researchers have contributed to the discussion surrounding specialist and nonspecialist sector treatment settings. Saxe and colleagues (1983) developed an overview of treatment settings as part of their review of the cost-effectiveness of treatment for alcohol problems. This effort was an important first step toward developing a taxonomy that can be used to match persons with alcohol problems with the appropriate type of care at each stage of recovery. The Saxe team described four types of settings: inpatient, outpatient, intermediate, and other. The discussion below uses the Saxe taxonomy to describe treatment settings found in the specialist alcohol problems treatment sector.

Inpatient Treatment Settings The inpatient setting in Saxe's taxonomy was further divided into hospital and freestanding residential categories. Three types of hospital settings were identified: general, psychiatric, and aversive conditioning. The general hospital category was subdivided even further by the type of unit—detoxification or rehabilitation. (The type of unit here corresponds to treatment stage as described in Chapter 3.) However, Saxe and his coworkers did not specify types of units for the other inpatient settings or for outpatient settings, a gap in their framework that should be addressed because setting and stage of treatment are not necessarily linked.

An additional hospital category is the alcoholism or chemical dependency hospital, which includes the aversion hospital noted by the Saxe team; 58 such hospitals were identified in a recent American Hospital Association (1987) survey. The survey also identified 874 general and other special hospitals that claimed distinct treatment units (15 percent of the total federal and nonfederal hospitals reporting) and 165 psychiatric hospitals with separate units (31 percent of those reporting). The largest number of hospital units were in California and Texas, although the states with the highest rates of beds per capita were New Hampshire and North Dakota (see Chapter 7).

Freestanding residential rehabilitation facilities, the second major type of inpatient setting described by the Saxe team, may carry out rehabilitation only, detoxification only, or a combination of both. Freestanding alcohol rehabilitation facilities vary in their relationship to hospitals as described in the NIAAA-sponsored classification discussed in Chapter 3 (Bast, 1984). They can be a wholly owned unit located offsite or in a separate building on the sponsoring general hospital's grounds. For example, California's Betty Ford Center is housed in a separate building on the grounds of the sponsoring community hospital; it is licensed as a specialty chemical dependency rehabilitation hospital, a category unique to California (J. Schwarzlose, Betty Ford Center, personal communication, December 18, 1987). Freestanding rehabilitation facilities can also be independently owned and maintain an agreement for backup by a hospital for detoxification and the treatment of acute medical problems. The rehabilitation center can carry out detoxification in a separate designated unit or as part of the rehabilitation unit.

Many of the states fund or operate freestanding detoxification centers that were initially developed to replace the jails in which public inebriates were placed to sober up (DenHartog, 1982; Diesenhaus, 1982; Finn, 1985). These facilities may follow either the medical model or the social model. Referral systems for detoxification vary from community to community as a function of the resources available and the community's level of acceptance of the social model or mixed medical and social model (see Chapter 7). Most communities, however, have two parallel systems, a dichotomy based primarily on whether the available funding sources recognize social model detoxification programs as eligible providers. Such a division also reflects the continued identification of social model centers with public inebriates, the homeless, and indigents (Diesenhaus, 1982; Sadd and Young, 1986).

In addition to their relationship to hospitals, freestanding alcohol detoxification and rehabilitation facilities also vary in their licensing status from state to state; in some states, freestanding facilities can now be licensed as specialty hospitals (e.g., California's chemical dependency rehabilitation hospitals). Some notable freestanding alcohol treatment centers (e.g., Hazelden in Minnesota; see Chapter 3) contain differentiated detoxification and rehabilitation units and in some instances have multiple licenses for their acute care units and their primary care units.

Outpatient Settings In recent years, the hospital-based or freestanding specialist outpatient clinic has become a major locus of treatment for alcohol problems. Outpatient treatment settings include traditional outpatient clinics that offer individual, group, and family therapy and clinics that offer fixed-length day or evening rehabilitation programs. These fixed-length primary care outpatient programs are often based on the traditional Minnesota model inpatient programs. Harrison and Hoffmann (1986) described three such programs as part of a study comparing the effectiveness of inpatient and outpatient primary rehabilitation. Outpatients attended 20 primary treatment sessions in the evening following work. Each session lasted approximately three hours and typically included a lecture and one or two group therapy sessions. Family participation varied somewhat, ranging from nightly participation in the program to one night per week involvement in family groups and other activities. "Aftercare" followed the completion of the primary care phase of treatment and consisted of weekly sessions for patients and "significant others" at the programs along with referral to Alcoholics Anonymous. The three programs differed in the amount of formal aftercare provided; one provided up to six months; another, a minimum of six weeks; and the third, a minimum of eight weeks.

Intermediate Settings The day treatment or intermediate setting noted by the Saxe team in its taxonomy has not been given sufficient attention by funders despite studies that have shown it can be used effectively at each stage of treatment (Lebenluft and Lebenluft, 1988). As a result, there is no standard definition of day treatment, although it has been differentiated from standard outpatient treatment. In general, day treatment has been suggested as an alternate setting for primary rehabilitation, although there have been instances in which its use has also been advocated for detoxification, extended care, and relapse prevention (e.g., Kolodner, 1977; McLachlan and Stein, 1982). In day treatment, persons with alcohol problems participate in a structured program for most of the working day (usually a minimum of four hours for a minimum of three days a week) for a set number of weeks. This schedule contrasts with those of most outpatient programs, in which the person generally attends one or two sessions a week for an open-ended period of time.

It is not known how many day treatment programs are currently in existence across the country. One reason for the paucity of information is that the day hospital category has been included in the outpatient category in the most recent National Drug and Alcohol Treatment Unit Survey (NDATUS; see the discussion later in this chapter) (USDHHS, 1987a). An earlier study by Frankel (1983) reported on a survey of 14 day treatment programs that were identified using the definition contained in the 1980 NDATUS (NIAAA, 1981). The programs Frankel reviewed were selected from the 156 day care programs identified in that survey and tended to fit the psychiatric variant of the medical model (i.e., have a psychological orientation and use psychotropic medications in treatment); indeed, 11 of the 14 programs used DSM-III concepts and criteria (see Chapter 2) for setting admission standards. The use of DSM-III diagnoses may have been related to the programs' apparent focus on employed adults with health insurance. (Many publicly funded social model specialty treatment programs that receive categorical state and block grant funds through the state alcoholism agency do not use DSM-III or ICD-9 diagnoses [Lawrence Johnson and Associates, Inc., 1983; Lewin/ICF, 1988a,b]). This informal survey revealed a great deal of program variation in program duration, which ranged from 11 days to 18 months. Shorter programs included an aftercare outpatient component; the specifics of the various aftercare programs were not reviewed by Frankel.

All 14 programs used a structured program schedule that included alcohol education through films and discussions, as well as individual, group, and family counseling. All of the programs also required or expected participation in Alcoholics Anonymous. The other components of the programs varied significantly, ranging from a highly behaviorally oriented program to more traditional Minnesota model primary care approaches. A number of the programs met at night in four-hour sessions so that the person in treatment could continue working during the day.

Several of the programs reviewed by Frankel were day treatment programs that were sponsored or operated by employee assistance programs (see the discussion under "Other Treatment Settings" later in this chapter). One such effort was the United Technologies Employee Assistance Program, which developed and operated its own day treatment program as an alternative to costly hospital-based primary rehabilitation programs and what it considered to be ineffective, one-session-per-week outpatient programs (Bensinger and Pilkington, 1983; Frankel, 1983). The program ran 5-1/2 days per week, offering an intensive course of seminars, psychotherapy, and AA meetings at the treatment facility (two per week) to selected employees who were identified and referred by EAP counselors as individuals whose needs were appropriate for this level of rehabilitation care. Two days per week in the program were designated as family days; significant family members were encouraged to participate, and a weekly Al-Anon meeting was held at the treatment facility. Clients and spouses were expected to attend additional outside AA or Al-Anon meetings while in the program and to continue in an AA group once they had been discharged. The planned "stay" was two weeks, but it could be shortened or lengthened according to individual needs. For those needing detoxification and medical treatment, coordinated services were available at an affiliated detoxification unit in a nearby general hospital. Aftercare consisted of work site meetings with the EAP counselor as well as participation in AA groups.

One of the great attractions of the day treatment concept, both for persons with alcohol problems and, indeed, for any psychiatric and medical patients, is its lower cost compared with inpatient treatment (whether in a hospital or in another residential setting). Day treatment or day care has also been proposed as an alternative to long-term care in a skilled or intermediate-level-care nursing home for the chronically physically and mentally impaired and for the frail elderly. Those who advocate use of the day-care alternative have developed similar formulations of the issues involved, whether the focus is treatment of the person with alcohol problems, or treatment of the physically or mentally ill. Dibello and colleagues (1982) suggested that psychiatric day-care programs, including those that serve people with alcohol problems exclusively, be classified into four major types according to which needs are served: (1) crisis support programs for individuals with acute phase disability who exhibit dramatic and serious symptoms and who require stabilization services to return to their presymptomatic state; (2) growth treatment programs for relatively stabilized persons with residual dysfunction who require habilitation/rehabilitation services to improve their interpersonal and vocational role performances; (3) maintenance-supportive treatment programs for persons with chronic problems who are stabilized and who require long term continuing care and support to prevent deterioration and relapse; and (4) diagnostic programs for persons who require direct observation over a significant period of time to identify problem areas and formulate a treatment plan.

The first three types of programs in the Dibello scheme are similar to the the three major stages or phases (acute intervention, rehabilitation, and maintenance) in the committee's model of the stages of treatment for alcohol problems described in Chapter 3. The fourth type, diagnostic programs, is also included (as a component of the assessment phase, a necessary part of the continuum of care and the committee's treatment stages model). The use of day care as a less expensive alternative to hospital care can be justified for "selected" individuals who need crisis stabilization (acute intervention) and growth treatment (rehabilitation). Day-care programs can also reduce costs by shortening the length of hospital stays when they are used as a transition from hospitalization to independent community living for patients who need maintenance-supportive care (extended care and relapse prevention) in order to avoid relapse.

Some day treatment efforts have been directed toward a particular special population (see Section IV). Zimberg (1974, 1983) described a pilot day-care program targeted to the needs and lifestyle of the "black socioeconomically deprived alcoholic" as part of a comprehensive program offering ambulatory and hospital detoxification, a halfway house, medical treatment, and vocational counseling. However, neither this model nor any of the other day treatment variants described above has been widely disseminated and replicated or evaluated, despite several studies suggesting that, for undifferentiated groups of persons needing treatment for alcohol problems, primary care in an intermediate, or day-care, setting is just as effective as inpatient primary care in a hospital or other type of residential setting.

One such study that became an important basis for policy development was a comparison of inpatient and outpatient treatment carried out on behalf of the Minnesota Chemical Dependency Program Division (Harrison and Hoffmann, 1986). Using a quasi-experimental design (because clinical realities and pragmatic considerations precluded the use of random assignment), this study contrasted four-week inpatient primary care at two facilities with four week-outpatient primary care at three facilities. All five of the programs reflected the Minnesota model of treatment and were organized around the philosophy and 12-step recovery program of Alcoholics Anonymous. They were also homogeneous in methods and intensity. Lectures and group sessions were the primary components of the rehabilitation approach; the AA variant of the disease model of chemical dependency was the source of the educational content of the lectures, films, and discussions. Total abstinence from all mood-altering chemicals was the goal of treatment for all five programs.

Harrison and Hoffmann found that there were no differences in outcome for subjects in the two conditions who were matched for number and severity of their alcohol-related symptoms and impairments. Despite some limitations as a result of sampling restrictions, the study's findings were an important contribution to the policy changes adopted by the Minnesota legislature in creating its consolidated funding strategy. This approach, which is discussed in Chapters 18 and 20, uses a single method to match persons to the appropriate level of care for treatment paid for with state-administered funds.

Similarly, Longabaugh and colleagues (1980, 1983) reported on the results of a study in which persons undergoing detoxification were randomly assigned to an inpatient or an equivalent partial hospitalization primary rehabilitation experience. Day hospital patients lived at home and commuted daily to the hospital to attend its Problem Drinker Program (PDP) (McCrady et al., 1985). Inpatients resided in one of the hospital's patient care units and walked to the same program; inpatients also participated in other activities in the unit's therapeutic program. The study found that persons treated in the partial hospitalization program functioned as well or better than their inpatient counterparts on all critical measures of treatment outcome.

The committee visited the program and found the PDP to be a highly structured, behaviorally oriented approach that uses the principles of social learning as its underlying theoretical basis. Like the majority of behavior therapy variants of the psychological model, the PDP begins with a thorough assessment of the behavioral patterns associated with drinking and with a functional analysis of the person's urges to drink and his or her drinking episodes (i.e., behavioral chains). The program uses group sessions to teach patients how to carry out the functional analysis and to set specific goals for behavioral change. Educational sessions and materials deal with the negative consequences of unwise alcohol consumption and common behavioral patterns that are associated with excessive drinking. Volunteers who have overcome serious drinking problems serve as role models, modeling specific behaviors that are designed to reduce drinking. Planned activities, contingency contracting, and social skills training offer practice in carrying out alternative behaviors. Married patients participate in couples groups; in addition, a relatives workshop focuses on reinforcing positive behavior, decreasing family protection of the patient's drinking, and coping with relapses. When appropriate, meetings are held with employers to establish specific contingencies (in terms of work consequences) that will result from drinking and non-drinking behavior.

The PDP is an ongoing program that receives reimbursement from most insurers but that has not been extensively replicated elsewhere despite its demonstration of potential cost savings (McCrady et al., 1986). The committee sees an expansion of intermediate care programs such as the PDP as an important element in increasing treatment availability. Efforts to replicate such programs are indicated but appear to require additional resources, as well as, a series of clinical trials with various populations and unit locations, to persuade practitioners and funders of their unique value. The combination of primary care, and extended care when needed, and maintenance in the same program seems to be related to successful outcome as shown in a number of studies and suggested by several researchers; however, translation to clinical practice may require additional clinical trials as well as modification of current financing mechanisms (McCrady et al., 1986).

Often, halfway houses are also considered to be intermediate care settings. They have most frequently been described as transitional residential living facilities for persons who have completed primary treatment but require additional support and treatment to maintain their initial gains (e.g., Rubington, 1974; Berman and Klein, 1977; Armor et al., 1978; Orford and Velleman, 1982; Pattison, 1985). In this sense, they tend to be used as extended care for less socially competent persons who require additional support to achieve and maintain a positive outcome. Confusion is created, however, because the same label had been applied to facilities that also offer primary care services and to extended care and maintenance services. New terms have been introduced to differentiate among the various services offered by these facilities (e.g., quarterway homes, domiciliaries, alcohol-residences, recovery homes).

Thus, there is no uniform definition among the states of the halfway house and the services it offers. Some states view it solely as a setting that provides a supportive, alcohol-free living environment; any ongoing formal treatment (extended care or maintenance) must be delivered elsewhere. Other states require that halfway houses be professionally staffed and provide formal treatment. Private and public health insurers tend not to recognize halfway houses or recovery homes (the term used primarily in California) as eligible providers, and they frequently do not provide coverage for primary care, transitional care, extended care, and maintenance activities provided by these facilities (see Chapter 18). Again, studies are needed of the service profiles and outcomes associated with different paths through the alcohol problems treatment system that will determine the appropriate role of such facilities and the propriety of coverage for their activities.

Other Treatment Settings The committee has chosen to discuss under this rubric several areas of treatment provision that cannot appropriately be subsumed under the earlier treatment setting categories (although these areas may include elements or components that characterize those settings). The treatment programs to be discussed include those operated by the Salvation Army; self-help groups—in particular, Alcoholics Anonymous; drinking driver programs; and employee assistance programs.

The treatment programs operated by the Salvation Army are one such example of the complex residential treatment services that have evolved to provide a continuum of care within one facility (Stoil, 1988). Originally thought of as halfway houses, these programs are a mixture of the social and medical models, although the Salvation Army tends to see itself more as a social service sector agency with a medical unit than as a specialty alcohol problems treatment sector agency. Its programs provide social support, vocational rehabilitation, and medical services, along with primary treatment, to those persons with alcohol problems who are seen as among the least socially competent and stable and who have the poorest prognosis. It is estimated that the Salvation Army treats more than 70,000 persons each year. Its Harbor Lights or Social Rehabilitation programs serve primarily men (often skid row residents or homeless persons) who have few personal or economic resources and for whom treatment must include additional supportive services. Salvation Army programs place a strong emphasis on vocational training and spiritual counseling and are still often viewed as halfway houses because of their target population and their emphasis on job placement and retention occurs concurrently with attempts to modify drinking behavior through various modalities (e.g., AA meetings, monitored Antabuse, alcohol education, group counseling). They typically offer a longer term intervention that comprises an initial primary care phase and an extended care program.

Self-help groups Self-help groups, primarily Alcoholics Anonymous (AA), Al-Anon, and Alateen, are a significant segment of the specialist sector. There are also several newer groups, such as Women for Sobriety and Drink Watchers (see Appendix C), that offer an alternative ideology and model of recovery. Although these groups are used by some persons, but do not yet have the acceptance or the worldwide distribution currently enjoyed by AA (J. Kirkpatrick, Women for Sobriety, personal communication, December 14, 1987).

AA was founded in 1935 by Bill W., a New York stockbroker, and Dr. Bob, an Akron surgeon, who met at Bill W.'s initiative to discuss their problems in abstaining from drinking alcoholic beverages (Alcoholics Anonymous World Services, Inc., 1955, 1959). (Consistent with AA's tradition of anonymity, the literature does not use last names, although Bill W. had participated quite publicly in the expansion of research, teaching efforts, and treatment services. He testified before Congress in 1970 at the hearings held by Senator Hughes regarding the need to develop a cohesive national policy and to establish the National Institute on Alcohol Abuse and Alcoholism.) Al-Anon is a network of similar self-help groups for the spouses of persons with alcohol problems; Alateen serves the same function for their children (Ablon, 1982; Al-Anon, 1986; Cermak, 1989).

AA has grown to be a worldwide organization while still maintaining its basic structure and traditions (Leach and Norris, 1977; Kurtz, 1979; Alibrandi, 1982; Rudy, 1986). Indeed, the use of AA principles and techniques has become an integral part of the majority of treatment programs in this country (Boscarino, 1980; Bradley, 1988). AA is the best-known alcohol problems treatment resource, and most laypersons consider it to be the most useful (Robinson and Henry, 1979).

Belonging to AA demands participation in a program of recovery, called by the organization "working the twelve steps." The twelve steps are guides to the process of personal change that is required to achieve sobriety. A program of recovery includes (a) participating in meetings in which members share the history of their problems caused by drinking and their experiences in maintaining sobriety; (b) obtaining help and support from other members in meeting the challenges that in the past have led to "slips" and a return to drinking; and (c) finding an AA member who will serve as a sponsor and provide guidance and help in times of crisis when the urge to return to drinking becomes overwhelming. Members typically attend at least one meeting a week; new members are encouraged to attend daily meetings ("ninety meetings in 90 days"). The AA program of recovery and its philosophy are described in a number of publications that are studied by all members. The fundamental text is the book *Alcoholics Anonymous,* published by AA's General Services Office (Jackson, 1988).

From AA's inception, its members have viewed their problems with alcohol as "alcoholism"—an illness that prevents those afflicted with it from controlling their drinking. In the organization's view "recovery" requires self-diagnosis and acceptance of the inability to control drinking and its inevitable consequences; therefore, according to AA, recovery requires abstinence.

The individual AA group and the meetings it holds are of central importance to the organization's functioning. Meetings have a common structure: one member is elected as chair for the meeting, and one or two members tell their stories—an account of their personal history, the development of drinking problems, the sufferings experienced and inflicted on others, the deceptions and lies, and finally "hitting bottom" and beginning to turn around. A description of their introduction to AA and the process of recovery within the "fellowship," with practical hints on "working the steps," completes the presentations. Although structured, the meetings are informal and friendly; the focus is on the sharing and common recognition of the problems that are faced by all who attend and participate in the discussion. Reference is frequently made to the 12 steps and to the meaning a given step has for a member and the effort that was required to achieve that step.

In addition to meetings there may be study groups and social gatherings held informally or at a central meeting place. At such events, AA literature will be discussed and passed around. As they develop, local groups become recognized and listed in the directories published by the local or central AA service office. Often, groups work together to form a local central office or intergroup association; there, volunteers will answer phone requests for information and serve on committees. There are also area and national conventions at which members meet to discuss the organization and "to continue to carry on the traditions of the fellowship."

The more experienced AA members engage in "twelfth-stepping"—serving as sponsors and working with new members to engage them in the recovery process. More experienced AA members may also serve on institution committees that arrange for meetings to be held in treatment facilities, make AA literature available to persons in treatment there, and arrange sponsorship for those in treatment. The members may volunteer to conduct the meetings at the institutions and to run orientation and study sessions.

In 1987, AA membership was estimated to be more than 1.5 million persons in more than 73,000 groups worldwide (Trice and Staudemeier, 1989). Membership in the United States and Canada was estimated by the AA General Services Conference to be about 800,000 affiliates. In the United States the largest numbers of members are to be found in California (18 percent of active members), New York (6 percent of active members), Illinois (5 percent), and Texas and Minnesota (4 percent each) (Jackson, 1988). The AA General Services Office conducts a survey of a sample of its membership every three years (Alcoholics Anonymous World Services, Inc., 1987). The most recent survey of 7,000 U.S. and Canadian affiliates was conducted in 1986. The survey found that men constituted the majority of members (66 percent), although the percentage of women had continued to increase from 30 percent in 1980 and 1983 to 34 percent in 1986. The majority of members continued to be in the 31-to-50 age bracket; the trend toward adding younger members, which was noted in earlier surveys, appeared to have leveled off (those in the 30-and-under age range constituted 21 percent in 1986 after an increase from 15 to 20 percent between 1980 and 1983). Sixty percent reported prior counseling. The average member attended four meetings per week. The average length of sobriety for members was 52 months, with 29 percent reporting sobriety for more than five years, 33 percent reporting sobriety for one to five years, and 33 percent reporting sobriety for less than one year.

The upward trend of member drug problems in addition to alcohol problems continued, with an increase from 31 percent in 1983 to 38 percent in 1986. AA does not see itself as serving those with only or primarily drug problems. To assist those persons, AA has offered assistance to other self-help groups modeled after AA that target persons with drug problems (Alcoholics Anonymous World Services, Inc., 1988).

AA can function in a number of ways for a person experiencing alcohol problems: as the main resource used for recovery, as part of a formal treatment plan, or as an aid in sustaining the recovery achieved through formal treatment (Diesenhaus, 1982; Hoffmann et al., 1987; USDHHS, 1987; Bradley, 1988; Anderson and Gilbert, 1989). A large number of persons with alcohol problems recover using AA alone or in conjunction with professional treatment, although the precise number of such individuals is not known with certainty (USDHHS, 1987). There is evidence that continuing attendance at AA meetings is positively correlated with the maintenance of abstinence, although it is not clear whether it is the attendance itself or the motivational factors leading to continued attendance that are the determining factors (Emrick, 1987).

Although AA does not view itself as a treatment modality (e.g., Jackson, 1988), it has been viewed as such for evaluation and planning purposes because of the prominent role it plays in the design and implementation of treatment programs in this country. There are two discrete elements to this role. The first aspect is the formal relationships that exist between the intergroup or local AA committees and treatment facilities or other institutions (e.g., prisons, jails). Procedures have been developed that allow AA volunteers who are doing "twelfth-step" work to serve on the institutional committees that arrange for meetings and sponsors. Experienced AA members may also visit the facility regularly to run an open meeting, develop and support an institutional group that is listed with the AA General Services Office, or meet potential affiliates seeking sponsors (Alcoholics Anonymous World Services, Inc., 1961, 1979). Continuation in AA after discharge from the institution is stressed; AA serves as the major aftercare mechanism for many primary treatment programs.

The second aspect of the AA role is the use of its philosophy, methods, and materials by professional and recovered staff in carrying out formal treatment programs (Laundergan, 1982; Nace, 1987; Weisner and Room, 1984; Bradley, 1988; Gallant, 1988). Many programs blend professional diagnostic and treatment activities with the 12-step AA recovery program, and there is strong emphasis on the use of "recovering alcoholics" as primary counselors to guide the person in treatment through a multidisciplinary program. For example, many treatment programs center their education and counseling around AA-approved publications, in particular, the "Big Book," requiring that it be read and discussed in group sessions. Many programs also use workbooks (e.g, the Hazelden Foundation's "Guide to the Fourth Step Inventory" and other similar publications) to guide the "stepwork" carried out in group and individual sessions. Treatment programs often hold AA orientation sessions and meetings at the treatment facility, which persons in treatment are encouraged or required to attend. Persons in treatment are also encouraged to find an AA sponsor prior to discharge, and continued involvement in AA is a major component of many facilities' aftercare planning. Programs that adhere to the Minnesota model often establish criteria for the completion of a treatment stage in terms of stepwork (e.g., discharge from primary rehabilitation in concert with taking the AA "Fifth Step" [Laundergan, 1982]).

AA as an organization does not consider itself to be a formal treatment program, but there are many individuals who use only AA, initially or after a relapse or slip, to recover. Affiliating with AA involves the same stages of treatment as a formal treatment program. Each stage can be carried out in either type of program, with movement back and forth, or conjointly, following the orientation of the Minnesota model and the California social model programs. Subacute detoxification can be and often is carried out at home with support, encouragement, and monitoring of physical status by other AA members. Primary rehabilitation coincides with "working the steps," just as in formal programs with an AA orientation. Continuing to attend meetings and working the program with a sponsor's guidance are equivalent to formal extended care and maintenance or relapse prevention. A person may use various techniques for relapse prevention. Increasing the number of meetings he or she attends, increasing study of the "Big Book" and other AA materials, and seeking more direct support from a sponsor and other AA members. Lifelong maintenance, or aftercare, is available by continuing to attend meetings, doing "twelfth-step" work, and volunteering for group and intergroup responsibilities. This reformulation of the AA program of recovery in the terms of the committee's classifying scheme does not attempt, as others have done (e.g. Khantzian and Mack, 1989), to analyze and explain how AA functions (based on a psychological or sociocultural theory). Rather, the committee wishes to present AA within the same framework as formal treatment to suggest the possibility of studying who can and should be matched with the AA program, either as the person's sole treatment modality or in conjunction with other treatments.

AA is considered by many lay persons and professionals to be the most successful treatment for persons with alcohol problems (Bradley, 1988), despite the lack of well-designed and well-executed studies that can be cited to support or negate the validity of this perception (Ogborne and Glaser, 1981; Glaser and Ogborne, 1982; Emrick, 1989b; Ogborne, 1989; Trice and Staudemier, 1989). Research has shown that not all who are introduced to AA, either as a component of a formal treatment program or as an alternative to formal treatment, affiliate with the organization and that not all who affiliate, benefit (Emrick, 1989a,b; Ogborne, 1989; Trice and Staudemier, 1989). It has been estimated that only 20 percent of persons with alcohol problems who are referred to AA ever attend meetings regularly. Additional research is needed to determine the characteristics of those who will affiliate and benefit so that matching criteria can be developed. Guidelines for such research have been suggested by Ogborne and Glaser (1981).

Like AA, drinking-driver (DWI) programs and employee assistance programs (EAPs) represent significant forces in the development and structuring of the specialist alcohol problems treatment sector (Weisner and Room, 1984). Although these programs are primarily thought of as referral and intervention programs, they can be said to provide treatment services as the committee defined treatment for alcohol problems in Chapter 3.

Drinking-driver programs Although the name may differ from state to state, DWI programs are specialty referral and treatment programs for drinking-and-driving offenders. In each state a network of specialized programs provides intervention and treatment services to persons who have been arrested for or convicted of an alcohol-related traffic offense. These programs now include a differentiation into first-offender and multiple-offender programs (California State Department of Alcohol and Drug Programs, 1988; McCarthy and Argeriou, 1988). Most admissions to such treatment are referred by the courts, either through a diversion program or as part of a sentencing arrangement, and these specialty programs must meet specific standards to qualify for receiving court referrals. The licensing arrangements vary from state to state and often involve the state alcoholism authority as well as agencies involved in public safety, highway safety, or the court and corrections (probation) systems. DWI programs are considered by some to be more a part of the corrections sector than the alcohol problems treatment sector (Weisner, 1986); these programs are discussed in more detail in Chapter 16 and Appendix D.

Employee assistance programs Employee assistance programs, or EAPs, are included in the specialty sector although they no longer deal exclusively with alcohol problems. Instead, most such programs have adopted a "broad-brush" philosophy that encompasses other personal problems that may be affecting job performance (Roman, 1981). Today, EAPs can be thought of as agencies that provide identification, intervention, diagnostic services, referral, and follow-up services to persons at their place of employment. In addition, EAPs provide primary prevention services to all employees and consult with supervisors and managers on ways to work with troubled employees. Increasingly, EAPs are also providing short-term outpatient counseling services as primary treatment (Sonnestuhl and Trice, 1986). EAPs may be internal, with services administered and provided by employees of the sponsoring company or government agency, or external, with services provided by an independent contractor.

EAPs generally are not classified as treatment programs but as prevention and intervention programs (USDHHS, 1987b). However, EAPs offer a variety of services, ranging from short-term counseling (intervention, primary rehabilitation) through day care (primary rehabilitation) to worksite aftercare groups (maintenance) (Roman and Blum, 1985; Sonnestuhl and Trice, 1986) and consequently, they are considered by some to be treatment providers. A recent survey of services offered by EAPs found that 74 percent of the 1,238 respondents provided "brief in-program counseling" and 10 percent provided "in-program treatment" (e.g., a "company run residential program") (Backer and O'Hara, 1988). More than 94 percent of the respondents reported that their EAPs also offered crisis intervention services. Although this survey focused on drug abuse services, given the approach used by most EAPs and the history of their development, it can be assumed that at least as many EAPs offer these treatment services for persons with alcohol problems.

EAPs are the outgrowth of the industrial alcoholism movement initiated in the 1940s (Roman, 1981; Trice and Schronbrun, 1981) and were originally established to deal exclusively with persons with alcohol problems. Although there are several historical antecedents to the development of work site programs to detect and refer employees whose job performance is negatively affected by their excess drinking, the explanation cited most often for the successful initiation of programs is the coalition of efforts between industrial physicians and recovered alcoholics who sought to bring AA principles to their coworkers (Roman, 1981; Trice and Schonbrun, 1981; Delaney, 1988). Other contributions included the efforts of the Yale Center for Alcohol Studies during the 1950s, of the National Council on Alcoholism's industrial services' program during the 1960s, and of the private Smither's Foundation. All three organizations obtained information on the programs operating in various companies and diffused that information to other executives and physicians. Joint efforts to develop programs cosponsored by unions and management were strengthened by the interest and involvement of the AFL-CIO community services program and the United Auto Workers.

EAPs have been important contributors to the development of the contemporary specialist alcohol problems treatment sector. When NIAAA was established in 1971, it adopted as one of its major priorities the identification and referral to treatment of employed persons with alcohol problems. Emphasis was placed on early intervention and identification by way of impaired job performance. A major goal during the 1970s was the development of treatment resources, both programmatic and financial, for the employed person with alcohol problems. Corporations and government agencies were encouraged to develop both EAPs and specific health insurance benefits for treating alcohol problems. The availability of third-party funding and referrals from EAPs, which shared the ideology underlying the Minnesota model of treatment, were major determinants of the nationwide spread of programs to treat persons with alcohol problems (Roman, 1982).

A State Perspective on Treatment Providers

Given this complex array of sectors and providers, it is understandable that individuals who are seeking help for their own alcohol problems or for someone they care about may have some difficulty identifying the program or person who would best be able to assist them. Each state and each community have developed their own formal and informal "mapping" of the treatment system and of individual providers, as well as their strengths and weaknesses. Many publish directories to guide persons seeking a referral, whether as a professional, a family member, or a candidate for treatment themselves. To better understand who provides which services and for whom, it is helpful to review the treatment system as described in one of the states, at the same time recognizing that there is some variation in the continuum of care among the states.

As described earlier (see Chapter 3), Minnesota has been considered a leader in the development of treatment services to persons with alcohol problems and uses a formulation of a continuum of care that includes stages and equivalent, alternate settings.

TABLE 4-1 Overview of the Current Continuum of Care for Minnesota Residents

Prevention/Intervention Services	Treatment Services
Prevention and education programs	Primary residential treatment programs
Information, diagonstic, and referral programs	Freestanding facilities
County social services agencies	Hospital-based Facilities
Mental health centers	State regional treatment centers
Other information and referral programs	Intermediate/Extended residential treatment
Self-help programs	programs
Employee assistance programs (EAPs)	Halfway houses
Driving while intoxicated clinics	Extended care facilities
Detoxification centers	Board and lodging facilities
	Nonresidential treatment programs
	Freestanding facilities
	Hospital-based facilities

SOURCE: *Directory of Chemical Dependency Programs* (Minnesota Chemical Dependency Program Division, 1987).

Several of the models reviewed in Chapter 3, including the model used as the basis for recommendations in the recent national plan (USDHHS, 1986), were derived from the Minnesota continuum of care. Because the committee has used developments in Minnesota elsewhere in the report as examples of trends, it seems consistent to use a description of the different kinds of programs available in Minnesota to portray the variety of treatment providers available across the country.

The programs listed are drawn from each of the general and specialist sectors discussed in the first part of this chapter and illustrate the increasing diversity in programs and funding sources that must be captured in national surveys if the evolving "de facto alcohol problems treatment system" is to be understood. Table 4-1 provides an overview of the current continuum of care available to Minnesota residents.

Each of the categories of intervention and treatment programs described in the directory are discussed below; the program descriptions are summaries of those in the directory.

> Information, diagnostic, and referral programs—These programs provide
> assessments of chemical use related problems for individuals, families, and
> concerned persons and refer them for appropriate treatment services.

There are 196 information, diagnostic, and referral centers listed in the Directory. The majority (86) are operated by county social services agencies; mental health centers operate the next largest group (32). A variety of other agencies (public health departments, family and human services agencies, alcohol and drug counseling agencies, hospitals, nursing homes, community action agencies, senior citizens programs, community centers, etc.) operate the remainder. Each county social service agency provides these services; some county social service agencies also offer direct treatment services. Many of the mental health centers and other information and referral programs also provide treatment services.

Self-help programs fall under this category and provide a range of services from information through aftercare. There are 11 self-help program offices listed in the Minnesota directory, including 2 AA intergroup offices; the others include Al-Anon,

Women for Sobriety, Narcotics Anonymous, and the Indian Health Board. The directory notes that there is no charge for the services of these groups.

The directory describes EAPs as programs that provide identification, intervention, diagnosis, referral, and, in some instances, direct counseling to persons at their place of employment. The directory notes that EAPs can be internal, operated by the work organization itself, or external, operated by a specialist under contract. Not all known EAPs are included; the directory lists only three of the major EAPs operated by companies or government agencies for their own employees and 15 consulting organizations that offer EAP services to companies and institutions.

> Driving while intoxicated clinics—These programs provide education for those individuals who are arrested, convicted, and referred by the court system for alcohol-related traffic offenses in an attempt to motivate the drinking driver to alter his drinking-and-driving behavior.

Minnesota's DWI clinics are specialty programs authorized by the state's Department of Public Safety to provide a defined course of education on the effects of alcohol on driving for individuals referred by the court system as the sentence or a part of the sentence following conviction for an alcohol-related driving offense. The course length must be no less than eight hours and no more than nine hours, usually divided into three or four different class sessions; the state specifies curricula and provides instructional presentation guidelines. DWI clinics are required to be nonprofit and must be part of a sponsoring organization such as a mental health center or a safety organization. They are supported by registration fees paid by the students. The persons served tend to be residents of the county of the court's jurisdiction because as part of the sentence there are geographic restrictions on the distance that can be traveled (no more than 35 miles from the student's residence).

> Detoxification centers—These programs provide subacute detoxification with minimal medical services provided onsite. Three categories of service are provided: (1) health observation during acute intoxication and withdrawal to ensure medically safe detoxification; (2) basic personal care, including provision of meals, clean clothing, and protection of the person and the person's belongings; and (3) assessment of the person's relation to chemicals and of his or her other problems, determination of service needs, and referral to appropriate community resources.

Minnesota decriminalized public intoxication in 1971 and mandated the establishment of detoxification centers by the counties. In 1987 there were a total of 37 freestanding and hospital-based subacute detoxification centers operating across the state, ranging in size from 1 to 88 beds. Typically, these subacute medical model centers have a consulting relationship with a physician, and there is at least one licensed nurse on the staff. Detoxification technicians who are trained onsite provide the majority of direct services. Larger centers have counseling components; smaller centers use counselors from the county chemical dependency program or elsewhere for this purpose. Larger centers usually have nurses on staff for all shifts and a physician who comes into the facility on a regular basis; smaller centers typically have a nurse on duty during the day and one on call for emergencies during off hours. Length of stay varies from 1 to 7 days, although one center offers care for as long as 21 days. The average length of stay is 2 to 4 days.

There are 18 freestanding and 16 hospital-based detoxification centers; there are two detoxification centers that are part of a community mental health center and one located in a correctional facility. Charges range from $80 to $198 per day. One of the six state hospitals (regional centers) also reports offering detoxification. The charge is given as $101 per day. Sources of funding vary among the centers; they include county government, state government, Medicare, Medicaid, private health insurance, client fees, private donations, Title XX (the social services block grant), county social service funds, state Medical Assistance, local government, and public welfare. Other characteristics of the centers surveyed that are noted in the directory are services provided, security (e.g., seclusion room), and patterns of medication use.

> Freestanding primary residential treatment—These programs provide intensive rehabilitative services (medical and psychological therapies) within a highly structured therapeutic living environment. Their efforts are aimed at helping individuals modify their behaviors related to chemical use and to develop the personal and social skills necessary to successfully reenter the community.

Minnesota's 24 licensed, freestanding primary residential treatment programs range in size from 13 to 197 beds. Charges range from $80 to $295 per day. Reported funding sources include fees, private health insurance, county funds, food stamps, state grants-in-aid, Title XX, United Way, the Indian Health Service, private foundations, and individual donors. Eleven programs report that they also provide detoxification services.

Six programs describe their target populations as adolescents who most often range in age from 12 to 18 years; 14 other facilities admit youth (under the age of 18) to their adult programs. There are two programs that report American Indians as their target population. All programs admit both men and women; there is one program that serves adult gay men and lesbian women.

> Hospital-based primary residential treatment programs—These programs provide intensive rehabilitative services (medical and psychological therapies) within a highly structured therapeutic living environment. Like the freestanding facilities, their aim is to help individuals modify those of their behaviors that are related to chemical use and to develop the personal and social skills necessary to successfully reenter the community.

There are 29 hospital-based primary treatment programs in Minnesota ranging in size from 10 to 97 beds. Two of the programs are in Veterans Administration hospitals, and one is in a university hospital. Charges range from $121 to $306 per day. Planned length of stay varies from 14 to 72 days for the 24 programs reporting a fixed-length program. Five programs describe their length of stay as variable or determined by the person's need. Six programs target adolescents and 10 others admit youth under the age of 18. All 29 programs report admitting both men and women.

The regional treatment centers are state hospital-based programs that provide a range of intensive rehabilitative services within a structured living environment. Their aim is to help individuals modify those of their behaviors that are related to chemical use and to develop the personal and social skills necessary to reenter the community successfully. The six state hospitals (regional centers) also report offering primary residential treatment. The charge given is $101 per day. The programs vary in their length of stay, orientation, and profile of services offered. One also offers detoxification, and another offers extended care.

> Halfway houses—These transitional living facilities provide a supportive environment and rehabilitative services for persons who have completed

primary treatment but who are not completely prepared to reenter the community without additional help.

There are 39 halfway houses listed in the 1987-1988 Minnesota *Directory of Chemical Dependency Programs;* 17 programs serve only men, whereas 4 admit only women. The facilities vary in size from 10 to 60 beds. Age limits vary considerably: 3 halfway houses specialize in working with adolescents, 1 specializes in helping young adults, and 17 of the 36 adult facilities also admit youth under the age of 18.

Six halfway houses are targeted at American Indians, and one is targeted at adult black Americans. Six report that they receive contract funding from the Veterans Administration. One of the facilities serves parolees and probationers. There are two facilities that report serving chemically dependent mentally ill individuals (commonly known as "dual-diagnosis patients").

Charges for halfway house stays in Minnesota range from $8 to $70 per day. The sources of funding listed in the directory include food stamps, county funds, the Indian Health Service, state appropriations, private health insurance, Title XX, and general assistance funds.

Extended care facilities—These programs provide long term residential treatment services within a structured living environment to severely chemically dependent individuals who have had prior treatment experiences.

The directory lists 12 extended care facilities. Two programs report that they serve only men, and two admit only women. The facilities vary in size from 10 to 60 beds. Age limits vary considerably with two facilities specializing in work with adolescents; one of the 11 adult facilities also admits youth under the age of 18. One facility is targeted at male veterans, another is targeted at men and women over the age of 55, and another specializes in work with chemically dependent mentally ill individuals.

The charges listed range from $31 to $125 per day. Sources of funding include food stamps, county funds, the Indian Health Service, state appropriations, private health insurance, Title XX, general assistance, client fees, Medicare, Medicaid, private donations, and child welfare funds.

Board and lodging programs—These programs serve the needs of the chronic alcoholic who is essentially homeless and indigent and has failed to maintain sobriety despite prior treatment; the purpose of the program is to provide humane care, basically food and shelter, within a warm safe environment that involves some personal responsibility and communal activities with the intent of improving the individual both physically and socially.

There are 20 board and lodging facilities listed in the Minnesota directory. (In the stage model of treatment suggested by the committee, these would be considered as maintenance facilities.) The facilities vary in size from 8 to 200 beds (at a Salvation Army adult rehabilitation center). The length of stay varies, with 10 facilities having no restrictions; others set limits of six months to one year. Admission requirements also vary. considerably, with four facilities specializing in working with men and two with older adults; one facility is located within a nursing home.

The charges listed range from no fee (a Salvation Army program) to $600 per month. Sources of funding include Supplemental Security Income, (SSI), United Way, county funds, the Veterans Administration, state appropriations, private health insurance, Title XX, Medicare, Medicaid, client fees, private donations, and general assistance.

Freestanding nonresidential treatment programs—These programs provide a range of rehabilitative services to less severely dependent individuals who are able to modify those of their behaviors that relate to chemical use while still functioning in the community.

There are 105 freestanding nonresidential treatment programs offering a wide range of programs: fixed-length, structured primary and extended care rehabilitation programs at a fixed cost ranging from $275 to $3,500, as well as more traditional outpatient psychotherapy with weekly sessions for a fixed or variable length of stay. The charges per session in this category range from $25 to $75. Funding sources vary considerably but include all those available to the residential programs.

Hospital-based nonresidential programs—These programs provide a range of intensive rehabilitative services to less severely dependent individuals who are able to modify those of their behaviors that relate to chemical use while they continue to function in the community.

There are 55 hospital-based, nonresidential treatment programs offering a wide range of programs: fixed-length, structured primary and extended care rehabilitation programs at a fixed cost ranging from no charge (Veterans Administration) through $900 to $1,850, as well as more traditional outpatient psychotherapy with weekly sessions for a fixed or variable length of stay with charges per individual session ranging from $38 to $85. Funding sources vary among the individual programs but include all those available to the residential programs.

Both freestanding and hospital-based nonresidential programs offer day and evening sessions, dividing their treatment episodes into phases; the most common division is a primary care phase followed by an aftercare phase. Some offer several programs with alternative durations and intensities (frequency and length of sessions). Various designators are used to describe the program and its phases. Lengths of stay for each phase and for the total treatment episode, hours of contact, and number of sessions per week differ. Most facilities identify their program as an intensive primary care program lasting about 5 weeks with four sessions per week followed by aftercare lasting 12 weeks with one session per week. Almost all structured programs include a family component (e.g., 5 weeks, two sessions per week while the person in treatment attends four sessions per week).

In terms of special populations (see Section IV), Minnesota reports that 30 of its programs provide specialized services to American Indians, 3 programs serve blacks and 3 serve Hispanic Americans. There are 16 halfway house programs that serve men only and 53 programs that provide specialized services to women. There are 66 programs that indicate the availability of special services to youth; 13 programs report offering specialized services to the elderly. There are 60 programs serving those with "dual disabilities"—mental illness and chemical dependency.

A Federal Perspective

Like the Minnesota and other state alcoholism authorities, the federal government is primarily a funder and regulator of treatment for alcohol problems. Yet the federal government also operates a number of very large, nationally dispersed intervention and treatment systems that share the diversity seen in the states. Similarly to the states, federal agencies operate or contract for EAPs to serve their employees under Office of Personnel Management guidance. There are also drinking-driver programs for military personnel, and there are treatment programs provided for selected employees and beneficiaries.

Through its Department of Medicine and Surgery, the Department of Veterans Affairs, previously known as the Veterans Administration (VA), operates the largest centrally directed health care system in the nation. The VA provides treatment for alcohol-related problems/disorders to all eligible veterans (VA, 1977; Macro Systems, Inc., 1980; NIAAA, 1983b). VA investigators also conduct alcohol-related basic, clinical, and services research (IOM, 1989). Treatment and rehabilitation for alcohol dependence first began in VA hospitals in 1957; in 1967 the VA established an office to operate alcohol and drug abuse treatment as special medical programs within its psychiatric services. The first separately funded alcohol dependence treatment units (ADTPs) were established in 1970. All VA hospitals have the capability to treat alcohol-related medical emergencies, either in a specialized unit or on the medical service.

By fiscal year 1986 the VA's 172 hospitals were operating 103 specialized ADTPs along with 51 drug dependence treatment programs (DDTPs). During that year the specialized ADTPs treated more than 53,000 inpatients; more than 44,000 veterans with alcohol problems were treated in psychiatric units or medical beds (VA, 1987). The average length of stay in the ADTPs was 21.1 days. The average length of stay of all those discharged with a principle diagnosis of alcohol dependence or alcohol abuse was 16.3 days. The occupancy rate for the approximately 3,600 specialized ADTP beds was 85.1 percent. When both the principal and associated diagnoses are considered, alcohol-related disorders (22 percent) are second only to heart disease (41 percent) as the most common diagnoses among patients discharged from VA hospitals. This finding suggests that approximately $2 billion of the VA's total health care budget of more than $9.5 billion constitute expenditures to deal with alcohol problems.

During fiscal year 1980 the VA was given the authority to contract with non-VA community programs for treatment and rehabilitation services for veterans with alcohol or drug dependence or abuse disabilities. Between fiscal years 1984 and 1986 the VA inpatient programs used this authority to place approximately 5,000 veterans in halfway houses for 60 to 90 days of extended care.

The VA has introduced a prospective payment methodology (see Chapter 18) to fund its hospitals and outpatient clinics; the alcohol and drug abuse treatment services are also included in this method of financing (Errera et al., 1985; Nightingale, 1986). There have been no studies to date, however, of the impact of the introduction of this new financing mechanism on the functioning of the ADTP or on the outcome of treatment for alcohol problems.

The Department of Defense (DOD) provides prevention and treatment and rehabilitation services for both its civilian and military work forces, as required by law. The assistant secretary of defense for health affairs is responsible for developing policy. DOD has developed a comprehensive public health approach to the control of alcohol and drug use that utilizes education, law enforcement, and treatment. Each of the military services and the Defense Department agencies manages its own program within the policy guidelines promulgated by the assistant secretary. The treatment programs vary among the services, but all stress education, detection, and rehabilitation (Orvis et al., 1981). Alcohol is considered to be the primary substance abuse problem. Both hospital-based and residential programs are used for those who are judged to be more severely impaired. The overall orientation of the DOD programs reflects a mixed medical-social model; AA concepts are integrated into the program philosophies. The department conducts periodic surveys to aid the evaluation of the effectiveness of its policies and to monitor the prevalence of alcohol and other drug problems. Urine testing is also conducted and is believed to deter abuse (Bray et al., 1985).

The Bureau of Prisons provides treatment for alcohol problems to inmates of federal penal institutions and makes arrangements for those who achieve community status (i.e., probation, parole, residing in a community center) to receive appropriate treatment or aftercare services. There is no centralized, formally organized alcohol problems treatment program administration; each institution designs and evaluates its own program. Similarly, there is no formally structured diversion or treatment program for detainees in the pretrial phase or for parolees in the community; individual placements are made, and community corrections facilities are required to provide a minimal level of aftercare. Combined chemical abuse treatment units housing inmates with both alcohol and drug problems constitute the majority of the programs within the institutions. AA meetings, coordinated by volunteers from the community, are a major component of these institutional programs.

The Indian Health Service (IHS), through its Office of Alcoholism, sponsored the operation of 309 alcohol problems treatment programs in fiscal year 1987 (IHS, 1988; Rhoades et al., 1988). Alcohol problems treatment is also provided in IHS hospitals and primary care clinics. The IHS Office of Alcoholism was established in 1978 as a result of the passage of Public Law 94-437 and was given the responsibility to administer the American Indian/Native American alcohol treatment programs that had originally been funded through the Office of Economic Opportunity and the NIAAA categorical grants (see Chapters 15 and 18). The agency has developed its own stages of treatment model, focusing its rehabilitation efforts on nonhospital alternatives. Detoxification is primarily the responsibility of the IHS nonspecialist health components. Treatment (rehabilitation), which is provided by contract agencies following IHS guidelines and specifications, is provided in three environments: primary residential, halfway house, and outpatient.

IHS conceptualizes these three environments as components along a continuum of care. The ideal course of treatment is one in which one of the 42 primary residential treatment centers (PRTCs) serves as the entry point for persons who need intensive counseling and education along with a very structured environment that is free of alcohol and other drugs. On successful completion of the first phase of rehabilitation in the PRTC, the patient moves on to the next stage of treatment in an outpatient counseling program or halfway house in his or her own community, either for continuing treatment or aftercare. Halfway house continuing treatment is for those patients who complete the primary residential treatment phase and require additional time in a drug-free structured environment as well as follow-up counseling. Outpatient continuing treatment is for those patients who are returning to a family and community environment that is supportive of recovery.

Outpatient treatment is also used as an alternative to inpatient (primary residential) treatment when a bed is not available or when the family and community will support the initial phase of primary treatment on an outpatient basis. Outpatient treatment is sometimes used as a stopgap measure while waiting for a PRTC or halfway house bed to become available.

A National Perspective

Another means of understanding the structure of the alcohol problems treatment system throughout the nation is by reviewing the data from national surveys. Since the early 1970s there has been an ongoing effort to provide state and federal policymakers with the information they require to manage the resources needed to provide treatment services for persons with alcohol problems. As a major part of this effort the National Institute on Drug Abuse (NIDA) and NIAAA have periodically conducted surveys of all known public and private treatment facilities, seeking data on such variables as capacity, staffing, funding, utilization, and services. Since 1979 this survey, which was originally known as the National Drug and Alcoholism Treatment Utilization Survey (NDATUS), has been conducted jointly by the two institutes and therefore contains responses from units that provide services only for persons with alcohol problems, as well as from units that provide treatment for persons with both alcohol and other drug problems (NIAAAa, 1983; Yahr, 1988). Now known as the National Drug and Alcoholism Treatment Unit Survey, the NDATUS is a survey of specialist facilities and programs that provide an organized program of alcohol and drug abuse services.

The NDATUS was originally conducted in 1974 by NIDA. In 1979, however, it was expanded to include alcoholism as well as drug abuse facilities. The 1984 survey, renamed the National Alcoholism and Drug Abuse Program Inventory (NDAPI), did not obtain the same information as previous NDATUS efforts; in fact, the amount of information collected from each reporting unit by the NDAPI was greatly reduced from that collected in earlier years. This reduction in collected data was part of the overall effort by Congress and the Reagan administration to streamline grant program management and reduce federal reporting requirements. These modifications were introduced with the advent of the alcohol, drug abuse and mental health services block grant in 1982 (Institute for Health and Aging, 1986).

Unlike the 1984 survey, the 1987 survey contained questions to solicit additional information that was seen by both federal and state policymakers as necessary to study the distribution of services (USDHHS, 1986). The survey was designed to meet several objectives: (a) the development of an updated listing of substance abuse units for an information and referral hotline operated by NIDA; (b) the provision of information to policymakers about the type of services provided by treatment units, their capacity and utilization, and their funding sources and levels; (c) the collection of aggregate data on selected characteristics of persons using the services (age, sex, and race). The 1987 NDATUS attempted to survey all known facilities and organized programs that provided any services to persons with alcohol and other drug-related problems. A treatment unit was defined as a facility that had (a) a formal structured arrangement for drug abuse or alcoholism treatment using specified personnel; (b) a designated portion of the facility (or its resources) set aside for treatment services; (c) an allocated budget for such treatment; and (d) treatment services provided directly at the facility. The NDATUS also provided a point prevalence survey of utilization (i.e., the number of persons enrolled in formal treatment on October 30, 1987, the date of the survey).

A unit was not included in the analysis if it did not provide some information on persons actually in treatment. As a result, there is a substantial amount of missing data and the committee has not been able to use the data as extensively as it had originally planned. In the 1987 NDATUS, in contrast to previous surveys, programs with satellite units were given the option of reporting at either the program or unit level. Therefore, the information that were collected represents an unknown mix of program and unit data (NIDA/NIAAA, 1989).

The 1987 NDATUS also obtained basic information for the NIDA hotline listing from prevention and other nontreatment units. Some of these units appear to provide intervention and assessment services that would be included in the broader definition of treatment being used by the committee. Although the 1987 NDATUS was expanded because the 1984 NDAPI did not provide sufficient information about the scope and characteristics of the treatment delivery system, the revised survey still does not contain all of the information obtained in prior years. The most notable missing information is staffing patterns.

The format and level of detail contained in these surveys have varied over the years, although an effort has been made to utilize common response categories and definitions whenever possible to enable comparisons with data collected in previous years and to describe trends. Because there have been differences in definitions, however, as well as in response rates among the states and between years, comparisons among them can only be seen as tentative and exploratory (Reed and Sanchez, 1986). Therefore, trend analysis has not been undertaken, and the NDATUS is used primarily to describe the current situation. Trend analysis is important in understanding the changes in treatment availability and should be undertaken in more comprehensive studies directed at the evolution of the specialty alcohol problems treatment sector. *NIAAA should develop an ongoing program for analysis of the NDATUS data, including analyses of carefully designed subsets of programs that have responded to the survey over the years.*

A total of 8,690 programs and units responded to the 1987 NDATUS (NIDA/NIAAA, 1989). The majority (6,866) described their functions as including treatment; 5,211 units described their functions as including prevention and education, and 3,844 units indicated other functions. There were 5,791 treatment units that reported providing treatment services to persons with alcohol problems, 1,708 (29 percent) of them described their orientation as providing alcoholism services, and 4,083 (71 percent) identified their orientation as combined alcoholism and drug services. There were 337,337 persons receiving services on the census date (October 30); with budgeted capacity at 416,337 in the 5,627 units that reported on their active patients, the utilization rate was 81 percent.

TABLE 4-2 Location of Units Providing Treatment to Persons with Alcohol Problems

Unit's Location	Units		Persons in Treatment October 30, 1987	
	Number	%	Number	%
Community mental health center	842	14	60,946	17
Hospital[a]	1,166	20	55,270	16
Correctional facility	60	1	2,945	1
Halfway house/recovery home[b]	698	12	12,838	4
Other residential facility	701	12	21,705	6
Outpatient facility	2,004	35	173,912	50
Other	319	6	22,973	6
Not reporting	1	_c	24	_c
Total	5,791	100	350,613	100

SOURCE: NIDA/NIAAA (1989:Table 7).
[a]Includes general hospitals, VA hospitals, alcoholism hospitals, mental/psychiatric hospitals, and other specialized hospitals.
[b]The *recovery home* classification was added to meet concerns expressed by providers who utilize the California social model of recovery.
[c]Less than one percent.

According to this survey, the majority of persons in treatment (61 percent) is now being seen in combined alcohol and drug units, although this percentage varies among the states. Many states now have an overwhelming majority of combined units reporting (e.g.,Pennsylvania, Louisiana, Michigan); only a few states have a greater number of alcoholism-only units reporting (e.g., New York, New Jersey, Rhode Island).

The "unit location" variable in the survey (Table 4-2) identifies the type of organization within which a treatment unit is placed or the name by which it would commonly be known in the community. The unit location cannot precisely define the sector of which a unit is a part or the ideology to which a unit subscribes, but it can serve as an indicator of which organizational factors may contribute to the orientation of the treatment regimens offered. Thus, units located in community mental health centers are most likely to use the psychological model, units located in halfway houses are most likely to use the social model, and units located in hospitals are most likely to use the medical model.

The survey used a matrix to obtain information on the types of treatment being received on the census date; "Facility Location" and "Type of Care" were the descriptors used. The two facility location categories that were available to respondents were hospital inpatient and nonhospital. The type of care is defined as the primary treatment approach or regimen to which staff have assigned the person seeking treatment. The definitions of the five types of care included in the 1987 NDATUS are as follows:

Inpatient/Residential

Detoxification (Medical)—The use of medication under the supervision of medical personnel to systematically reduce or eliminate the effects of alcohol in the body in a hospital or other 24-hour-care facility.

Detoxification (Social)—The systematic reduction or elimination of the effects of alcohol in the body (returning the person to a drug-free state), in a specialized nonmedical facility by trained personnel with physician services available when required.

Rehabilitation/Recovery—An approach that provides a planned program of professionally directed evaluation, care, and treatment for the restoration of functioning for persons impaired by drug abuse or alcoholism. In some states, this type of care is referred to as treatment or recovery (excluding detoxification).

Custodial/Domiciliary—Provision of food, shelter, and assistance in routine daily living on a long-term basis for persons with alcohol or other drug-related problems.

Outpatient/Nonresidential—Treatment/recovery/aftercare or rehabilitation services provided by a unit in which the person receiving treatment does not reside. The person may receive drug or alcoholism treatment services with or without medication, including counseling and supportive services. Day care is included in this category.

Four of the types of care (medical and social detoxification, rehabilitation/recovery, and custodial domiciliary) are portrayed as taking place within 24-hour-care environments with persons residing at the treatment facility; only one (outpatient/nonresidential) is described as taking place in a setting where the persons in treatment do not reside. In keeping with current practice, detoxification is clearly identified as a separate stage and is further differentiated into social and medical model approaches. Rehabilitation is not differentiated in this manner. In general, the NDATUS definitions acknowledge the variations among the states in defining the continuum of care and the elements that constitute it. The definitions also include the recovery conceptualization, which is preferred in California as more accurately reflecting that state's nonmedical or social model of treatment (see Chapter 18).

Although the NDATUS is the major survey instrument available for gathering data on the treatment of alcohol problems, its usefulness is limited by the breadth of its categories and definitions. The type of care classification mixes what has been identified in this report as the orientation, stage, and setting of treatment. Consequently, the NDATUS data do not reveal which model was used for a particular individual's treatment or the stage of treatment of a person on the day of the census, even though (as discussed in Chapter 3) these are increasingly important distinctions for level of care placement and cost-efficient treatment. For example, the NDATUS differentiates between social and medical model for only the detoxification stage. The survey does not differentiate by orientation the rehabilitation and custodial/domiciliary types of care, although these variations exist (Borkman, 1986). The available survey data also do not fully differentiate among the types of beds being utilized by persons in treatment on the day of the survey. Although detoxification is clearly distinguishable, the rehabilitation and maintenance stages are partially combined in the definition of hospital/residential rehabilitation/recovery type of care. The short-term rehabilitation unit and the halfway house or extended care facility cannot always be distinguished. Thus, the beds belonging to the type of care defined as rehabilitation/recovery could appropriately be in use for either primary rehabilitation and extended care or transitional care (halfway house).

Another consequence of the construction of the survey is that it lumps together in the outpatient setting persons who are in differing stages of treatment. Individuals could have been in any of the stages on the census date. Moreover, the day-care, or intermediate, setting is not reported separately, but is included in the outpatient rehabilitation category, even though (as discussed in Chapter 3) day treatment is seen as an increasingly important cost-effective approach to both detoxification and primary care and can be used for maintenance and relapse prevention as well (e.g., Longabaugh et al., 1983; Frankel, 1983). Similarly, the outpatient environment slots could be in use for ambulatory detoxification, primary rehabilitation, extended care, or relapse prevention and supportive maintenance, as well as for treatment of those medical or psychiatric complications that can be dealt with in an ambulatory status.

Of the individuals reported in the survey, the majority (299, 679, or 85 percent) was enrolled in the outpatient/nonresidential rehabilitation/recovery type of care. The remainder was enrolled in one of the four inpatient programs: 10,507 in detoxification (4,015 in the 390 units that reported offering medical detoxification; 6,492 in the 939 social detoxification units); 37,739 in the 2,185 rehabilitation/recovery programs; and 2,688 in the 182 custodial/domiciliary programs. The data also show that there are units offering medical model detoxification in every state except Vermont; there are social model detoxification units reported in all states except the District of Columbia, Maine, North Dakota, West Virginia, and Wyoming. Every state has units offering outpatient and inpatient/residential rehabilitation. There are custodial/domiciliary units in all but eight states: Delaware, Hawaii, Michigan, Montana, New Jersey, North Dakota, West Virginia, and Wyoming.

As noted earlier, the NDATUS data do not show whether an individual was in outpatient detoxification, primary treatment, or aftercare on the day of the census. To compensate for this kind of aggregation some outpatient units appear to have attempted at least to categorize some of their clients in a detoxification status: 15 outpatient units reported providing social model detoxification for 69 persons and 8 outpatient units reported providing medical model detoxification for 105 persons. The actual level and geographic distribution of ambulatory detoxification or rehabilitation services are not available because of the overly broad definitions for facility location and type of care used. Any attempt to define and organize the various types of treatment or care available for persons with alcohol problems must recognize that any given form of organization can provide different stages of care in each setting using any single treatment modality or a mixture of modalities. *The NDATUS should be redesigned to reflect actual practice more accurately and to identify clearly which types of treatment are being provided.*

The term *ownership* is used in the NDATUS to describe the type of organization that is legally responsible for the unit's operation. The survey uses four categories: (1) for profit, which includes individuals, partnerships, and corporations; (2) not for profit, which includes church-related groups, nonprofit corporations, or other forms of nonprofit organization; (3) state and local government, which includes all forms of such organization; and (4) the federal government, which includes any federal agency. The NDATUS ownership category is similar to the ownership category in the American Hospital Association's (1987) annual survey of hospitals; in that survey, ownership is divided into federal and nonfederal groupings including state and local government, nongovernment/not for profit, and investor owned/for profit. Substantial differences in the models of services offered and the types of persons treated in programs in each of these ownership groups have been suggested (Jacobs, 1985; Miller and Hester, 1986: Yahr, 1988; see Appendix D).

Privately operated units constituted the majority (81 percent) of the respondents in the 1987 NDATUS (16 percent were private/for profit, and 66 percent were private/not for profit). The third largest category (16 percent) was state- and local-government-operated programs. The trends noted in prior surveys continued: there was an increase in the proportion of private programs (both for-profit and not-for-profit types) and a decrease in the proportion of public (both state and federal government) programs (Reed and Sanchez, 1986; Yahr, 1988). This trend must be interpreted very cautiously, however, because there is a substantial and as yet unexplained drop in the total number of programs that responded to the 1987 survey when compared with those responding to the 1984 NDAPI and with the number of programs estimated to be active from the 1987 survey of programs receiving funding from the state alcoholism authorities (Butynski and Canova, 1988). The "underreporting" is seen in both the 17 percent drop in the total number of programs responding to the survey (from 6,963 in 1984 to 5,791 in 1987) and in the 2 percent drop in the number of facilities responding to the question on ownership (from 5,791 to 5,667). There are several possible reasons for the drop. The extensive outreach efforts conducted for the 1984 survey may have resulted in a higher response rate. There are also some changes in the 1987 survey in the way multisite programs are reported that may have contributed to the decrease in the number of units. In addition, despite its lack of specificity in other definitional areas, the 1987 NDATUS provided a more stringent definition of a treatment unit than that used in 1984 (NIDA/NIAAA, 1989).

Treatment Personnel

Any discussion of the settings and organizations in which treatment services are provided must also deal with the personnel who perform the specific services and the levels of training, education, and experience that are needed to carry out the necessary treatment and administrative activities. Human resources utilization in the treatment of alcohol problems tends to be a matter of some controversy (Gunnerson and Feldman, 1978; Mitnick, 1978; USDHHS, 1981; Camp and Kurtz, 1982; Rosenberg, 1982; Saxe et al., 1983; Blum and Roman, 1985; Lewis et al., 1987; Bowen and Sammons, 1988; McGovern, 1988).

The major sources of this controversy are the historical failure of traditional health and mental health professionals to work effectively with people with alcohol problems and the filling of this void by lay persons, primarily recovering alcoholics, who had by the 1960s begun to develop their own programs using the principles of Alcoholics Anonymous (D. J. Anderson, 1981; Bissell, 1982; McGovern and Armstrong, 1986). The net result of these two phenomena is that, along with the development of nontraditional treatment programs in the specialty sector, there has been a shift in the usual alignment of roles and responsibilities in the treatment of alcohol problems that has not yet been consolidated into a singular approach to human resources planning and training.

During the 1970s, the field went through an initial rapid expansion in the role of and reliance on the alcoholism counselor as the primary therapist, or case manager, and program administrator. Alcoholism counselors became the dominant treatment staff working in organized programs funded by NIAAA and the states. However, Saxe and colleagues (1983) noted the change that has taken place in recent years: a reinfusion of psychologists and psychiatrists into the alcohol treatment work force in the late 1970s after the development of the network of nonmedical programs in the 1960s and early 1970s. In those programs, counselors had occupied the roles of primary therapist, administrator, milieu management and support staff, outreach worker, diagnostician, and advocates for development. Today, given the need to develop programs that could receive third-party health insurance funding, program accreditation standards often require that physicians take on supervisory and administrative responsibility for clinical operations and that treatment be carried out only by primary therapists who meet specific educational or licensing standards. This shift has led to a transitional period in which many of the personnel working in the field are identified as "alcoholism counselors" regardless of their original discipline and training, and in which the nondegreed, recovering person who has become a counselor or administrator is feeling shunted aside by the professionals and the funding agencies.

There was no national policy or program for developing a coherent human resources system for the treatment of alcohol problems until 1979 when NIAAA's State Manpower Development Program was initiated (Camp and Kurtz, 1982; Ziener, 1988). This program provided categorical grant funding to each of the state alcoholism authorities to develop a manpower plan and to conduct training of treatment providers. The program ended with the incorporation of all NIAAA categorical grants into a block grant in 1982 (see the discussion in Chapter 18); the block grant does not require states to continue this effort and most states no longer produce a plan (W. Butynski, National Association of State Alcohol and Drug Abuse Program Directors, personal communication, 1988; B. Meyers, Colorado State, Alcohol and Drug Abuse Division, personal communication, 1988; Horizons Technology Inc., 1988). During the years of its implementation, however, the State Manpower Development Program produced an annual human resources plan for alcohol treatment, using information collected by the states from treatment providers on their needs for personnel and for training activities. An assessment was also made of the demographic makeup of the work force to determine its representativeness and compatibility with the persons being served (Macro Systems, Inc., 1980).

Currently, each state and each involved discipline develop their own policies, and the degree of activity among the states and disciplines varies considerably. Among the most active are the American Medical Society on Alcoholism and Other Drug Dependencies (Galanter and Bean-Bayog, 1989), the American Psychiatric Association (Galanter et al., 1989), the Association for Medical Education and Research in Substance Abuse, and the National Association of Alcoholism and Drug Abuse Counselors (McGovern, 1988).

The most recent national survey of personnel employed in facilities that offer treatment for alcohol problems was conducted in 1982 (NIAAA, 1983a). (After a hiatus of seven years, questions to solicit these data will again be included in the 1989 NDATUS.) In 1982 there were 44,098 total paid and volunteer staff working in the 2,734 alcoholism-only treatment units reporting. There were a total of 31,520 paid, full-time employees (generally referred to as FTEs, or full-time equivalents, for the purposes of quantification). The three largest general categories of workers in treatment programs were counselors, nurses, and administrative and support staff.

Administrative and support staff accounted for 26 percent of the FTEs reported in the 1982 survey, and direct care staff accounted for the remaining 74 percent. The distribution of direct care employees was analyzed by discipline rather than by function or role. The largest direct care staff group was counselors (34 percent). The majority of the counselors (20 percent of the total) did not have a related academic degree; the remainder (14 percent) had either a counseling degree or some type of certification for counseling training. Physicians made up about 3 percent of the total staff and were most likely to be part time. Registered nurses constituted about 11 percent of the total staff pool, whereas other medical disciplines (e.g., licensed practical and vocational nurses, orderlies, pharmacists, and physicians' assistants) accounted for an additional 9 percent. Psychologists made up almost 3 percent and social workers, 4 percent. The remaining 12 percent were other direct care staff who were not identified with a discipline.

In addition to physicians, doctoral-level psychologists were more likely to be part-time employees whereas counselors, master's-level psychologists, nurses, and social workers were more likely to be full-time employees.

The 1982 survey showed that counselors, many of whom were recovering persons, had become the primary treatment service providers in many of the specialist programs and that they functioned with considerable autonomy in those settings. This situation is still the norm today. Although still identified as "alcoholism counselors" (or, increasingly, as "addictions counselors"), these personnel perform a variety of roles previously reserved for the other professional disciplines. In a given program an individual trained as a counselor may fill an administrative role (e.g., program director, unit supervisor), a clinical role (e.g., case manager, primary therapist, group therapist, psychodrama leader, family counselor, intake worker), or a milieu management role (e.g., residence supervisor, activity therapist, group leader).

The widespread use of physicians to provide medical services in inpatient detoxification and rehabilitation programs has continued. A common pattern in freestanding residential rehabilitation programs and rehabilitation units in general hospitals is to have a single physician, or a physician group, serve as the medical director of the program or unit and assume the responsibility of attending physician for all those who are admitted. The physician is responsible for the development of the multidisciplinary treatment plan and for ensuring that the appropriate physical examinations and laboratory tests are carried out and that medications, if needed, are correctly administered and monitored. Psychiatrists perform these required medical functions in VA and psychiatric hospitals. Psychiatrists also provide consultations and specific services to persons in other settings who have coexisting psychiatric disorders.

Nurses play key roles in staffing and administering medical model detoxification and rehabilitation programs. Nurses primarily provide direct services to persons admitted to inpatient detoxification and rehabilitation settings; they manage the medical treatment prescribed by the physician, retaining responsibility for the nursing care plan and management of the unit milieu. Nurses working in an inpatient unit participate in the alcohol education sessions and are often responsible for providing lectures on the physical consequences of excessive alcohol use. They also provide supportive counseling. Other nurses, with training in psychotherapy and family counseling, have moved into counseling and administrative roles in all settings. The program director for a rehabilitation unit in a general hospital is often a nurse.

Doctoral-level clinical psychologists are generally used on a part-time basis as diagnostic consultants, group therapists, and individual therapists. Master's-level psychologists may function in a similar fashion, but they are more likely to be full-time employees of the program rather than consultants. In a given program, an individual trained as a psychologist may also fill an administrative role (e.g., program director, director of clinical services) as well as a clinical or milieu management role.

Social workers and counselors with master's degrees are widely used as primary therapists or case managers. Primary therapists coordinate the provision of services to an individual from intake (the admission evaluation) to follow up. They generally provide any individual therapy or counseling the person receives. In addition, social workers are also increasingly found in administrative roles as well as in clinical and milieu management roles.

Many hospital and residential programs, if they are large enough, further differentiate counseling roles. There may be an intake counselor, a primary counselor during the inpatient stay, and an aftercare counselor who is responsible for postdischarge follow-up. Increasingly there may also be a designated family counselor who leads family groups and works with individual families. Outpatient programs ordinarily do not have such a division of labor.

The disciplines licensed for independent practice in their speciality (e.g., internal medicine, psychiatry, nursing, social work, marriage and family counseling, psychology) may also provide services within a private practice setting, in which they carry out the more traditional roles of diagnostician, case manager, and therapist as defined by their speciality. There are no data available on the number of private practice professionals who devote their entire practice to the treatment of persons with alcohol problems. Moreover, there are no data on the percentage of time that is devoted to treating persons with alcohol problems by the disciplines for whom such treatment is a part of their practice.

Which discipline fills the various clinical, supervisory, and administrative roles in the operation of an organized treatment program depends on the program's philosophy and orientation (Kole and Mitnick, 1978). In medical settings the functions or roles generally reflect the traditional medical hierarchy (Camp and Kurtz, 1982). In nonmedical settings there is more shifting of responsibilities among personnel and many tasks that are seen as appropriate to personnel with different initial training, experience, and credentials. For example, the role of the physician as the primary treatment provider and supervisor has been challenged by advocates of the social model of detoxification and rehabilitation (Borkman, 1986). In halfway houses and recovery homes, physicians and other professionals often serve as consultants or providers of a specific discipline-limited service rather than as care givers who are responsible for the overall treatment plan. Indeed, social model detoxification and rehabilitation programs and halfway houses are likely to be staffed with counselors who have varying degrees of experience and education.

The key role played by alcoholism counselors in the administration and delivery of treatment in publicly supported programs has created problems in financing such treatment through traditional public and private insurance mechanisms (Camp and Kurtz, 1982; Lawrence Johnson and Associates, Inc., 1983). Efforts to develop credentialing for alcoholism counselors were a key part of the federal strategy to obtain stable funding for the treatment of alcohol problems and were actively pursued until the shift to block grant funding in 1982. At that time, with federal assistance, more than 34 states had developed mechanisms for certifying counselors, either through the state alcohol agency or through a statewide voluntary association. Since 1982 there have been sporadic efforts aimed at developing a national credentialing system, but they have met with little success. This effort is now continuing under the leadership of the National Association of Drug and Alcohol Counselors (McGovern, 1988).

Present estimates are that approximately twenty thousand professionals describe themselves as alcoholism or alcoholism and drug abuse counselors. The National Association of Alcoholism and Drug Abuse Counselors currently has a membership of 11,000 persons who work in treatment programs in a variety of educational, corrections, health care, and other settings. Counselors, rehabilitation therapists, administrators, social workers, psychologists, nurses, and physicians, including psychiatrists, constitute the association's membership. A survey conducted as part of an NIAAA-sponsored effort to develop model standards for credentialing counselors (see the discussion later in this chapter) reported the following breakdown of professions under the umbrella of alcoholism counseling: counselors—60 percent, rehabilitation therapists—7 percent, administrators—4 percent, social workers—9 percent, psychologists—7 percent, nurses—6 percent, and physicians—0.4 percent (Birch and Davis Associates, Inc., 1984) .

The two disciplines that have been most active in the last several years in attempting to continue these early credentialing efforts have been counselors and physicians. For alcoholism counselors the aim has been to gain legitimization and acceptance as a professional discipline. For physicians the aim has been to both increase the amount of training that all physicians receive so that fewer persons with alcohol problems will go undetected in primary care settings (USDHHS, 1986; Cotter and Callahan, 1987; Lewis et al., 1987; Bowen and Sammons, 1988) and to develop an acceptance of the treatment of alcohol problems as an area of specialization (Galanter and Bean-Bayog, 1989).

J. E. Royce (1981) traced the origins of the new profession of alcoholism counseling to the incorporation of recovered alcoholics into the treatment team at the Yale Plan Clinic in 1944. The role of the counselor was further developed at Minnesota's Willmar State Hospital in the early 1950s in a program in which recovered alcoholics with native counseling ability were used to provide treatment. The role of the alcoholism counselor continued to be refined as part of the development of the Minnesota model (see Chapter 3) at Willmar State Hospital and its subsequent use at the Hazelden Treatment Center (D. J. Anderson, 1981; Emanuel, 1984). In 1954 the Minnesota Civil Service Commission, designated the alcoholism worker or counselor as a formal employment category, a step D. J. Anderson (1981) considered to be a significant achievement in the development of counseling during this period. There were parallel developments in other parts of the country as more and more programs began to use recovering persons to provide treatment (Camp and Kurtz, 1982). The growth of community mental health centers and community health centers, both of which used nondegreed workers in community outreach programs, greatly influenced the acceptance of the alcoholism worker (counselor) as a paraprofessional (Kole and Mitnick, 1978; Mitnick, 1978) during a time when the established helping professionals showed little interest in the field of alcohol problems. As a result more and more of the treatment enterprise was born by the recovered alcoholism worker.

Staub and Kent (1973) describe in detail the development of the role of the alcoholism worker as a paraprofessional. The increasing responsibility for carrying out treatment assumed by these recovered persons was not unquestioned. The Krystal-Moore controversy (Krystal and Moore, 1963) regarding the personnel qualified to treat the person with alcohol problems is illustrative of the tension that existed between degreed professionals and nondegreed workers in the field. Krystal's position was that only trained professionals were qualified to treat persons with alcohol problems. He argued that alcoholism was a symptom of an underlying emotional problem that required psychotherapy conducted by professionals with additional specialized training. Moore's position was that individual psychotherapy was not the most effective form of treatment for the vast majority of persons with alcohol problems; rather, treatment for alcohol problems required the involvement of all disciplines in seeking the appropriate use of their skills through more effective techniques. Many psychiatrists agreed with Moore that counselors who were recovering persons had an important role to play in the treatment of alcohol problems (Lemere et al., 1964).

C. M. Rosenberg (1982) described the typical paraprofessional alcoholism counselor in 1971 as a 40-year-old man who was addicted to alcohol but who had gained significant sobriety through involvement with Alcoholics Anonymous. Rosenberg considered such a person a paraprofessional, owing to limited education and the lack of formal academic and clinical qualifications in one or the other of the health professions. The rapid growth of a cadre of paraprofessionals (counselors) who were often without formal education credentials but who were trained in counseling skills that met the needs of their clients in task-oriented group environments was a remarkable feature of the development of all human services in the 1960s and 1970s and not just the treatment of alcohol problems (Mitnick and Kole, 1978; D. J. Anderson, 1981). The negative attitudes of established health care professionals (physicians, nurses, social workers, and clergy) toward working with the "alcoholic" paradoxically fostered the growth of the new profession.

The passage of alcoholism counseling from a paraprofessional to a somewhat more professional standing is reflected in a report to NIAAA that was commissioned to develop proposals for national standards for alcoholism counselors (Roy Littlejohn Associates, Inc., 1974). The Littlejohn study described the counselor as a key member of a prevention/-treatment/rehabilitation team in programs where persons with alcoholism problems receive help. Alcoholism counseling, according to the Littlejohn study, was a "new profession" that embraced a wide range of tasks: intake, crisis intervention, individual and group counseling, education and prevention, and program development and consultation. Counselors were now seen as full-time paid professionals who were distinguishable from members of lay or volunteer organizations such as AA.

The 1970s brought the development of state and national counselor organizations together with the emergence of certification and credentialing initiatives (Kole and Mitnick, 1978; Birch and Davis Associates, Inc., 1984). By the end of the 1970s counselors were providing most of the direct counseling services to persons with alcohol problems and their families. In their professional role, counselors functioned as essential members of multidisciplinary teams in a variety of settings. Nondegreed counselors performed many of the case management and psychotherapy functions that had previously been seen as reserved for physicians, psychologists, and social workers.

Much of the effort in the alcohol counseling arena during the 1980s has been centered on the development of professional standards and procedures for credentialing counselors. At the national and state levels, various components of the alcohol problems field have addressed this issue. Currently, in 34 states, counselors are credentialed by either the state alcoholism authority or by a voluntary organization. Although the standards and procedures are similar, there has been no success achieved in developing a single set of standards to be used in all states or in having all the states recognize those individuals who are credentialed in other states. A uniform plan for credentialing that guarantees reciprocity among the states has been developed by the groups that constitute the Certification Reciprocity Consortium—Alcohol and Other Drug Abuse. In addition, the National Commission on Credentialing of Alcoholism and Drug Abuse Counseling represents key constituency groups that share a common interest in facilitating the implementation of a national competency-based credentialing system. The acceptance and implementation of such national standards may be the critical issue that ultimately determines the professional status and growth of alcoholism counseling (McGovern, 1988).

The Birch and Davis Associates report (1984), the outcome of the NIAAA initiative to develop model professional standards for counselors, is of great significance in this area. As part of the larger project, two national surveys of practicing alcoholism and drug counselors were conducted; counselors were asked to identify which activities were the core tasks of their job and what knowledge and skills were required to carry out those tasks. The respondents to the Birch and Davis survey, regardless of differences in practice settings, work experience, educational background, and life experiences consistently agreed in the ranking of the tasks, knowledge, and skills appropriate to alcoholism counseling. Two separate validation studies produced three major core products: (1) a set of counselor job tasks, (2) a body of knowledge and skills that reflects the competencies the counseling field expects of its practitioners, and (3) guidelines on techniques to assess the competencies of individuals seeking a counselor credential.   Competencies in core functions, which are identified as screening, intake, orientation, assessment, treatment planning, individual group and significant other counseling, case management, crisis intervention, client education, referral, reports and recordkeeping, and consultation with other professionals in regard to client treatment services, were defined as requirements for certification.

One consequence of the credentialing and professionalizing efforts of the past decades are dramatic changes that have occurred in the counseling field over the past 10 years. At the end of the 1970s most counselors were male, 45 years old, in recovery, and with little formal education beyond high school. Today's counselors are younger, with a higher representation of women, and are more likely to have academic training; fewer are in recovery (60 percent), and they have higher rates of certification (Birch and Davis Associates, Inc., 1984; Blum and Roman, 1985; McGovern, 1986, 1988). Another debate of the 1970s was whether a counselor had to be a recovering alcoholic to be effective. Now, many more treatment settings use recovered counselors and nonalcoholic counselors, and McGovern and Armstrong (1986) argue that recovered and nonalcoholic counselors now espouse common goals born of a common philosophy of treatment. Studies show that both groups are equally effective, given appropriate training (Blum and Roman, 1985; McGovern and Armstrong, 1986).

In addition to the movement toward credentialing and professionalizing counselors, independent efforts have been proceeding to develop both specialized training and credentialing mechanisms for each of the major academic disciplines involved in the treatment of alcohol problems (Galanter and Bean-Bayogg, 1989).   A variety of professional associations has arisen to bring together workers from the various disciplines who specialize in treating persons with alcohol problems. Each of these groups has taken positions on what they consider to be the optimal configuration of treatment services and personnel, and some have been involved in developing their own credentialing procedures.

In particular, the training of physicians as specialists in the treatment of alcohol problems and as generalists who are sensitive to alcohol problems has long been an NIAAA priority, and there has been significant progress in the development of physician training programs in diagnosis and referral for alcohol problems. One of the initial efforts in this area was the Career Teacher Program, launched in 1971 and sponsored by NIAAA and NIDA (Lewis, 1989). This program laid the groundwork for nationwide changes that are now occurring in medical education about alcohol problems. It provided a shared experience for participating faculty members throughout the country in curriculum content and issues of effective teaching, as well as in ways to overcome the negative attitudes of students, faculty, and institutions toward treating persons with alcohol problems.   Its products included teaching monographs, educational materials, and the development of curriculum objectives. Surveys on the impact of the program, which ended in 1981, showed that elective courses in substance abuse tripled at Career Teacher schools, but required courses still remained at fewer than 1 percent of the total curriculum.

The federal initiative was renewed again in 1985 with support for a national conference sponsored jointly with the Association for Medical Education and Research in Substance Abuse (AMERSA), which grew out of the Career Teacher Program. The conference was organized as a consensus activity to define the minimal knowledge and skills that various medical disciplines should possess (e.g., pediatricians, internal medicine, family medicine) and also to define the minimal knowledge and skills all physicians should possess in diagnosis and referral for alcohol and other drug problems (Alcohol, Drug Abuse, and Mental Health Administration, 1985). It attracted medical leaders from universities, national professional societies, and the Public Health Service and formed a consensus that was the basis for a new federal contract program to develop and implement model curricula for medical students and residents. As a result of these efforts, there is now a clearer understanding of the curricular content needed (and the most effective means of teaching this content) to develop the essential alcohol problems-related knowledge and skills for all physicians across specialities and in particular for the disciplines of pediatrics, family medicine, and internal medicine. In addition, contracts have recently been awarded to schools of nursing to define that profession's teaching needs and to develop a model nursing curriculum. NIAAA and NIDA have also launched a new grant program that establishes a medical and nursing faculty fellows program to enlarge and improve alcohol- and drug-related clinical training. All of these recent efforts by the federal government are in response to a growing interest among the general public and medical professionals concerning these training issues (Bowen and Sammons, 1988).

Part of the renewed interest in medical training related to alcohol problems has come from groups interested in primary care, including such national professional societies as the Society of General Internal Medicine, the Society of Teachers of Family Medicine, and the Ambulatory Pediatric Association. These organizations, which are committed to providing quality primary care of common problems, recognize the pervasiveness and heterogeneity of alcohol problems and the sorts of interventions that may be effective, including the kind of brief advice and treatment discussed elsewhere in this report (see Chapter 9). These national professional societies have formed active task forces and have joined with the American Medical Association as cosponsors of the annual AMERSA national conference. All of these developments in medicine and nursing point to a new breed of practitioner who will have received formal education about alcohol problems and who will be able and willing to identify and treat alcohol problems or to refer individuals for specialist treatment.

This new breed of practitioners will join the cadre of trained professionals— physicians, nurses, counselors, social workers, and clinical psychologists—already at work providing treatment for alcohol problems. Unfortunately, the dimensions of this cadre are unclear because there is a serious lack of accurate, timely work force data at the national level. This lack of data compromises efforts to plan for future training and professional needs. Fundamental questions for each of the disciplines involved cannot be answered: for example, the backgrounds and characteristics of persons working in the field, whether they are working in the specialty alcohol problems treatment sector or in the related primary health, corrections, education, mental health, or social services sectors; the nature of their long-term career opportunities; and whether there is currently growth or constriction in the number of specialized training programs. As a consequence, it is not possible to formulate a forward-looking work force training policy.

Currently, there is no national group or agency charged with gathering work force data and with formulating an appropriate policy on training and credentialing. During the process of completing the report the committee learned that staffing information was to be added to the NDATUS. This addition is a positive development but will only provide data for the specialty treatment sector. Such data needs also to be collected from the nonspecialist sector. Recent federal legislation (the Anti-Drug Abuse Act of 1988) gives the clinical training responsibility for counselors and health professionals to ADAMHA's Office of Substance Abuse Prevention (OSAP), suggesting that there will be a renewed federal interest and effort (Horizons Technology, Inc., 1988). Under an interagency agreement, OSAP will focus on the training of counselors and health professionals already in the field, and NIAAA and NIDA will continue and expand their efforts to educate health professionals at the the graduate school and continuing education levels.

Given the lack of concerted, coordinated human resources planning and the questions that continue to be raised about the roles each discipline should play in delivering and in administering treatment for alcohol problems, *there appears to be a need to reestablish a unified work force planning effort*. The first steps in such planning should be accurate determinations of the staffing in existing specialist programs and the role or roles currently played by each discipline.

Summary and Conclusions

Persons with alcohol problems receive care in a wide variety of generalist organizations, as well as in organizations that specialize in treating alcohol problems. A description of either the specialist service delivery system or the generalist system is difficult because there has not yet been an acceptable comprehensive classification that fully incorporates the developments of the last 20 years. One major development has been the tremendous expansion of institutional and community-based treatment programs, both within traditional agencies (e.g., general hospitals) and nontraditional agencies (e.g., freestanding social setting detoxification centers). There also appear to be an increasing number of private practitioners working in the field of alcohol problems. Treatment is provided by personnel from a variety of disciplines including physicians, social workers, counselors, and psychologists. There have been redefinitions of the roles played by each discipline in more traditional health care facilities, but, in all of the organized settings, alcoholism counselors have become the major providers of treatment.

Even though there has been a major effort to obtain increased acceptance of the treatment for alcohol problems as belonging within the mainstream of health care services, many of these newer agencies are not in traditional health care settings and do not follow what have become the established patterns of staffing and functioning. This variation has contributed to problems in describing who is providing what kind of treatment to whom. Some of the agencies focus on providing one type of care (e.g., social setting detoxification, hospital-based rehabilitation); others attempt to offer comprehensive health and social services during all stages of treatment to a special population (e.g., the Salvation Army, Indian Health Service). The dominant historical influence on the field has been its origins in the integration of Alcoholics Anonymous philosophy and professional concepts now known as the Minnesota model and exemplified by the pioneering work at Willmar State Hospital, the Hazelden Foundation, and the Yale Plan Clinics. Alcoholics Anonymous itself continues as the best-known provider of support and treatment for alcohol problems.

Although is possible to draw a broad outline of the service delivery system for the treatment of alcohol problems and to describe some of its components, it is not possible to accurately identify who provides what types of treatment to whom because of the lack of systematic surveys and studies. The evolving network of service providers (both programs and personnel) and the relationship of provider characteristics to the availability, conduct, and outcome of treatment have not been adequately described or studied (Gilbert and Cervantes, 1988; Wallen, 1988). *An expanded research program is needed to investigate the social ecology of the treatment system* (Weisner and Room, 1984; Weisner, 1986). In developing its analysis of the treatment system, the committee has been hampered by the lack of studies on a number of important topics: the impact of the organizational, ideological, and financial characteristics of treatment providers; their interrelationships; their relationships to referral sources; and the impact of various funding strategies on the organization, utilization, and outcome of treatment. More research is needed; examples of studies that should be replicated and expanded are (a) examination of the trends in the profiles of offered services that are associated with ownership type (Yahr, 1988), (b) examination of the utilization of different services by the various special population groups (Gilbert and Cervantes, 1988), and (c) examination of trends in reimbursement sources for different types of specialty programs (Creative Socio-Medics Corporation, 1981). Performing such studies will require surveys that are better designed and better conducted than the major vehicle now available, the National Drug and Alcohol Treatment Unit Survey.

Studies of service profiles and of the outcomes associated with different paths through the treatment system are also needed. Specifically, research should investigate the value of providing increased intermediate care (day-care) options at each stage of treatment and of providing social model treatment. Private and public health insurance tend not to recognize day-care programs, halfway houses, or recovery homes as eligible providers, thus cutting off from coverage those persons needing such care. These programs generally are a mixture of the social and medical models, offering social support, vocational rehabilitation, and medical services along with primary treatment. *The committee sees an expansion of intermediate care programs as an important element in increasing treatment availability and effectiveness.*

Any studies of the organizations in which treatment services are provided must also analyze who performs the specific services. Human resources utilization in the treatment of alcohol problems continues to be somewhat controversial. One of the major aspects of this controversy is whether recovering persons, who in many cases have developed their own programs outside the health care mainstream, should continue to fill the void left by traditional health and mental health professionals in treating people with alcohol problems. Along with the development of nontraditional treatment programs in the specialty sector, there has been a shift in the usual alignment of staff roles and responsibilities that has not yet been consolidated into a single approach to human resources planning, training, and credentialing. Without a national policy or program for developing such an approach, each state and involved discipline currently develop their own policies. The degree of activity and the particular mechanisms used vary considerably among these bodies.

Given the lack of concerted, coordinated human resources planning and the questions that continue to be raised about the roles each discipline should play in delivering and administering treatment for alcohol problems, there appears to be a need to reestablish a unified manpower planning effort. The first step in such planning is accurate determinations of the staffing in existing specialist programs and of the role or roles currently played by each discipline in programs in both the specialist and nonspecialist sectors. Additional research is required to determine the nature and level of treatment services being provided by each of the disciplines in the generalist health, social services, education, and corrections sectors as well as in the specialist alcohol problem treatment sector.

REFERENCES

Ablon, J. 1982. Support system dynamics of Al-Anon and Alateen. Pp. 987-995 in Encylopedic Handbook of Alcoholism, E. M. Pattison and E. Kaufman, eds. New York: Gardner Press.

Al-Anon. 1986. First Steps: Al-Anon . . . 35 Years of Beginnings. New York: Al-Anon Family Group Headquarters.

Alcohol, Drug Abuse, and Mental Health Administration (ADAMHA). 1985. Consensus Statement from the Conference on Alcohol, Drugs, and Primary Care Physician Education: Issues, Roles, Responsibilities, Rancho Mirage, California, November 12-15. Rockville, Md.: ADAMHA.

Alcoholics Anonymous World Services, Inc. 1955. Alcoholics Anonymous: The Story of How Many Thousands of Men and Women Have Recovered from Alcoholism. New York: Alcoholics Anonymous World Services, Inc.

Alcoholics Anonymous World Services, Inc. 1959. Alcoholics Anonymous Comes of Age: A Brief History of AA. New York: Alcoholics Anonymous World Services, Inc.

Alcoholics Anonymous World Services, Inc. 1961 (rev., 1987). A.A. in Treatment Facilities: How and Why A.A. Members Carry the Message into Treatment Facilities. New York: Alcoholics Anonymous World Services, Inc.

Alcoholics Anonymous World Services, Inc. 1979. A Members-Eye View of Alcoholics Anonymous. New York: Alcoholics Anonymous World Services, Inc.

Alcoholics Anonymous World Services, Inc. 1987. A.A. surveys its membership: A demographic report. About AA: A Newsletter for Professional Men and Women Fall:1-2.

Alcoholics Anonymous World Services, Inc. 1988. Singleness of purpose is central to recovery in A.A. About A.A.: A Newsletter for Professional Men and Women Spring:1.

Alibrandi, L. A. 1982. The fellowship of Alcoholics Anonymous. Pp. 979-986 in Encylopedic Handbook of Alcoholism, E. M. Pattison and E. Kaufman, eds. New York: Gardner.

American Hospital Association (AHA). 1987. Hospital Statistics. Chicago: American Hospital Association.

Anderson, D. J. 1981. Perspectives on Treatment: The Minnesota Experience. Center City, Minn.: Hazelden Foundation.

Anderson, G. L. 1979. The Student Assistance Program: An Overview. Madison, Wisc.: Wisconsin Bureau of Alcohol and Other Drug Abuse.

Anderson, J. G., and F. S. Gilbert. 1989. Communication skills training with alcoholics for improving performane of two of the Alcoholics Anonymous recovery steps. Journal of Studies on Alcohol 50:361-367.

Armor, D. J., J. M. Polich, and H. B. Stambul. 1978. Alcoholism and Treatment. Santa Monica, Calif.: John Wiley and Sons.

Backer, T. E., and K. O'Hara. 1988. A national study on drug abuse services and EAPs. The ALMACAN 18(8):24-25.

Bast, R. J. 1984. Classification of Alcoholism Treatment Settings. Rockville, Md.: National Institute on Alcohol Abuse and Alcoholism.

Bayer, A., ed. 1980. A Health Planner's Guide to Planning and Evaluating Alcoholism Services. Bethesda, Md.: Alpha Center for Health Planning.

Bensinger, A., and C. F. Pilkington. 1983. An alternative method in the treatment of alcoholism: The United Technologies Corporation day treatment program. Journal of Occupational Medicine 25:300-303.

Berman, H., and D. Klein. 1977. Project to Develop a Comprehensive Alcoholism Benefit Through Blue Cross: Final Report of Phase I. Prepared for the National Institute on Alcohol Abuse and Alcoholism. Chicago: Blue Cross Association.

Birch and Davis Associates, Inc. 1984. Development of Model Professional Standards for Counselor Credentialling. Prepared for the National Institute on Alcohol Abuse and Alcoholism, Washington, D.C. (reprinted 1986: Dubuque, Ia.: Kendall/Hunt Publishing).

Bissell, L. 1982. Recovered alcoholic counselors. Pp. 810-817 in Encyclopedic Handbook of Alcoholism, E. M. Pattison and E. Kaufman, eds. New York: Gardner Press.

Blum, T. C., and P. M. Roman. 1985. The social transformation of alcoholism intervention: Comparisons of job attitudes and performance of recovered alcoholics and non-alcoholics. Journal of Health and Social Behavior 26:365-378.

Borkman, T. 1986. The Alcohol Services Reporting System (ASRS) Revision Study. Prepared for the California State Department of Alcohol and Drug Programs, Health and Welfare Agency. Sacramento, Calif.

Boscarino, J. 1980. A national survey of alcoholism treatment centers in the United States: A preliminary report. American Journal of Drug and Alcohol Abuse 7:403-413.

Bowen, O. R., and J. H. Sammons. 1988. The alcohol abusing patient: A challenge to the profession. Journal of the American Medical Association 260:2267-2268.

Bradley, A. M. 1988. Keep coming back: The case for a valuation of Alcoholics Anonymous. Alcohol Health and Research World 12:192-199.

Bray, R. M., M. E. Marsden, L. L. Guess, S. C. Wheeless, D. K. Pate, G. H. Dunteman, and V. G. Innacchione. 1985. Highlights of the 1985 Worldwide Survey of Alcohol and Nonmedical Drug Use Among Military Personnel. Prepared for the Assistant Secretary of Defense (Health Affairs), Department of Defense. Research Triangle Park, N.C.: Research Triangle Institute.

Brown University Center for Alcohol Studies. 1984. Care for the Chronic Inebriate: Analysis and Recommendations. Prepared for the Rhode Island Department of Mental Health, Retardation, and Hospitals, Division of Substance Abuse. Providence, R.I.: Brown University Center for Alcohol Studies.

Brown University Center for Alcohol Studies. 1985. Substance Abuse Treatment in Rhode Island: Population Needs and Program Development. Prepared for the Rhode Island Department of Mental Health, Retardation, and Hospitals and the Department of Health. Cranston, R.I.: Rhode Island Department of Mental Health, Retardation, and Hospitals.

Butynski, W., and D. Canova. 1988. Alcohol problem resources and services in state supported programs, FY 1987. Public Health Reports 103:611-620.

Butynski, W., N. Record, P. Bruhn, and D. Canova. 1987. State Resources and Services Related to Alcohol and Drug Abuse Problems: Fiscal Year 1986. Prepared for the National Institute on Alcohol Abuse and Alcoholism and the National Institute on Drug Abuse. Washington, D.C.: National Association of State Alcohol and Drug Abuse Program Directors.

Cahalan, D. 1987. Understanding America's Drinking Problem: How to Combat the Hazards of Alcohol. San Francisco: Jossey-Bass.

California State Department of Alcohol and Drug Programs. 1988. California Alcohol Program State Plan: Fiscal Year 1987-1988. Sacramento: California State Department of Alcohol and Drug Programs.

Camp, J. M., and. N. R. Kurtz. 1982. Redirecting manpower for alcoholism treatment. Pp. 371-397 in Prevention, Intervention and Treatment: Concerns and Models, J. de Luca, ed. Washington, D.C.: U.S. Government Printing Office.

Cermak, T. L. Al-Anon and recovery. 1989. Pp. 91-104 in Recent Developments in Alcoholism: Emerging Issues in Treatment, vol. 7, M. Galanter, ed. New York: Plenum Press.

Cleary, P. D., M. Miller, B. T. Bush, M. M. Warburg, T. L. Delbanco, and M. D. Aronson. 1988. Prevalence and recognition of alcohol abuse in a primary care population. American Journal of Medicine 85:466-471.

Cotter, F., and C. Cahallan. 1987. Training primary care physicians to identify and treat substance abuse. Alcohol Health and Research World 11(4):70-73.

Creative Socio-Medics Corporation. 1981. An Analysis of Third-Party Funding in the Alcoholism Treatment Delivery System of the United States. Prepared for the National Institute on Alcohol Abuse and Alcoholism. Vienna, Va.: Creative Socio-Medics.

Davis, K. 1987. The organization and financing of alcohol and drug abuse services. Presented to the Annual Meeting of the Institute of Medicine, Washington, D.C., October 21, 1987.

Delaney, T. 1988. Statement presented to the open meeting of the Committee for the Study of Treatment and Rehabilitation Services for Alcoholism and Alcohol Abuse, Institute of Medicine, January 25.

DenHartog, G. L. 1982. "A Decade of Detox": Development of Non-hospital Approaches to Alcohol Detoxification—A Review of the Literature. Substance Abuse Monograph Series. Jefferson City, Miss.: Division of Alcohol and Drug Abuse.

Dibello, G. A. W., G. W. Weitz, D. Poynter-Berg, and J. L. Yurmak. 1982. Handbook of Psychiatric Partial Hospitalization. New York: Bruner-Mazel.

Diesenhaus, H. I. 1982. Current trends in treatment programming for problem drinkers and alcoholics. Pp. 219-290 in Prevention, Intervention, and Treatment: Concerns and Models, J. de Luca, ed. Washington, D.C.: U.S. Government Printing Office.

Diesenhaus, H. I., and R. Booth, eds. 1977. Cost-Benefit Study of State Hospital Drug and Alcohol Treatment Programs. Report submitted to the Joint Budget Committee, Colorado State Legislature, Denver. December.

Emrick, C.D. 1987. Alcoholics Anonymous: Affiliation processes and effectiveness as treatment. Alcoholism: Clinical and Experimental Research 11:416-423.

Emrick, C. D. 1989a. Alcoholics Anonymous: Emerging concepts. Pp. 3-10 in Recent Developments in Alcoholism: Emerging Issues in Treatment, vol. 7, M. Galanter, ed. New York: Plenum Press.

Emrick, C. D. 1989b. Alcoholics Anonymous: Membership characteristics and effectiveness as treatment. Pp. 37-53 in Recent Developments in Alcoholism: Emerging Issues in Treatment, vol. 7, M. Galanter, ed. New York: Plenum Press.

Errera, P., E. Nightingale, J. O. Lipkin, and M. L. F. Ashcroft. 1985. DRGs and psychiatry: Work in progress. General Hospital Psychiatry 7:316-320.

Finn, P. 1985. Decriminalization of public drunkenness: Response of the health care system. Journal of Studies on Alcohol 46:7-22.

Frankel, G. 1983. Alcoholism treatment in the partial hospital or day program. Alcohol Health and Research World 7(3):32-36.

Galanter, M., and M. Bean-Bayog. 1989. A study of physicians certified in alcohol and drug dependence. Alcoholism: Clinical and Experimental Research 13:1-2.

Galanter, M., E. Kaufman, Z. Taintor, C. B. Robinowitz, R. E. Meyer, and J. Halikas. 1989. The current status of psychiatric education in alcoholism and drug abuse. American Journal of Psychiatry 146:35-39.

Gallant, D. M. 1988. Alcoholism: A Guide to Diagnosis, Intervention, and Treatment. New York: Norton.

Gilbert, M. J., and R. C. Cervantes. 1986. Alcohol services for Mexican Americans: A review of utilization patterns, treatment considerations and prevention activities. Hispanic Journal of Behavioral Sciences 8:1-60.

Gilbert, M. J., and R. C. Cervantes. 1988. Alcohol treatment for Mexican Americans: A review of utilization patterns and therapeutic approaches. Pp. 199-231 in Alcohol Consumption among Mexicans and Mexican Americans: A Binational Perspective, M. J. Gilbert, ed. Los Angeles: Spanish Speaking Mental Health Research Center, University of California, Los Angeles.

Glaser, F. G., and A. Ogborne. 1982. Does A. A. really work? British Journal of Addictions 72:123-129.

Grad, F. P., A. L. Goldberg, and B. A. Shapiro. 1971. Alcoholism and the Law. Dobbs Ferry, N.Y.: Oceana Publications.

Gunnersen, U., and M. L. Feldman. 1978. Alcohol and Alcoholism Programs:. A Technical Assistance Manual for Health Systems Agencies. San Leandro, Calif.: Human Services, Inc.

Harrison, P. A., and N. G. Hoffmann. 1986. Chemical Dependency Inpatients and Outpatients: Intake Characteristics and Treatment Oucome. Prepared for the Chemical Dependency Program Division, Minnesota State Department of Human Services. St. Paul, Minn.: St. Paul-Ramsey Foundation.

Harwood, H. J., P. Kristiansen, and J. V. Rachal. 1985. Social and economic costs of alcohol abuse and alcoholism. Issue Report No. 2. Research Triangle Institute, Research Triangle Park, N.C.

Horizons Technology, Inc. 1988. Prevention Training: Final Report. Prepared for the Office of Substance Abuse Prevention of the Alcohol, Drug Abuse, and Mental Health Administration. Oakton, Va.: Horizons Technology, Inc., October 3.

Indian Health Service (IHS). 1989. A Progress Report on Indian Alcoholism Activities: 1988. Rockville, Md.: IHS.

Institute for Health and Aging. 1986. Review and Evaluation of Alcohol, Drug Abuse and Mental Health Services Block Grant Allotment Formulas: Final Report. Prepared for the Alcohol, Drug Abuse, and Mental Health Administration. San Francisco.

Institute of Medicine (IOM). 1989. Prevention and Treatment of Alcohol Problems: Research Opportunities. Washington, D.C.: National Academy Press.

Jacobs, O. 1985. Public and Private Sector Issues on Alcohol and Other Drug Abuse: A Special Report with Recommendations. Prepared for the Alcohol, Drug Abuse, and Mental Health Administration (ADAMHA). Rockville, Md.: ADAMHA.

Jackson, J. 1988. Testimony presented before the U. S. Senate Governmental Affairs Committee regarding the causes of and governmental responses to alcohol abuse and alcoholism, Washington, D.C., June 16.

Khantzian, E. J., and J. E. Mack. 1989. A.A. and contemporary psychodynamic theory. Pp. 67-89 in Recent Developments in Alcoholism, vol. 7, M. Galanter, ed. New York: Plenum Press.

Kissin, B. 1977. Theory and practice in the treatment of alcoholism. Pp. 1-51 in Treatment and Rehabilitation of the Chronic Alcoholic. Vol. 5 of The Biology of Alcoholism, B. Kissin and H. Begleiter, eds. New York: Plenum Press.

Kissin, B., and M. Hansen. 1985. Integration of biological and psychosocial interventions in the treatment of alcoholism. Pp. 63-103 in Future Directions in Alcohol Abuse Treatment Research, B. S. McCrady, N. E. Noel, and T. D. Nirenberg, eds. Washington, D.C.: U.S. Government Printing Office.

Kole, D. M., and L. Mitnick. 1978. Utilization and substitutability of alcohol, drug abuse, and mental health personnel. Pp. 107-118 in Working Papers and Other Supporting Documents. Vol. 2 of the Report of the ADAMHA Manpower Policy Analysis Task Force, D. M. Kole, ed. Rockville, Md.: Alcohol, Drug Abuse, and Mental Health Administration.

Kolodner, G. 1977. Ambulatory detoxification as an introduction to treatment. Pp. 311-317 in Currents in Alcoholism, vol. 1, F. A. Sexias, ed. New York: Grune and Stratton.

Krystal, H., and R. A. Moore. 1963. Who is qualified to treat the alcoholic: A discussion. Quarterly Journal on Studies of Alcoholism 24:705-718.

Kurtz, E. 1979. Not God: A History of Alcoholics Anonymous. Garden City, Minn.: Hazelden Foundation.

Laundergan, J. C. 1982. Easy Does It: Alcoholism Treatment Outcomes, Hazelden and the Minnesota Model. Minneapolis: Hazelden Foundation.

Lawrence Johnson and Associates, Inc. 1983. Evaluation of the HCFA Alcoholism Services Demonstration: Final Evaluation Design. Prepared for the Office of Research and Demonstrations, Health Care Financing Administration. Washington, D.C.

Leach, B., and J. L. Norris. 1977. Factors in the development of Alcoholics Anonymous. Pp. 441-543 in Treatment and Rehabilitation of the Chronic Alcoholic. Vol. 5 of The Biology of Alcoholism, B. Kissin and H. Begleiter, eds. New York: Plenum Press.

Lebenluft, E., and R. F. Lebenluft. 1988. Reimbursement for partial hospitalization: A survey and policy implications. American Journal of Psychiatry 145:1514-1520.

Lemere, F., R. J. Williams, E. M. Scott, R. G. Bell, D. B. Falkey, and D. J. Myerson. 1964. Who is qualified to treat the alcoholic? Comment on the Krystal-Moore discussion. Quarterly Journal of Studies on Alcoholism 25:558-572.

Lewin/ICF. 1989a. Analysis of State Alcohol and Drug Data Collection Instruments, vols.1-6. Prepared for the Office of Finance and Coverage Policy, National Institute on Drug Abuse. Washington, D.C., March.

Lewin/ICF. 1989b. Feasibility and Design of a Study of the Delivery and Financing of Drug and Alcohol Services. Prepared for the National Institute on Drug Abuse of the Alcohol, Drug Abuse, and Mental Health Administration. Washington, D.C., April 26.

Lewis, D. C., and A. J. Gordon. 1983. Alcoholism and the general hospital: The Roger Williams intervention program. Bulletin of the New York Acadamy of Medicine 59:181-197.

Lewis, D. C., R. G. Niven, D. Czechowicz, and J. G. Trumble. 1987. A review of medical education in alcohol and other drug abuse. Journal of the American Medical Association 257:2945-2948.

Longabaugh, R. 1980. The Cost-Effectiveness of Partial Hospitalization vs. Continued Inpatient Treatment in the Treatment of Alcoholism. Prepared for Blue Cross and Blue Shield of Rhode Island. Providence, R.I.: Butler Hospital.

Longabaugh, R., B. S. McCrady, E. Fink, R. Stout, T. McCauley, and D. McNeill. 1983. Cost effectiveness of alcoholism treatment in partial versus inpatient settings: Six month outcomes. Journal of Studies on Alcohol 44:1049-1071.

Macro Systems, Inc. 1980. Final Report: Federal Activities on Alcohol Abuse and Alcoholism: FY 1978. Prepared for the National Institute on Alcohol Abuse and Alcoholism. Silver Spring, Md.: Macro Systems, Inc.

McAuliffe, W. E., P. Breer, N. White, C. Spino, L. Goldsmith, S. Robel, and L. Byam. 1988. A Drug Abuse Treatment and Intervention Plan for Rhode Island. Cranston, R.I.: Rhode Island Department of Mental Health, Retardation, and Hospitals.

McCarthy, D., and M. Argeriou. 1988. Rearrest following residential treatment for repeat offender drunken drivers. Journal of Studies on Alcohol 49:1-6.

McCrady, B. S., L. Dean, E. Dubreil, and S. Swanson. 1985. The Problem Drinkers Program: A programmatic application of social learning based treatment. Pp. 417-471 in Relapse Prevention, G. A. Marlatt and J. Gordon, eds. New York: Guilford Press.

McCrady, B. S., R. Longabaugh, E. Fink, R. Stout, M. Beatie, and A. Ruggeri-Authelet. 1986. Cost effectiveness of alcoholism treatment in partial versus inpatient settings: 12-month outcomes. Journal of Consulting and Clinical Psychology 54:708-713.

McGovern, T. F. 1986. Our professional identity—birth, infancy, and adolescence of our profession. The Counselor 4(4):7-9, 30.

McGovern, T. F. 1988. Executive summary: Issues in the training and credentialing of substance abuse counselors. Prepared for the Committee for the Study of Treatment and Rehabilitation Services for Alcoholism and Alcohol Abuse., May.

McGovern, T. F., and D. Armstrong. 1986. Comparison of recovering and non-alcoholic counselors: A survey. Alcoholism Treatment Quarterly 4(1):43-60.

McLachlan, J. F. C., and R. L. Stein. 1982. Evaluation of a day clinic for alcoholics. Journal of Studies on Alcohol 43:261-272.

Miller, W. R., and R. K. Hester. 1986. Inpatient alcoholism treatment: Who benefits? American Psychologist 41:794-805.

Minnesota State Chemical Dependency Program Division. 1987. Biennial Report to the Governor and the Minnesota Legislature. St. Paul: Minnesota State Department of Human Services.

Minnesota State Chemical Dependency Program Division. 1987. Directory of Chemical Dependency Programs in Minnesota: 1987/1988. St. Paul: Minnesota State Department of Human Services.

Minnesota State Chemical Dependency Program Division. 1989. Report to the State Legislature on the Status of the Consolidated Chemical Dependency Treatment Fund. St. Paul: Minnesota State Department of Human Services.

Mitnick, L. 1978. Manpower issues in community alcoholism programs. Pp. 159-169 in Report of the ADAMHA Manpower Policy Analysis Task Force. Vol. 2, Working Papers and Other Supporting Documents, D. M. Kole, ed. Rockville, Md.: Alcohol, Drug Abuse, and Mental Health Administration.

Mitnick, L., and D. M. Kole. Credentials. Pp. 119-123 in Report of the ADAMHA Manpower Policy Analysis Task Force. Vol. 2. Working Papers and Other Supporting Documents, D. M. Kole, ed. Rockville, Md.: Alcohol, Drug Abuse, and Mental Health Administration.

Morehouse, E. R. 1984. Preventing Alcohol Problems Through a Student Assistance Program. Washington, D.C.: U.S. Government Printing Office.

Nace, E. P. 1987. The Treatment of Alcoholism. New York: Bruner-Mazel.

National Council on Alcoholism (NCA). 1987. A Federal Response to a Hidden Epidemic: Alcohol and Other Drug Problems Among Women. New York: NCA.

National Institute on Alcohol Abuse and Alcoholism (NIAAA). 1983a. National Drug and Alcoholism Treatment Utilization Survey. Executive Report. Rockville, Md: NIAAA.

National Institute on Alcohol Abuse and Alcoholism (NIAAA). 1983b. Report to the United States Congress on Federal Activities on Alcohol Abuse and Alcoholism. Rockville, Md.: NIAAA.

National Institute on Alcohol Abuse and Alcoholism/National Institute on Drug Abuse (NIAAA/NIDA). 1989. Health Professions Education Program. Rockville, Md.: NIAAA/ NIDA.

National Institute on Drug Abuse/National Institute on Alcohol Abuse and Alcoholism (NIDA/NIAAA). 1989. Highlights from the 1987 National Drug and Alcoholism Treatment Unit Survey (NDATUS). Rockville, Md.: NIDA/NIAAA.

New York State Division of Alcoholism and Alcohol Abuse (NYDAAA). 1989a. DAAA Awards Grants to 11 Hospitals to Improve Ways to Refer Patients for Alcoholism Treatment. Albany, N.Y.: NYDAAA.

New York State Division of Alcoholism and Alcohol Abuse (NYDAAA). 1989b. Five Year Comprehensive Plan for Alcoholism Services in New York State: 1989-1994. Albany, N.Y.: NYDAAA.

Nightingale, E. J. 1986. Experience with prospective payment in the Veterans Administration. American Psychologist 41:70-72.

Ogborne, A. C. 1989. Some limitations of Alcoholics Anonymous. Pp. 55-65 in Recent Developments in Alcoholism: Emerging Issues in Treatment, vol. 7, M. Galanter, ed. New York: Plenum Press.

Ogborne, A. C., and F. B. Glaser. 1981. Characteristics of the affiliates of Alcoholics Anonymous: A review of the literature. Journal of Studies on Alcohol 42:661-675.

Orvis, B. R., D. J. Armor, C. E. Williams, A. J. Barras, and D. S. Schwarzbach. 1981. Effectiveness and Cost of Alcohol Rehabilitation in the United States Air Force. Santa Monica, Calif.: RAND Corporation.

Pattison, E. M. 1974. Rehabilitation of the chronic alcoholic. Pp. 587-658 in Clinical Pathology. Vol. 3 of The Biology of Alcoholism, B. Kissin and H. Begleiter, eds. New York: Plenum Press.

Pattison, E. M. 1977. Ten years of change in alcoholism treatment and delivery systems. American Journal of Psychiatry 134:261-266.

Pattison, E. M., M. B. Sobell, and L. C. Sobell. 1977. Emerging Concepts of Alcohol Dependence. New York: Springer Publishing Company.

Pattison, E. M. 1985. The selection of treatment modalities for the alcoholic patient. Pp. 189-294 in The Diagnosis and Treatment of Alcoholism, 2d ed., J. H. Mendelson and N. K. Mello, eds. New York: McGraw-Hill.

Pattison, E. M., R. Coe, and H. O. Doer. 1978. Population variation among alcoholism treatment facilities. International Journal of the Addictions 8:199-229.

Plaut, T. F. A., ed. 1967. Alcohol Problems: A Report to the Nation. New York: Oxford University Press.

Regier, D. A., I. D. Goldberg, and C. A. Taube. 1978. The de facto U.S. mental health services system: A public health perspective. Archives of General Psychiatry 35:685-693.

Reed, P. G., and D. S. Sanchez. 1986. Characteristics of Alcoholism Services in the United States-1984: Data from the September 1984 National Alcoholism and Drug Abuse Program Inventory. Rockville, Md.: National Institute on Alcohol Abuse and Alcoholism.

Rhoades, E. R., R. Mason, P. Eddy, E. M. Smith, and T. R. Burns. 1988. The Indian Health Service approach to alcoholism among American Indians and Alaskan Natives. Public Health Reports 103:621-627.

Robinson, D., and S. Henry. 1979. Alcoholics Anonymous in England and Wales: Basic results from a survey. British Journal of Alcohol and Alcoholism 13(1):36-44.

Roman, P. M. 1981. From employee alcoholism to employee assistance. Journal of Studies on Alcohol 42:244-272.

Roman, P. M. 1982. Employee alcoholism programs in major corporations in 1979: Scope, change, and receptivity. Pp. 177-200 in Prevention, Intervention, and Treatment: Concerns and Models, J. de Luca, ed. Washington, D.C.: U.S. Government Printing Office.

Roman, P. M., and T. C. Blume. 1985. The core technology of employee assistance. The ALMACAN 15(3):8-1.

Rosenberg, C. M. 1982. The paraprofessionals in alcoholism treatment. Pp. 802-809 in Encyclopedic Handbook of Alcoholism, E. M. Pattison and E. Kaufman, eds. New York: Gardner Press.

Roy Littlejohn Associates, Inc. 1974. Proposed National Standards for Alcoholism Counselors--Final Report. Prepared for the National Institute on Alcohol Abuse and Alcoholism. Washington, D.C.

Royce, J. E. 1981. Alcoholic Problems and Alcoholism. New York: Collier-Macmillan.

Rudy, D. 1986. Becoming Alcoholic: Alcoholics and the Reality of Alcoholism. Carbondale, Ill.: Southern Illinois University Press.

Sadd, S., and D. W. Young. 1986. A Controlled Study of Detoxification Alternatives for Homeless Alcoholics. New York: Vera Institute of Justice.

Saxe, L., D. Dougherty,. K. Esty, and M. Fine. 1983. The Effectiveness and Costs of Alcoholism Treatment. Washington, D.C.: U.S. Congress, Office of Technology Assessment.

Sonnestuhl, W. J., and H. M. Trice. 1986. Strategies for Employee Assistance Programs: The Crucial Balance. Ithaca, N.Y.: ILR Press.

Staub, G. E., and L. M. Kent, eds. 1973. The Paraprofessional in the Treatment of Alcoholism. Springfield, Ill.: Charles C. Thomas.

Stinson, D. J., W. G. Smith, I. Amidjaya, and J. Kaplan. 1979. Systems of care and treatment outcomes for alcoholic patients. Archives of General Psychiatry 36:535-539.

Stoil, M. 1987. Salvation and sobriety. Alcohol Health and Research World 11(3):14-17.

Tournier, R. 1979. Alcoholics Anonymous as treatment and ideology. Journal of Studies on Alcohol 40:230-239.

Trice, H. M., and M. Schonbrun, 1981. A history of job-based alcoholism programs. Journal of Drug Issues 11:171-198.

Trice, H. M., and W. J. Staudemeier. 1989. A sociocultural history of Alcoholics Anonymous. Pp. 11-95 in Recent Developments in Alcoholism: Emerging Issues in Treatment, vol. 7, M. Galanter, ed. New York: Plenum Press.

U.S. Department of Health and Human Services (USDHHS). 1981. Fourth Special Report to the U. S. Congress on Alcohol and Health. Rockville, Md.: National Institute on Alcohol Abuse and Alcoholism.

U.S. Department of Health and Human Services (USDHHS). 1985. Fifth Special Report to the U.S. Congress on Alcohol and Health. Rockville, Md.: National Institute on Alcohol Abuse and Alcoholism.

U.S. Department of Health and Human Services (USDHHS). 1986. Toward a National Plan to Combat Alcohol Abuse and Alcoholism. Report Submitted to the United States Congress. Rockville, Md.: National Institute on Alcohol Abuse and Alcoholism.

U.S. Department of Health and Human Services (USDHHS). 1987a. 1987 National Drug and Alcoholism Treatment Unit Survey: NDATUS Instruction Manual for States and Reporting Units. Rockville, Md.: National Institute on Drug Abuse and National Institute on Alcohol Abuse and Alcoholism.

U.S. Department of Health and Human Services (USDHHS). 1987b. Sixth Special Report to the U.S. Congress on Alcohol and Health. Rockville, Md.: National Institute on Alcohol Abuse and Alcoholism.

U.S. Department of Health, Education, and Welfare (USDHHS). 1971. First Special Report to the U.S. Congress on Alcohol and Health. Rockville, Md.: National Institute on Alcohol Abuse and Alcoholism.

Veterans Administration (VA). 1977. Mental Health and Behavioral Sciences Service Program Guide: Alcohol Dependence Treatment Program. Washington, D.C.: VA.

Veterans Administration (VA). 1987. Annual Report, 1986. Washington, D.C.: U.S. Government Printing Office.

Wallen, J. 1988. Alcoholism treatment service systems: a health services research perspective. Public Health Reports 103:605-611.

Weisner, C. 1986. The social ecology of alcohol treatment in the United States. Pp. 203-243 in Recent Developments in Alcoholism, vol. 5, M. Galanter, ed. New York: Plenum Press.

Weisner, C., and R. Room. 1984. Financing and ideology in alcohol treatment. Social Problems 32:167-184.

Williams, C. N., D. C. Lewis, J. Femino, L. Hall, K. Blackburn-Kilduff, R. Rosen, and C. Samella. 1985. Overcoming barriers to identification and referral of alcoholics in a general hospital setting: One approach. Rhode Island Medical Journal 68:131-138.

Wilson, R., and P. Hartsock. 1981. Current Practices in Alcoholism Treatment Needs Estimation: A State-of-the-Art Report. Prepared for the National Institute on Alcohol Abuse and Alcoholism. Gaithersburg, Md.: Alcohol Epidemiologic Data System.

Yahr, H. T. 1988. A national comparison of public- and private-sector alcoholism treatment delivery system characteristics. Journal of Studies on Alcohol 49:233-239.

Ziener, G. 1988. Surf and turf: A historical perspective on past alcohol and drug abuse training systems. Pp. B1-B10 in Prevention Training: Final Report, Horizons Technology, Inc. Prepared for the Office of Substance Abuse Prevention of the Alcohol, Drug Abuse, and Mental Health Administration. Oakton, Va.: Horizons Technology, Inc.

Zimberg, S. 1974. Evaluation of alcoholism treatment in Harlem. Quarterly Journal of Studies on Alcohol 35:550-557.

Zimberg, S. 1983. Comprehensive model of alcoholism treatment in a general hospital. Bulletin of the New York Academy of Medicine 59(2): 222-229.

5 Does Treatment Work?

A potential hazard of framing simple questions is that they may evoke simplistic answers. The committee has nevertheless entitled this chapter "Does Treatment Work?" because "this question is put to us by patients, legislators, referring physicians, social planners, and many others" (Gottheil, 1985). Some have chosen to answer the question as it stands, usually with an unqualified affirmative. The committee, however, concurs with the opinion of Sanchez-Craig (1986) that "both the question and its answer are exceedingly complex" and believes that a more helpful and productive answer will be forthcoming if the question is reframed.

Reframing the Question

An examination of several problems inherent in the usual form of this question is instructive and can guide the reframing process. As it stands, the question seems to imply that there is a single or unitary phenomenon that is to be dealt with; however, as discussed in Chapter 1, alcohol problems are multiple and diverse. The question also focuses only on the problems themselves and not on the individuals who manifest them. It appears to overlook the reality of the current therapeutic effort, which consists of many treatments rather than a single standardized form of treatment (see Chapter 3).

In addition, the question seems to imply a "one-shot" approach to the treatment of alcohol problems, in which a single episode of treatment is the exclusive focus of attention. Some individuals may achieve lasting positive results from such an episode, but for others a satisfactory outcome hinges on many episodes of treatment, often of different kinds and often delivered over an extended period of time. As a useful (albeit limited) analogy, some forms of cancer may be effectively dealt with by a single treatment episode, but other cancers may require repeated episodes of care, as well as combinations or sequences of several treatments (surgery, radiation, and chemotherapy).

The simple form of the question "Does treatment work?" also places too much weight on treatment; it does not put the treatment process into an appropriate perspective. As has been particularly emphasized in the work of Rudolf Moos and his associates (Cronkhite and Moos, 1978, 1980; Moos et al., 1982; Moos et al., 1990), treatment is only one of many factors that contribute to outcome. Among the others are the characteristics of the individual who manifests the problem, the characteristics of the problem itself, and the characteristics of the individual's posttreatment experiences. For example, the probability of a positive outcome in a psychotic, homeless individual presenting for treatment with delirium tremens is likely to be lower than that for a mildly anxious, socially stable individual presenting in a sober state without withdrawal symptoms, even assuming that each person receives appropriate treatment.

Finally, there is an implication in the question that there may be a uniform criterion for "working," that is, some absolute standard for outcome. In a very general sense, one could say that such goals as "health" or "increased well-being" or "reduction or elimination of alcohol consumption" represent such standards. Clinicians, however, are aware of the need for flexible goals adapted to individual circumstances. A goal of no further episodes of delirium tremens in the first individual mentioned in the preceding paragraph would represent a major achievement for him but would be totally irrelevant for the second individual.

For these as well as other reasons, the question as it stands requires elaboration. Reframing questions of this kind is an approach that has been taken in other areas of therapeutics such as psychotherapy, in which the simple question "Does psychotherapy work?" has given rise to similar problems (Kiesler, 1966; Paul, 1967). Here, the expanded question may be framed as follows: Which kinds of individuals, with what kinds of alcohol problems, are likely to respond to what kinds of treatments by achieving what kinds of goals when delivered by which kinds of practitioners? (Cf. Pattison et al., 1977.)

Answering the Reframed Question: Methods

If there has been a tendency to frame and to respond in a simplistic manner to questions regarding whether treatment works, there has also been a similar tendency in operation with respect to choosing the appropriate *method* for making such determinations. To wit: to determine whether treatment works, one conducts a randomized controlled trial (RCT).

The Randomized Controlled Trial

The RCT has an important and even crucial role to play in the overall process of examining the results of treatment. Nevertheless, it is only a partial role; realistically, the RCT should be seen as only one of a number of methods for exploring the results of treatment. Given the complexity of treatment, such a perspective should not be surprising, but there has been a tendency to view the RCT as the "gold standard" for all judgments regarding treatment outcome. Perhaps it should be viewed more as a bronze standard, that is, as a significant part of an alloy that has other important constituents as well.

In a randomized controlled trial, individuals who manifest the target problem are randomly assigned either to the treatment method being studied or to a control (no-treatment) or comparison (other-treatment) condition or conditions. A number of methods may be used for implementing random assignment, such as tables of random numbers, the drawing of lots, or even the flipping of a coin; what is crucial is that every subject in the study have an equal probability of being assigned to each group in the study. The purpose of the random assignment is to make any differences between the treatment group(s) and the control or comparison group(s) chance differences rather than systematic differences. Outcome is then determined for all groups. Because there are no systematic differences relevant to outcome between the groups (because of the randomization procedure), and because one group has received the treatment being examined and the other (or others) has not, differences in outcome beyond what might be expected by chance alone can with some confidence be attributed to the effects of the treatment.

This methodology can be used to address a wide variety of issues that arise in treatment. In one study, for example, individuals seen at a treatment center without access to inpatient beds were referred elsewhere when it seemed indicated but were invited to return following their inpatient experience. Because many did not do so, it was felt that "a personal letter expressing concern for the patient's well-being and repeating our invitation for further assistance" might increase the rate of return. To test this idea, half of the next 100 patients were selected at random to receive such a letter. Of the group that received the letter, 50 percent returned; only 31 percent of those who did not receive the letter returned. Because this result was well beyond what could have been expected on the basis of chance, it was concluded that the letter was effective in promoting further contact with the program (Koumans and Muller, 1965).

Although this example seems both straightforward and useful, RCTs have not been widely utilized in clinical treatment programs. Furthermore, when they have been used, it has often been to examine only the outcome of treatment rather than to examine other issues.   The reasons for such restricted use of what is clearly a broadly applicable methodology have not been systematically studied.   They seem to lie partly in the method itself but, significantly, in the social ecology of treatment and research as well.

Even though taking therapeutic action with respect to a given problem and observing the effects of that action would seem to be closely related activities—perhaps even two aspects of the same activity—they are not always perceived as such.   The activities of clinicians and researchers have sometimes been viewed as antagonistic: clinicians treat, and researchers observe.   The pathways to becoming a clinician and to becoming a researcher have in like manner been perceived as sharply divergent.   One becomes a clinician, it is sometimes argued, through experience; one becomes a researcher through study.   Treatment is a practical discipline; research is an academic discipline.   The clinician's knowledge is intuitive; the researcher's knowledge is experimental.   Although these dichotomies may be artificial and exaggerated, and the activities involved may in fact be complementary (cf. Blackburn, 1971), with few exceptions the gulf between clinician and researcher is a regrettable reality in the treatment of alcohol problems (cf. Kalb and Propper, 1976; Cook, 1985).

Differing "cultures" have grown up around the treatment of alcohol problems on the one hand and research on such problems on the other.   These cultures shape the actions of those who are part of them.   The RCT is part of the culture of research; it is not part of the culture of treatment.   Regrettably, it seems a common perspective that RCTs are carried out by researchers and not by clinicians.   The committee believes these cultural differences have much to do with the relative absence of RCTs from clinical settings in the field of alcohol treatment.

Yet there are also practical reasons for the absence of RCTs from the clinical setting.   The conduct of such trials involves the exercise of a level of methodological sophistication that is beyond the capability of many clinical treatment programs.   That no treatment at all might be as effective as the treatment they offer is understandably not a proposition most clinical programs will readily entertain; in addition, because most do not offer alternative interventions (cf. Glaser et al., 1978), comparison studies often are not feasible.   There is evidence that many persons who seek treatment do not understand the process of random assignment, even when it has been extensively explained (Appelbaum et al., 1983).   At the same time there is evidence that those who volunteer for random assignment to treatment have a systematically poorer prognosis than those who decline to volunteer (Longabaugh and Lewis, 1988).

Deeply felt ethical concerns may make it difficult for clinicians to entertain the possibility of referral to controlled trials.   Clinicians are sought out for their informed opinions as to what kind of treatment might be best for a particular individual.   As they often have definite opinions on such questions, whether substantiated by well-controlled studies or not, they may feel remiss if they do not provide their personal view, albeit in a highly qualified form, when it is urgently solicited.   A medical ethicist has commented on this problem:

> One could readily concede that the preference of a physician, unsupported
> by adequate scientific evidence, is relatively unreliable, but one might
> nevertheless insist that patients are entitled to know of such preferences
> (accompanied by appropriate warnings as to their merely intuitive nature).
> For a physician to withhold such information would be to violate his
> patient's right to the best possible care. (Schafer, 1982:723)

Under these circumstances, referral to a trial in which treatment is selected by chance alone is quite unlikely to ensue (cf. Marquis, 1983; Angell, 1984; Taylor et al., 1984).

There is a further problem regarding the generalizability of results from RCTs. Although the subjects of controlled trials can certainly be individuals who are enrolled in standard treatment programs (as in the example given above), in many instances they tend to be highly selected. This selectivity is often introduced with the intent of making the results of the study more clear-cut and understandable. It nevertheless involves a distortion of the usual clinical situation that may limit the applicability of the study.

For example, researchers with the Cardiovascular Disease Databank at Duke University Medical Center, which contains information on all patients with suspected coronary artery disease seen at the center, compared the characteristics of their patients with the eligibility criteria of three large randomized trials of coronary bypass surgery. They found that (respectively) only 13 percent, 8 percent, and 4 percent of their patients met these criteria. The researchers concluded that "the results of these RCTs. . .apply directly to only a small fraction of the patients with coronary disease, and it is uncertain whether one can extrapolate from the results in a highly selected subgroup to the general population of patients" (Hlatky et al., 1984:377).

Even in instances in which such selection is not a problem, generalization may still be difficult. The RCT has proven to be an indispensable method of documenting the effectiveness of drugs and procedures in general medicine. Such procedures, however, and especially such medications are highly likely to be uniform across different treatment settings. Treatments of the sort generally used to deal with alcohol problems are much less likely to be uniform. Without special efforts of the kind that are becoming increasingly common in most areas of behavioral research (see Chapter 11), such interventions as group therapy, individual psychotherapy, and even Alcoholics Anonymous meetings are likely to be highly variable from one setting to the next. Although the comparability of medications cannot be taken for granted (Koch-Weser, 1974), two standard doses of, for example, insulin, are much more likely to be comparable than two sessions of "usual" group therapy.

Thus, there are difficulties in the application of RCTs to clinical treatment programs. Some of these problems have to do with the inherent attributes of the methodology itself, such as its complexity and the difficulties experienced by persons seeking treatment in understanding the concept of randomization. Many other problems have to do with factors external to the methodology, such as the way in which it tends to be used. The committee regrets that RCTs are not more frequently utilized in clinical settings to explore critical issues, and it favors efforts to assist in the more frequent deployment of this methodology. But it views these efforts as necessarily long-term and believes that, in the shorter term, alternative methodologies that avoid some of the problems noted above (although they may be subject to other difficulties) could usefully be broadly deployed in clinical treatment programs as an important complement to RCTs.

Defining some of the terms employed in discussing the results of treatment may be a useful way of placing the RCT in perspective. Among the more prominent are efficacy and effectiveness. *Efficacy* refers to the probability of benefit to individuals in a defined population from a treatment provided for a given problem under ideal conditions of use (modified from Lohr et al., 1988). A test of efficacy answers the question "*Can* treatment work?" *Effectiveness* reflects the probability of benefit when the treatment is applied under ordinary conditions by the average therapist to a typical individual requiring treatment (modified from Lohr et al., 1988). A test of effectiveness answers the question "*Does* treatment work?"

In terms of methodology the RCT is the method that can most convincingly demonstrate either efficacy or effectiveness. It has in general been used to demonstrate efficacy, which is another way of saying that it has tended to be used in research settings by academically trained clinical researchers. Although it could be used by clinicians in clinical settings to demonstrate effectiveness, and the committee would strongly support its use in this manner, there are many difficulties in the way (see above) that are not likely to be readily resolved. *An alternative course is to deploy a methodology in treatment settings that, if not as powerful as the RCT, nevertheless provides data that are useful in themselves, that speak to the issue of effectiveness, and that complement what can be learned from RCTs conducted in other settings.*

As will be discussed further in Chapter 12, systematic monitoring of the outcome of treatment is such a method. To know that a high percentage of individuals who pass through a particular treatment program subsequently achieve a positive outcome is knowledge worth having for its own sake. Because in the usual outcome monitoring study there is no identical comparison group, this type of study does not prove that the good results observed were due to the treatment provided, although it does suggest that the program *may* be effective. However, if randomized controlled trials have suggested that the method of treatment being provided is effective, a greater level of confidence can be entertained that the treatment provided in the program monitored is efficacious—that it may have been a significant factor in producing the positive outcomes that were observed.

Although outcome monitoring is a far less complex methodology than the conduct of RCTs, it has not been widely used in examining the treatment of alcohol problems. There are, however, signs that this is changing, both in the public sector (e.g., the state of Minnesota requires all publicly funded programs to participate in some form of outcome monitoring) and in the private sector (e.g., the Chemical Abuse/Addictions Treatment Outcome Registry, or CATOR, an outcome-monitoring service, is increasingly subscribed to by private treatment programs). The committee applauds such efforts and considers the broad application of outcome monitoring to be both feasible and desirable. (See Chapter 12 for a more detailed discussion.) If coupled with a more general use of RCTs in research settings (IOM, 1989), regular outcome monitoring in clinical settings would represent a highly significant advance in the treatment of alcohol problems.

The Role of Quality Assurance

For a convincing demonstration of efficacy or effectiveness to occur, mechanisms should be in place to assure "truth in packaging"—that the treatment allegedly being delivered is actually being delivered and that it is being delivered appropriately. Accomplishing this assurance involves such activities as the selection, training, and monitoring of treatment staff. (These activities and others like them are part and parcel of RCTs, but the term *quality assurance* is usually applied only to realistic treatment situations.)

The necessity for quality assurance activities arises from long experience. Not all alcohol treatment programs succeed in providing what they claim to be providing (Moffett et al., 1975). Programs vary. Key staff leave; new staff are hired. Various staff differ considerably in background, training, orientation, personal characteristics, and so forth. In the absence of quality assurance mechanisms the treatment activities of individual staff members may evolve in differing and idiosyncratic therapeutic directions. The need for quality assurance is not unique to the treatment of alcohol problems but is common to all therapeutic situations (cf. Eddy and Billings, 1988; Lohr et al., 1988; Roper et al., 1988).

Other Methods

In addition to the RCT and outcome monitoring, there are other methods that can yield useful and important information regarding the impact of treatment on persons with problems. The individual case study is an example. Surveys of consumer satisfaction are another. In recent years much attention has been given to quasi-experimental methods of studying treatment. In short, many methods are available that can add to our understanding of the results of treatment, and they may all be required to fully comprehend so complex an undertaking. A single method, by itself, will not suffice.

Answering the Reframed Question: Results

Workers in the alcohol treatment field have done yeoman service in attempting to answer questions of treatment efficacy and effectiveness. One estimate is that more than 600 treatment outcome studies have been completed, about half of which have been completed in the 1980s; among these there have been approximately 200 comparative clinical trials, about two-thirds of which have employed random assignment (Miller, 1988; IOM, 1989). In addition to these original studies, the subject has been repeatedly reviewed over the last four decades (cf. Bowman and Jellinek, 1941; Voegtlin and Lemere, 1942; Hill and Blane, 1967; Pattison, 1974; Baekeland et al., 1975; Emrick, 1975; Clare, 1976; Baekeland, 1977; Emrick, 1979; Diesenhaus, 1982; Miller and Hester, 1986; Annis, 1987; IOM, 1989). This body of work represents a commendable and important effort.

What conclusions can be drawn? As with any large and diverse body of information, the data admit of differing interpretations. During the course of the present study the assembly and analysis of information on treatment efficacy and effectiveness was undertaken jointly by this committee and IOM's Committee to Identify Research Opportunities for the Prevention and Treatment of Alcohol-Related Problems. The results appear as part of this second committee's report (IOM, 1989). The relevant chapter of that report is reproduced here as Appendix B for the convenience of the reader.

Many of the conclusions noted in the appended material are directly applicable to the work of this committee; a few are specifically responsive to our sister committee's charge and are therefore beyond the purview of this group. Other conclusions have been modified to reflect accurately the particular views of the committee for the present study. Its somewhat modified conclusions, which are supported by the material and the citations to be found in the appendix, are as follows:

1. *There is no single treatment approach that is effective for all persons with alcohol problems.* A number of different treatment methods show promise in particular groups. Reason for optimism in the treatment of alcohol problems lies in the range of promising alternatives that are available, each of which may be optimal for different types of individuals.

For example, a series of studies on heterogeneous treatment populations has shown no overall advantage in terms of outcome for residential or inpatient treatment over outpatient treatment. Each treatment setting may be most appropriate for particular persons. Specifically, nonhospital residential care may be most appropriate for individuals who are socially unstable (i.e., who are homeless, unemployed, etc.) but who do not have coexisting acute medical or severe psychiatric problems. Inpatient hospital care may be most appropriate for persons with coexisting acute medical or severe psychiatric problems, regardless of their level of social stability. Outpatient care may be indicated for socially stable individuals who do not have coexisting acute medical or severe psychiatric problems.

2. *The provision of appropriate, specific treatment modalities can substantially improve outcome.* A variety of specific treatment methods for alcohol problems has been associated with increased improvement, relative to no treatment or alternative treatments, in controlled studies.

3. *Brief interventions can be quite effective compared with no treatment, and they can be quite cost-effective compared with more intensive treatment.* For some people with alcohol problems, relatively minimal interventions have been shown to be significantly more effective than no intervention and on a cost-effectiveness basis may compare favorably with more intensive treatment (see Chapter 9). The low cost and simple nature of brief interventions render them accessible to a broad range of persons with alcohol problems who might otherwise not receive treatment.

4. *Treatment of other life problems related to drinking can improve outcome in persons with alcohol problems.* Posttreatment problems and experiences have been shown to be important determinants of outcome. Social skills training, marital and family therapy, antidepressant medication, stress management training, and the community reinforcement approach all show promise for promoting and prolonging favorable outcome. Such broad-spectrum strategies seem to affect outcome by helping to resolve other significant life problems that, if left untreated, could precipitate relapse.

5. *Therapist characteristics are determinants of outcome.* Treatment is not offered by neutral agents. Therapist skills and attributes can be important factors in influencing treatment outcome. The interaction of therapist variables with treatment variables and with variables of the individuals manifesting alcohol problems, as well as the more direct effects (main effects) of therapist characteristics, has been shown to account for a substantial amount of variance in motivation, drop-out, compliance, and outcome.

6. *Outcomes are determined in part by treatment process factors, posttreatment adjustment factors, the characteristics of individuals seeking treatment, the characteristics of their problems, and the interactions among these factors.* Individual difference variables that are nonspecific (e.g., resistance to treatment) or specific to particular approaches (e.g., the establishment of a conditioned aversion response) have been shown to predict treatment outcome. Recent research on pretreatment matching likewise indicates that responses to a particular treatment may depend on the personal and problem characteristics of those seeking treatment.

7. *People who are treated for alcohol problems achieve a continuum of outcomes with respect to drinking behavior and alcohol problems and follow different courses of outcome.* Drinking behavior following treatment ranges from an increase in drinking, to no change in drinking, to a reduction in drinking but with continuing problems, to problem-free drinking, to total abstinence. Alcohol problems may increase or decrease following treatment. Some treated individuals show initial improvement with subsequent deterioration ("faders"). Others show a gradual increase in improvement ("sleepers"). Still others oscillate between outcomes (e.g., between abstinence and problem-free drinking or between abstinence and problem drinking).

8. *Those who significantly reduce their level of alcohol consumption or who become totally abstinent usually enjoy improvement in other life areas, particularly as the period of reduced consumption becomes more extended.* Treatment for alcohol problems thus wisely emphasizes the importance of significantly reducing or eliminating alcohol consumption.

The committee views these conclusions as somewhat tentative but highly encouraging. They are tentative both because additional replications of completed studies are needed and because many treatment methods have not been evaluated under a range of circumstances—for example, with many different kinds of persons. Moreover, new treatment methods are constantly being developed, and various combinations and sequences of treatment methods require exploration. There is no foreseeable end to the need for information regarding the impact of treatment. Its investigation is part and parcel of the provision of treatment (see Chapter 12).

The conclusions are viewed as highly encouraging because they suggest that treating people with alcohol problems is an endeavor that can produce very positive results. Although it is not realistic to expect outstanding results in every instance, some such results will occur, and most persons can be helped in some way. The conclusions contain many important indications of improvements that might be made in current treatment practices. These suggestions will be dealt with in more detail in the balance of this report.

Summary and Conclusions

The simplistic question "Does treatment work?" needs to be reframed. In its stark, albeit common, form, it does not reflect accurately the complexities of the therapeutic situation or current understanding of the results of treatment research. A preferable version of the question is the following: Which kinds of individuals, with what kinds of alcohol problems, are likely to respond to what kinds of treatments by achieving what kinds of goals when delivered by which kinds of practitioners?

The ongoing effort to provide appropriate answers to this reframed question requires the deployment of a variety of investigative methods. Although the randomized controlled trial (RCT) has many advantages and should be more broadly used to answer questions of clinical relevance, it has disadvantages that tend to limit its widespread application in clinical treatment settings. Alternative methodologies, if less powerful in terms of the demonstration of treatment efficacy, may nevertheless be more widely applicable and can provide information to complement that derived from RCTs.

Based on treatment research efforts to date, which should be continued and extended, the committee believes that some necessarily tentative but highly encouraging conclusions may be drawn. Although no single treatment has been identified as effective for all persons with alcohol problems, a variety of specific treatment methods has been associated with positive outcomes in some groups of persons seeking treatment. Brief interventions have been shown to be effective compared with no treatment and compared with more complex treatments.

Although it is important to approach alcohol problems directly, dealing with other life problems can also contribute to positive outcomes. Treatment outcomes are affected by a multiplicity of factors, both within the treatment situation (e.g., the skills and attributes of therapists) and outside the treatment situation (e.g., the posttreatment experiences of the individual). A significant, extended reduction or elimination of alcohol consumption is usually associated with improvement in other areas of living; as in the treatment of other human problems, however, a variety of outcomes is to be expected.

REFERENCES

Angell, M. 1984. Patients' preferences in randomized clinical trials. New England Journal of Medicine 310:1385-1387.

Annis, H. M. 1987. Effective treatment for drug and alcohol problems: What do we know? Presented to the Annual Meeting of the Institute of Medicine, Washington, D.C., October 21.

Appelbaum, P. S., L. H. Roth, and C. Lidz. 1983. The therapeutic misconception: Informed consent in psychiatric research. International Journal of Law and Psychiatry 5:319-329.

Baekeland, F. 1977. Evaluation of treatment methods in chronic alcoholism. Pp. 385-440 in Treatment and Rehabilitation of the Chronic Alcoholic. Vol. 5 of The Biology of Alcoholism, B. Kissin and H. Begleiter, eds. New York: Plenum Press.

Baekeland, F., L. Lundwall, and B. Kissin. 1975. Methods for the treatment of chronic alcoholism: A critical appraisal. Pp. 247-327 in Research Advances in Alcohol and Drug Problems, vol. 2, R. J. Gibbins, Y. Israel, H. Kalant et al., eds. Toronto: John Wiley and Sons.

Blackburn, T. R. 1971. Sensuous-intellectual complementarity in science. Science 172:1003-1007.

Bowman, K., and E. M. Jellinek. 1941. Alcohol addiction and its treatment. Quarterly Journal of Studies on Alcohol 2:98-176.

Clare, A. W. 1976. How good is treatment?   Pp. 279-289 in Alcoholism: New Knowledge and New Responses, G. Edwards and M. Grant, eds. Baltimore: University Park Press.

Cook, D. R. 1985. Craftsman vs. professional: Analysis of the controlled drinking controversy. Journal of Studies on Alcohol 46:433-42.

Cronkhite, R. C., and R. H. Moos. 1978. Evaluating alcoholism treatment programs: An integrated approach. Journal of Consulting and Clinical Psychology 46:1105-1119.

Cronkhite, R. C., and R. H. Moos. 1980. Determinants of the posttreatment functioning of alcoholic patients: A conceptual framework. Journal of Consulting and Clinical Psychology 48:305-316.

Diesenhaus, H. I. 1982. Current trends in treatment programming for problem drinkers and alcoholics. Pp. 219-290 in Prevention, Intervention, and Treatment: Concerns and Models, J. de Luca, ed. Washington, D.C.: U.S. Government Printing Office.

Eddy, D. M., and J. Billings. 1988. The quality of medical evidence: Implications for quality of care. Health Affairs 7:19-32.

Emrick, C. D. 1975. A review of psychologically oriented treatment of alcoholism. II. The relative effectiveness of different treatment approaches and the effectiveness of treatment versus no treatment. Journal of Studies on Alcohol 36:88-108.

Emrick, C. D. 1979. Perspectives in clinical research: Relative effectiveness of alcohol abuse treatment. Family and Community Health 2:71-88.

Glaser, F. B., S. W. Greenberg, and M. Barrett. 1978. A Systems Approach to Alcohol Problems. Toronto: ARF Books.

Gottheil, E. 1985. Introduction. Pp. 1-8 in Summaries of Alcoholism Treatment Assessment Research, D. J. Lettieri, M. A. Sayers, and J. E. Nelson, eds. Rockville, Md.: National Institute on Alcohol Abuse and Alcoholism.

Hill, M. J., and H. T. Blane. 1967. Evaluation of psychotherapy with alcoholics: A critical review. Quarterly Journal of Studies on Alcohol 28:76-104.

Hlatky, M. A., K. L. Lee, F. E. Harrell, Jr., et al. 1984. Tying clinical research to patient care by use of an observational data base. Statistics in Medicine 3:375-384.

Institute of Medicine. 1989. Prevention and Treatment of Alcohol Problems: Research Opportunities. Washington, D.C.: National Academy Press.

Kalb, M., and M. S. Propper. 1976. The future of alcohology: Craft or science?   American Journal of Psychiatry 133:641-645.

Kiesler, D. J. 1966. Some myths of psychotherapy research and the search for a paradigm. Psychological Bulletin 65:110-136.

Koch-Weser, J. 1974. Bioavailability of drugs. New England Journal of Medicine 291:233-237,503-506.

Koumans, A. J. R., and J. J. Muller. 1965. Use of letters to increase motivation for treatment in alcoholics. Psychological Reports 16:1152.

Lohr, K. N., K. D. Yordy, and S. O. Thier. 1988. Current issues in quality of care. Health Affairs 7:5-18.

Longabaugh, R., and D. C. Lewis. 1988. Key issues in treatment outcome studies. Alcohol Health and Research World 12:168-175.

Marquis, D. 1983. Leaving therapy to chance. The Hastings Center Report 13(4):40-47.

Miller, W. R. 1988. The effectiveness of treatment for alcohol problems: Reasons for optimism. Presented at the conference "Drug Abuse and Alcohol: New Prospects for Recovery," at the Royal Society of Medicine, London, May 10.

Miller, W. R., and R. K. Hester. 1986. The effectiveness of alcoholism treatment: What research reveals. Pp. 121-174 in Treating Addictive Behaviors: Processes of Change, W. R. Miller and N. Heather, eds. New York: Plenum Press.

Moffett, A. D., S. W. Greenberg, and F. B. Glaser. 1975. Nonprograms in the management of drug and alcohol abuse. Pp. 617-627 in Developments in the Field of Drug Abuse: National Drug Abuse Conference, 1974, E. Senay, V. Shorty, and H. Alksne, eds. Cambridge, Mass.: Schenkman Publishing Company.

Moos, R. H., R. C. Cronkhite, and J. W. Finney. 1982. A conceptual framework for alcoholism treatment evaluation. Pp. 1120-1139 in Encyclopedic Handbook of Alcoholism, E. M. Pattison and E. Kaufman, eds. New York: Gardner Press.

Moos, R. H., J. W. Finney, and R. C. Cronkhite. 1990. Alcoholism Treatment: Context, Process, and Outcome. New York: Oxford University Press.

Pattison, E. M. 1974. Rehabilitation of the chronic alcoholic. Pp. 587-658 in Clinical Pathology. Vol. 3 of The Biology of Alcoholism, B. Kissin and H. Begleiter, eds. New York: Plenum Press.

Pattison, E. M., M. B. Sobell, and L. C. Sobell. 1977. Emerging Concepts of Alcohol Dependence. New York: Springer Publishing Company.

Paul, G. L. 1967. Strategy of outcome research in psychotherapy. Journal of Consulting Psychology 31:109-118.

Roper, W. L., W. Winkenwerder, G. M. Hackbarth, et al. 1988. Effectiveness in health care: An initiative to evaluate and improve medical practice. New England Journal of Medicine 319:1197-1202.

Sanchez-Craig, M. 1986. The hitchhiker's guide to alcohol treatment. British Journal of Addiction 81:597-600.

Schafer, A. 1982. The ethics of randomized clinical trials. New England Journal of Medicine 307:719-724.

Taylor, K. M., R. Margolese, and C. L. Soskolne. 1984. Physicians' reasons for not entering eligible patients in a randomized clinical trial of surgery for breast cancer. New England Journal of Medicine 310:1363-1367.

Voegtlin, W. L., and F. Lemere. 1942. The treatment of alcohol addiction: A review of the literature. Quarterly Journal of Studies on Alcohol 2:717-803.

6   Is Treatment Necessary?

Faced with this chapter's title question, one is tempted to respond reflexively, with both urgency and gruffness, "Of course it is! How can one seriously question the necessity of treatment for problems that destroy hundreds of thousands of lives and cost our country hundreds of millions of dollars each year?" Yet the diversity of alcohol problems (see Chapter 2) requires that this question be considered more thoughtfully.

In the previous chapter, which is supplemented by the material in Appendix B, the considerable evidence that some people with alcohol problems respond in a definite and gratifying manner to some treatments has been extensively presented. In this chapter the committee addresses some additional facts that serve to fill out a more comprehensive and at the same time more complex picture of response to treatment. These include the findings that *(a) some people with alcohol problems overcome them without any formal treatment experience; (b) some people who receive formal treatment have worse drinking problems afterward; and (c) some people who are coerced into treatment do not fare better than those who receive no treatment.*

Improvement in Alcohol Problems
Without Formal Treatment

The phenomenon of improvement without treatment is characteristically referred to as "spontaneous remission," a label that is misleading with respect to both of its two terms (Stall and Biernacki, 1986). Available data suggest that the resolution of alcohol problems without recourse to formal treatment (Tuchfeld, 1981) is neither spontaneous (it often occurs as a consequence of readily identifiable antecedents) nor best viewed as a remission (it often is not a temporary hiatus in the natural course of a relentlessly progressive problem). In this report, therefore, the phenomenon will be referred to as "improvement in alcohol problems without formal treatment." That such improvement does in fact occur is beyond serious doubt, although (as will be seen) many questions about the phenomenon remain unanswered.

The reversal of disease states without formal therapeutic intervention is well known in medicine. Specifically effective medical interventions have in general been available only during the twentieth century, yet humanity has survived. Furthermore, a decline of mortality rates from many diseases long preceded the introduction of specific treatment, probably as a result of such nonspecific factors as improved diet (McKeown, 1976). It was at one time customary for medical students entering their training to be congratulated on choosing their profession wisely because a significant proportion of the problems they would be called on to address would take care of themselves.

Walter B. Cannon (1871-1945) coined the term *homeostasis* to reflect the tendency of the human organism to return itself to a dynamic steady state following various kinds of perturbations, including illnesses. Multiple mechanisms, such as the production of antibodies to potentially harmful invading organisms on the physical level or the development of various defense mechanisms on the psychological level, subserve this purpose. Wound healing is an important example. When extravagantly praised for his therapeutic efforts on the battlefield, Ambroise Pare (1517-1590), the father of modern surgery, commented: "I dressed the wound; God healed it."

So powerful is the tendency for human problems to revert to normal unaided by intentional therapeutics that special means must be employed in therapeutic evaluations to take reversions that are not due to treatment into account. The randomized controlled trial (RCT) described in the previous chapter is commonly used for this purpose. Rigorous testing of efficacy is required even in instances in which success seems likely or is critically important (e.g., in tests of vaccines or of anticancer agents), in large measure because of the reality of improvement without formal treatment.

Given the foregoing, it should not be surprising that improvement without formal treatment may also occur in alcohol problems. A number of lines of evidence suggest that it does. One is clinical observation. The first North American treatise on alcohol problems, prepared by Benjamin Rush (1745-1813), contains a number of examples of the cessation of alcohol problems in the absence of formal intervention. Two are presented here.

> A farmer in England, who had been many years in the practice of coming home intoxicated, from a market town, one day observed appearances of rain, while he was in market. His hay was cut, and ready to be housed. To save it, he returned in haste to his farm, before he had taken his customary dose of grog. Upon coming into his house, one of his children, a boy of six years old, ran to his mother, and cried out, "O mother, father is come home, and he is not drunk." The father, who heard this exclamation, was so severely rebuked by it, that he suddenly became a sober man.

> A noted drunkard was once followed by a favorite goat, to a tavern, into which he was invited by his master, and drenched with some of his liquor. The poor animal staggered home with his master, a good deal intoxicated. The next day he followed him to his accustomed tavern. When the goat came to the door, he paused: his master made signs to him to follow him into the house. The goat stood still. An attempt was made to thrust him into the tavern. He resisted, as if struck with the recollection of what he suffered from being intoxicated the night before. His master was so much affected by a sense of shame, in observing the conduct of his goat to be so much more rational than his own, that he ceased from that time to drink spirituous liquors. (Jellinek, 1943:339)

Most contemporary evidence for improvement without formal treatment comes from studies of alcohol problems in the general population. By definition, it is not possible to study the phenomenon in a population undergoing formal treatment. However, this does *not* mean that so-called spontaneous remission does not occur in treatment populations. Although improvement that occurs in an individual in treatment is characteristically attributed to the treatment provided, it may in fact be due to other causes. It is just such a possibility that RCTs and other research designs are used to explore.

The results of a large number of studies in general populations and their implications for the understanding of improvement without formal treatment have been extensively summarized by Fillmore and her associates (1988) in a review prepared for the use of this committee. In general, two types of studies have been done: cross-sectional and longitudinal. In the first the status of alcohol problems of individuals in a large population has been examined at one point in time. In the second the status of alcohol problems of individuals in a smaller population has been examined at more than one point in time (usually two points). Although these studies do not directly examine improvement without formal treatment, a relatively consistent picture emerges from them.

First, the prevalence of alcohol problems declines with age. People in younger age categories are more likely to have alcohol problems. As they grow older, their alcohol problems are likely to decrease in severity or to cease altogether. Excess mortality from alcohol problems accounts for some proportion of this observation but not for all of it. The commonly advanced explanation for this "maturing out" of alcohol problems is the tendency of the young to "sow their wild oats" and subsequently, with increasing experience, to conform to social expectations. "Maturing out" is a pattern that has also been observed in persons with drug problems (Winick, 1962).

Second, although these changes with age occur in both men and women, the prevalence of alcohol problems among women is substantially less than among men. For example, the prevalence of "alcohol abuse and/or dependence" during the year prior to interview in the five-site Epidemiological Catchment Area (ECA) survey was 11.9 percent for men and 2.2 percent for women (Helzer and Burnham, in press). Correspondingly, the rate of "spontaneous remission" is higher among women (see esp. Fillmore, 1987). Here, the explanation tends to be that the drinking of alcohol is more consistent with the traditional social definition of the male role than of the female role; "the most obvious reason is that there are positive norms for heavy drinking among men, but not among women. Heavy drinking is considered appropriate masculine behavior" (Ferrence, 1980:117). Therefore, there is less social pressure on females to begin drinking and more pressure on them to stop.

Third, improvement without formal treatment is not a minor or insignificant phenomenon. In the population-based ECA study, for example, "remission" rates for all cases meeting DSM-III criteria for "alcoholism" averaged between 45 and 55 percent at all five sites (Helzer and Burnham, in press). A summary statement on age, sex, and improvement without formal treatment, drawn from all currently available information, is that there is

> a higher prevalence of problems in youth, but erratic and non-chronic with a 50-60 percent chance of remission both in the long and short term among men and more than 70 percent chance of remission among women; in middle age, a much lower prevalence, but chronic with a 30-40 percent chance of remission among men and about a 30 percent chance of remission among women; in older age, a great deal lower prevalence of problems, which were more likely chronic, with a 60-80 percent chance of remission among men and a 50-60 percent chance of remission among women. (Fillmore et al., 1988:29)

Fourth, although these general patterns are both clear and have been relatively stable across time and across jurisdictions, they are by no means universally descriptive. Not all persons with alcohol problems "mature out" of them, and some women do have very severe and very persistent alcohol problems. Although age and sex do seem to have an effect on the course of alcohol problems, there are many variations in such courses within each sex and age group.

For example, in one longitudinal study that looked at drinking problems at two points in time (age 18 and age 31), 63.4 percent of the sample had a different problem status at age 31, but 36.6 percent of the sample had the same problem status (Temple and Fillmore, 1985). In another longitudinal study (Vaillant, 1983) that looked at a population sample at multiple points in time, four separate courses were observed among those who had developed severe alcohol problems. In short, the drinking problems of some persons change over time, becoming worse or better or fluctuating; the drinking problems of other persons do not change over time.

Fifth, at present it is not possible to predict with certainty whether the alcohol problems of a given individual will or will not improve over time. One reason is that, although relatively adequate data are available on the course of alcohol problems by age and by sex, there appear to be a large number of additional variables that affect whether or not such problems persist and on which relatively few data are available.   These variables may include such factors as social class, social stability, social setting, significant life events, severity of the alcohol problem, ethnicity, and comorbidity (the concurrent presence of other problems, especially psychiatric disorders and drug problems).

The systematic study of the impact of these variables on the course of alcohol problems is a task for the future.   If (as is probable) they prove to be important determinants, their number and variety underscore the probability of divergent courses for different individuals.   Another way of saying this is that improvement without formal treatment is not a unitary phenomenon that uniformly affects all persons with alcohol problems.   Rather, it is a heterogeneous phenomenon that affects different persons in a highly variable manner and for many different reasons.

Thus, although formal treatment is helpful to some persons with alcohol problems, others improve without it.   Formal treatment is not always necessary, but in our current state of knowledge it is not possible to predict for whom it is and for whom it is not necessary.   Another significant consideration is that treatment is not only at times unnecessary but may actually be harmful.

Deterioration in Alcohol Problems with Formal Treatment

When an individual recognizes his or her alcohol problem and actively seeks assistance in resolving it, treatment is often viewed as a moral imperative and is considered by some to be a right (cf. Fried, 1975).   It has been argued that this is so whether or not the treatment has been shown to be effective (Halmos, 1966).   But what if the treatment being offered carries a significant risk of harming the person?   In this circumstance, treatment is not simply unnecessary but can result in matters becoming worse than they would have been if no treatment or a different treatment had been provided.   The point is that *all treatment must be considered within the context of a risk/benefit analysis* (cf. Institute of Medicine, 1989).

Risks are understood to accompany many forms of medical treatment.   Penicillin, as well as other highly effective drugs, may result in sensitivity reactions or other side effects in some proportion of individuals.   Nor are treatment risks necessarily limited to the individual under treatment; the adverse effects on unborn children of thalidomide and of the use of estrogens to prevent miscarriages come to mind.   Some surgical procedures carry with them significant hazards.   General anesthesia itself carries a small but definite risk of mortality.   As with medical and surgical treatment, it is clear that there are numerous potential negative effects of treatment for alcohol problems (Emrick, 1988).

Potentially harmful alcohol treatment interventions include the use of vigorous negative confrontation techniques with individuals who lack the means to cope with the confrontation in a constructive manner (Annis and Chan, 1983; Miller and Sovereign, 1985).   Focusing on an individual's drinking problem to the exclusion of other disorders that require direct treatment (e.g., coexisting psychiatric disorders) may also be harmful. The routine rather than the selective use of antialcohol medications can be fraught with difficulty, and in general the rigid application of a treatment philosophy or a technical intervention without due consideration for individual differences is hazardous.

Potentially harmful characteristics or behaviors of the treaters of alcohol problems also constitute a risk factor.   For example, dependent individuals may be exploited to satisfy the needs of the therapist or of the treatment program.   Other common difficulties attributable to treaters include being rejecting, cold, impersonal, unsupportive, or actually hostile with individuals in treatment, or insisting that the individual is just like the therapist and can only improve by doing exactly what the therapist has done to overcome his or her alcohol problems. Certain characteristics or behaviors of the individual in treatment may also contribute to harmful treatment effects; some examples include low self-esteem, low involvement in or compliance with treatment, a lack of interpersonal skills, or reliance escape as a method of coping with stress.

Inasmuch as alcohol treatment can result in harm, a reflexive "yes" to the question "Is treatment necessary?" may not only result in the wasteful use of treatment resources (through the delivery of unnecessary or ineffective treatment) but may actually lead to injury, albeit unintentioned. Treatment is therefore not to be undertaken lightly. Once again the absence of data does not permit a prediction of who will be harmed by treatment, anymore than it permits a prediction of who will not require formal treatment.

Coerced Treatment for Alcohol Problems

Perhaps the question "Is treatment necessary?" would not be so crucial were it not for the fact that many individuals who are currently being treated for alcohol problems are forced to receive treatment (Boscarino, 1980; Furst, 1981; Weisner, 1987; State of Connecticut Drug and Alcohol Abuse Criminal Justice Commission, hereafter referred to as State of Connecticut, 1988). Because of the major and increasing role played by coercion in the treatment of alcohol problems, the committee has included as Appendix C to its report a review of the topic prepared by one of its members. Much of the following discussion is based on this document. It is worth noting that a consideration of "statutory and voluntary mechanisms" for the provision of treatment was a specific element of the congressional charge to the committee.

Coerced treatment has become an important issue not only in the United States but at an international level as well. A World Health Organization study found that 20 of the 43 countries investigated had some kind of diversion legislation allowing treatment to serve as an alternative to judicial action (Curran et al., 1987). Moreover, criminal justice referrals in particular jurisdictions may be extensive; a study in one state found that, if all such referrals were accepted by alcohol treatment programs, they would occupy 64 percent of the total available rehabilitation beds (State of Connecticut, 1988).

Most prominent among the coerced at present are those who are sent to treatment by the courts for drunken-driving offenses (Fillmore and Kelso, 1987). For example, one state experienced a 400 percent increase of driving while intoxicated (DWI) offenders into treatment programs for alcohol problems during 1986-1987 (State of Connecticut, 1988). In some jurisdictions arrested drinking drivers are given their choice of alcohol treatment or criminal justice sanctions; in others they are automatically referred to treatment programs for alcohol problems (U.S. Department of Transportation, 1976; Weisner, 1986; Stewart et al., 1987). Without denying that drunken driving is a critical social problem, it must nevertheless be emphasized that those persons who drink and drive constitute a group that overlaps with but is not identical to the group of individuals who have serious alcohol problems (Donovan et al., 1983; Vingilis, 1983; Wilson and Jonah, 1985; Perrine, 1986).

Other important sources of referral to treatment under coercion include civil commitment, diversion from the criminal justice system for public drunkenness and crimes other than DWI offenses in which alcohol has played a role, workplace referrals ("constructive coercion"), and referrals that come about as a result of carefully structured and highly confronting small group sessions (Johnson, 1973, 1986). Presumably, the sum total of these referrals constitutes a very large and rapidly growing number. Unfortunately, there are at present no reliable data on this number for the country as a whole.

Studies that have been carried out on the effects of treatment with coerced individuals vary greatly in terms of comparison groups and the outcome measures that are used. Drawing conclusions is not an easy matter. The committee's sense of the available information is that, although certain groups of individuals (e.g., professionals, the regularly employed) may benefit on the whole from coerced treatment, and although certain types of coercion are more effective than others (e.g., effective coercion often involves severe penalties for failure to comply with treatment—so-called contingencies—that are an invariable consequence of that failure), involuntary treatment is by no means uniformly beneficial and in some instances may actually be harmful (Wells-Parker, 1989. Even when forced treatment proves to be beneficial, it may not be the most efficient way to resolve the problems at issue. For some individuals it may be unnecessary to provide more than a minimally coercive intervention to reach maximum effectiveness (Peck et al., 1985), yet coerced treatment characteristically involves much more than a minimal intervention.

Coerced treatment also presents particularly difficult ethical and even legal issues (cf. Marco and Marco, 1980). For example, are the individual's basic civil liberties endangered? Is the person being inappropriately labeled through a particularly aggressive coercion effort? Are coerced individuals treated with as much dignity and diligence as are persons who undertake treatment voluntarily? What of the issue of informed consent when persons are coerced into treatment? If people are treated against their will and harm ensues, who is liable?

These and other ethical and legal considerations underscore the complexities that surrounds the forced treatment of any person with an alcohol problem. Treatment must be handled thoughtfully, objectively, and compassionately. An unthinking "yes" to the question "Is treatment necessary?" places one at considerable risk for making improper treatment interventions.

Implications for Treatment

To review: many people with alcohol problems improve without formal treatment. Some people with alcohol problems are made worse by treatment. Compulsory treatment of alcohol problems is not always helpful. These findings are not surprising, and they apply to treatment situations other than the treatment of alcohol problems. Although they hardly require the abandonment of the therapeutic effort, they do make it clear that, as with all such efforts, a guiding principle should be to *proceed with caution.*

For example, treatment should be considered only if the existence of an alcohol problem is highly probable. This dictum places a premium on the careful assessment of all individuals who are seeking treatment (see Chapter 10) but is especially pertinent for those acting under coercion. When the existence of an alcohol problem is uncertain, primary or secondary prevention efforts (see Chapter 9) or other measures (e.g., general psychotherapy, revocation of a driver's license) may prove to be more appropriate than treatment directed at alcohol problems.

In addition, it is important to take care to find the optimal treatment for the particular problem of a given individual (see Chapter 11). Due account should be taken of the potential negative effects of all treatments; any treatment with the power to help is likely to possess the power to harm when injudiciously deployed. Furthermore, if a given intervention proves to be ineffective, an alternative intervention should be considered.

Appropriate caution can also take the form of favoring interventions that fall short of the most intensive and costly treatment methods but that are effective for some individuals. Conservative palliation in many instances is to be preferred to radical intervention. Particular consideration is wisely given to less utilization of intensive and costly intervention for those groups, such as the young, the female, and the elderly, in which improvement outside of formal treatment is more likely. For such groups, emphasis may more reasonably be placed on supporting nontreatment factors that promote improvement (e.g., employment, recreation, interpersonal ties, other social supports).

Further understanding and documentation of how people with alcohol problems improve without formal treatment should be helpful in approaching treatment in a cautious and logical manner. There is the intriguing possibility that such understanding may encourage the development of novel approaches to treatment itself. In this sense improvement with treatment and improvement outside of treatment are not adversaries but collaborators.

Treatment Based on Knowledge of Improvement Without Treatment

Therapy based on a knowledge of factors that are believed to be critical in producing improvement without formal treatment has been proposed in the field of smoking cessation (Marlatt et al., 1988; IOM, 1989). A similar approach has been taken in the treatment of alcohol problems. In developing what came to be called a community reinforcement approach, its originators set out to "examine the natural deterrents of alcoholism and . . . alter these natural deterrents to maximize their effectiveness" (Hunt and Azrin, 1973:91-92). Their understanding of such natural deterrents was that "[i]n the alcoholic state, one may incur social censure from friends as well as from one's family. Discharge from one's employment is likely. Pleasant social interactions and individual recreational activities cannot be performed as satisfactorily, if at all, when one is alcoholic" (p. 92).

They therefore set about enhancing their subjects' social, marital, familial, vocational, and recreational activities by providing specific counseling (e.g., job-seeking skills) as well as additional supports (e.g., a non-alcohol-related social club meeting on Saturday nights). However, they also took steps to ensure that these aids would be swiftly and certainly withdrawn if the individual resumed drinking. For example, if recourse to drinking caused marital difficulties, the spouse was advised to move out of the house until the individual being treated became sober and requested that he or she return. In a word, both the carrot and the stick were judiciously applied (Hunt and Azrin, 1973).

Its developers note that "[this] procedure does not require hospitalization except as a means of helping the patient through his withdrawal symptoms and physical disability, if any" (Hunt and Azrin, 1973:99). Thus, the approach is in accord with the contemporary deemphasis on inpatient (hospital or freestanding residential) treatment (Saxe et al., 1983; Annis, 1986; Miller and Hester, 1986) and the importance of environmental variables in outcome (Cronkhite and Moos, 1978; Moos et al., 1979). Controlled trials of the community reinforcement approach, as well as its individual components (Azrin, 1976; Azrin et al., 1982; Mallams et al., 1982; Sisson and Azrin, 1986) have been positive, and a major replication study is under way (W. R. Miller, University of New Mexico, personal communication, January, 1989).

Another therapeutic approach has been developed that complements the community reinforcement approach. Rather than dealing with those naturally occurring factors that facilitate the remission of alcohol problems, this approach deals with the naturally occurring factors that make them worse. It has been called relapse prevention (Marlatt and Gordon, 1985; Annis, 1986b; Annis and Davis, 1988).

Relapse prevention is based on the notion that the treatment strategies that will keep a person with alcohol problems from drinking once he or she has stopped may differ from the strategies that will enable him or her to stop drinking in the first place. There is evidence that a wide variety of techniques are effective in producing at least short-term elimination or reduction of alcohol consumption (Miller, 1988). Relapse prevention builds on such an initial success and attempts to extend the elimination or reduction into the future. Alcoholics Anonymous and other self-help groups are often used therapeutically in this manner and in some senses at least could also be thought of as relapse prevention measures.

In one such approach (Annis, 1986b; Annis and Davis, 1988) a painstaking inventory is taken of those naturally occurring situations in which relapse to drinking is likely to occur. The therapist then helps the individual learn other ways of coping with such dangerous situations rather than by drinking. When the individual learns successfully to negotiate situations that previously resulted in relapse, the probability of relapse is lessened. One alternative coping strategy to resist drinking that has been explored is the use of an antialcohol drug, Temposil (citrated calcium carbimide), which is not currently available for therapeutic use in the United States (Peachey and Annis, 1985). It is felt that, ideally, such a strategy would give way to more complex and psychosocially based treatment.

Treatments that evolve along these lines may prove to be quite effective. Whether from the community reinforcement approach or the relapse prevention approach, or from other approaches that are yet to be developed, an important contribution to the treatment of alcohol problems may arise (along the lines suggested by Ambroise Pare) from encouraging the individual to come increasingly under the sway of naturally occurring factors that will facilitate the resolution of his or her problem. Pare helped nature along by inventing the surgical ligature (Vaillant, 1983). In like manner the answer in the alcohol field to the title question of this chapter may be that treatment is sometimes a necessary supplement to natural healing processes.

Summary and Conclusions

There is ample evidence that a significant number of individuals who develop alcohol problems will be able to deal with those problems without undergoing formal treatment. As well, some persons have less positive outcomes as a result of treatment. The coercion of persons into treatment is an increasingly common phenomenon but is not invariably associated with positive outcome.

It is also true, of course, that many persons benefit greatly from appropriate treatment (the previous chapter and Appendix B provide copious documentation that this is so) and that they may do so even under coercion and in some instances only under coercion. Yet each of these sets of facts must be balanced against the other in trying to respond to the title question of this chapter. Is treatment necessary? The committee believes the answer is a qualified "yes" that must take into account the complexities of the issues involved in our current state of knowledge.

How should one proceed? Cautiously, the committee believes, and with humility. Treatment for alcohol problems, like other treatments, should be applied judiciously, with due consideration given to individual differences. Treatment should not be foresworn, because it is helpful to many; but neither should it be provided as a matter of course, because for some it is not necessary and for others it may be harmful. The extremes of unbridled therapeutic enthusiasm on the one hand and thoroughgoing therapeutic nihilism on the other must be avoided. In addition, improvement outside of formal treatment, negative therapeutic reactions, and the fact of coercion should be seen not only as complicating factors but as opportunities for learning more about treatment. Such strategies as the community reinforcement approach and relapse prevention are illustrative.

We especially need to learn a great deal more about how to predict who does not need treatment, who will be harmed by treatment, and who will benefit from treatment only under coercion. The directions and recommendations provided by the committee in Section III of this report are in keeping with this goal. If implemented, the difficulties in making appropriate therapeutic decisions should diminish over time. In the meantime the guiding admonition of Hippocrates must be kept firmly in mind: ***primum non nocere***—the first duty of the treater is to do no harm.

REFERENCES

Annis, H. M. 1986a. Is inpatient rehabilitation of the alcoholic cost effective? Con position. Advances in Alcohol and Substance Abuse 5:175-190.

Annis, H. M. 1986b. A relapse prevention model for treatment of alcoholics. Pp. 407-433 in Treating Addictive Behaviors: Processes of Change, W. R. Miller and N. Heather, eds. New York: Plenum Press.

Annis, H. M., and D. Chan. 1983. The differential treatment model: Empirical evidence from a personality typology of adult offenders. Criminal Justice and Behavior 10:159-173.

Annis, H. M., and C. S. Davis. 1988. Assessment of expectancies. Pp. 82-111 in Assessment of Addictive Behaviors, G. A. Marlatt and D. Donovan, eds. New York: Guilford Press.

Azrin, N. H. 1976. Improvement in the community-reinforcement approach to alcoholism. Behavior Research and Therapy 14:339-348.

Azrin, N., R. W. Sisson, R. Meyers, et al. 1982. Alcoholism treatment by disulfiram and community reinforcement therapy. Journal of Behavior Therapy and Experimental Psychiatry 13:105-112.

Boscarino, J. 1980. A national survey of alcoholism centers in the United States: A preliminary report. American Journal of Drug and Alcohol Abuse 7:403-413.

Cronkhite, R. C., and R. H. Moos. 1978. Evaluating alcoholism treatment programs: An integrated approach. Journal of Consulting and Clinical Psychology 46:1105-1119.

Cronkhite, R. C., and R. H. Moos. 1980. Determinants of the posttreatment functioning of alcoholic patients: A conceptual framework. Journal of Consulting and Clinical Psychology 48:305-316.

Curran, W. J., A. E. Arif, and D. C. Jayasuriya. 1987. Guidelines for Assessing and Revising National Legislation on Treatment of Drug and Alcohol-Dependent Persons. Geneva: World Health Organization.

Donovan, D., G. A. Marlatt, and P. Salzberg. 1983. Drinking behavior, personality factors, and high-risk driving. Journal of Studies on Alcohol 44:395-428.

Emrick, C. D. 1988. Executive summary: Negative treatment effects. Prepared for the IOM Committee for the Study of Treatment and Rehabilitation Services for Alcoholism and Alcohol Abuse, March.

Ferrence, R. G. 1980. Sex differences in the prevalence of problem drinking. Pp. 69-124 in Alcohol and Drug Problems in Women, O. J. Kalant, ed. New York: Plenum Press.

Fillmore, K. M. 1987. Women's drinking across the life course as compared to men's. British Journal of Addiction 82:801-811.

Fillmore, K. M., and D. Kelso. 1987. Coercion in alcoholism treatment: Meanings for the disease concept of alcoholism. Journal of Drug Issues 17:301-319.

Fillmore, K. M., E. Hartka, B. M. Johnstone, R. Speiglman, and M. T. Temple. 1988. Spontaneous remission from alcohol problems: A critical review. Prepared for the IOM Committee for the Study of Treatment and Rehabilitation Services for Alcoholism and Alcohol Abuse, June.

Fried, C. 1975. Rights and health care—beyond equity and efficiency. New England Journal of Medicine 293:241-245.

Furst, C., L. Beckman, C. Nakamura, and M. Weiss. 1981. Utilization of Alcohol Treatment Services in California. Los Angeles: University of California Alcohol Research Center, Neuropsychiatric Institute.

Halmos, P. 1966. The Faith of the Counsellors: A Study in the Theory and Practice of Social Casework and Psychiatry. New York: Schocken Books.

Helzer, J. E., and A. Burnham. In press. Alcohol abuse and dependence. In Psychiatric Disorders in America, L. N. Robins and D. A. Regier, eds. New York: The Free Press.

Hunt, G. M., and N. H. Azrin. 1973. A community-reinforcement approach to alcoholism. Behavior Research and Therapy 11:91-104.

Institute of Medicine. 1989. Prevention and Treatment of Alcohol Problems: Research Opportunities. Washington, D.C.: National Academy Press.

Jellinek, E. M. 1943. Benjamin Rush's "An inquiry into the effects of ardent spirits upon the human body and mind, with an account of the means of preventing and of the remedies for curing them." Quarterly Journal of Studies on Alcohol 4:321-341.

Johnson, V. E. 1973. I'll Quit Tomorrow. New York: Harper and Row.

Johnson, V. E. 1986. Intervention: How to Help Someone Who Doesn't Want Help. Minneapolis, Minn.: Johnson Institute Books.

Mallams, J. H., M. D. Godley, G. M. Hall, et al. 1982. A social-systems approach to resocializing alcoholics in the community. Journal of Studies on Alcohol 43:1115-1123.

Marco, C. H., and J. M. Marco. 1980. Antabuse: Medication in exchange for a limited freedom--is it legal? American Journal of Law and Medicine 5:295-330.

Marlatt, G. A., and J. R. Gordon, eds. 1985. Relapse Prevention: Maintenance Strategies in the Treatment of Addictive Behaviors. New York: Guilford Press.

Marlatt, G. A., S. Curry, and J. R. Gordon. 1988. A longitudinal analysis of unaided smoking cessation. Journal of Consulting and Clinical Psychology 56:715-720.

McKeown, T. 1976. The Modern Rise of Population. London: Edward Arnold.

Miller, W. R. 1988. The effectiveness of treatment for alcohol problems: Reasons for optimism. Prepared for the conference "Drug Abuse and Alcohol: New Prospects for Recovery," at the Royal Society of Medicine, London, May 10.

Miller, W. R., and R. K. Hester. 1986. Inpatient alcoholism treatment: Who benefits? American Psychologist 41:794-805.

Miller, W. R., and R. G. Sovereign. 1985. A comparison of two styles of therapeutic confrontation. Presented at the 34th International Congress on Alcoholism and Drug Dependence, Calgary, Alberta, September.

Moos, R. H., E. Bromet, V. Tsu, et al. 1979. Family characteristics and the outcome of treatment for alcoholism. Journal of Studies on Alcohol 40:78-88.

Peachey, J. E., and H. M. Annis. 1985. New strategies for using the alcohol-sensitizing drugs. Pp. 199-216 in Research Advances in New Psychopharmacological Treatments for Alcoholism, C. A. Naranjo and E. M. Sellers, eds. Amsterdam: Excerpta Medica.

Peck, R. C., D. D. Sadler, and M. W. Perrine. 1985. The comparative effectiveness of alcohol rehabilitation and licensing control actions for drunk driving offenders: A review of the literature. Alcohol, Drugs, and Driving: Abstracts and Reviews 1:15-39.

Perrine, B. 1986. Varieties of drunken and of drinking drivers: A review, a research program, and a model. Alcohol, Drugs, and Traffic Safety-T86: Proceedings of the 10th Annual International Conference on Alcohol, Drugs, and Traffic Safety, Amsterdam, September 9-12.

Saxe, L., D. Dougherty, K. Esty, and M. Fine. 1983. The Effectiveness and Costs of Alcoholism Treatment. Washington, D.C.: U.S. Congress, Office of Technology Assessment.

Sisson, R. W., and N. H. Azrin. 1986. Family-member involvement to initiate and promote treatment of problem drinkers. Journal of Behavior Therapy and Experimental Psychiatry 17:15-20.

Stall, R., and P. Biernacki. 1986. Spontaneous remission from the problematic use of substances: An inductive model derived from a comparative analysis of the alcohol, opiate, tobacco, and food/obesity literatures. International Journal of Addictions 2:1-23.

State of Connecticut Drug and Alcohol Abuse Criminal Justice Commission. 1988. The Drug and Alcohol Abuse Crisis within the Connecticut Criminal Justice System. State of Connecticut Drug and Alcohol Abuse Criminal Justice Commission, Hartford, Conn., March.

Stewart, K., L. G. Epstein, P. Gruenewald, et al. 1987. The California First DUI Offender Evaluation Project: Final Report. Prepared for the California Office of Traffic Safety. Walnut Creek, Calif.: Pacific Institute for Research and Evaluation, February.

Temple, M. T., and K. M. Fillmore. 1985. The variability of drinking patterns and problems among young men, ages 16-31: A longitudinal study. International Journal of Addictions 20:1595-1620.

Tuchfeld, B. 1981. Spontaneous remission in alcoholics: Empirical observations and theoretical implications. Journal of Studies on Alcohol 42:626-641.

U.S. Department of Transportation. 1976. Description of ASAP Diagnosis, Referral, and Rehabilitation Functions. Vol. 1 of Program Level Evaluation of ASAP Diagnosis, Referral, and Rehabilitation Efforts. Washington, D.C.: National Highway Traffic Safety Administration.

Vaillant, G. E. 1983. The Natural History of Alcoholism: Causes, Patterns, and Paths to Recovery. Cambridge, Mass.: Harvard University Press.

Vingilis, E. 1983. Drinking drivers and alcoholics: Are they from the same population? Pp. 299-342 in Research Advances in Alcohol and Drug Problems, vol. 7, R. E. Smart, F. B. Glaser, Y. Israel, et al., eds. New York: Plenum Press.

Weisner, C. 1986. The transformation of alcohol treatment: Access to care and the response to drinking-driving. Journal of Public Health Policy 7:78-92.

Weisner, C. 1987. Studying alcohol treatment as a system: Research issues and data sources. Presented at the Alcohol Treatment Service Systems Research Panel, Alcohol and Drug Problems Association National Conference, St. Louis, Missouri, September.

Wells-Parker, E., B. J. Anderson, D. L. McMillen, and J. W. Landrum. 1989. Interactions among DUI offender characteristics and traditional intervention modalities: A long-term recidivism follow-up. British Journal of Addiction 84:381-390.

Wilson, J., and B. Jonah. 1985. Identifying impaired drivers among the general driving population. Journal of Studies on Alcohol 46:531-536.

Winick, C. 1962. Maturing out of narcotic addiction. Bulletin on Narcotics 14:1-7.

7 Is Treatment Available?

Among the questions which the committee has attempted to address has been whether all those who wish to receive treatment for alcohol problems are able to receive the treatment of their choice. The heterogeneity of alcohol problems necessitates a variety of widely available treatment settings, orientations, and modalities so that persons with different sets and severities of alcohol problems can be successfully matched with the appropriate treatment regimens. One means of examining this question is to determine whether there is an even distribution of specialist treatment resources throughout the nation and whether alternative forms of treatment are available.

Distribution of Resources for Alcohol Problems Treatment

It can be assumed that, given an equal distribution of all types of care, those persons who are in need of treatment have an equal chance of being matched to the appropriate level and modality of treatment at each of the various treatment stages. Yet the committee's reviews of the literature and discussions with researchers, state alcoholism authority staff, practitioners, and federal administrators of treatment programs indicated that there have been no recent compilations of information about the distribution of treatment resources for the nation as a whole. The committee's investigation also revealed that there have not been any recent national studies of the level of available resources relative to the level of need or demand for treatment (i.e., the number of persons determined by themselves or others to require treatment for an alcohol problem).

Other data areas also reveal a lack of attention. There have been few recent studies of the resources available and accessible to those in need of treatment within different sections of the country or resources available to different subgroups or special populations. A recent noteworthy exception is the work of Gilbert and Cervantes (1986, 1988), which has looked at both the availability and accessibility of treatment for Mexican Americans. These investigators conducted secondary analyses of data collected by several state alcoholism authorities on persons receiving treatment in state-funded agencies to examine the level of utilization and the types of referrals for this special population. They found a high level of service utilization related to coercive referrals. This effort provides a model for the type of studies required to investigate differential availability and accessibility of treatment resources for persons with alcohol problems.

The committee's analysis focuses on availability. In health planning, the availability of treatment services typically refers to the supply and mix of health resources and services relative to the needs or demands of a given individual or community. Availability is not the same thing as accessibility. Accessibility typically refers to the degree to which the health care system inhibits or facilitates the ability of an individual or group to gain entry and to receive appropriate services, when services are available (Aday and Anderson, 1983). Determining whether services are "appropriate" is a matter of no small complexity; a judgment of appropriateness indicates that a match has been made between the specific needs of the "client"—whether an individual, a group, or a community—and the services and resources available and utilized (Gunnersen and Feldman, 1978; NIAAA, 1980; Brown University Center for Alcohol Studies, 1985; Gilbert and Cervantes, 1988; McAullife et al., 1988; New York Division of Alcoholism and Alcohol Abuse, 1989). Data on accessibility to treatment for alcohol problems are even sparser than those for availability; additional studies of accessibility are needed before a more comprehensive review can be undertaken.

A benefit of addressing the question of treatment availability, however, is that it can serve as one of the indexes by which accessibility can be determined. Barriers to accessibility are usually described in terms of physical, cultural, linguistic, geographic, and financial constraints. Physical accessibility often refers to the architectural structure of the treatment setting and the limitations it may pose to the mobility of the physically handicapped; it also refers to the availability of appropriate transportation from a person's home to the facility. Cultural accessibility is most often dealt with by the use of bilingual, bicultural treatment staff within standard or traditional services; efforts to increase cultural accessibility have also stressed the need for culturally sensitive, culturally relevant treatments and for administrative control of the program by members of the cultural group that is the target population (see Section IV). Geographic accessibility implies that treatment services are located within a reasonable distance of the individual's residence. Financial accessibility implies that the cost of the service is reasonable and there is no disincentive to use needed services because of their costs or the method of reimbursement (see Chapters 8, 18, and 20).

The lack of sufficient resources to meet requests for service has been termed "programmatic" barriers to accessibility and is measured by the incompleteness of the continuum of care, where some components exist and others do not (Brown University Center for Alcohol Studies, 1985). When components are missing, backups occur in which case people must wait for treatment or treatment is terminated prematurely; in both instances there is a higher probability of relapse. Examples of missing components that have been identified in the continuum of care for treatment of alcohol problems are the lack of long-term custodial/domiciliary beds to provide maintenance services for chronically disabled public inebriates who are recycled through detoxification centers (e.g., Shandler and Shipley, 1988a,b; see Chapter 16), and the lack of formal relapse prevention programs for persons who complete primary rehabilitation and who are not good candidates for AA affiliation (see Chapter 3). These structural constraints have also been called "program design" barriers in cases in which a program developed for one subgroup is applied to another without modifications that accommodate critical differences (e.g., the failure to provide child care services for mothers of small children who may be in need of inpatient primary rehabilitation [Beckman and Kocel, 1983; USDHHS, 1984]).

The state alcoholism authorities have struggled with the issue of treatment availability from the vantage point of resource allocation. In response to the federal formula grant requirement that each state have a procedure to determine priorities for treatment resource development, several states (e.g., New Jersey, Nebraska, Massachusetts, Colorado, New York) had developed sophisticated resource allocation models based on a consideration of the different needs of individuals at different stages of treatment (Wilson and Hartsock, 1981). Some of these states (e.g., Colorado, New York) have continued to routinely do such comparisons of needs and resources available in determining resource allocation priorities, even though the federal requirement was discontinued in 1982. However, there appears to have been a decrease in the states' overall efforts to use comparisons of prevalence indicators and utilization data in planning for treatment services. Formerly states were required to develop a comprehensive annual plan for services that included such a comparison to qualify for federal formula grant funds. With the ending of the formula grant program, many states no longer prepare an annual services plan and states vary in their perception of the need to have a formal method for resource allocation. Interest remains, however, in determining the relationship of the level of need to the treatment available, although a great deal of this effort may be driven as much by the need for a methodology to conduct certificate of need reviews (i.e., reviews required if inpatient services are to be expanded) as by the need to plan and allocate treatment funds (Brown University Center for Alcohol Studies, 1985; New York Division of Alcoholism and Alcohol Abuse, 1988). Still, several states (e.g., Maryland, New York, Rhode Island) have undertaken to develop improved methods of treatment needs estimation and resource allocation (New York Division of Alcoholism and Alcohol Abuse, 1983, 1987; Sheridan, 1986; Rush, 1988); The most recent such effort is that undertaken by Indiana (J. Mills, Indiana Division of Addiction Services, personal communication, December 15, 1987). None of the federal agencies that operate their own treatment systems has a formal resource allocation model in place.

Given the absence of recent studies on which to base judgments about the differential availability of treatment, the committee decided to use whatever published data were available to look at the distribution of alcohol problems treatment resources across the country. There are a number of problems in conducting such a national analysis because there are no consensually accepted methods for determining either the prevalence of alcohol problems or for projecting the appropriate level of treatment resources that will be required (Wilson and Hartsock, 1981; Brown University Center for Alcohol Studies, 1985; Institute for Health and Aging, 1986). In addition, as discussed in Chapter 3, there is no consensually accepted taxonomy, or model, for describing the resources (settings and modalities of treatment) to be planned for (Saxe et al., 1983; Bast, 1984) and no agreement on the components that make up a comprehensive treatment delivery system. The current situation is much the same as that described 10 years ago in an NIAAA-sponsored guide for health planners:

> The terminology used to describe alcoholism service configurations varies considerably throughout the country. Generally, the terminology is descriptive of either the environment/setting (e.g., hospital, halfway house) in which treatment takes place or the service (e.g., outpatient, inpatient) provided within the environment. Often, descriptions are reliant upon the treatment modalities (therapeutic orientations, e.g., A.A., aversive conditioning) implemented within a service. Occasionally the descriptions are mixed, causing environments to be confused with services and services to be confused with modalities. (Gunnersen and Feldman, 1978:45)

There is also no single inventory that captures the utilization of treatment services, both in terms of the wide variety of current facilities and programs and the individual practitioners that provide treatment for alcohol problems (see Chapter 4).

The last available comprehensive review of the methods used by the individual states to estimate and plan for treatment resource needs was undertaken in 1980 by the NIAAA-sponsored Alcohol Epidemiologic Data System (AEDS) project (Wilson and Hartsock, 1981). The study found that states and territories used many different methods of prevalence estimation, needs and demand forecasting, and resource description and allocation. AEDS project staff developed and proposed for national adoption a normative model for providing county-level estimates of persons needing treatment and the resources required (AEDS, 1982).

The AEDS normative approach produced estimates of the treatment resources needed to meet projected demand for services in a given service area or county (e.g., detoxification beds, halfway house beds, outpatient episodes). The estimates were derived, first, from the utilization history of the county captured by the NDATUS. These allocations were than adjusted, taking into account prevalence estimates; sociodemographic indexes including sex, race, and age; and local use patterns (AEDS, 1985). In the AEDS model, prevalence was estimated through the use of two composite weighted indexes: the Chronic Health Index and the Alcohol Casualty Index (both are mortality- and morbidity-based prevalence estimators).

The AEDS normative model was not adopted by the federal government or by any of the states. It was not perceived as an advance because it used primarily a demand-based or rates under treatment approach to project resource needs. In health planning and health economics, need is differentiated from demand. Need typically refers to an objectively determined index of the number of individuals with the particular condition, problem, or illness for which a given service is required (i.e., the prevalence or number of "cases"). Demand is used to describe the expressed desire for a particular service, which can be independent of objectively determined need, and is more related to subjective and economic factors (e.g., advertising, price of services, geographic proximity, attractiveness of facilities, stigmatization of persons identified as needing the treatment, etc.). Utilization—services actually used—is sometimes considered an index of need and at other times an index of demand.

In planning for treatment of alcohol problems the utilization of treatment services is often considered an index of need and has been used as such by particular states and health systems agencies to project future need for alcohol problems treatment resources (Gunnersen and Feldman, 1978; Bayer, 1980; Ford, 1980; AEDS, 1982; McGough and Hindman, 1986). In the AEDS study, states that were reported as projecting future needs for alcohol treatment services from historical utilization included Nebraska, Connecticut, Maine, and Missouri (Wilson and Hartsock, 1981). Although demand-based planning is commonly used by state alcohol authorities for planning and budgeting, it is not generally accepted by health planners, who prefer population-based approaches (e.g., community surveys) (MacStravic, 1978; NIAAA, 1980). Since the AEDS normative model also has a demand-based component, its suggested use as a national standard may also be questioned.

A more recent review of needs estimation methods was undertaken by the Institute of Health and Aging (1986) as part of a study to determine whether a more equitable formula could be found for allocating the alcohol, drug abuse, and mental health services block grant among the states and territories. The institute's review of the literature on the current status of prevalence estimation methods led to several conclusions: (a) there is no single, best approach to prevalence estimation; (b) the various indexes used to estimate the prevalence of mental health, alcohol, and drug abuse problems are not highly intercorrelated; and (c) the adoption and use of any model or set of measures as a national standard remains controversial within both the scientific and planning communities. Given this lack of consensus on and acceptance of a specific model for estimating prevalence (and in turn for allocating monies among the states accorded to need), the institute recommended that Congress continue to use population size, weighted by age and gender to reflect high-risk groups, as the need factor in the allocation formula, rather than introducing a more specific prevalence index.

Given the absence of recent research and further refinement of methods, it is likely that whatever methodology is used to assess the level of treatment resources currently available and the extent to which the prevalence of alcohol problems is the determinant of the availability of treatment, questions will be raised about the validity and appropriateness of the analysis. *This is an area in which the committee suggests further study and consensus development. A replication of the original AEDS review of the methods in use by the states for both needs estimation and determining resource availability is indicated and would be useful for future planning and resource allocation if the states could agree on a common methodology.*

Despite the important gaps noted above, there are nonetheless several data sources that can provide a rough first comparison of available treatment resources and the prevalence of alcohol problems which can be used as a preliminary answer to the question: "Is treatment for alcohol problems equally available throughout the United States?" The assumptions underlying this analysis are that treatment resources should either be distributed equally throughout the nation or, if there is variation from a national rate, should be dispersed geographically to reflect the actual distribution (prevalence) of alcohol problems across the states and territories. The principle guiding the analysis is that there should be the same availability of treatment resources in each of the states and territories.

Similar assumptions were used in assessing the level of services available throughout Pennsylvania's counties (Glaser and Greenberg, 1975; Glaser et al., 1978) and in the previously mentioned Institute of Health and Aging's 1986 evaluation of the formula for allocating the block grant funds. These are also the assumptions commonly used in many of the studies on the availability of health and mental health services where the distribution among counties or states of some resource (e.g., number of physicians or other health service providers per 100,000 persons; number of acute care hospital or nursing home beds per 100,000 persons) (see MacStravic, 1978; Bayer, 1980; Aday and Anderson, 1983; Knesper et al., 1984; Harrington et al., 1988).

There are two surveys conducted periodically by the federal and state governments specifically to determine current levels of services and funding for the treatment of alcohol problems that the committee originally thought would be useful in conducting such an analysis. The first, the National Drug and Alcoholism Treatment Utilization Survey (NDATUS), is designed to be a census of all known facilities and programs that provide a distinct organized program of alcohol and drug abuse services. The second, now known as the State Alcohol and Drug Abuse Profile (SADAP), is a survey of the funding and services provided in state supported programs. The committee found that both surveys were not achieving the level of coverage of providers contemplated in their design. Other surveys, such as those conducted by the American Hospital Association, the National Institute of Mental Health, and the National Center for Health Statistics, capture some information on services provided within general hospitals, psychiatric hospitals and clinics, and by private practitioners in office settings (e.g., psychiatrists, internists, social workers, clinical psychologists, and counselors) that may not be covered by these surveys of organized programs. However, the surveys do not use common definitions so that there is no single or aggregate source of data that can be used as a measure of the available level of services. *A more complete analysis of the availability of treatment for alcohol problems would also involve an attempt to determine the availability of treatment in these specialist and nonspecialist practice settings. The committee suggests that such studies be undertaken so that future policy reviews of treatment availability can be more complete.*

Recognizing these limitations, the committee initially examined data from these two sources (the NDATUS and SADAP) to determine whether the states and territories varied in the availability of treatment for alcohol problems and, in cases in which wide variation was found, to attempt to understand the determinants of such variation. The committee found wide differences among the states in both surveys; however, only that variation found in the NDATUS is reported here. SADAP is an annual survey of state resources and services which is conducted by the National Association of State and Drug Abuse Directors (NASADAD), on behalf of the Department of Health and Human Services (Butynski et al., 1987). The SADAP was not used because of several problems. First, the SADAP data do not provide a measure of capacity but rather of utilization. A second problem with these data is that alcohol services funding information cannot be separated from the data on funding on other drug abuse services; the SADAP data are not differentiated because the majority of states has now combined what were formerly separate agencies for alcohol and drug abuse, and expenditures are not always identified categorically. In addition, the SADAP expenditure data do not differentiate among the types of activity (prevention, treatment, or administration and planning) for which expenditures are made. The SADAP is also limited to those treatment agencies that receive funding from the state alcoholism authority and does not include many private sector and federal government programs. In contrast, the NDATUS is a survey of all known treatment units and seeks to differentiate expenditures for treatment of alcohol problems from treatment for problems with other drugs. The committee also examined the American Hospital Association's annual survey of hospitals.

The National Drug and Alcoholism Treatment Unit Survey

As part of its agency mission, NIAAA has been engaged in an ongoing effort to provide state and federal policymakers with the information they require to manage the resources which are needed for providing treatment services for persons with alcohol problems. As part of this effort, NIAAA has periodically conducted surveys of known public and private treatment facilities, seeking data on such variables as capacity, staffing, funding, utilization, and services offered. Since 1979, the major survey, now known as the National Drug and Alcoholism Treatment Unit Survey (NDATUS), has been conducted jointly with the National Institute on Drug Abuse; consequently, the NDATUS surveys two kinds of units that offer services to persons with alcohol problems: (1) those that provide services only for persons with alcohol problems and (2) those that provide treatment for persons with both alcohol and other drug problems (NIAAA, 1983; Yahr, 1988).

The original survey format was discontinued in 1983, and an abbreviated survey, renamed the National Alcoholism and Drug Abuse Program Inventory (NADAPI), was conducted in 1984. The NDAPI collected much less information from each reporting unit than had been collected in earlier years by the NDATUS. The reduction in data collected was part of the overall effort to streamline program administration and reduce federal reporting requirements that was introduced with the advent of the alcohol, drug abuse and mental health services block grant in 1982 (Institute for Health and Aging, 1986). However, because the data collected in 1984 was insufficient to meet the data needs of the sponsoring agencies, the survey conducted in 1987 was very similar in coverage to the 1982 NDATUS survey, and it contained additional items to capture information that was seen as necessary by both federal and state policymakers (USDHHS, 1987a).

The NDATUS is now an ongoing census of all known facilities and organized programs that provide any specialist services to persons with alcohol and other drug problems. In 1984, the survey had been expanded to include nontreatment facilities and units. In 1987 the survey was distributed by the state agency responsible for administering the ADMS block grant. Responses were received from 2,132 "alcoholism only" (28 percent) and 5,360 "combined alcoholism and drug abuse" units (72 percent) in 1987. The total of 7,492 "alcoholism services units" responding included 5,891 units that provided treatment services and 1,601 units that provided primary prevention activities, education activities, central intake activities, and other types of services (NIDA/NIAAA, 1989).

The NDATUS provides an estimate of the specialist resources available throughout the nation and is the most comprehensive data set readily available for use in carrying out a comparison of the distribution of treatment resources currently available among the states and territories. The survey obtained information on the number of persons in treatment on October 30, 1987 and on the capacity of the units in which that treatment was provided (USDHHS, 1987a). Thus, for the purposes of this exploratory analysis, the committee has assumed that the NDATUS variable, "budgeted treatment capacity," can serve as an index of the availability of treatment for alcohol problems.

As shown in Table 7-1, a total of 5,627 alcoholism treatment units completed the 1987 survey; data on persons in treatment were obtained from 1,664 "alcoholism only" (30 percent) and 3,963 "combined alcoholism and drug abuse" units (70 percent). More than 337,000 persons were reported to be in treatment in all units on the date of the survey; budgeted capacity was 416,337, yielding a utilization rate of 81 percent.

The 1987 NDATUS requested each treatment unit to provide information according to the "type of care" it offered. Type of care was defined as ". . . the primary treatment approach or regimen assigned to the client by the treatment unit staff" (USDHHS, 1987a:A-8). The survey provided a matrix for the program to report the number of active clients in treatment on the census date and the budgeted capacity of the

TABLE 7-1 Number of Alcohol Problems Treatment Units, Number of Persons in Treatment, Budgeted Capacity, and Utilization Rate of Units by Type of Care on October 30, 1987

Type of Care	Units	Persons in Treatment	Budgeted Capacity	Utilization Rate (%)
Inpatient/residential				
Medical detoxification	939	6,391	10,353	62
Social detoxification	390	4,015	6,154	65
Rehabilitation/recovery	2,185	37,501	50,615	74
Custodial/domiciliary	2,168	2,688	3,822	70
Total	5,682	50,595	70,944	71
Outpatient/nonresidential	3,701	287,333	345,393	83
Total inpatient and outpatient	5,627	337,928	416,337	81

SOURCE: Based on data from the 1987 National Drug and Alcoholism Treatment Utilization Survey (NIDA/NIAAA, 1989)

unit (i.e., the maximum number of individuals who could be enrolled as active clients given the unit's staffing, funding, and physical facility at the time of the census). Five types of care were identified: (1) medical detoxification, which was defined as involving the use of medication under the supervision of medical personnel in either a hospital or other 24-hour-care facility; (2) social detoxification, involving procedures other than medication carried out by trained personnel with physician services available when required in a specialized nonmedical facility; (3) inpatient/residential rehabilitation/recovery, a planned program of professionally directed evaluation, care, and treatment in either a hospital or other 24-hour-care facility; (4) custodial/domiciliary care, defined as the provision of food, shelter, and assistance in routine daily living on a long-term basis; and (5) outpatient/ nonresidential rehabilitation, which was any form of treatment (detoxification, rehabilitation, recovery, or aftercare) in which the person does not reside in a treatment facility.

For the four types of inpatient and residential care, budgeted capacity means the maximum number of beds a facility has in operation on the survey's census date. The comparable term for outpatient capacity is "slots," that is, the number of persons who can be seen by existing staff on an outpatient basis. The figure does not necessarily refer to licensed capacity. Particularly in the case of outpatient services, the given capacity could be seen as a conservative estimate of potential availability because additional slots could easily be added if there were a demand for services and if funding was available. Future surveys should use a standard definition of capacity to determine capacity and utilization rate (e.g., the number of licensed and staffed beds and slots). An improved survey would more clearly differentiate among orientation, stage, and setting. *The committee suggests that there be an effort to develop a type-of-care categorization which fully captures the range of facilities and programs available for treatment of alcohol problems.*

The types of care identified in the NDATUS correspond roughly to the stages of treatment outlined in Chapter 3, but the NDATUS categorization mixes settings with stages and orientation. In the NDATUS outpatient care includes all three of the major stages identified by the committee: acute intervention (detoxification), rehabilitation, and maintenance (aftercare). Inpatient care is divided into the three major stages and detoxification is further divided into the two major orientations. The outpatient slots similarly could be used for ambulatory detoxification, primary treatment and rehabilitation, continuing treatment, or relapse prevention and supportive maintenance, as well as for treatment of those medical/psychiatric complications that can be dealt with in an ambulatory status.

Because the committee was interested in variations in the availability of treatment for alcohol problems across the 50 states and two jurisdictions (District of Columbia and Puerto Rico) for which data from the 1987 NDATUS are available, the number of slots for outpatient care and the number of beds for each of the four types of inpatient care were converted into a rate per 1,000 persons for each state or jurisdiction. (The conversion used estimates of the drinking-age population on July 1, 1987). It is assumed, for the purposes of this analysis, that the percentage of units reporting in each state does not vary significantly. The data should be interpreted with some caution because there are indications that there were differences across the states in both facilities to which the survey was sent and in the return rate.

The Distribution of Treatment Capacity

The results of the conversion discussed above appear in Table 7-2, which presents by state or jurisdiction, the rates per 1,000 persons in the general population for total treatment capacity, for each of the five types of care, and for total inpatient/residential care. Nationally, there is capacity for 1.7 persons per thousand to be in treatment for alcohol problems. The national rate for budgeted treatment capacity for outpatient care was 1.41 persons per thousand. The national treatment capacity rates for the four types of care identified as only taking place in an inpatient setting were as follows: 0.04 for medical detoxification, 0.03 for social detoxification, 0.21 for rehabilitation, and 0.02 for domiciliary care. The national treatment capacity rate for the four inpatient types of care together was 0.29 per 1,000 persons. The national rate for the two detoxification orientations together was 0.07 per 1,000 persons in the general population.

An examination of the variation among the states for each type of care suggests that there is not equal treatment availability for alcohol problems as measured by the number of beds per 1,000 persons in the general population. Treatment capacity for what the NDATUS categorizes as inpatient/residential rehabilitation and recovery services would conform most closely to what is considered the standard treatment regimen for alcohol problems; that is, the fixed-length inpatient rehabilitation program. For this type of care the range among the states is from a high of 0.49 beds per 1,000 persons in the District of Columbia to a low of 0.07 in Puerto Rico. Other states with high rates are Alaska (0.48), Minnesota (0.43), Montana (0.39), New Hampshire (0.37), and Rhode Island (0.36). Other states with low rates are West Virginia (0.09), South Carolina (0.10), and Georgia, Indiana, and Illinois (0.11).

Detoxification is the only type of care for which reporting is differentiated by treatment philosophy or orientation as well as by treatment stage. The range among the states for treatment using the social detoxification model is from zero to 0.10 beds per 1,000 persons. There are five states (West Virginia, Maine, Wyoming, North Dakota, and the District of Columbia) in which no units reported operating social detoxification beds. Another 28 states have rates less than the national rate (.003). States with a high rate of social detoxification capacity are New York (0.10), Colorado (0.09) Arizona (0.08), South Dakota (0.07), and Nevada and New Mexico (0.06). Medical detoxification has a similar range from zero to 0.14. Only one state (Vermont) has no units reporting medical detoxification beds. It should be noted, however, that medical detoxification can also take place in "scatter beds" in a general or psychiatric hospital and not be reported on the NDATUS. (Scatter beds are those beds in a either a medical-surgical ward or psychiatric ward which are used for detoxification but are not part of an organized program.) States

TABLE 7-2 Budgeted Alcohol Problems Treatment Capacity by State and by Type of Care (rate per 1,000 persons)

State	Inpatient/Residential					Out-patient	Total In- & Out-patient
	Medical Detox.	Social Detox.	Rehab./ Recovery	Custodial/ Domiciliary	Total		
Alabama	0.016	0.004	0.172	0.025	0.217	0.195	0.412
Alaska	0.054	0.002	0.481	0.064	0.601	0.029	3.860
Arizona	0.033	0.083	0.277	0.032	1.425	1.023	1.448
Arkansas	0.041	0.007	0.177	0.022	0.247	0.445	0.692
California	0.022	0.027	0.337	0.003	0.389	2.302	2.691
Colorado	0.018	0.089	0.166	0.027	0.300	3.338	3.638
Connecticut	0.055	0.018	0.220	0.010	0.302	0.881	1.183
Delaware	0.049	0.027	0.171	0.000	0.246	2.116	2.362
Dist. of Columbia	0.102	0.000	0.489	0.146	0.738	1.260	1.998
Florida	0.056	0.047	0.198	0.034	0.335	0.739	1.074
Georgia	0.055	0.001	0.109	0.010	0.175	0.896	1.071
Hawaii	0.002	0.014	0.260	0.000	0.275	0.514	0.789
Idaho	0.065	0.031	0.232	0.008	0.336	1.347	1.682
Illinois	0.018	0.033	0.111	0.017	0.178	0.929	1.108
Indiana	0.019	0.014	0.105	0.014	0.153	1.107	1.260
Iowa	0.026	0.011	0.283	0.029	0.348	1.216	1.565
Kansas	0.021	0.029	0.205	0.009	0.264	1.082	1.346
Kentucky	0.015	0.015	0.117	0.016	0.163	1.375	1.538
Louisiana	0.008	0.004	0.119	0.002	0.133	0.940	1.074
Maine	0.072	0.000	0.190	0.024	0.286	2.852	3.138
Maryland	0.031	0.002	0.167	0.047	0.306	2.315	2.621
Massachusetts	0.136	0.002	0.287	0.005	0.429	1.985	2.415
Michigan	0.030	0.002	0.144	0.000	0.176	1.702	1.878
Minnesota	0.039	0.017	0.430	0.020	0.506	3.390	0.896
Mississippi	0.042	0.035	0.198	0.017	0.291	1.706	1.997
Missouri	0.030	0.027	0.202	0.007	0.266	0.802	1.069
Montana	0.012	0.016	0.385	0.000	0.414	1.509	1.923
Nebraska	0.011	0.044	0.269	0.012	0.336	2.810	3.147
Nevada	0.010	0.057	0.266	0.000	0.333	0.586	0.919
New Hampshire	0.141	0.038	0.371	0.013	0.563	1.423	1.986
New Jersey	0.063	0.007	0.246	0.048	0.364	1.190	1.986
New Mexico	0.031	0.056	0.347	0.000	0.434	2.324	1.554
New York	0.052	0.101	0.143	0.008	0.303	1.882	2.758
North Carolina	0.020	0.039	0.124	0.008	0.190	0.851	2.185
North Dakota	0.107	0.000	0.336	0.000	0.570	2.862	1.141
Ohio	0.029	0.004	0.158	0.019	0.215	1.220	3.433
Oklahoma	0.008	0.014	0.153	0.001	0.176	0.834	1.010
Oregon	0.035	0.037	0.302	0.035	0.410	2.661	3.071
Pennsylvania	0.123	0.006	0.288	0.004	0.421	1.500	1.921
Puerto Rico	0.002	0.013	0.071	0.006	0.092	1.285	1.377
Rhode Island	0.081	0.020	0.364	0.012	0.478	2.996	3.473
South Carolina	0.023	0.033	0.099	0.002	0.157	3.164	3.320
South Dakota	0.040	0.068	0.306	0.095	0.510	2.144	2.654
Tennessee	0.012	0.008	0.143	0.003	0.166	0.569	0.735
Texas	0.055	0.008	0.178	0.007	0.248	0.300	0.548
Utah	0.026	0.014	0.227	0.062	0.329	2.186	2.514
Vermont	0.000	0.018	0.144	0.029	0.192	2.082	2.274
Virginia	0.041	0.011	0.151	0.017	0.220	1.185	1.405
Washington	0.059	0.006	0.197	0.006	0.268	2.365	2.632
West Virginia	0.007	0.000	0.086	0.000	0.094	0.205	0.344

TABLE 7-2 *continues*

TABLE 7-2 (Continued)

State	Inpatient/Residential					Out-patient	Total In- & Out-patient
	Medical Detox.	Social Detox.	Rehab./ Recovery	Custodial/ Domiciliary	Total		
Wisconsin	0.062	0.005	0.222	0.023	0.313	1.301	1.614
Wyoming	0.062	0.000	0.245	0.000	0.477	2.175	2.652
National Total	0.042	0.025	0.207	0.016	0.289	1.409	1.699

SOURCE: Committee analysis of data from the 1987 NDATUS (NIDA/NIAAA, 1989)

with high rates of capacity for medical detoxification are New Hampshire and Massachusetts (0.14), Pennsylvania (0.12), and North Dakota (0.11). Others with low rates are Hawaii, Puerto Rico, West Virginia, Louisiana and Oklahoma (all with rates of less than 0.01).

For all four types of inpatient care the range of beds per 1,000 persons was from a low of 0.09 in Puerto Rico and West Virginia to a high of 0.74 in the District of Columbia. The median is 0.31. Other states with high rates are Alaska (0.60), North Dakota (0.57), New Hampshire (0.56), and South Dakota and Minnesota (0.51). Other states with low rates are Louisiana (0.13), Indiana (0.15), South Carolina (0.16), and Kentucky (0.17).

Treatment capacity for undifferentiated outpatient care among the states ranges from a low of 0.20 in Alabama to a high of 3.34 in Colorado. The median is 1.32. Other states with a high outpatient treatment capacity are Alaska (3.26), South Carolina (3.16) and Rhode Island (3.00). Other states with low rates are West Virginia (0.21), Texas (0.30), Minnesota (0.39), and Arkansas (0.44).

There is wide variation among the states on all of these indexes, with no easily discernible pattern in the variation among the states. Certain states have a high level of one or more types of care and lesser levels of other types of care. Several states have either a higher level of overall treatment capacity (e.g., Alaska, North Dakota, Rhode Island) or a low level of capacity in all types of care (e.g., Alabama, Hawaii, and West Virginia). Pearson product moment correlations were computed to describe the extent to which the five types of care were related (Table 7-3). The strongest relationships were found between the rehabilitation bed and medical detoxification capacities (r = .34) and rehabilitation and custodial/domiciliary care (r = .40). Although this pattern would suggest that there were moderate positive associations among the types of care available, there were only very weak relationships between the four inpatient types and outpatient care. The correlation between the total of the four inpatient types and the rate for outpatient care is only .17.

Table 7-3 also shows a negative correlation between the rate for medical detoxification and the rate for social detoxification (r = -.17). Every state except Vermont had specialist units that reported providing medical detoxification. Five states had no units reporting social detoxification beds.

As shown in Table 7-2, the rate for total budgeted treatment capacity ranges from a low of 0.34 beds per 1,000 persons in West Virginia to a high of 3.86 for Alaska. The median is 1.7 slots and beds available per 1,000 persons. There are 25 states in which total treatment capacity exceeds the national level. In addition, total treatment capacity in eight

TABLE 7-3 Pearson Product Moment Correlations Between Indexes for Types of Care Available in Each State (rates per 1,000 persons)

Type of Care	Social Detoxification	Rehabilitation Recovery	Domiciliary/ Custodial	Total Inpatient	Total Outpatient
Medical detox.	- .17	.34	.16	.47	.11
Social detox.		.01	.01	.09	.17
Rehab./Recov.			.40	.74	.14
Domic./custod.				.50	.12
Total inpatient					.17
Total outpatient					

states is greater than 3.0 per 1,000 persons (Alaska, Colorado, Rhode Island, North Dakota, South Carolina, Nebraska, Maine, and Oregon), whereas capacity reported in seven states is below 1.0 per 1,000 persons (Nevada, Minnesota, Hawaii, Tennessee, Arkansas, Texas, Alabama, and West Virginia). There is a slight tendency for the smaller states to have a higher level of treatment capacity ($r = -.18$).

Thus, on the basis of this review of the 1987 NDATUS data, the answer to the initial question of whether treatment for alcohol problems is equally available throughout the United States must be answered in the negative. Moreover, there is rather wide variation in the capacity available among the 50 states and two jurisdictions analyzed by the committee. Using the 1987 NDATUS data it appears that any type of specialty treatment is 11 times more available in Alaska than it is in West Virginia. The pattern of wide variation among the states and territories is just as extreme for each of the types of care.

Expenditure Data

Another way to establish whether there are variations in capacity among the states is to review the level of funding available for treatment of alcohol problems. The 1987 NDATUS asked each treatment unit to provide data on the sources and total expenditures for alcohol and drug abuse services during the fiscal year which included the NDATUS census date (October 30, 1987) (USDHHS, 1987a). These data can also be used to provide a rough indication of the relative availability of services. Even with the limitations that can be expected when using programs' self reports of funding, the committee has assumed that the NDATUS level of expenditures can be used as another estimate of the level of effort to provide services in a given state and therefore, when expressed as a per capita rate, can serve as a comparative index for the differential availability of services.

The expenditures reported by treatment units in the 1987 NDATUS have been summarized and expressed in Table 7-4 as a per capita rate for each state. Total expenditures for the treatment of alcohol problems as reported in the 1987 NDATUS were $1.712 billion (NIDA/NIAAA, 1989), which translates into a per capita expenditure for treatment in specialty units of $6.99 for the nation as a whole. There is wide variation among the states in the per capita expenditure reported for treatment for all types of care. The total per capita expenditures range from highs of $23.54 reported for Rhode Island and $22.70 for North Dakota to lows of $2.36 and $1.33 reported for Oklahoma and Puerto Rico, respectively. The median is $5.44. Thirty six states have a per capita expenditure treatment of alcohol problems that is below the national median.

It should be noted that this median figure does not represent only the amount of expenditures made by the state governments to purchase services for their residents but rather the total expenditures within a state from all sources of funds, public and private. Also included are expenditures made on behalf of residents from other states who seek out a specific treatment center.

Regardless of the determinants of the variation, the important finding in the committee's analysis of the 1987 NDATUS information is the extreme variation among the states in the per capita expenditure of funds for the treatment of alcohol problems, a finding that suggests that there is extremely differential availability of treatment resources across the country. Of significance is the lack of recent analyses and studies of this variation.

TABLE 7-4 Hospital Bed Rates, Per Capita Total Expenditures, and Problem Indexes by State

State	Alcohol/CD Hospital Beds[a] (per 1,000 persons)	Per Capita Total Expenditure[b]	Age-adjusted Death Rate: Cirrhosis[c]	Per Capita Alcohol Consumption (gallons)[d]
Alabama	0.12	2.23	8.85	1.91
Alaska	0.07	22.29	16.59	3.52
Arizona	0.08	9.52	11.90	3.15
Arkansas	0.11	1.98	7.09	1.64
California	0.13	15.92	15.47	3.12
Colorado	0.12	8.22	9.72	2.88
Connecticut	0.16	7.81	9.22	2.8
Delaware	0.00	5.37	9.52	3.13
District of Columbia	0.28	3.15	30.25	5.67
Florida	0.09	4.28	12.24	2.97
Georgia	0.13	6.19	10.35	2.44
Hawaii	0.02	3.60	5.76	2.89
Idaho	0.03	2.40	9.09	2.33
Illinois	0.16	4.33	11.12	2.68
Indiana	0.21	4.55	7.41	2.15
Iowa	0.24	8.35	6.22	2.05
Kansas	0.26	3.56	6.68	1.89
Kentucky	0.07	3.53	8.18	1.85
Louisiana	0.15	3.15	8.43	2.43
Maine	0.16	5.89	11.53	2.56
Maryland	0.13	7.70	8.58	2.76
Massachusetts	0.11	6.55	10.55	2.97
Michigan	0.11	4.92	12.57	2.57
Minnesota	0.34	9.79	7.02	2.56
Mississippi	0.17	2.28	6.62	2.05
Missouri	0.22	3.67	7.83	2.37
Montana	0.12	16.31	10.56	2.74
Nebraska	0.32	9.95	6.98	2.28
Nevada	0.10	3.03	14.67	5.07
New Hampshire	0.58	13.36	8.67	4.52
New Jersey	0.07	5.44	11.52	2.78
New Mexico	0.11	9.99	13.40	2.70
New York	0.09	11.40	15.33	2.55
North Carolina	0.10	4.39	9.44	2.16
North Dakota	0.52	22.70	7.25	2.40
Ohio	0.14	6.65	8.71	2.18
Oklahoma	0.15	2.36	8.62	1.81
Oregon	0.16	7.85	8.91	2.54
Pennsylvania	0.11	5.37	9.32	2.23
Rhode Island	0.07	23.54	10.70	2.87
South Carolina	0.09	5.53	8.90	2.50
South Dakota	0.17	5.63	5.00	2.24
Tennessee	0.16	2.66	7.16	1.96

TABLE 7-4 *continues*

TABLE 7-4 (continued)

State	Alcohol/CD Hospital Beds[a] (per 1,000 persons)	Per Capita Total Expenditure[b]	Age-adjusted Death Rate: Cirrhosis[c]	Per Capita Alcohol Consumption (gallons)[d]
Texas	0.17	3.68	8.61	2.63
Utah	0.10	5.43	8.71	1.58
Vermont	0.16	4.49	10.84	3.18
Virginia	0.10	6.02	8.65	2.53
Washington	0.16	5.44	9.81	2.66
West Virginia	0.13	2.84	8.48	1.64
Wisconsin	0.18	6.84	7.54	3.16
Wyoming	0.24	4.60	10.37	2.64
National total	0.13	6.99	10.58	2.58

[a]SOURCE: Committee analysis of data from the 1986 AHA Annual Survey of Hospitals (American Hospital Association, 1987).
[b]Committee analysis of data from the 1987 NDATUS (NIDA/NIAAA, 1989).
[c]These data represent age-specific death rates per 100,000 persons in a particular age group. See Table 1 *Age-Adjusted Death Rates for Alcohol-Related Causes by States, 1975-1982: Chronic Liver Disease and Cirrhosis* (Colliver and Malin, 1986).
[d]Data taken from Table XX *Apparent Per Capita Ethanol Consumption (in gallons) by States, 1986* (Steffens et al., 1988).

American Hospital Association Annual Survey of Hospitals

Each year the American Hospital Association (AHA) surveys individual hospitals in the United States and its territories. In one of its special reports to Congress on alcohol and health, DHHS noted the increase in the availability of specialist treatment units in community hospitals that is documented in these surveys (USDHHS, 1987b). In addition, concern has been expressed regarding the proliferation of high-cost medical treatment which such diffusion represents (Miller and Hester, 1986; Yahr, 1988). The number of hospitals offering treatment for alcohol and drug problems in a designated unit was reported to have increased from 465 (16,005 beds) in 1978 to 829 units (25,981 beds) in 1984 (USDHHS, 1987b). In 1986, 1,097 of the 6,296 hospitals (17 percent) responding to the survey reported either a designated unit (1,039 hospitals with 29,058 beds) or being totally devoted to the treatment of "alcoholism and chemical dependency" (58 hospitals and 3,486 beds). Hospitals with specialist programs were reported in each state except Delaware. There were 1,342 hospitals that reported that they had a specialist outpatient service for the treatment of alcohol problems (AHA, 1987).

To look at the availability of specialist treatment from a more conventional perspective, the committee converted these data to a rate per 1,000 persons. No distinction is made in the AHA survey as to stage—units could be offering acute intervention only, rehabilitation only, or both acute intervention and rehabilitation. The results of this transformation are presented in column 1 in Table 7-4. Nationally, in designated hospital units there are 0.13 specialty beds per 1,000 persons. There is wide variation among the states, ranging from no beds reported in Delaware and a rate of 0.03 beds per 1,000 persons in the general population in Hawaii and in Idaho to a high rate of 0.52 beds in North Dakota and 0.58 beds in New Hampshire. There are 24 states with a rate greater than the national rate noted in the table.

The rate per 1,000 persons for specialty beds in hospitals is only moderately related to the rate for the types of care as found in the NDATUS. There is a correlation of .27 between the medical detoxification rate and the hospital rate and a correlation of .20

between the hospital rate and the rehabilitation rate. There are small negative correlations between the hospital bed rate and the rate for social detoxification ($r = -.10$) and outpatient care ($r = -.08$). There may be several explanations for this pattern of correlations. The AHA data do not distinguish between beds used to treat persons with alcohol problems and those used to treat persons with other drug problems. Reimbursement opportunities may determine which type of program is initiated. Differences in practice patterns and in ideological beliefs in the effectiveness of a given treatment strategy, which could be determinants in the development of units, have not been studied. Differences among communities in hospital overcapacity leading to new uses for medical-surgical beds have been discussed as a reason for the increase in the number of designated units, but there have been no published empirical studies of this hypothesis.

Relationship Between Treatment Availability and the Prevalence of Alcohol Problems

To assess whether there was any relationship between the distribution of treatment resources and the prevalence of alcohol problems within the various states, the committee computed Pearson product moment correlations between the treatment capacity rates and two commonly used indirect indexes of the prevalence of alcohol problems that require treatment: apparent per capita consumption of beverage alcohol (Williams et al., 1986; Steffens et al., 1988) and age-adjusted death rates for chronic liver disease and cirrhosis (Colliver and Malin, 1986) (see Table 7-5). These indexes are readily available estimates of the prevalence of alcohol problems and can provide reliable substitutes for the more complex composite indexes or survey data that are often used to estimate the number of persons in need of treatment (Popham, 1970; Schmidt, 1977; AEDS, 1982). These indexes are traditionally included in more complex formulas that have been used to estimate the size of the population in need of treatment services. The two indexes have been used by NIAAA to assess trends in evaluating the nation's efforts to curb alcohol problems (Colliver and Malin, 1986; USDHHS, 1986; Williams et al., 1986).

Apparent per capita consumption of alcoholic beverages is often used as an indirect prevalence measure in research and policy analysis. This index, which is derived from beverage alcohol sales and excise tax data, must be interpreted with a certain amount of caution, however, because the reports do not take into account such factors as alcoholic beverages purchased in one state and consumed in another, unreported sales, purchases and consumption by tourists, consumption of home-brewed beverages, and purchased but unconsumed beverages (Popham, 1970; USDHHS, 1986). Even with these limitations, apparent per capita consumption is one of the few indirect measures of prevalence for which data are readily available for use in an interstate comparison (Williams et al., 1986). The data on consumption included in Table 7-4 and used in this analysis are drawn from the work of Steffens and colleagues (1988) and represent the total per capita consumption of beer, wine, and spirits for the population aged 14 and older. There is wide variation among the states in apparent per capita consumption. Among the states with the highest rates of consumption are the District of Columbia, Nevada, New Hampshire, Alaska, and Vermont; those with the lowest rates included Utah, West Virginia, Arkansas, Oklahoma, Kentucky, and Alabama.

Age-adjusted death rates for chronic liver disease and cirrhosis are the second commonly used index of the level of alcohol problems in a community. Cirrhosis of the liver is one of the leading causes of death in the United States and is estimated to involve alcohol in 41 to 95 percent of cases. Official reports of mortality from liver cirrhosis provide the foundation for the Jellinek estimation formula, which is the best known and, historically most widely used method for estimating prevalence of clinical alcohol problems

TABLE 7-5   Pearson Product Moment Correlations Between Alcohol Problem Indicators and Treatment Availability Indicators

Treatment Availability Indicators	Problem Indicators	
	Per Capita Consumption	Age-adjusted Death Rate/ Cirrhosis
NDATUS Type of Care		
Medical detoxification	.21	.15
Social detoxification	.14	.05
Rehabilitation/recovery	.35	.27
Custodial/domiciliary	.35	.48
Total inpatient	.31	.26
Outpatient	-.08	.00
Total	.02	.04
NDATUS per capita expenditure	.14	.10
AHA bed capacity	.02	-.21

(Popham, 1970; Marden, 1980).   In a sense, cirrhosis mortality is the most conservative estimate, because it focuses on the delineation of the subgroup with the most severe alcohol problems (Marden, 1980).   Local differences in reporting practices are of the most concern in looking at interstate comparisons.   The data on the cirrhosis mortality rate included in Table 7-4 and used in this analysis are drawn from the work of Colliver and Malin (1986).   There is also wide variation among the states in age-adjusted death rates for chronic liver disease and cirrhosis.   Among the states with the highest rates are the District of Columbia, Alaska, California, New York, and New Hampshire; those with the lowest rates included South Dakota, Hawaii, Iowa, Mississippi, and Kansas.

For the 50 states and the District of Columbia, the correlation between apparent per capita consumption and the NDATUS rate of budgeted capacity for treatment is .02, which suggests that there is no relationship between this index and the availability of specialist treatment for alcohol problems.   The correlation between the cirrhosis mortality rate and the NDATUS total per capita budgeted treatment capacity is .04, again suggesting that there is no association between treatment resources and the level of alcohol problems.   However, these analyses should only be seen as preliminary; their greater value is an indication of the need to develop a regular program for monitoring the level of available treatment and for conducting detailed studies on the organization, utilization, and financing of treatment alternatives.

In any realistic study of the reasons for variation among the states in treatment availability, there are many other factors that may be at work which must be attended to: the state's population size, level of poverty, taxing power, fiscal capacity, fiscal effort, regulatory climate, beverage alcohol availability, insurance mandates, citizen advocacy, ethnic composition, drinking patterns, and age distribution.   Studies using multiple regression analyses will be required to determine whether there are meaningful relationships among the many variables that are currently thought to impact on treatment availability. What the literature review and this preliminary analysis highlight is the lack of such studies on the distribution of treatment resources in relation to need (i.e., prevalence), studies that are needed to inform the decisions of policymakers regarding the organization and financing of treatment for alcohol problems.

Summary and Conclusions

Concerned whether all those who wish to receive treatment for alcohol problems are able to receive the treatment of their choice, the committee attempted to determine whether there is a widespread distribution of treatment resources across the United States. Through review of the scant literature and committee analysis of the most relevant data available from the NDATUS and AHA surveys of providers, the committee found that specialist treatment is not equally distributed throughout the country. There is wide variability between jurisdictions in total available treatment capacity. There are also differences in the distribution of each of the types of care and in per capita expenditure of funds. The cause or causes of this variability are unknown and largely unstudied. The variation does not appear to be related to the differences in the prevalence of alcohol problems among the states when prevalence is estimated by two commonly used indexes.

When reviewing the level of resources available in a given jurisdiction, it is difficult to determine what constitutes overcapacity or undercapacity in any of the types of care for which NDATUS or AHA data are available, without an accepted national standard for each type of care (e.g., the number of beds and the number of outpatient slots needed per 1,000 persons in the general population, in total and for each stage of treatment). A starting point for development of such standards would be to utilize the deviation from the observed national rate for each type of care as found in the NDATUS data, or some comparable data set, and to examine the circumstances in the individual states which fall at the extremes of the distribution of rates. *Such comprehensive studies of the possible causes in the variation of development of each state's treatment delivery system should be undertaken to aid our understanding of the changes required to bring about a more equitable distribution of alcohol problems treatment resources across states and across treatment settings or types of care.*

There has been concern in recent years that the number of beds being used in the treatment of alcohol problems is increasing inordinately (Miller and Hester, 1986; Saxe et al., 1983; Saxe and Goodman, 1988; Yahr, 1988). Yet, the data presented earlier in the chapter would suggest that there may be an insufficient number of beds in a number of states. It should be noted that this type of analysis of survey data cannot determine whether the available beds are being used appropriately for the clinically necessary procedure and level or type of care required by a person's clinical status. Determining appropriateness of use is a critical element of studies of availability and access to treatment (MacStravic, 1978). There are few studies of this nature, even though the appropriate use of the inpatient setting for detoxification and for rehabilitation continues to be a major policy issue for the field and for third-party payers.

Several states (e.g., Colorado, Nebraska, New York, Massachusetts, Maryland, Rhode Island) have developed specific estimates of the number of beds or slots that would be required for each treatment setting, treatment stage, treatment modality, or type of care to meet the needs of their "target population". Although usually not stated in terms of a rate per 1,000 persons, the target population estimates can be translated into such rates. Again, it should be noted that there is no consistency among the states in defining settings, types of care, and modalities, and that the types of care included in NDATUS do not conform to individual state definitions. (See Chapters 4 and 18 for the definitions used by Minnesota, Oregon, and Colorado.) There is also no consistency in the estimates of need used by the various states or in the proportion of persons with alcohol problems who require treatment at each stage in a given setting or with a given modality (AEDS, 1982; Brown University Center for Alcohol Studies, 1985).

The committee suggests that there should be the development and testing of a comprehensive model for describing the treatment delivery system for persons with alcohol problems. Such a model should capture all of the existing state variations for use in ongoing analyses of the availability of appropriate types of treatment. Without a consensually developed model to guide such studies, there will be little progress toward defining an appropriate level of services. Policymakers must have access to information on the treatment services being provided that is comprehensive, detailed, timely, and accurate. Currently there are very few meaningful aggregate data available for decisionmaking regarding resource needs and allocation.

Improved surveys are needed that truly capture the relevant data on treatment activities, providers, and costs so that planning, budgeting, and policymaking can proceed in an appropriately informed manner (Weber, 1987; Robertson, 1988; Mintzes, 1988). Reintroduction of the NDATUS items that were designed to collect data on persons in treatment, capacity, funding, and staffing is a step in the right direction, but the NDATUS alone is an insufficient tool for understanding the factors that determine availability of treatment. Another strategy to be encouraged is the development of uniform definitions for items in a minimal data set that can be used by the federal, state, and county governments to collect comparable data on the persons seen in treatment from the programs they fund. These data can than be easily aggregated to permit national and interstate comparisons (Lewin/ICF, 1989a,b). The development of standard demographic, diagnostic, referral source and treatment data items is currently being reviewed by the state alcohol and drug agencies and the Alcohol, Drug Abuse, and Mental Health Administration. Having such data collected in such a standardized manner across jurisdictions would make surveys like NDATUS and SADAP more useful and would allow researchers to carry out the needed in-depth studies of availability and accessibility within and across states using comparable data on the persons assigned to various treatments.

It is clear that there is sufficient variation in treatment resources across the states to conclude that equal availability to specialist treatment for alcohol problems does not exist in this country. The variation does not appear to be related to the differences in the prevalence of alcohol problems among the states. *The committee suggests that there be extensive study of the reasons for these differences in order to develop strategies for equalizing availability of all types of care and to begin addressing questions of accessibility. Ongoing monitoring of the availability of treatment resources should be instituted; it can then be expanded into monitoring of accessibility.*

REFERENCES

Aday, A. L., and R. M. Anderson, 1983. Equity of access to medical care: An overview. Pp. 19-54 in Appendices: Empirical, Legal and Conceptual Studies. Vol. 3 of Securing Access to Health Care: A Report on the Ethical Implication of Differences in the Availability of Health Services, President's Commission for the Study of Ethical Problems in Medicine and Biomedical and Behavioral Research. Washington, D.C.: U.S. Government Printing Office.

Alcohol Epidemiologic Data System (AEDS). 1982. Procedures for Assessing Alcohol Treatment Needs: Administrative Document. Prepared for the National Institute on Alcohol Abuse and Alcoholism. Gaithersburg, Md.: Alcohol Epidemiologic Data System.

Alcohol Epidemiologic Data System, NIAAA. 1985. County Problem Indicators: 1975-1980, U.S. Alcohol Epidemiological Data Reference Manual, Vol. 3. Rockville, Md.: U.S. Department of Health and Human Services.

American Hospital Association (AHA). 1987. Hospital Statistics. Chicago: American Hospital Association.

Bast, R. J. 1984. Classification of Alcoholism Treatment Settings. Rockville, Md.: National Institute on Alcohol Abuse and Alcoholism.

Bayer, A. 1980. Introduction. Pp. 1-2 in A Health Planner's Guide to Planning and Reviewing Alcoholism Services: Selected Readings, A. Bayer, ed. Bethesda, Md.: Alpha Center for Health Planning.

Beckman, L. J., and K. M. Kocel. 1983. The treatment delivery system and alcohol abuse in women: Social policy implications. Journal of Social Issues 38:139-151.

Brown University Center for Alcohol Studies. 1985. Substance Abuse Treatment in Rhode Island: Population Needs and Program Development. Providence, R.I.: Rhode Island Department of Mental Health, Retardation, and Hospitals and Department of Health.

Butynski, W., N. Record, P. Bruhn, and D. Canova. 1987. State Resources and Services Related to Alcohol and Drug Abuse Problems: Fiscal Year 1986. Prepared for the National Institute on Alcohol Abuse and Alcoholism and the National Institute on Drug Abuse, Washington, D.C.: National Association of State Alcohol and Drug Abuse Directors, Inc.

Colliver, J. D., and H. Malin. 1986. State and national trends in alcohol-related mortality: 1975-1982. Alcohol Health and Research World 10(3):60-64.

Ford, W. E. 1980. A data-based technique for projecting alcoholism services. Pp. 24-34 in A Health Planner's Guide to Planning and Reviewing Alcoholism Services: Selected Readings, A. Bayer, ed. Bethesda, Md.: Alpha Center for Health Planning.

Gilbert, M. J., and R. C. Cervantes. 1986. Alcohol services for Mexican Americans: A review of utilization patterns, treatment considerations and prevention activities. Hispanic Journal of Behavioral Sciences 8:1-60.

Gilbert, M. J., and R. C. Cervantes. 1988. Alcohol treatment for Mexican Americans: A review of utilization patterns and therapeutic approaches. Pp. 199-231 in Alcohol Consumption Among Mexicans and Mexican Americans: A Binational Perspective, M. J. Gilbert, ed. Los Angeles: Spanish Speaking Mental Health Research Center, University of California, Los Angeles.

Glaser, F. B., and S. W. Greenberg. 1975. Relationship between treatment facilities and prevalence of alcoholism and drug abuse. Journal of Studies on Alcohol 36:348-358.

Glaser, F. B., S. W. Greenberg, and M. Barrett. 1978. A Systems Approach to Alcohol Treatment. Toronto: Addiction Research Foundation.

Gunnersen, U. and M. L. Feldman. 1978. Alcohol and Alcoholism Programs: A Technical Assistance Manual for Health Systems Agencies. San Leandro, Calif.: Human Services, Inc.

Harrington, C., J. H. Swan, and L. A. Grant. 1988. Nursing home bed capacity in the United States, 1979-1986. Health Care Financing Review 9:81-97.

Institute for Health and Aging. 1986. Review and Evaluation of Alcohol, Drug Abuse and Mental Health Services Block Grant Allotment Formulas: Final Report. Prepared for the Alcohol, Drug Abuse, and Mental Health Administration. San Francisco, Calif.: University of California, San Francisco.

Knesper, D. J., J. R. C. Wheeler, and D. J. Pagnucco. Mental health service providers' distribution across counties in the United States. American Psychologist 1984:1424-1934.

Lewin/ICF. 1989a. Analysis of State Alcohol and Drug Data Collection Instruments, vols. 1-6. Prepared for the Office of Finance and Coverage Policy, National Institute on Drug Abuse. Washington D.C.: Lewin/ICF.

Lewin/ICF. 1989b. Feasibility and Design of a Study of the Delivery and Financing of Drug and Alcohol Services. Prepared for the National Institute on Drug Abuse. Washington, D.C.: Lewin/ICF.

Marden, P. G. 1980. Efforts to estimate the prevalence of alcohol abuse. Pp. 14-21 in A Health Planner's Guide to Planning and Reviewing Alcoholism Services: Selected Readings, A. Bayer, ed. Bethesda, Md.: Alpha Center for Health Planning.

McAuliffe, W. E., P. Breer, N. White, C. Spino., L. Goldsmith, S. Robel, and L. Byam. 1988. A Drug Abuse Treatment and Intervention Plan for Rhode Island. Cranston, R. I.: Rhode Island Department of Mental Health, Retardation, and Hospitals.

McGough, D. P., and M. Hindman. 1986. A Guide to Planning Alcoholism Treatment Programs. Rockville, Md.: National Institute on Alcohol Abuse and Alcoholism.

MacStravic, R. E. 1978. Determining Health Needs. Ann Arbor, Mich.: Health Administration Press.

Miller, W. R., and R. K. Hester. 1986. Inpatient alcoholism treatment: Who benefits? American Psychologist 41:794-805.

Mintzes, B. 1988. Statement presented at the open meeting of the IOM Committee for Treatment and Rehabilitation Services for Alcoholism and Alcohol Abuse, Washington, D.C., January 25.

National Institute on Alcohol Abuse and Alcoholism (NIAAA). 1980. Health Planning Technical Assistance Manual for Alcohol and Drug Abuse Agencies. Rockville, Md.: U.S. Department of Health and Human Services.

National Institute on Alcohol Abuse and Alcoholism (NIAAA). 1983. Executive Report: Data from the September 30, 1982 National Drug and Alcoholism Treatment Utilization Survey. Rockville, Md.: National Institute on Alcohol Abuse and Alcoholism. April.

National Institute on Drug Abuse/National Institute on Alcohol Abuse and Alcoholism (NIAAA/NIDA). 1989. Highlights from the 1987 National Drug and Alcoholism Treatment Unit Survey (NDATUS). Rockville, Md.: National Institute on Drug Abuse/National Institute on Alcohol Abuse and Alcoholism. February.

New York Division of Alcoholism and Alcohol Abuse (NYDAAA). 1983. Five Year Comprehensive Plan for Alcoholism Services in New York State: 1984-1989. Albany, N.Y.: NYDAAA.

New York Division of Alcoholism and Alcohol Abuse (NYDAAA). 1987. Five Year Comprehensive Plan for Alcoholism Services in New York State: 1984-1989, Final 1987 Update. Albany, N.Y.: NYDAAA.

New York Division of Alcoholism and Alcohol Abuse (NYDAAA). 1988. Long Range Comprehensive Plan for Alcoholism Services in New York State: Long Range Plan-1988. Albany, N.Y.: NYDAAA.

New York Division of Alcoholism and Alcohol Abuse (NYDAAA). 1989. Five Year Comprehensive Plan for Alcoholism Services in New York State: 1989-1994. Albany, N.Y.: NYDAAA.

Popham, R. E. 1970. Indirect methods of alcoholism prevalence estimation: A critical evaluation. Pp. 678-685 in Alcohol and Alcoholism, R.E. Popham, ed. Toronto: University of Toronto Press.

Robertson, A. D. 1988. Federal and state support for alcohol and drug abuse services. Testimony on behalf of the National Association of State Alcohol and Drug Abuse Directors presented to the U. S. Senate Committee on Governmental Affairs hearing regarding an overview of federal activities on alcohol abuse and alcoholism, National Association of State Alcohol and Drug Abuse Directors, Washington, D.C., May 25.

Rush, B. 1988. A systems approach to estimating the required capacity of alcohol treatment services. Addictions Research Foundation Community Programs Evaluation Center, London, Ontario, December.

Saxe, L., D. Dougherty, K. Esty, and M. Fine. 1983. The Effectiveness and Costs of Alcoholism Treatment. Washington: U.S. Congress, Office of Technology Assessment.

Saxe, L., and L. Goodman. 1988. The effectiveness of outpatient vs. inpatient treatment: Updating the OTA report. Boston University Center for Applied Social Science, Boston.

Schmidt, W. 1977. Cirrhosis and alcohol consumption: an epidemiological perspective. Pp 15-47 in Alcoholism: New Knowledge and Responses, G. Edwards and M. Grant, eds. London: Croom Helm.

Shandler, I. W., and T. E. Shipley. 1987a. New focus for an old problem: Philadelphia's response to homelessness. Alcohol Health and Research World 2(3):54-56.

Shandler, I. W., and T. E. Shipley. 1987b. Policy, funding, resources are needed. Alcohol Health and Research World 2(3):88.

Sheridan, J. R. 1986. The extent of alcohol and drug abuse in the State of Maryland and resource allocation methods. Prepared for the Maryland Alcoholism Control/Drug Abuse Administration, Baltimore, Md., July.

Steffens, R. A., F. S. Stinson, C. G. Freel, and D. Clem. 1988. Surveillance Report No. 10: Apparent Alcohol Consumption: National, State and Regional Trends, 1977-1986. Rockville, Md.: National Institute on Alcohol Abuse and Alcoholism, Division of Biometry and Epidemiology, Alcohol Epidemiologic Data System.

U.S. Department of Health and Human Services (USDHHS). 1984. Fifth Special Report to the U.S. Congress on Alcohol and Health. Rockville, Md.: National Institute on Alcohol Abuse and Alcoholism.

U.S. Department of Health and Human Services (USDHHS). 1986. Toward a National Plan to Combat Alcohol Abuse and Alcoholism: Report Submitted to the U.S. Congress. Rockville, Md.: National Institute on Alcohol Abuse and Alcoholism.

U.S. Department of Health and Human Services (USDHHS). 1987b. Sixth Special Report to the U.S. Congress on Alcohol and Health. Rockville, Md.: National Institute on Alcohol Abuse and Alcoholism.

U.S. Department of Health and Human Services (USDHHS). 1987a. 1987 National Drug and Alcoholism Treatment Unit Survey: NDATUS Instruction Manual for States and Reporting Units. Rockville, Md.: National Institute on Drug Abuse and National Institute on Alcohol Abuse and Alcoholism.

Weber, R. 1987. Advocacy Group Data Needs and Researcher Responsibilities. Presented at the National Council on Alcoholism Forum, Cleveland, Ohio, April 24.

Williams, G. D., D. Doernberg, F. Stinson, and J. A. Noble. 1986. Epidemiologic Bulletin 12: State, regional, and national trends in apparent per capita consumption. Alcohol Health and Research World 10(3):60-63.

Wilson, R., and P. Hartsock. 1981. Current Practices in Alcoholism Treatment Needs Estimation: A State-of-the-Art Report. Prepared for the National Institute on Alcohol Abuse and Alcoholism. Gaithersburg, Md: Alcohol Epidemiologic Data System.

Yahr, H. T. 1988. A national comparison of public- and private-sector alcoholism treatment delivery system characteristics. Journal of Studies on Alcohol 49:233-239.

8   Who Pays for Treatment?

One of the continuing concerns voiced by those active in the treatment of alcohol problems is that financial barriers may prevent individuals who need help from receiving appropriate treatment. In testimony at its public hearing and in written responses to its request for delineation of issues, the committee heard clearly that the expressed goal of many in the field is that persons who require treatment for alcohol problems have access to the same set of financing options that are available for treatment of persons with physical illnesses. Another concern that is often expressed is that only a small proportion of those who need treatment have received it. It is not clear whether these concerns reflect a failure to identify and refer such individuals (D. C. Lewis, 1987), inadequate treatment capacity, or financial barriers to receiving needed care (Fein, 1984; Davis, 1987; Morrisey and Jensen, 1988). A criticism often made by representatives of the field is that inadequate benefits for treatment are provided through the health insurance mechanisms that are available for other illnesses (e.g., T. Daugherty, Recovery Centers of America, Inc., personal communication, January 21, 1988; Ford, 1988; Shulman, 1988).

These concerns raise the question of who is paying for treatment of persons with alcohol problems and what is the relative contribution of each of the various funders to the overall funding support for each of the specific treatment stages and settings.

Until the early 1970s the major sources of funding for treatment of persons with alcohol problems were state and local governments that provided these services as part of their mental health, public health, and criminal justice programs. Emergency care for public inebriates in jails and in public hospital emergency rooms and medical wards and custodial care for chronic alcoholics in state mental hospitals were the major resources available (Glasscote et al., 1967; Plaut, 1967; Boche, 1975). Health insurance was not available, although many persons were treated for the physical complications of chronic, excessive alcohol use under other diagnoses (Rosenberg, 1968; Hallan, 1972; USDHEW, 1974, 1978; Fein, 1984).

Because of the evidence that funding was not available for the treatment of alcohol problems in community hospitals and other health and social service settings, the voluntary associations and governmental agencies involved in the alcohol field have concentrated on shifting support to a broad range of funding sources and developing a stable financing base through specific categorical funding and health insurance coverage (USDHEW, 1974; Regan, 1981; USDHHS, 1981; J. S. Lewis, 1982; Butynski, 1986; USDHHS, 1986). Traditionally, financing for the treatment for alcohol problems was seen as belonging under the rubric of mental health services and as such has suffered from the same negative, stigmatizing perceptions of health insurers, employers, and the community at large that have bedeviled mental health funding (Sharfstein et al., 1984). It was not until the early 1960s that a movement developed for separate funding mechanisms and organizations for treatment of mental disorders, alcohol problems, and drug abuse problems (Plaut, 1967; President's Commission on Mental Health, Task Panel on Alcohol Related Problems, 1978; J. S. Lewis, 1982; Weisman, 1988).

Since its establishment in 1971 NIAAA has sponsored studies of the impact of treatment of alcohol problems on subsequent health care costs (e.g., Holder and Hallan, 1983; Holder, 1987) as well as studies on the effectiveness of treatment. These studies have been used to encourage the expansion of both public and private sources of funds for treating alcohol problems (Saxe et al., 1983; Fein, 1984; Luckey, 1987; USDHHS, 1987). The results of these studies have been used by the field to demonstrate to legislators, employers, and insurers the benefits of such treatment. The research has focused on several hypotheses: (1) that the treatment of alcohol problems has positive outcomes; (2) that the addition of a specific benefit for treatment of alcohol problems will not increase insurers' payouts because of the offsets to be achieved through reductions in the high medical costs of untreated alcohol-dependent persons (Jones and Vischi, 1979; Fein, 1984; Davis, 1987; Holder, 1987); and (3) that early case finding and treatment of alcohol problems would help to reduce other social costs (e.g., lost productivity, automobile and other accidents, criminal justice processing and incarceration costs, and welfare transfer payments (Fein, 1984).

Attempts by leaders in the field to obtain consideration for treatment of alcohol problems as a primary disorder, and not simply a symptom of mental illness, have included efforts to develop separate model benefit packages that would encourage insurers to provide coverage for state-of-the-art treatment. Such models have been presented by the voluntary organizations involved in seeking expanded treatment resources (National Council on Alcoholism Task Force on Health Insurance, 1974; Flavin, 1988) as well as by insurers like the Blue Cross-Blue Shield Association (Berman and Klein, 1977; Leyland et al., 1983), and the Group Health Association (Plotnick et al., 1982). Although there are those who question the wisdom of moving in the direction of depending primarily on health insurance for a stable source of funding, given the sociocultural model of treatment which they endorse (Borkman, 1988; Reynolds, 1988), the field's major emphasis continues to be on efforts to move financing of treatment for alcohol problems into the mainstream of health care financing. Active support of legislative efforts to obtain mandated private health insurance benefits is seen as a major means to accomplish this goal (Butynski, 1986; Luckey, 1987; Flavin, 1988).

The result of these efforts has been a steady increase in the number of public and private sources of financing. Many third-party payers now have specific, discrete reimbursement policies for the treatment of alcohol withdrawal, or detoxification, and treatment of excessive alcohol consumption, or rehabilitation (Jacob, 1985; Davis, 1987; USDHHS, 1987; Gordis, 1987; Morrisey and Jensen, 1988). Yet the attempt to separate funding and organizational structures to support specialty, high-quality treatment of alcohol problems has been only partially and inconsistently successful. Treatment for alcohol problems is still considered to belong in the "nervous and mental disorders" category by most public and private health third-party payers, including Medicaid and Medicare, a policy that creates difficulties in obtaining data on actual expenditures and in developing an independent body of research on financing and its relation to practice (Burton, 1984; Sharfstein et al., 1984; Muszynski, 1987).

There is no single survey currently in use that captures data on the amount of money being spent for the treatment of alcohol problems (Muszynski, 1987; Robertson, 1988). There is also no compendium of the recent trends in financing treatment services. This is an area of health services research which has been severely neglected for the past eight years (Wallen, 1988). Recently, however, an initiative has been developed to expand the study of the organization and financing of treatment for alcohol problems (NIAAA, 1989). The studies to be carried out under this initiative may begin to generate some of the information needed by policymakers.

Shifts in the loci of treatment in recent years have contributed to the difficulties in tracking expenditures. Treatment is now provided in a diverse network of traditional and nontraditional settings including hospitals, freestanding residential facilities, private practitioners' offices, and outpatient clinics (see Chapter 4). The growth of the specialty sector for treating alcohol problems has seen a concomitant increase in the number of specialized hospital units that provide detoxification or rehabilitation or both; such growth has also fostered the development of freestanding detoxification and primary care and extended care rehabilitation facilities which are not licensed or registered as hospitals and thus are not included in more traditional surveys of health facilities (e.g., those carried out by the American Hospital Association and the National Center for Health Statistics). There has also been a veritable explosion of organized specialty outpatient clinics that also are not covered in the traditional health care facility surveys (Reed and Sanchez, 1986).

Many of these nontraditional agencies receive federal and state categorical funds (dedicated to the treatment of alcohol problems) through the state alcoholism authorities. There is an increasing trend, however, to combine under the substance abuse/chemical dependency rubric the funding and organization of services for persons experiencing problems with alcohol with services for persons experiencing problems with other drugs (Butynski and Record, 1983). One of the difficulties created by this combination is the failure to obtain reporting from the states on their distribution of both state funds and federal alcohol, drug abuse, and mental health services block grant funds that are specifically earmarked for the treatment of alcohol problems. The State Alcohol and Drug Abuse Profile (SADAP), which serves as the key report on the use of state and federal funds for the treatment of alcohol problems, does not disaggregate the funds being spent specifically for treatment of alcohol problems. Rather, the SADAP reports total expenditures, which include administrative oversight, planning and regulation, and primary prevention as well as for treatment (Butynski and Record, 1983; Butynski and Canova, 1988).

These considerations make it difficult to obtain current, precise data on the sources of funding specific to the treatment of alcohol problems. Recognizing these limitations, the committee has nonetheless attempted to identify the major funding sources and to present what is known about who pays for the treatment of alcohol problems in both traditional and nontraditional treatment settings.

Who Are the Payers?

There are a number of different sources of payment for the treatment of alcohol problems, and these payers can be thought of as falling into three major categories: (1) the individual seeking treatment and his or her family; (2) a health insurance company acting on behalf of individuals or employers who purchase insurance; or (3) a government agency. Health insurers and government agencies are generally referred to, respectively, as private or public third-party payers. Through the years, the major source of financing for treatment of alcohol problems has been third-party payers, as is the case for all health services.

Public and private third-party payers differ primarily in the beneficiaries they serve (defined by client eligibility criteria), the methods used to finance their payments (taxes or premiums), and the type of oversight or regulation to which they are subject. Private third-party payers may be insurance companies that are organized either as a special type of nonprofit corporation (e.g., the Blue Cross Association plans and labor union trusts) or as for-profit commercial carriers. Private third-party payers may also be prepaid group health plans or health maintenance organizations (HMOs), either nonprofit or for-profit, that provide insurance and deliver care (see Chapter 18). Private third-party payers offer coverage to subscribers or customers, either through group plans, which are purchased by an employer on behalf of its employees or by an association on behalf of its members, or through plans purchased directly by an individual. An increasing number of employers are choosing to become self-insured; that is, employers bear the cost of the claims directly rather than by purchasing insurance from an insurance carrier although they may purchase "stop-loss" insurance for major illnesses to lessen their total exposure. Self-insured health insurance plans are administered in the same manner as those purchased from an insurance company. Benefit plans and premium levels are designed to meet the needs of the individuals to be covered, and they use actuarial techniques which reflect the health status of the insured to project the levels of service that will be needed and the costs anticipated. Such plans generally use professional or governmental accreditation or licensing standards to identify eligible providers (organizations and practitioners), as well as procedures that will be eligible for reimbursement. Alternatively, third-party payers may develop their own standards (Gibson, 1988).

Private third-party insurers are funded through the premiums paid by purchasers; premiums are adjusted periodically based on the claims made by the subscriber group and the benefit design of the specific insurance policy. The coverage minimums, benefit designs, and premiums of private third-party payers are regulated by the states through their insurance departments; the exception is self insured plans which come under the federal Employment, Retirement, and Income Security Act of 1974 (ERISA). Currently, it is estimated that self-insured plans cover approximately 42 percent of the work force.

Medicaid and Medicare are generally thought of as the public third-party payers for health care services, although, any state or local government agency (as well as a federal government agency) that purchases health care services for a defined group of eligible beneficiaries can be a public third-party payer. Government agencies generally limit coverage to a special population that has been identified through legislation: the economically disadvantaged, the medically indigent, the mentally ill, the physically disabled, the aged, the military, the drug abuser, the person with alcohol problems, veterans, the public inebriate, high-risk pregnant women, families with dependent children, the blind, the homeless, and so on. The benefits to be provided (i.e., the services to be purchased) are also authorized through legislation and are refined through the regulations and appropriations processes. Government agencies may provide reimbursement either through a unit of service purchase system, or a program budget contract or grant system, or a prospective payment system modeled after Medicare's, just as private insurers do. Eligible providers are identified, either through legislation or regulation, using the same methods adopted by private insurers.

The federal government as a third-party payer funds treatment for alcohol problems through a variety of mechanisms including the direct operation of treatment programs in federal facilities for various categories of federal beneficiaries, the purchase of services provided in a variety of public and private facilities through its public health insurance programs, and the provision of funds for the development and support of treatment programs at other levels of government and in the private sector through categorical and block grant programs (NIAAA, 1984). Agencies that operate their own networks of programs for treatment of alcohol problems are the Veterans Administration, the military services within the Department of Defense, the Bureau of Prisons, and the Indian Health Service (see Chapter 4). Agencies that provide funding through insurance are the Health Care Financing Administration (Medicare and Medicaid), the Department of Defense (CHAMPUS), the Veterans Administration (CHAMP-VA), and the Office of Personnel Management (Federal Employees Health Benefits Plan). Agencies that provide block grant funding are the Alcohol, Drug Abuse, and Mental Health Administration and the Office of Human Services. Other agencies administer programs that may provide funding used in the treatment of persons with alcohol problems although such treatment is not their primary focus (e.g., the Department of Agriculture's food stamp program).

State and local government agencies provide both categorical funds, targeted for treatment of alcohol problems and administered by a specialty agency, or funds that are part of a larger medical services or social services program for the disabled or for the indigent. State and local governments may also operate treatment programs directly, either through an agency specializing in the treatment of alcohol problems or as part of their mental health or public health treatment agencies, or through all three mechanisms.

Funding practices and program administration vary considerably among the states and territories (Akins and Williams, 1982; Butynski and Record, 1983; Butler and Littlefield, 1985; Butynski and Canova, 1988). Although each state and territory has an agency that is responsible for funding and monitoring treatment activities, this agency may not be the only state entity to expend such funds. State Medicaid, vocational rehabilitation, and social services agencies are also likely to be providing funds for treatment or supportive services for persons with alcohol problems.

Individuals with no private or public health insurance or with insurance that does not include a benefit for the treatment of alcohol problems make up the largest group of persons being treated in programs supported by state and federal categorical funds, which are administered by the states through their specialist state alcoholism agencies. Persons treated in publicly operated or funded programs tend to be socioeconomically disadvantaged (Costello, 1980, 1982; Costello and Hodde, 1981; Pattison, 1985; Weisner and Room, 1984; Weisner, 1986; Weisman, 1988). Socially disadvantaged persons seeking treatment for alcohol problems report serious disruptions in many life areas; they also tend to have high rates of unemployment, poor work histories, and few job skills so that treatment requires a mix of medical and social support services. State and local alcoholism agencies have recognized these needs in their funding policies and will often support the delivery of both treatment and social services in nonhospital primary care and extended care facilities (see Chapters 3 and 4). The agencies typically serve a broker role in arranging for the necessary social services to provided to persons in treatment (Akin and Williams, 1982).

Typically, public payers are funded through general tax revenues. The federal government's programs are primarily funded through in this manner; however, Medicare is funded through a combination of a specific tax on earnings, general revenues, and premiums. States and local governments typically finance their obligations through general revenue taxes. Through the years, several states have adopted dedicated, or earmarked, taxes or license fees (or both) that are used to pay for treatment for alcohol problems. In several states (e.g., Minnesota, Colorado) persons arrested for driving while intoxicated are legally required to pay fees for court-ordered diagnostic, treatment, education, and supervision services.

Increasingly, public third-party payment plans have been redesigned to resemble private insurance with deductibles, copayment requirements, and episode, benefit period, annual, or lifetime limits on reimbursement. These changes have led most state and local agencies to require that the community-based agencies with which they contract for services have in place a sliding fee scale (generally based on income and necessary expenses) as a copayment mechanism. Many public payers now have a procedure for the coordination of benefits, with the government agency serving as a secondary payer after public or private insurance has been exhausted. These same coordination of benefits requirements apply when an individual is treated in a state or local government-operated detoxification or rehabilitation program.

Third-party payers can also be differentiated in terms of which components of treatment they will pay for. Public and private health insurers clearly confine their benefits to services that are identified as medical and that meet specific standards of medical necessity. An individual provider who is eligible to receive reimbursement under a health insurance plan generally must be either a physician, a health care professional licensed for independent practice, or a health care worker providing a service under the supervision of a physician or other licensed health care professional. Facilities (e.g., hospitals, clinics) must be licensed as health care institutions to receive reimbursement. Categorical programs administered by state alcoholism agencies are more likely to cover supportive services (e.g., sheltered living) and treatment delivered by nontraditional personnel in nontraditional facilities, (e.g., alcoholism counselors, halfway houses).

Who Pays for Treatment in Specialty Programs?

As noted in the previous chapter, the National Drug and Alcohol Treatment Utilization Survey (NDATUS) is periodically administered by NIAAA (in conjunction with NIDA) to obtain data on a number of aspects of treatment for alcohol problems in this country, including the sources of funding in specialty programs. As part of its data collection activities NIAAA has conducted studies on the sources of funding available to specialty programs, the barriers to be overcome in achieving stability in funding, and the characteristics of the treatment delivery system. Despite certain limitations, this survey remains the best source of data on the sources of funding for treatment of alcohol problems in specialist programs.

The most recent NDATUS survey to provide data on the cost of alcohol problems treatment was carried out in 1987 (NIDA/NIAAA, 1989), and it reported total expenditures for treatment of alcohol problems $1.712 billion (Table 8-1). Before the 1987 survey, the last NDATUS to contain cost data was carried out in 1982 (NIAAA, 1983); total spending of $1.123 billion was reported in that study.

As shown in Table 8-1 the 1987 NDATUS gathered information on 11 broad categories of funding sources; the data are not broken down according to the amounts received from major sources such as commercial health insurance, Blue Cross/Blue Shield, and HMOs in the private third-party category or Medicaid, CHAMPUS, and Medicare in the public third-party pay category. Seven of the categories are for governmental sources. Four of the categories capture information on funds received from a state or local governmental agency (33 percent of the total), and three are federal government sources

TABLE 8-1 Sources of Funding for Specialty Units Providing Treatment for Alcohol Problems in 1982 and 1987, Based on Data from the National Drug and Alcoholism Treatment Unit Survey (in thousands of dollars)

Funding Sources	1982 Amount	1982 Percentage	1987 Amount	1987 Percentage
State government program funds	235,751	21.1	345,023	20.2
Local government program funds	108,254	9.6	107,660	6.3
State/local government fees for service	45,413	4.0	78,830	4.6
Public welfare	18,257	1.6	27,778	1.6
Public health insurance	77,922	6.9	145,746	8.5
Alcohol, drug abuse, and mental health block grant	50,910	4.5	N/A[a]	-
Social services block grant	13,959	1.2	N/A[b]	-
Other ADAMHA support	12,133	1.1	9,440	0.6
Other federal funds	112,456	10.0	76,957	4.5
Private health insurance	296,419	26.4	592,470	34.6
Private donations	28,754	2.6	26,906	1.6
Client fees	110,272	9.8	236,531	13.8
Other	12,677	1.1	64,752	3.8
Total	1,123,175[c]	100.0	1,712,069	100.0

SOURCE: NIAAA (1983); NIDA/NIAAA (1989).
[a] Included in the state government program funds category.
[b] Included in the public welfare category.
[c] Totals may not add because of rounding.

(13 percent). The nongovernmental sources include private health insurance (33 percent), private donations (2 percent), and out-of-pocket payments (14 percent). A residual category ("other") represents 4 percent of the total. The contribution of each major source of funds for each state and territory included in the NDATUS is presented in Table 8-2.

TABLE 8-2 Major Sources of Funding for Specialty Units Providing Treatment for Alcohol Problems by State, Including Puerto Rico and the District of Columbia, Based on Data from the 1987 National Alcoholism and Drug Treatment Unit Survey (in percent)

| State | Percentage of total | | | | | |
	State and Local Govt.	Federal Govt.	Public Third Party	Private Third Party	Client Fees	Other and Donations
Alabama	28.2	1.4	8.0	44.0	9.0	9.4
Alaska	67.6	9.4	0.1	9.9	4.8	8.3
Arizona	30.2	7.4	2.4	42.4	11.9	5.6
Arkansas	47.2	1.4	5.4	19.4	4.1	22.5
California	12.9	4.2	4.7	57.9	18.9	1.4
Colorado	39.8	0.1	7.7	26.0	22.8	3.6
Connecticut	53.1	1.5	7.1	15.5	18.4	4.4
Delaware	57.0	0.1	0.0	0.0	38.1	4.8
Dist. of Col.	97.1	0.0	0.0	1.5	1.3	0.0
Florida	45.4	9.0	6.9	22.6	12.0	4.1
Georgia	41.9	2.7	4.3	14.8	36.3	0.1
Hawaii	42.7	10.0	0.1	1.8	16.6	28.8
Idaho	56.8	4.2	0.6	12.0	23.7	2.7
Illinois	52.8	3.9	3.5	25.3	9.9	4.6
Indiana	25.4	12.7	6.8	34.0	10.7	10.5
Iowa	47.9	15.8	8.2	21.2	3.3	3.6
Kansas	34.4	0.9	8.3	39.0	13.9	3.4
Kentucky	50.1	2.6	13.8	20.1	7.6	5.8
Louisiana	38.0	2.0	13.5	12.2	27.5	3.0
Maine	52.0	13.3	5.8	9.2	12.2	6.8
Maryland	49.4	4.7	19.1	8.2	15.4	3.1
Massachusetts	56.2	4.3	6.9	13.3	10.4	8.5
Michigan	35.1	4.0	7.8	33.2	9.7	10.2
Minnesota	38.0	8.9	7.7	28.7	12.6	4.2
Mississippi	54.7	15.5	4.2	11.4	10.4	3.8
Missouri	46.1	11.8	3.7	23.8	7.2	7.4
Montana	29.9	3.5	1.6	42.4	17.4	5.1
Nebraska	27.5	12.0	1.3	17.5	36.4	5.3
Nevada	65.0	11.0	0.3	2.5	13.5	7.8
New Hampshire	19.8	2.6	4.6	51.5	4.0	1.5
New Jersey	27.7	6.7	1.1	43.2	11.9	9.3
New Mexico	56.4	15.1	4.1	8.7	11.9	3.9
New York	41.8	1.2	22.5	19.7	9.2	5.5
North Carolina	59.6	3.5	2.9	9.8	15.1	9.1
North Dakota	44.4	0.3	9.3	30.0	13.3	2.7
Ohio	24.9	2.9	10.9	46.1	8.5	6.6
Oklahoma	39.3	17.8	8.4	16.3	11.5	6.8
Oregon	45.2	10.0	2.0	16.2	19.7	6.9
Pennsylvania	29.4	2.3	18.3	39.2	6.0	4.8
Puerto Rico	75.8	0.2	0.0	0.0	0.1	23.9
Rhode Island	18.2	0.8	6.2	67.5	6.5	0.8

TABLE 8-2 *continues*

TABLE 8-2 (continued)

| State | Percentage of total | | | | | |
	State and Local Govt.	Federal Govt.	Public Third Party	Private Third Party	Client Fee	Other and Donations
South Carolina	50.8	9.3	4.3	15.6	15.3	4.6
South Dakota	38.9	27.4	0.3	20.6	10.7	2.1
Tennessee	33.1	18.9	10.7	23.6	9.7	4.0
Texas	15.3	4.6	9.3	38.5	10.8	21.5
Utah	53.3	9.0	2.0	10.1	19.3	6.3
Vermont	61.9	0.9	8.2	13.4	11.4	4.1
Virginia	31.9	12.3	4.3	30.6	9.2	11.8
Washington	35.5	4.7	6.6	28.5	15.9	8.9
West Virginia	65.5	0.4	9.1	11.1	7.0	6.8
Wisconsin	38.6	6.7	12.4	30.5	6.3	5.6
Wyoming	62.1	4.2	2.3	17.4	10.4	3.5
National[a]	32.7	5.0	8.5	34.6	13.8	5.4

SOURCE: NIDA/NIAAA (1989).

[a] Row totals may not sum to 100 percent because of rounding.

The first category, state government program funds, are so-called categorical funds that are appropriated specifically to provide treatment services on a program or unit level and are not necessarily tied to reimbursement for specific services to a given individual. In 1987 federal funds provided to a state through the alcohol, drug abuse, and mental health services block grant were included in this category. The Omnibus Budget Reconciliation Act of 1981 created a number of health and social services block grants to states with the intention of simplifying federal funding requirements by combining and replacing a number of categorical project and formula grant programs to states, local governments, and community based agencies (U.S. General Accounting Office, 1985). The alcohol, drug abuse, and mental health services block grant consolidated the formula grant and project grant and contract programs administered by the National Institute on Alcohol Abuse and Alcoholism with similar programs administered by the National Institute on Drug Abuse and the National Institute of Mental Health. At the same time, the administration of these funds was transferred from the Institutes to their parent agency, the Alcohol, Drug Abuse, and Mental Health Administration.

The block grant is administered consistent with congressional intent and administration policy to provide the states with flexibility in setting and carrying out local priorities and to avoid burdensome reporting requirements. The basic premise of block grants is that states (and territories) should be free to target resources and to design administrative mechanisms to meet the needs of their citizens (ADAMHA, 1984; U.S. General Accounting Office, 1984).

The bulk of the block grant is passed through by the state alcoholism agency to local governments or to nonprofit contract agencies that deliver direct services. States allocate the funds according to whatever policies they use to contract for services. There are several restrictions on the ways funds can be used. A limit is set on the amount of money which can be used for state administrative activities. In addition 20 percent of the funds are to be used for prevention. Two further restrictions are that block grant treatment funds may not be spent for services in a hospital and a specific percentage must be spent to increase services to women (U.S. General Accounting Office, 1984; National Council on Alcoholism, 1987).

Recently, additional funding was provided through the alcohol and drug abuse treatment and rehabilitation (ADTR) block grant, authorized by the Anti-Drug Abuse Act of 1986 as emergency two year funding to begin in federal fiscal year 1987. The ADTR block grant was established to: (1) increase the availability and outreach of existing centers; (2) expand the capacity of alcohol and drug abuse treatment and rehabilitation programs to serve persons who have been refused treatment elsewhere because of a lack of facilities and personnel; and (3) provide access to vocational training, job counseling, and educational programs for persons receiving treatment for alcohol and drug problems (Alcohol, Drug Abuse, and Mental Health Advisory Board, 1987). Initially, the ADTR block grant was seen as a short-term, emergency measure to counter the decline in treatment capacity that occurred following the original 25 percent cut in alcohol, drug abuse, and mental health services block grant funds (J. S. Lewis, 1988). The ADTR block grant funds have now been continued as part of the revised services block grant.

Local government program funds, the second funding source on Table 8-1, are those revenues received by a reporting unit from a local government agency on a program or unit level, under either a contract or a grant. A third category, state and local government fees for service, represents funds received as reimbursement for services provided to specific individuals. Public welfare is the fourth category in which a state or local government agency is the funding source; it includes all medical or social services payments received through general assistance or general relief funds. The public welfare category also includes federal funds distributed to a state for its community and social services and food stamp programs.

Another important source of funds for the treatment of low income and disabled persons with alcohol problems was established through the Title XX social services grant-in-aid program. The Title XX program, which was instituted with the passage of Public Law 93-647, the Social Services Amendments of 1974, consolidated and controlled the costs of funding social services, while increasing state flexibility in administering and allocating funds (Booz-Allen and Hamilton, Inc., 1978; Morrison, 1978). Under the 1981 Omnibus Budget Reconciliation Act the program was later changed into a block grant determined by population with no matching requirement and is now known as the community services block grant. The program gives the states broad authority, consistent with federal guidelines, to define social services and who receives them. The state agency administering the block grant can provide services to eligible persons with alcohol problems either by transferring funds to the state alcoholism agency which then contracts with eligible treatment providers; by contracting directly with treatment providers; or by including persons with alcohol problems among those eligible to receive needed supportive services in other agencies. Certain states (e.g., South Carolina, Minnesota, Massachusetts) have used Title XX funds to cover alcohol problem treatment programs or services that do not meet the federal or private health insurance definitions for medical services (e.g., quarterway houses, non-hospital social setting detoxification, alcohol problems counseling). In these states, the community services block grant remains a relatively important source of funds and is reported in the public welfare category.

The table shows that in 1982 and 1987 state government program funds, including the alcohol, drug abuse, and mental health services block grant, were the second largest single source of funds: 20 percent of the total revenues in 1987. It seems appropriate to combine the four categories used for state and local funds because they are primarily alternative methodologies for distributing funds (e.g., program budgets and fees for service; matching funds) rather than different funding sources. Together, state and local government funds represent 33 percent of the total revenues in 1987, down slightly from

35 percent in 1982. The 1987 total includes the alcohol, drug abuse, and mental health services block grant, while the 1982 total does not, suggesting a possible decline in either state or local funding. The importance of state and local funds, including the alcohol, drug abuse, and mental health services block grant, varies substantially among the states, ranging from a high of 97 percent in the District of Columbia to a low of 12 percent in California. Thirty nine of the states fell above the national level of 33 percent. The median is 44 percent.

A category that showed a substantial increase between 1982 and 1987 was the amount of client fees received (Table 8-1). This figure was up 114 percent in dollars and increased from 10 percent to 14 percent of the total funding. Again substantial state variation is seen, with a range from less than 1 percent of total funding in Puerto Rico to over 36 percent in Nebraska. Thirty-four of the states fell below the national level of 14 percent. The median was 11 percent.

There are two categories in Table 8-1 that represent funds received directly from the federal government. The ADAMHA Program Support category includes all funds received directly from one of the component institutes (NIAAA, NIDA, or NIMH) of the Alcohol, Drug Abuse, and Mental Health Administration through a project grant or contract. The other federal funds category includes funds from any federal agency that contracts with local treatment providers for services to its beneficiaries (e.g., the Indian Health Service, Veterans Administration) or operates its own treatment programs (e.g., the Veterans Administration, Bureau of Prisons). In 1987 ADAMHA program support funds make up less than 1 percent of the total funding for alcohol problems treatment; they are primarily for research projects. Other federal funds made up approximately 5 percent of national revenues and are directed primarily at programs operated by federal agencies.

The pattern of state, local, and federal government funding has changed somewhat since the 1982 NDATUS survey, in part because of changes in the reporting format. As noted on Table 8-1, the information previously reported separately for the alcohol, drug abuse, and mental health services block grant has been combined with the state government program funds category and the information on the social services block grant (formerly Title XX) has been combined with the public welfare category. These changes led to a substantial decrease in the percentage of total funds coming directly to a provider from any federal agency—from 17 percent in 1982 to 5 percent in 1987. This decrease is not simply a reporting artifact but a real change from the federally directed use of federal funds to state-determined use of federal tax dollars with minimum federal requirements.

Additional federal funds are included in the public health insurance category. These funds may originate directly from a federal agency to purchase specific services on behalf of identified beneficiaries (e.g., Medicare, the U.S. military's CHAMPUS), or they may be channeled through a joint federal-state program like Medicaid. Although Medicaid is a federal-state program like the ADAMHA and social services block grants, it carries more federal requirements on how the money is to be expended than do the block grants, and there is much variation among the states in whether treatment for alcohol problems is covered. Income from the Federal Employees Health Benefits Program is not considered to be a specific source of funds but is included in the private health insurance category.

As shown in Table 8-1, public third-party payers accounted for 8 percent of the total funding for programs surveyed by the 1987 NDATUS that provided specialty treatment for alcohol problems. The public third-party funds category included Medicare, Medicaid, CHAMPUS and CHAMP-VA, and Supplemental Security Income. Each is a distinct financing program that has different eligibility criteria for beneficiaries and has its own benefit plan for treatment of alcohol problems.

Medicare is a public health insurance program that covers most elderly Americans, aged 65 and over, and certain disabled individuals under the age of 65 who meet specific criteria or have chronic kidney disease. The Medicare program for the elderly retired was established in 1966 under Title XVIII of the Social Security Act; coverage for disabled individuals began in 1974. Medicare was originally designed primarily to protect its aged and disabled beneficiaries against the cost of health care for acute illnesses. Recently, expanded coverage for chronic illnesses has been added.

Treatment for alcohol problems is available in accordance with general Medicare coverage rules and the limitations that apply because alcohol intoxication and alcohol dependence are classified as mental disorders (Noble et al., 1978). Medicare does not provide a specific benefit for the treatment of alcohol problems because its benefit package is structured according to specific health care settings rather than on the basis of specific diagnoses. There are two distinct programs, Part A, Hospital Insurance (HI) and Part B, Supplementary Medical Insurance (SMI).

Part A, Hospital Insurance (HI), covers inpatient hospital services, posthospital care in skilled nursing facilities when medically necessary, hospice care, and care provided in patients' homes. HI is a compulsory program financed primarily by Social Security payroll taxes. The hospital treatment of alcohol problems under Medicare is included in the general category of psychiatric health services along with mental disorders and drug abuse; in contrast to Medicare's more liberal benefit available for physical illnesses, coverage for inpatient care within a psychiatric hospital is limited to 190 lifetime days. The 190-day lifetime limit on inpatient psychiatric hospital services was originally included in the Medicare benefit design to ensure that only active treatment under a physician's supervision and evaluation—and not "custodial care"—would be covered.

In federal fiscal year 1986, HI covered 31 million enrollees, and benefits amounted to about $49 billion; the bulk of these expenditures ($46 billion, or 93 percent) went for inpatient hospital services. In 1986 Medicare was billed for 62,672 episodes of in-hospital treatment of persons with alcohol involved principal diagnoses. Billed charges were $274 million for 775,735 days of care (Cowell, 1988). Because expenditures were less than billed charges, however, the exact amount paid out for these episodes is not known. The majority of the episodes were for persons with a diagnosis of alcohol dependence (59 percent); another 6 percent had a principal diagnosis of alcohol abuse, and 13 percent had a principal diagnosis of alcoholic psychosis. The remaining 22 percent of the episodes involved treatment of an alcohol-involved physical disorder, with the largest group having a principal diagnosis of chronic liver disease and cirrhosis (17 percent). (Similar data is not available for expenditures under SMI.) These figures suggest that, although Medicare is seen by the field as an important source of financing of services for the aged and disabled, it is not a major contributor. Medicare's impact as the nation's largest single insurer is seen by the field as a major policy influence on all insurers, who frequently follow its lead in benefit restrictions.

Medicaid is a jointly financed federal-state welfare program. The federal government contribution is considered to be a federal grant-in-aid to state governments to provide medical assistance to low-income persons who meet certain additional eligibility requirements. Medicaid is administered by the states within broad federal guidelines establishing required and optional services. Grant funds are allocated to participating states on an open-ended formula basis and provide a minimum of 50 percent share in the cost of covered medical services and a varying share of certain administrative costs (Burton, 1984). All states participate in Medicaid, although Arizona has developed an alternative program and has received waivers of some federal requirements. Medicaid is financed by general tax revenues.

Medicaid was established in 1965 as Title XIX of the Social Security Act to provide access to health care for the categorically needy (those individuals who are receiving cash assistance through a federal program such as Aid to Families with Dependent Children), the medically needy (those whose income is below a certain level after deduction of medical costs, but who still do not qualify for public assistance); and any other group of needy persons that a given state elects to cover. Generally, those persons who receive cash assistance under the Aid to Families with Dependent Children or Supplemental Security Income programs are eligible for Medicaid. In addition, there is a special subset of needy aged and disabled individuals who are enrolled in both Medicaid and Medicare and are called "crossovers." Medicaid serves approximately 24 million low income children and adults who are aged, blind or disabled; these persons make up approximately 41 percent of all those who fall below the poverty line. This suggests greater need to coordinate the two programs. Strictly speaking, Medicaid is not an insurance program but a welfare entitlement program. Yet, states administer Medicaid as if it were an insurance program, even though there are no premiums and the third parties who are "at risk" for covered care are the governments which provide tax revenues to finance the program.

Each state designs its own unique Medicaid program, and the coverage of alcohol problems treatment varies from state to state. Federal statutes and regulations spell out the program's basic eligibility, reimbursement, and coverage policies, and there is a set of federally mandated services (e.g., hospital inpatient and outpatient care; early and periodic screening, diagnosis, and treatment of physical and mental defects for individuals under the age of 21; physicians' services; nurse-midwives services; and so forth). States may elect to provide Medicaid coverage for additional optional categories of service beyond the mandated hospital and outpatient services; examples of optional services include home health services, clinic services, inpatient psychiatric facility services for individuals under the age of 21, and intermediate care facility services for individuals aged 65 or older in specified institutions.

Like Medicare, Medicaid does not have a specific benefit for the treatment of alcohol problems. Medicaid, like Medicare and other health insurance plans, still categorizes the treatment of alcohol problems under the mental disorders rubric. Coverage for inpatient hospital treatment of alcohol-related diagnoses is federally mandated except in institutions for mental disorders or for tuberculosis; however, a state can include physician-supervised nonhospital residential services and outpatient care in its optional services, and some have done so (Cooper, 1979). Medicaid does not necessarily provide coverage for the educational, vocational, and psychosocial services that are considered by most treatment providers and state alcoholism agencies as an essential part of rehabilitation and maintenance (relapse prevention).

The need for Medicare and Medicaid to have a specific benefit which recognizes nontraditional professionals and facilities has been an issue for a number of years. An unfinished demonstration project has been studying whether Medicare and Medicaid benefits should become available for treatment by nonhospital providers which utilize a mixed medical and social model for detoxification and rehabilitation (Saxe et al., 1983; Lawrence Johnson and Associates, Inc., 1986). Although project data collection was completed several years ago, funding and analytic problems have delayed the final results.

Medicaid coverage of outpatient treatment for alcohol problems does not appear to be a significant funding resource in most states. There are exceptions—for example, New York in which the state has elected to cover patients in state-aided and state-operated alcohol problems counseling outpatient programs. There have been no recent detailed studies of the states' benefits for and limitations on the treatment of alcohol problems; routine reporting of services available state by state does not include this level of description. In many states, reporting on treatment of alcohol problems is included in reporting on psychiatric expenditures. Indeed, because Medicaid was originally designed as a decentralized program, there have been few detailed data available at the national level to monitor performance and expenditures (Howell et al., 1988).

The Civilian Health and Medical Program of the Uniformed Services (CHAMPUS) operates as a health insurance program for its enrollees, who are dependents of active-duty, retired, and deceased military personnel and retirees. The difference between CHAMPUS and a private insurer is that enrollees do not pay premiums, although beneficiaries do have copayments and other benefit design constraints and limits. CHAMPUS pays for treatment by approved facilities and providers, operating through private insurers who act as intermediaries to process and pay claims. Whenever possible, enrollees must also receive hospital care at military medical facilities. In recent years CHAMPUS has adopted a number of cost-containment measures and has experimented with alternative delivery systems, in part out of concern for the overuse of inpatient psychiatric and chemical dependency hospitals and residential treatment facilities by adolescent dependents.

CHAMPUS has had a specific benefit package for the treatment of alcohol problems that includes hospital care for detoxification; inpatient rehabilitation and such other services as partial care and outpatient care are covered under the psychiatric benefit. There are limitations on the benefit, however, and nontraditional, social model programs are not eligible providers. CHAMPUS is currently undertaking a review of its alcohol and drug treatment benefit package.

The range of proportions of total funding for treatment of alcohol problems provided by public third-party payers is from zero in 3 states (Delaware, District of Columbia, and Puerto Rico) to 18 percent in Pennsylvania, 19 percent in Maryland and 22 percent in New York (Table 8-2). The national total is 8.5 percent. The median is 5.6 percent. For treatment programs surveyed by the 1982 NDATUS public health insurance provided 7 percent of the total funding with a range from zero in 10 states to 17 percent in Maryland and 18 percent in New York. It is likely that the majority of the funds reported in this category are Medicaid reimbursements, given the size of the three major federal programs included in the reporting category, their provider eligibility criteria, and the states which show a substantial level of reimbursement (e.g., New York, Maryland, and Pennsylvania that have created specific Medicaid benefits for treatment of alcohol problems).

In 1987 the largest single source of funding for all specialty units treating alcohol problems continues to be private third-party payers at 35 percent of the total, up from 26 percent in 1982. The level of private insurance available nationally (35 percent) was greater than one might expect, given the concerns that were expressed to the committee at its public hearing regarding insurers' resistance to the inclusion of coverage for treatment of alcohol problems. Nevertheless, according to the 1987 NDATUS, interstate variation in the proportion of the total accounted for by private health insurance income was substantial. There were only 11 jurisdictions (Table 8-2) in which the level of private insurance was at or above this level the national level of 35 percent. The median was 20 percent. States with very high levels of private health insurance in relation to other sources of funding were Rhode Island, California, New Hampshire, and Ohio. Jurisdictions with very low levels of private health insurance for alcohol problems treatment are Delaware, Puerto Rico, District of Columbia, Hawaii, Nevada, and Maryland. Five states, with 34 percent of the nation's total population, alone accounted for 63 percent of the private health insurance reimbursement. California, which had the largest number of programs reporting, itself accounted for 42 percent of the total private health insurance reimbursement. Similar variation was found in the 1982 NDATUS. As indicated above, although private insurance accounted for 26 percent of the funding nationally in 1982, the range was from less than 5 percent in Hawaii and Wyoming to over 50 percent in North Dakota and Ohio (NIAAA, 1983:Table A-11).

This pattern of variation among states indicates a need for further study of the determinants of coverage in each state. There should also be further study of the availability of third-party funds from private and public insurance in each state. A study using data from the 1979 NDATUS found that private insurance accounted for approximately 20 percent of all revenues reported by specialty programs in 1980, whereas public insurance accounted for 7 percent (Creative Socio-Medics Corporation, 1981). There was an increase of 6 percent for private insurance and no increase in the proportion of public insurance funding (primarily Medicaid and Medicare) over the two year period between the 1980 and the 1982 NDATUS surveys. In the 5-year period between the 1982 and the 1987 NDATUS, there was no substantial shift in the relative importance of public health insurance as a source of funds (there was a gain of slightly more than 1 percent) but there was a substantial increase (8 percent) in the contribution of private health insurance. This growth can be considered an indicator of the degree of success that has been achieved in moving toward the goal of increased health insurance availability and coverage for treatment of alcohol problems. However, it should be noted that the gain has not been achieved uniformly throughout the nation, and there are still 27 states in which the level of private health insurance reimbursement is below 20 percent.

Further study is required to determine which programs in which states that have what kinds of population and what kind of insurance environments have shared in the increase. (The issue of mandating benefits for treatment of alcohol problems to stimulate coverage is discussed in Chapter 18.) A comparison of the 1982 and 1987 NDATUS data for the proportion of private health insurance funding received by the different types of providers suggests that the increases that are seen may not be uniform among the various types of providers. In 1982 ownership was a significant factor: private nonprofit providers reported that 30 percent of their funding came from private health insurance, private for-profit units reported 67 percent from private insurance, and units operated by state and local governments reported 16 percent (NIAAA, 1983: Table 15). The 1987 NDATUS data also suggest that the various sources of funding are concentrated in specific types of organizations and care. The specialist units operated by for-profit organizations report receiving the majority of their funds from private third-party payers (64 percent), client fees (21 percent), and public third-party payers (10 percent). Less than 2 percent of their revenue is received from state and local government sources. In contrast, units operated by private nonprofit organizations received only 34 percent of their funds from private third-party payers, 14 percent from client fees, and 9 percent from public third-party payers. State and local government sources provide 34 percent of their funds. The units operated by state and local governments received the majority of their funds from state and local government sources (77 percent). Health insurance reimbursement for services operated by these units is quite limited: with 4 percent of their total funding from private insurers and 8 percent from public insurers. Similarly, the major source of funding (83 percent) for units operated by federal agencies is federal revenues.

From the NDATUS data, it is possible to identify those units that are hospital based, that are located in freestanding residential facilities, or that are primarily outpatient clinics. These units vary in the sources of funding which they receive. According to the 1987 NDATUS, the hospital-based units, which served 39 percent of the total admissions for treatment of alcohol problems, received 78 percent of the private health insurance reimbursement available; private health insurance accounted for 47 percent of the hospital-based programs' total revenues. In contrast, the units located in freestanding residential facilities served 18 percent of all admissions and received only 12 percent of the private health insurance monies available, for 20 percent of their total revenue. The outpatient units served 44 percent of the admissions but received only 10 percent of the private health insurance available, for 5 percent of their total revenue.

In the case of available public health insurance funds, hospital-based units received 81 percent of these monies, making up 12 percent of their total revenue. Residential units received only 5 percent of the public health insurance dollars available, or 2 percent of their total revenue. Outpatient-based programs received 14 percent of the public health insurance funds available, accounting for 6 percent of their revenue.

The pattern differs for state and local government funds. Hospital-based units received 34 percent of the total available, for 20 percent of their revenues. Residential facilities received 33 percent of the state and local government funds, for 52 percent of their total revenue. Outpatient-based facilities received 43 percent of the state and local government dollars, for 48 percent of their revenue.

The findings from this review of the NDATUS data are consistent with those from the few other existing surveys on treatment funding. All of these studies show significant differences between the sources of funding available to specialty programs which are supported primarily by state and federal governments and the sources of funding available to privately operated generalist and specialty programs. Additional targeted studies are required, however, to determine more precisely the sources of funding for each provider type (i.e., unit location and ownership), setting (hospital, residential, outpatient) and type of care. Such studies should investigate funding sources both nationally and within each state because variations in provider eligibility among both public and private insurance benefit plans may be a major determinant of the variation among states in funding from these sources. Other potential sources of variation are the employment status and insurance status of the persons seen for treatment. The NDATUS does not gather information from the units on these characteristics of persons treated.

Sources of Funding in Public-Sector Specialty Programs

The NDATUS findings on differential funding are supported by data gathered directly from those programs that receive government funding from the state alcoholism agency. The State Alcohol and Drug Abuse Profile (SADAP) is an annual survey of state resources and services conducted by the National Association of State Alcohol and Drug Abuse Directors (NASADAD), on behalf of the Department of Health and Human Services (Butynski et al., 1987; Butynski and Canova, 1988). The survey was initiated in 1982 with the advent of federal alcohol, drug abuse, and mental health services block grant funding as a replacement mechanism for obtaining information on financing that had previously been gathered by NIAAA through its State Alcohol Profile Information System (SAPIS), the NDATUS, and the National Alcoholism Program Information System (NAPIS). (NAPIS was a client-based information and evaluation data collection system which had provided data on the revenues for individual NIAAA grantees. It was discontinued with the advent of the block grant).

The SADAP is carried out each year under the guidance of a joint federal-state advisory committee (Butynski and Record, 1983). Each state agency responsible for administering the alcohol and drug abuse portion of the alcohol, drug abuse, and mental health services block grant (the SA/DAA) voluntarily submits data on the sources of funding and total expenditures for alcohol and drug abuse services in state supported programs during their state fiscal year. The initial SADAP survey was conducted in 1983 and covered fiscal years 1982 and 1983. Significant changes in the cost-reporting methodology (e.g., a shift from allocations to expenditures) were made for the fiscal year 1985 survey; as a result, comparison with the first three years of the survey is not meaningful. The most recent report, however, contains data that can be used to draw a partial picture of the relative availability of the various funding sources to programs that serve predominantly low-income persons, both nationally and in a given state. Despite certain limitations the SADAP data constitute the most complete body of information currently available on the sources of financing for treatment of alcohol problems in publicly supported programs.

States report on expenditures only for those programs which received at least some funds administered by the SA/DAA. The states vary in the extent to which the SA/DAA administers the state and federal funds which are used by programs that provide treatment for alcohol problems. Most SA/DAAs do not administer Medicaid funds; some SA/DAAs administer social services as well as alcohol, drug abuse, and mental health services block grant funds. The data therefore do not include information on programs and private practitioners that do not receive SA/DAA-administered funds but may receive other public funds. For example, the following are excluded: programs operated by the Department of Defense, Veterans Administration, and Indian Health Services; most private for-profit hospital-based and freestanding detoxification and rehabilitation facilities; and most detoxification and rehabilitation units in general hospitals, whether nonprofit or for-profit, that receive Medicaid and Medicare funds. There is considerable variation among the states in the proportion of known units that are covered in the profile. State agencies provided an estimate of the percentage of total known alcohol and/or drug treatment units in the state or territory that received any funds administered by the SA/DAA; these estimates ranged from a high of 100 percent in Guam and Puerto Rico to a low of 17 percent in Minnesota. Among the larger states, Texas reported an estimate of 26 percent; New York, 81 percent, California, 60 percent; Illinois 45 percent; and Pennsylvania, 68 percent.

The SADAP data are collected for six very broad categories of funds and do not disaggregate the amounts received from such major sources as patient payments, type of health insurance (e.g., private, public, Medicare, Blue Cross, HMO, Medicaid), and other government agencies (e.g., the social services block grant, vocational rehabilitation, county general funds). Total expenditures in those programs which received at least some state administered funds for treatment of alcohol problems in fiscal year 1987 were $1.8 billion (Table 8-3). This total included $819 million (45 percent) from SA/DAA sources, $104 million (6 percent) from other state agency sources, $272 million (15 percent) from the ADAMHA and ADTR block grants, $51 million (3 percent) from other federal government sources, $164 million (9 percent) from county or local agency sources, and $396 million (22 percent) from other sources including reimbursement from private health insurance, fees, and court assessments imposed on drinking drivers.

Treatment expenditures made up the bulk of all expenditures (76 percent of the national total), although there is some interstate variation in the distribution of funds among program activities. The other program activities for which expenditures are reported are prevention services (13 percent) and administration, training, and research (11 percent).

Because the states do not break down their reporting of expenditures by the type of patient served (that is with either an alcohol problem or a drug problem), NASADAD has used the proportion of treatment episodes involving a person with an alcohol problem and the proportion of funding for treatment to estimate the amount of funds being spent on alcohol treatment (W. Butynski, NASADAD, personal communication, November, 1988). A total of 1,317,473 admissions for treatment of alcohol problems were reported during the year. This distribution of treatment funds and of patient care episodes suggests that the expenditures from all sources for the treatment of alcohol problems in publicly supported programs was slightly over $1 billion in 1987. However, a multiple regression analysis of the variation among states in expenditures and episodes reported on the SADAP that was carried out by IOM staff suggests that the cost per episode varies for those receiving alcohol treatment and those receiving drug treatment. The multiple regression analysis yields an estimate of $400 as the average cost per episode and total expenditures for the treatment of alcohol problems in publicly supported programs as $526 million. The discrepancy between the estimates using the NASADAD methodology and the IOM methodology suggests that the SADAP as currently constructed is not a useful data collection tool for policymakers interested in determining the relative contribution of various sources of funding for treatment of alcohol problems. The survey should be reconfigured to get directly at the amount of funds expended for treatment of alcohol prob-

TABLE 8-3   Comparison of Major Sources of Funds Over Fiscal Years (FY) 1985, 1986, and 1987 for Expenditures in State Alcohol/Drug Abuse Agency-Supported Programs, Based on Data Collected in the State Alcohol and Drug Abuse Profile (in percent)

Source of Funds	FY 1985	FY 1986	FY 1987
State alcohol/drug agencies	48	46	46
Other state agencies	4	6	6
Alcohol/drug abuse/mental health block grants	17	16	15
Other federal sources	3	3	3
County/local agency	6	9	9
Other (fees, insurance, etc.)	21	21	22
Total expenditures	$1.3 billion	$1.6 billion	$1.8 billion
Treatment expenditures			
NASADAD estimate	$834 million	$914 million	$1.0 billion
IOM estimate	$464 million	$488 million	$0.5 billion
Admissions	1,159,588	1,220,331	1,317,473

SOURCE: Adapted from Butynski et al. (1987:Table 1) and from Butynski and Canova (1988:Table 1).

lems. Another shortcoming of the SADAP is that there can be no direct comparison with NDATUS because the two surveys use different categories and definitions. The committee suggests that these surveys, if continued, use the same categories and definitions.

The SADAP data for fiscal year 1987 suggest that 79 percent of the total funds available for alcohol problems treatment came from state, local, or federal sources, whereas only 21 percent were from other nongovernmental sources. The largest source of funds was the SA/DAA itself (46 percent), with the alcohol, drug abuse, and mental health services block grant contributing an additional 15 percent. Other state agencies provide 6 percent; and county agencies, 9 percent. Other federal agencies contribute 3 percent. There is no further breakdown of the 21 percent received from other sources; this SADAP category includes reimbursement from private health insurance, fees, and court assessments imposed on drinking drivers.

Review of the SADAP data for the last three years (see Table 8-3) suggests that the pattern of funding among these six major sources has been fairly consistent. National expenditures increased over the three years, although eight states reported a decrease in total expenditures between fiscal years 1985 and 1987 (Butynski and Canova, 1988). NASADAD cautions that the differences over time must be interpreted carefully because any increases or decreases in specific proportions may reflect an improvement or deterioration in the reporting system rather than a real change. Although there was growth in all six categories, their relative contributions change: there is a decrease in the proportion contributed by the federal block grants to the states, as well as a decrease in the proportion of funds coming from the states, and there is an offsetting increase in the proportion of county and local funds.

The states vary widely in their distribution patterns and in their dependence on federal funds. Only six states—Alabama, Arkansas, Minnesota, Mississippi, North Dakota, and Texas—reported federal sources exceeding state sources. As reported in the 1987 SADAP, the contribution of federal funds to the revenues of specialty programs that receive at least some funding from the SA/DAA ranged from lows of 10 percent in New York and

12 percent in South Carolina to highs of 60 percent in Alabama, 60 percent in Texas, and 59 percent in Minnesota.

Even though NASADAD qualifies the interpretation of these data as possibly slightly underestimating the amount of funding from the other sources, the committee's conclusion is that for all states combined and for most states and territories individually, state revenues, including the alcohol, drug abuse, and mental health services block grant provide the single largest source of funding for treatment of alcohol problems in the publicly funded specialty sector. As described in the following section, a very different picture of the sources of funding for treatment is seen for specialty programs in the private sector.

Sources of Funding in Private Sector Specialty Programs

The National Association of Addiction Treatment Programs, or NAATP (until 1987, the National Association of Alcoholism Treatment Programs) is the trade association to which many specialty programs belong (Ford, 1988). In a 1986 survey of almost 11,000 patients discharged from 230 member inpatient treatment facilities, NAATP found that more than 67 percent of the patients were covered by a private health insurance plan (ICF, Inc., 1987). NAATP members are for the most part private for-profit or not-for-profit organizations. Few if any receive funds through state, local, or federal grants or contracts. Treatment programs in both hospital-based and freestanding settings were included in the survey, although freestanding facilities and some specialty hospitals are not eligible to receive reimbursement from some commercial insurers and, under most circumstances, from Medicare and Medicaid.

Like the majority of data available on the costs of alcohol problems treatment, there are limitations to the data from this survey which need be noted. First, because NAATP conducted the survey primarily to obtain information on the charges associated with the substance abuse DRG categories used for reimbursement by the Health Care Financing Administration, no distinction is made between alcohol- and drug-related diag-

TABLE 8-4 Comparison by Primary Payer Category for a Sample of Member Facilities of the National Association of Addiction Treatment Programs

Payer	Percent	Average Charges ($)	Average Length of Stay (Days)
Medicare	4.1	5,259	16.5
Medicaid	4.5	4,511	15.4
Commercial insurance	30.6	6,614	24.7
Blue Cross	24.9	6,140	24.0
Health maintenance	5.0	5,608	21.8
Preferred provider	0.5	6,857	25.5
Self-insured	6.1	7,022	24.9
Self-pay	11.3	4,803	20.0
Other	11.0	5,812	24.0
Unknown	2.0	N/A	N/A
Total	100.0	6,030	23.0

SOURCE: ICF, Inc. (1987:Table 9).
[a] Charges for all substance abuse diagnostic-related groups, all settings, and all ages.

noses. Rather, it is assumed that given the history of NAATP and the predominantly alcohol-focused programs of its members, the vast majority of the discharges constituted alcohol-related diagnoses. Second, only 39 percent of NAATP's member facilities provided data. Third, data were provided only on sources of funding for admissions to hospital or freestanding residential inpatient settings; some of the facilities did report on independently offered outpatient services, but the sample was considered too small for analysis.

In contrast to the SADAP findings for programs that receive some of their support from the state alcoholism agency, the providers who belong to NAATP reported that 67 percent of their inpatient admissions have private insurance coverage. As can be seen in Table 8-4, the primary payer for the largest percentage of patients was commercial insurance, followed by Blue Cross. Public health insurance (CHAMPUS, Medicare, and Medicaid) is identified as the primary payer for only 9 percent of the discharges. Other sources of public funds (e.g., state and local government grants or contracts, etc.) were not listed as separate categories; even if they are included in the other and unknown funding categories, public funds would at most represent the primary payer for 22 percent of the admissions. There is a relatively high proportion of self-pay admission. Hospital-based programs reported receiving Medicare reimbursement for 11 percent of their discharges, whereas freestanding facilities reported only 1 percent coverage by Medicare. The growth of the managed care industry is given as the interpretation of the finding that for approximately 6 percent of the NAATP admissions the primary payer was an HMO or a preferred provider organization (PPO).

Similar findings emerge for two groups of patients in treatment centers that participate in the Chemical Abuse/Addiction Treatment Outcome Register (CATOR). In a sample of Minnesota programs the vast majority (more than 75 percent) of adults admitted for treatment of alcohol problems had the cost of their treatment covered by health insurance (Hoffmann and Harrison, 1987). Private health insurance (either commercial, Blue Cross, or an HMO) was available to 77 percent of these individuals and public health insurance (Medicare, Medicaid) was available to 16 percent. Self payers constituted almost 6 percent of the sample, leaving only 5 percent in the "other" category which presumably could include state, local, and federal government grants or contracts. In a national sample of adolescent programs, more than 63 percent of those admitted for treatment had private health insurance coverage; only 9 percent of the admissions were reported to be covered through government assistance (Harrison and Hoffmann, 1988).

Who Pays for Treatment of All Health Care?

As can be seen in Table 8-5 the pattern of funding sources for specialist treatment of alcohol problems varies somewhat from that for all health care (Levit and Freeland, 1988). Private insurance payments constitute the largest funding source for both alcohol problems treatment and total health care costs (35 percent and 32 percent, respectively). However, state/local government is the next largest funding source for specialist units (33 percent) in contrast to the 8 percent contribution of this source to all health care. Public health insurance is a larger contributor in the greater health arena. Another category with a major difference is direct patient or out-of-pocket expenditures. Direct patient payments were 25 percent for all services and 14 percent for treatment of alcohol problems.

In the table the federal role is somewhat understated for the specialist treatment of alcohol problems because the data come from the 1987 NDATUS in which federal block grants were included as state contributions. (The specific contribution of the several block grants is unknown because there is no other source that tracks block grant funds used for the treatment of alcohol problems.) The major difference between federal government expenditures in the specialist sector and in the general health services sector is in Medicare expenditures. Medicare provides 17 percent of expenditures for all health care services and, perhaps 1 percent to 3 percent of expenditures for treatment of alcohol problems. Medicaid provides another 11 percent of the expenditures for all health care services, 6 percent of which comes from the federal government and 5 percent from state governments. At most Medicaid contributes 8 percent of the total costs of treatment of alcohol problems.

What Does Treatment of Alcohol Problems Cost?

Because the treatment of alcohol problems can be undertaken in a variety of settings that range from walk-in facilities with minimum staffing (e.g., social model nonresidential neighborhood recovery centers) to acute care general hospital units, there is considerable variation in treatment costs among programs even when the same treatment modalities are used (Holder and Hallan, 1983). These variations in costs are an issue that has been the subject of discussion in both the professional literature and the popular press (e.g., Holden, 1987).

Differences in costs are largely a function of the stage of treatment, the setting in which treatment takes place, the intensity of treatment, the staffing pattern required to accomplish treatment goals, and treatment duration (length of stay or number of sessions). Setting refers both to the physical facility, in which the cost is largely determined by the capital costs of the original construction of the facility and its debt service and to organizational characteristics. Capital costs can vary as a function of fire, life, and safety code standards included in licensure requirements. (For example, acute care hospitals serving bedridden persons must meet more rigorous standards than residential facilities serving ambulatory persons.) Because of these factors, detoxification and rehabilitation programs in general hospitals have on the average the highest facility costs; psychiatric hospitals and alcoholism hospitals will have slightly lower facility costs, residential programs will have slightly lower costs yet, and freestanding outpatient clinics or offices will have the lowest facility costs.

TABLE 8-5 Sources of Funding for Specialty Units Treating Alcohol Problems and for All Health Care (percentage of total funds)

Source of Funds	Alcohol Problems[a]	All Health Care[b]
State/local government[c]	33	8
Federal government	5	7
Private health insurance	35	32
Public health insurance[d]	8	27
Direct patient payments	14	25
Private donations/other	5	2
Total	100.0	101.0[e]

[a]Data taken from the IOM analysis of the 1987 NDATUS (NIDA/NIAAA, 1989).
[b]Information taken from Levit and Freeland (1988:Exhibit 3).
[c]This category excludes the state share of Medicaid but includes block grant funds for alcohol problems.
[d]This category includes Medicare and Medicaid but excludes CHAMPUS and CHAMP-VA for all health care.
[e]Does not sum to 100 percent because of rounding.

Staff costs are a function of the staff required to provide supervision and observation and to carry out treatment. Staffing pattern is determined by the specific modalities or procedures to be used as well as by licensure standards or payer eligibility standards. Staff coverage requirements can be for 24 hours a day, 7 days a week, as in inpatient hospital and residential programs; 4 to 8 hours a day, 5 days a week, as in daycare or intermediate setting programs; or 1 hour a week for outpatient counseling. Treatment models, licensure standards, or payer eligibility requirements can dictate the number and type of staff required, as well as their disciplines and experience levels. Hospital and residential facilities will have the highest staff costs per person served because of the need for 24 hour staff coverage and prescribed levels of staff needed to meet licensure standards. Hospitals that require specific professional nurse-to-patient ratios will have higher costs than residential facilities that do not have such requirements.

Duration refers to the length of the treatment episode expressed as the number of days for hospital and residential settings and the number of visits or sessions for intermediate or outpatient settings. Many programs offer fixed-length stays for rehabilitation, leading to comparisons of costs for a "treatment episode" that can range from $2,500 to $20,000, depending on the setting and length of stay.

Few recent studies have included the costs of treatment in comparisons of the effectiveness of alternative settings and modalities. Moreover, there have been very few published scientific analyses or surveys of the differential costs that reflect the full range of existing settings. Many surveys have been conducted by insurers or employers and published in the popular press; these surveys demonstrate the wide variance among providers, but they contain little analysis and few efforts to develop general models of the treatment episode and the treatment system, similar to those proposed in this report (see Chapter 3).

Holder and his team (1988) have attempted to place these costs in perspective, bringing together the data reported in a number of studies to demonstrate the variation among settings and payer sources. In the absence of representative data from a national data base organized in terms of their proposed model, they have utilized data from several studies and several years, standardized to a base year (1986) and drawn from a variety of facilities and programs throughout the country. Costs ranged widely across settings in their composite, from $8 per outpatient visit for California social model neighborhood recovery centers to $457 per day for general acute care hospitals in the Midwest.

Costs also varied within a setting category. In the Holder team's composite, hospital inpatient per-day costs ranged from a low of $148 in Minnesota hospitals receiving Blue Cross reimbursement to $457 in Chicago hospitals providing services to a large, self-insured manufacturer. Within this category the range of costs reflected regional as well as institutional differences in facility capital, staffing, administrative, and other operating costs. Because costs vary as well with the level of care within a hospital, different rates per day can be expected for different alcohol problems.

This variation can be seen in the charges to Medicare for hospital inpatient treatment of persons with alcohol-involved principal diagnoses (see the discussion earlier in this chapter) (Cowell, 1988). Overall, average charges were $4,373 per stay and $353 per day. Average billed charges varied by diagnosis. For alcohol dependence the average charge per episode was $3,768 for an average length of stay of 11.9 days and an average per diem charge of $317. For alcohol abuse the average charge per episode was $2,897 for an average length of stay of 9.9 days and an average per diem charge of $292. For alcoholic psychosis the average charge per episode was $4,411 for an average length of stay of 19.5 days and an average per diem charge of $226. For chronic liver disease and cirrhosis the average charge per episode was $7,365 for an average length of stay of 11.5 days and an average per diem charge of $662.

Similar variation among DRGs can be seen in the national survey of NAATP members (ICF, Inc., 1987). Overall, average charges were $6,046 per stay and $263 per day. For DRG 435, detoxification with dependence, the average charge per episode was $2,052 for an average length of stay of 5 days and an average per diem charge of $410. For DRG 436, rehabilitation with dependence, the average charge per episode was $5,897 for an average length of stay of 27 days and an average per diem charge of $216.

Differences in average cost per day are also seen between stages of treatment among social model residential programs (Holder et al., 1988). In a sample of San Diego County programs, the average cost per day for detoxification facilities was projected to be $86; for short-term recovery the cost per day was $54; and for recovery home services it was $28. (Short-term recovery corresponds to primary care and recovery home to extended care in the committee's proposed stages of treatment model [see Chapter 3]).

Overall, detoxification charges ranged from $86 per day in a social model program to $410 per day in a hospital. However, systematically collected data on the cost of detoxification are lacking. A recent study that compared the cost-effectiveness of inpatient and outpatient medical model detoxification for persons with mild to moderate withdrawal symptoms found that costs varied significantly (Hayashida et al., 1989). For outpatient detoxification lasting an average of 6.5 days, the cost per episode was estimated as ranging between $175 to $388; for inpatient detoxification lasting an average of 9.2 days at the same Veterans Administration hospital unit, costs were estimated as ranging from $3,319 to $3,665 per episode. The range reported by these investigators is a function of the assumptions and definitions used in calculating costs. The low estimate can be seen to represent the cost of adding episodes to an existing program so that no new start-up costs are incurred, whereas the high estimate can be seen as represent the cost if a new or expanded unit is required. Similar cost comparisons in other systems would be needed; generalization from a VA sample to other segments of the treatment system is difficult because of the unique characteristics of the persons served and the method of financing.

Similarly, costs for the intermediate care programs reviewed by Holder and colleagues (1988) ranged from $72 per day to $132 per day. In the national survey of NAATP members, programs providing intensive treatment that corresponds to short-term nonresidential primary care in the committee's model reported an average cost of $72 per session for an average "stay" of 21 visits (ICF, Inc., 1987). Programs providing intermediate care in a variety of settings in Iowa had costs ranging from $81 to $138 (Holder et al., 1988).

The 1989 directory of Minnesota chemical dependency programs yielded an average cost of $146 per day for detoxification, $184 per day for primary rehabilitation, $97 per day for extended care, and $24 for outpatient treatment (Minnesota Chemical Dependency Program Division, 1989).

Again, there is a lack of systematically collected data about the costs of treatment on a national basis for use in policymaking. The committee suggests that NIAAA carry out such a national survey of a representative sample of programs as a substudy within the annual NDATUS data collection effort.

Summary and Conclusions

There is no single survey that collects data on the total amount of funds currently being spent on the treatment of alcohol problems. Nevertheless, it is possible to utilize the data that are available to reach some conclusions regarding the changes that have occurred in the financing of such treatment and about the current funding situation.

There has been a steady increase in the number of public and private sources of financing. Efforts to develop distinct funding sources and discrete reimbursement policies have been moderately successful. Success in efforts to separate the funding of treatment for alcohol problems from the stigma and uncertainty that still surrounds mental disorders has been variable: such efforts have been more successful in the private insurance sector than in the public insurance sector. Nationally, private health insurance is now the largest single source of funding, having reached a level comparable to that for all health care (35 percent and 32 percent, respectively). Yet, the level of funding varies so greatly among the states that it cannot be concluded that we have reached the goal of obtaining coverage that is nondiscriminatory and equivalent to that provided for other illnesses. While some of the desired improvements in obtaining coverage seem to have taken place, private health insurance funding appears to be concentrated in hospital-based inpatient programs in the private sector and to be less available for the outpatient and intermediate care programs.

Further study is required of the determinants of funding for the treatment of alcohol problems in each state. There are significant differences in the sources of funding available to specialty programs that are supported directly by state and federal grants and contracts and to privately operated generalist and specialty programs. Targeted studies could determine more precisely the sources of funding for each provider type (i.e., unit location; ownership), settings (hospital, residential, outpatient) and types of care (medical model, social model). These studies are particularly important because variations in provider eligibility for reimbursement among both the public and private insurance benefit plans may be a major determinant of the variation in treatment alternatives availability among the states.

Although the proportion of funding provided by private health insurance has grown substantially, the largest source of total funding for the treatment of alcohol problems continues to be public funds (state, county, or local general fund revenues or dedicated taxes and fees; federal block grants; federal health insurance mechanisms in the form of Medicare, Medicaid, and CHAMPUS; or federal direct services through the Department of Defense, Indian Health Services, Veterans Administration, and Bureau of Prisons). The overall pattern of funding for specialist settings varies from that found for all health care settings. For specialist alcohol treatment, state and local governments are the most prominent source providing more than 33 percent of revenues as compared with 8 percent provided by these bodies for all health care. There is a lower proportion of direct patient payments and of federal public insurance (Medicare and Medicaid) available for the treatment of alcohol problems.

Systematically collected data on the sources of funding and the costs of treatment for alcohol problems that can be used for policymaking are lacking. There is no agency or association that has assumed the responsibility for carrying out such surveillance. In addition, there is no compendium of recent trends in financing alcohol problems treatment services because this area of health services research which has been severely neglected.

Shifts in the locus of treatment and in the role of the federal and state governments in providing and monitoring funding for treatment, as well as the increasing trend of combining funding and the organization of treatment for both alcohol and drug problems, have all contributed to the difficulties one experiences in tracking expenditures. Treatment is now provided through a diverse network of traditional and nontraditional facilities. Many of the nontraditional facilities are not included in more traditional surveys and many of the traditional facilities are not covered in either NDATUS or SADAP. There is an increasing trend to combine under the substance abuse/chemical dependency rubric reports on funding for services to persons experiencing problems with both alcohol and other drugs. This combination makes its difficult to obtain consistent and clear reporting from treatment providers and the states on their expenditures for treatment services to persons with alcohol problems through the two major national surveys specifically developed to aid policymakers: the National Drug Alcohol Treatment Survey (NDATUS) and the State Alcohol and Drug Abuse Profile (SADAP). *These surveys should be modified to provide consistent more useful information both about the funding sources and about the costs for treatment of alcohol problems in the full range of traditional and nontraditional treatment settings. Additional surveys and studies should be undertaken to provide more detailed information about funding sources and costs within each state and among the various types of care.*

REFERENCES

Akins, C., and D. Williams. 1982. State and local programs on alcoholism. Pp. 325-352 in Prevention, Intervention, and Treatment: Concerns and Models, J. de Luca, ed. Washington, D.C.: U.S. Government Printing Office.

Alcohol, Drug Abuse, and Mental Health Adminstration. 1984. Alcohol and Drug Abuse and Mental Health Services Data: Report to Congress, January, 1984. Rockville, Md.: Alcohol, Drug Abuse, and Mental Health Administration.

Alcohol, Drug Abuse, and Mental Health Advisory Board. 1987. First Report to Congress, April 1987. Rockville, Md.: Alcohol, Drug Abuse, and Mental Health Administration.

Berman, H., and D. Klein. 1977. Project to Develop a Comprehensive Alcoholism Benefit through Blue Cross: Final Report of Phase I. Prepared for the National Institute on Alcohol Abuse and Alcoholism. Chicago: Blue Cross Association.

Boche, H. L., ed. 1975. Funding of Alcohol and Drug Programs: A Report of the Funding Task Force. Washington, D.C.: Alcohol and Drug Problems Association of North America.

Booz-Allen and Hamilton, Inc. 1978. The Alcoholism Funding Study: Evaluations of the Sources of Funds and Barriers to Funding Alcoholism Treatment Programs. Prepared for the U.S. Department of Health Education and Welfare. Washington, D. C.: Booz-Allen and Hamilton, Inc.

Borkman, T. 1988. Executive summary: Social model recovery programs. Prepared for the IOM Committee for the Study of Treatment and Rehabilitation Services for Alcoholism and Alcohol Abuse, May.

Burton, J. L. 1984. Coverage Policies for Alcohol, Drug Abuse, and Mental Health Care under Major Health Care Financing Programs. Prepared for the ADAMHA Reimbursement Task Force. Rockville, Md.: Alcohol, Drug Abuse, and Mental Health Administration.

Butler, P., and C. Littlefield. 1985. Health Care Cost Containment in the Alcohol and Drug Abuse Division. Prepared for the Alcohol and Drug Abuse Division. Colorado Department of Health, Denver, Col., December.

Butynski, W. 1986. Private health insurance coverage for alcoholism and drug dependency treatment services-- state legislation that mandates benefits or requires insurers to offer such benefits for purchase. NASADAD Alcohol and Drug Abuse Report Special Report January/February:1-28.

Butynski, W., and D. Canova. 1988. Alcohol problem resources and services in state supported programs, FY 1987. Public Health Reports 103:611-620.

Butynski, W., and N. Record. 1983. State Resources and Needs Related to Alcohol and Drug Services. Prepared for the National Institute on Alcohol Abuse and Alcoholism and the National Institute on Drug Abuse. Washington, D.C.: National Association of State Alcohol and Drug Abuse Directors.

Butynski, W., N. Record, P. Bruhn, and D. Canova. 1987. State Resources and Services for Alcohol and Drug Abuse Problems: Fiscal Year 1986—An Analysis of State Alcohol and Drug Abuse Profile Data. Prepared for the National Institute on Alcohol Abuse and Alcoholism and the National Institute on Drug Abuse. Washington, D.C.: National Association of State Alcohol and Drug Abuse Directors.

Cooper, M. L. 1979. Private Health Insurance Benefits for Alcoholism, Drug Abuse, and Mental Illness. Washington, D.C.: Intergovernmental Health Policy Project, George Washington University.

Costello, R.M. 1980. Alcoholism aftercare and outcome: Cross-legged panel and path analysis. British Journal of Addictions 75:49-53.

Costello, R. M. 1982. Evaluation of alcoholism treatment programs. Pp. 1197-1210 in Encyclopedic Handbook of Alcoholism, E. M. Pattison and E. Kaufman, eds. New York: Gardner Press.

Costello, R. M., and J. E. Hodde. 1981. Costs of comprehensive alcoholism care for 100 patients over 4 years. Journal of Studies on Alcohol 42:87-93.

Cowell, C. 1988. Treatment of alcohol disorders: The Medicare exerience--analysis of unpublished data from the Medpar files (memorandum). Financing and Coverage Policy Branch, National Institute On Drug Abuse, Rockville, Md., September.

Creative Socio-Medics Corporation. 1981. An Analysis of Third Party Funding in the Alcoholism Treatment Delivery System in the United States. Prepared for the National Institute on Alcohol Abuse and Alcoholism. Vienna, Va.: Creative Socio-Medics Corporation.

Davis, K. 1987. The organization and financing of alcohol and drug abuse services. Presented at the annual meeting of the Institute of Medicine, Washington, D.C., October 21.

Fein, R. 1984. Alcohol in America: The Price We Pay. Newport Beach, Cal.: CareInstitute.

Flavin, D. 1988. Health insurance coverage for alcoholism and other drug dependencies. Testimony presented before the House of Representatives Committee on Energy and Commerce, Subcommittee on Commerce, Consumer Protection, and Competitiveness hearing on insurance coverage of drug and alcohol abuse treatment, Washington, D. C., September 8.

Ford, M. 1988. Statement presented to the open meeting of the IOM Committee for the Study of Treatment and Rehabilitation Services for Alcoholism and Alcohol Abuse. Washington, D.C., January 25.

Gibson, R. W. 1988. The influence of external forces on the quality assurance process. Pp. 247-264 in Handbook of Quality Assurance in Mental Health, G. Stricker and A. Rodriquez, eds. New York: Plenum Press.

Glasscote, R. M., T. F. A. Plaut, D. W. Hammersley, F. J. O'Neil, M. E. Chaefetz, and E. Cumming. 1967. The Treatment of Alcohol Problems: A Study of Programs and Problems. Washington, D.C.: Joint Information Service of the American Psychiatric Association and the National Association of Mental Health.

Gordis, E. 1987. Accessible and affordable health care for alcoholism and related problems: Strategy for cost containment. Journal of Studies on Alcohol 48:579-585.

Hallan, J. B. 1972. Health Insurance Coverage for Alcoholism. Prepared for the National Institute on Alcohol Abuse and Alcoholism. Rockville, Md: National Institute on Alcohol Abuse and Alcoholism.

Harrison, P. A., and N. G. Hoffmann. 1988. CATOR 1987 Report: Adolescent Residential Treatment: Intake and Follow-Up Findings. Saint Paul, Minn.: Chemical Abuse/Addiction Treatment Outcome Registry, Ramsey Clinic.

Hayashida, M., A. I. Alterman, A. T. McLellan, C. P. O'Brien, J. J. Purtill, J. R. Volpicelli, A. H. Raphaelson, and C. P. Hall. 1989. Comparative effectiveness and costs of inpatient and outpatient detoxification of patients with mild-to-moderate alcohol withdrawal syndrome. New England Journal of Medicine 320:358-365.

Hoffmann, N. G., and P. A. Harrison. 1987. CATOR 1986 Report: Findings Two Years After Treatment. Saint Paul, Minn.: Chemical Abuse/Addiction Treatment Outcome Registry, Ramsey Clinic.

Holder, H. H. 1987. Alcoholism treatment and potential health care cost saving. Medical Care 25:52-71.

Holder, H. D., and J. B. Hallan. 1983. Development of Cost Simulation Study of Alcoholism Insurance Benefit Packages. Prepared for the National Institute on Alcohol Abuse and Alcoholism. Rockville, Md.: National Institute on Alcohol Abuse and Alcoholism.

Holder, H. D., R. Longabaugh, and W. R. Miller. 1988. Cost and effectiveness of alcoholism treatment using best available information. Prepared for the IOM Committee for the Study of Treatment and Rehabilitation Services for Alcoholism and Alcohol Abuse.

Howell, E. M., M. Rymer, D. K. Baugh, M. Ruther, and W. Buczko. 1988. Medicaid tape-to-tape findings: California, New York, and Michigan, 1981. Health Care Financing Review 9(4):1-29.

ICF, Inc. 1987. Analysis of Treatment for Alcoholism and Chemical Dependency. Prepared for the National Assoication of Addiction Treatment Providers. Irvine, Calif.: National Association of Addiction Treatment Providers.

Jacob, O. 1985. Public and Private Sector Issues on Alcohol and Other Drug Abuse: A Special Report with Recommendations. Prepared for the National Institute on Alcohol Abuse and Alcoholism. Rockville, Md.: Alcohol, Drug Abuse, and Mental Health Administration.

Lawrence Johnson & Associates, Inc. 1986. Evaluation of the HCFA Alcoholism Services Demonstration: Final Second Analytic Report. Prepared for the Health Care Financing Administration. Washington, D.C.

Jones, K. R., and T. R. Vischi. 1979. Impact of alcohol, drug abuse and mental health treatment on medical care utilization: A review of the research literature. Medical Care 17(12, Suppl.):1-82.

Levit, K., and M. Freeland. 1988. National medical care spending. Health Affairs 7(5):124-136.

Lewis, D. C. 1987. Education and training of health professionals to intervene in drug and alcohol problems. Presented at the Institute of Medicine annual meeting, Washington, D.C., October 21.

Lewis, J. S. 1982. The federal role in alcoholism research, treatment and prevention. Pp. 385-401 in Alcohol, Science and Society Revisited, E. Gomberg, H. White, and J. Carpenter, eds. Ann Arbor, Mich. and New Brunswick, N.J.: University of Michigan Press and Center of Alcohol Studies, Rutgers University.

Lewis, J. S. 1988. Congressional rites of pasage for the rights of alcoholics. Alcohol Health and Research World 12:241-251.

Leyland, A. Jr., V. Paukstys, and T. Raichel. 1983. Substance Abuse Treatment Benefits: A Guide for Plans. Chicago: Blue Cross and Blue Shield Association.

Luckey, J. W. 1987. Justifying alcohol treatment on the basis of cost savings: The offset literature. Alcohol Health and Research World 12(1):8-15.

Minnesota Chemical Dependency Program Division. 1989. Directory of Chemical Dependency Programs in Minnesota. St. Paul: Minnesota Department of Human Services.

Morrisey, M. A., and G. A. Jensen. 1988. Employer-sponsored insurance coverage for alcoholism and drug abuse treatments. Journal of Studies on Alcohol 49: 456-461.

Morrison, L. 1978. Title XX Handbook for Alcohol, Drug Abuse, and Mental Health Treatment Programs. Prepared for the Alcohol, Drug Abuse, and Mental Health Administration. Washington, D.C.: U. S. Government Printing Office.

Muszynski, I. L. 1987. Trends and issues in the reimbursement of chemical dependency treatment programs. Paper presented at the National Association of Addiction Treatment Providers Conference, Houston, Texas, September 15.

National Council on Alcoholism (NCA). 1987. A Federal Response to a Hidden Epidemic: Alcohol and Other Drug Problems Among Women. New York: NCA.

National Council on Alcoholism, Task Force on Health Insurance. 1974. Recommendations for Health Insurance Coverage for Alcoholism (memorandum). National Council on Alcoholism, Washington, D.C., January 11.

National Institute on Alcohol Abuse and Alcoholism (NIAAA). 1983. National Drug and Alcoholism Treatment Utilization Survey: Executive Report. Rockville, Md: NIAAA.

National Institute on Alcohol Abuse and Alcoholism (NIAAA). 1984. Report to the U.S. Congress on Federal Activities on Alcohol Abuse and Alcoholism: FY 1981 and FY 1982. Rockville, Md.: NIAAA.

National Institute on Drug Abuse/National Institute on Alcohol Abuse and Alcoholism (NIDA/NIAAA). 1989. Highlights from the 1987 National Drug and Alcoholism Treatment Unit Survey (NDATUS). Rockville, Md: NIDA/NIAAA.

Noble, J. A., P. Widem, H. Malin, and J. R. Coakley. 1978. Medicare Coverage for the Treatment of Alcoholism: Excerpts from DHEW's 1978 Report to Congress on the Advantages and Disadvantages of Extending Medicare Coverage to Mental Health, Alcohol, and Drug Abuse Centers. Rockville, Md.: National Institute on Alcohol Abuse and Alcoholism.

Pattison, E. M. 1985. The selection of treatment modalities for the alcoholic patient. Pp. 189-294 in J. H. Mendelson and N. K. Mello, eds. The Diagnosis and Treatment of Alcoholism, 2nd ed. New York: McGraw-Hill.

Plaut, T.F.A., ed. 1967. Alcohol Problems: A Report to the Nation. New York: Oxford University Press.

Plotnick, D. E., K. M. Adams, H. R. Hunter, and J. C. Rowe. 1982. Alcoholism Treatment Programs within Prepaid Group Practices: A Final Report. Rockville, Md.: National Institute on Alcohol Abuse and Alcoholism.

President's Commision on Mental Health, Task Panel on Alcohol Related Problems. 1978. Report of the Liaison Panel on Alcohol Related Problems. Pp. 2078-2092 in Appendix: Task Panel Reports. Vol. 4 of the Report to the President from the President's Commission on Mental Health. Washington, D.C.: U.S. Government Printing Office.

Reed, P. G., and D. S. Sanchez. 1986. Characteristics of Alcoholism Services in the United States--1984. Rockville, Md.: National Institute on Alcohol Abuse and Alcoholism.

Regan, R. 1981. The role of federal, state, local, and voluntary sectors in expanding health insurance coverage for alcoholism. Alcohol Health and Research World 5(4):22-26.

Reynolds, R. I. 1988. Executive Summary: Social model services as an alternative to medical/clinical model services in San Diego county. Prepared for the IOM Committee for the Study of Treatment and Rehabilitation Services for Alcoholism and Alcohol Abuse, February.

Robertson, A. D. 1988. Federal and state support for alcohol and drug abuse services. Testimony on behalf of the National Association of State Alcohol and Drug Abuse Directors presented to the U. S. Senate Committee on Governmental Affairs hearing regarding an overview of federal activities on alcohol abuse and alcoholism, National Association of State Alcohol and Drug Abuse Directors, Washington, D.C., May 25.

Rosenberg, N. 1968. Survey of Health Insurance for Alcoholism. Prepared for the National Center for Prevention and Control of Alcoholism. Bethesda, Md.: National Institute of Mental Health.

Saxe, L., D. Dougherty, K. Esty, and M. Fine. 1983. The Effectiveness and Costs of Alcoholism Treatment. Washington, D.C.: U.S. Congress, Office of Technology Assessment.

Sharfstein, S. S., S. Muszynski, and E. Meyers. 1984. Health Insurance and Psychiatric Care: Update and Appraisal. Washington, D.C.: American Psychiatric Association Press.

Shulman, G. D. 1988. Statement presented to the Open Meeting of the IOM Committee for the Study of Treatment and Rehabilitation Services for Alcoholism and Alcohol Abuse. Washington, D.C., January 25.

U.S. Department of Health and Human Services (USDHHS). 1981. Fourth Special Report to the U.S. Congress on Alcohol and Health. Rockville, Md.: National Institute on Alcohol Abuse and Alcoholism.

U. S. Department of Health and Human Services (USDHHS). 1986. Toward a National Plan to Combat Alcohol Abuse and Alcoholism. Report submitted to the United States Congress. Rockville, Md.: National Institute on Alcohol Abuse and Alcoholism.

U. S. Department of Health and Human Services (USDHHS). 1987. Sixth Special Report to the U.S. Congress on Alcohol and Health. Rockville, Md.: National Institute on Alcohol Abuse and Alcoholism.

U.S. Department of Health, Education, and Welfare (USDHEW). 1971. First Special Report to the U.S. Congress on Alcohol and Health. Rockville, Md.: National Institute on Alcohol Abuse and Alcoholism.

U.S. Department of Health, Education, and Welfare (USDHEW). 1974. Second Special Report to the U.S. Congress on Alcohol and Health. Rockville, Md.: National Institute on Alcohol Abuse and Alcoholism.

U.S. Department of Health, Education, and Welfare (USDHEW). 1978. Third Special Report to the U.S. Congress on Alcohol and Health. Rockville, Md.: National Institute on Alcohol Abuse and Alcoholism.

U.S. General Accounting Office (USGAO). 1984. States Have Made Few Changes in Implementing the Alcohol, Drug Abuse, and Mental Health Services Block Grant. Washington, D.C.: U.S. General Accounting Office.

U.S. General Accounting Office (USGAO). 1985. Block Grants: Overview of Experiences to Date and Emerging Issues. Report to Congress. Washington D.C.: U.S. General Accounting Office.

Wallen, J. 1988. Alcoholism treatment services systems: A health research perspective. Public Health Reports: 103:605-611.

Weisner, C. 1986. The social ecology of alcohol treatment in the United States. Pp. 203-243 in Recent developments in Alcoholism, vol. 5, M. Galanter, ed. New York: Plenum Press.

Weisner, C., and R. Room. 1984. Financing and ideology in alcohol treatment. Social Problems 32:167-184.

Weisman, M. N. 1988. Musings on the art of treatment. Alcohol Health and Research World 12:282-87.

9 The Community Role: Identification, Brief Intervention, and Referral

In responding to the fundamental questions raised in the first section of this report, the committee has developed the premises on which its discussion of treatment for alcohol problems is based. Among these is a definition of the target population of the treatment enterprise that includes not only those who manifest the more severe sorts of alcohol problems but those with less severe problems. Indeed, as noted in Chapter 1, the target population for treatment comprises all who experience or who are likely to experience any sort of problem arising in connection with their use of beverage alcohol. Another premise, as noted in Chapter 2, is a definition of treatment that includes not only the therapeutic activities of those who specialize exclusively in dealing with individuals manifesting alcohol problems but any activity which has to do with the reduction of alcohol consumption and its consequences in members of the target population.

Most of the balance of this report focuses on the management of more severe alcohol problems in the specialized treatment sector. In this chapter, however, the focus is upon the other end of the spectrum. Perhaps because of the historical development of the field (see the Introduction and Summary), which reflects the natural tendency to divert the lion's share of initial attention to the most obvious problems, less is known about effective ways to deal with alcohol problems of lesser magnitude. A recent review has described this effort as being "still in its early stages" (Babor et al., 1987a). Nevertheless, dealing with mild and moderate alcohol problems is of great importance even at present and is likely to become even more important as further knowledge develops.

It is the view of the committee that the appropriate location for the effort directed at mild and moderate problems lies not within the specialized treatment sector but within community agencies that provide general services to various populations. The specialized treatment sector most appropriately addresses itself to substantial or severe alcohol problems; thus a collaborative effort between community agencies and the specialized treatment sector is required in order to have a significant positive impact upon the broad spectrum of alcohol problems.

In this effort the role of community agencies in the treatment of alcohol problems is threefold. First, it involves the identification of individuals with alcohol problems. Second, it involves the provision of therapeutic attention in the form of brief intervention to those with mild or moderate alcohol problems. Third, it involves the referral of those with substantial or severe problems, or those for whom brief intervention does not suffice, to the specialist sector for therapeutic attention. The reasons for this approach and the manner in which it might be undertaken are the subjects of this chapter.

An Orientation to the Community Role in Treatment

To orient the reader the committee offers a simple diagram of its view of the spectrum of interventions for alcohol problems (Figure 9-1) (Skinner, 1988). The area included within the triangle represents the general population. On the right the apex of the triangle represents that proportion of the population with substantial or severe alcohol problems, for whom specialized treatment is appropriate. (Dotted lines are used to indicate that such categorical distinctions, although useful, are not to be considered as hard and fast distinctions in the real world.)

211

On the left of the diagram the base of the triangle represents those persons in the population who do not manifest alcohol problems. Primary prevention is shown as being directed principally toward this segment of the population; it was defined in a recent review as "policies or programs that affect whole (or substantial parts of) communities with the

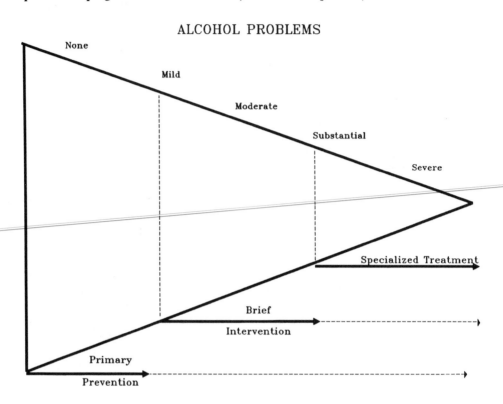

FIGURE 9-1 A spectrum of responses to alcohol problems. The triangle represents the population of the United States, with the spectrum of alcohol problems experienced by the population shown along the upper side. Responses to the problems are shown along the lower side (based on Skinner, 1988). In general, specialized treatment is indicated for persons with substantial or severe alcohol problems; brief intervention is indicated for persons with mild or moderate alcohol problems; and primary prevention is indicated for persons who have not had alcohol problems but are at risk of developing them. The dotted lines extending the arrows suggest that both primary prevention and brief intervention may have effects beyond their principle target populations. The prevalence of categories of alcohol problems in the population is represented by the area of the triangle occupied; most people have no alcohol problems, many people have a few alcohol problems, and some people have many alcohol problems.

intention of reducing the incidence of problems experienced by individuals" (Moskowitz, 1989:54). The dotted portion of the primary prevention line indicates that, although primary prevention activities are directed toward the population of individuals without alcohol problems (represented by the solid portion of the line) and are designed to prevent them from developing such problems, they nevertheless have important effects on individuals who have already developed problems. Such programs tend to "operate generally throughout the society . . . drinkers in many patterns of consumption are affected" (Moore and Gerstein, 1981:53-54).

For example, primary prevention measures that are taken to reduce the supply of alcohol are principally intended to keep those without problems from developing them. Yet such measures will also tend to reduce the consumption of other drinkers, including drinkers with varying kinds of alcohol problems (cf. Popham et al., 1975). Although primary prevention is of great interest and concern, it has been extensively considered in a recent report detailing a research agenda for this important area (IOM, 1989) and will not receive major emphasis here.

The middle section of the triangle represents persons who exhibit mild or moderate alcohol problems. "Brief intervention" is the term used (in Figure 9-1 and in this report) to designate those activities that are employed to deal with this group; what these activities might consist of will be discussed further below. The objective of brief intervention is to reduce or eliminate the individual's alcohol consumption in a timely and efficient manner, with the goal of preventing the consequences of that consumption. Other terms that are generally synonymous include "secondary prevention" (to contrast with primary prevention efforts directed at noncases and tertiary prevention efforts directed at severe cases), "early intervention," and "prompt intervention."

Although directed toward persons who manifest mild or moderate alcohol problems, brief intervention approaches also have some significance for those with more serious problems (indicated by the dotted line for brief intervention in the diagram). Most persons who experience substantial or severe alcohol problems neither seek nor receive formal treatment for them. Current information suggests that, at minimum, this statement applies in North America to four out of five such individuals (Hingson et al., 1982; McEvoy et al., 1987), though figures from older studies have been even higher (Baekeland and Lundwall, 1977; Smart et al., 1980). Similar findings have been reported outside of North America in a variety of settings, suggesting that problems of the availability of service are not a significant cause of the general failure of such individuals to seek treatment (see Appendix C).

The principal reason for not seeking treatment even in the face of substantial or severe alcohol problems seems to be a belief that such problems do not require assistance and will take care of themselves (Hingson et al., 1982; McEvoy et al., 1987). The persistence of such a belief, together with additional factors including the denial of problems and the stigma that an individual may perceive as being attached to his or her identification as someone with alcohol problems and to the seeking of treatment, may result in the continuing failure of many persons with substantial or severe alcohol problems to seek specialized treatment. A broadly based program of brief intervention, appropriately situated, can be viewed as in some measure responsive to this need.

Many of those who have substantial or severe alcohol problems but do not seek treatment for them will nevertheless seek assistance for other problems of many kinds that may be either related or unrelated to their consumption of alcohol. In this process they will come into contact with a variety of health, social services, and other community agencies. While ideally such persons upon being identified would accept referral to the specialized treatment sector, some proportion in fact will not do so. The availability of brief intervention within the community agency itself would assure that at least a degree of therapeutic attention is provided to these individuals and to their problems.

In this introductory section, the committee has provided, through a diagram and its accompanying text, an overview of what it believes might constitute the community role in treatment. Details of this role and how it might be implemented are provided below. First, however, the committee considers it necessary to indicate why the community role in treatment is of fundamental importance in the overall response to alcohol problems.

A Paradox and Its Implications

Let us return to Figure 9-1 and examine an aspect of it that has not yet been fully elaborated. As noted earlier, that portion of the population manifesting substantial or severe alcohol problems is represented on the right by the apex of the triangle. On the left are those with no problems, and in the center, those with mild or moderate problems. Simple inspection suggests that the number of persons in each category declines as one moves from left to right in the diagram, with the smallest number of persons being in the substantial or severe problems portion of the diagram. What the diagram suggests is that most people have no alcohol problems, many people have some alcohol problems, and a few people have many alcohol problems.

This suggestion has a substantial basis in empirical data. A national survey carried out more than 20 years ago (in 1964-1965 and 1967) on a carefully drawn household probability sample (Cahalan, 1970) looked in detail at specific alcohol problems. The survey found, first, that during the 3 preceding years, 57 percent of the men and 79 percent of the women in the study reported having none of the eleven actual or potential problems specifically asked about in the survey questionnaire. Second, 43 percent of the men and 21 percent of the women reported having some degree of one or more of these problems. Third, 28 percent of the men and 17 percent of the women had experienced a moderate level of problems. Fourth, 15 percent of the men and 4 percent of the women had experienced a high level of problems.

These data are consistent with the general shape of the diagram and are substantiated by the most recent version of the same survey (Hilton, 1987), which was again conducted on a nationwide sample. In this survey, however, two kinds of "drinking problems" were separately examined. One was "problematic drinking," which "consists of a set of drinking behaviors and immediate sequelae of drinking which, although not necessarily problematic in themselves, are thought to be indicative of alcohol dependence" (cf. the discussion of the alcohol dependence syndrome in Chapter 2). Examples included the inability to cut down on drinking, memory loss or tremors after drinking, and morning or binge drinking. The second kind of drinking problems surveyed was "tangible consequences," that is, "specific problems that can arise because of drinking." Examples included problems with one's spouse, problems on the job, problems with the police, and health problems. The 1984 survey specifically asked about 13 items of "problematic drinking" and 32 "tangible consequences." All items of the earlier survey are included in the later survey, but the list in the later survey is obviously considerably expanded.

In the committee's somewhat broader definition, all 45 of the items surveyed would be considered to be indicative of alcohol problems. Although the two categories in the survey are separately reported, both manifest the type of distribution indicated by Figure 9-1. Thus, 20 percent of current drinkers endorsed one or more "problematic drinking" items; 11 percent endorsed two or more; 7 percent, three or more; 4 percent, four or more; 3 percent, five or more, and 2 percent, six or more. Similarly, 21 percent endorsed one or more "tangible consequences" items; 15 percent endorsed two or more; 10 percent, four or more; 7 percent, six or more; 5 percent, 8 or more; 3 percent, 12 or more; and 1 percent, 16 or more (Hilton, 1987).

These data indicate that the form of the diagram has held relatively constant over the last two decades in terms of the nation as a whole. Some additional data reflect that this tendency may hold for local samples as well. In a household probability sample of the population in Contra Costa County, California, in 1987, a total of 1,980 persons was asked to respond specifically to 10 "alcohol related problematic events," a combination of what were called in the Hilton survey "problematic drinking" and "tangible consequences" items. It was found that 96 percent of the respondents had experienced none of these consequences in the last year; 3 percent had experienced one consequence; and 1 percent had experienced two consequences (C. M. Weisner, Alcohol Research Group, University of California, Berkeley, personal communication, May, 1989).

A hazard of citing such data as the foregoing is that figures will be taken out of context to calculate an exact number of persons with alcohol problems for the country at large. The committee could preclude this error only by not citing the data, but it considers the information to be relevant to this study. Perhaps the best course is to repeat a caution voiced by one of the principal researchers in this field:

> The problem distributions . . . are quite gradual. The gradient between drinkers with few problems and those with many is such that the data themselves never suggest a convenient, empirically derived dividing line that can be used to separate problematic from nonproblematic drinkers. Instead, analysts must rely on arbitrarily chosen cutpoints and prevalence estimates will vary accordingly. Given this state of affairs, it must be recognized that it is not possible to give a simple answer to the question "What is the prevalence of problem drinking in the United States?" on the basis of survey data. The answer depends heavily on the cutpoints that are chosen. (Hilton, 1987:171)

Data on other parameters are also consistent with the diagram. For example, in an examination of alcohol consumption based on seven national surveys, it was found that 35 percent of the population were abstainers, 32 percent light drinkers (up to three drinks weekly), 22 percent moderate drinkers (up to two drinks daily), and only 11 percent were heavy drinkers (more than two drinks daily). The authors observed: "[I]t is remarkable how much of the population either is completely abstinent or drinks very little. We calculate that close to two-thirds of the adult population drinks three or fewer drinks per week" (Moore and Gerstein, 1981:28). They go on to comment on alcohol problems as follows:

> [W]hile chronic drinkers with high consumption both cause and suffer far more than their numerical share of the adverse consequences of drinking, their share of alcohol problems is still only a fraction—typically less than half—of the total. Alcohol problems occur *throughout* the drinking population. They occur at lower rates but among much greater numbers as one moves from the heaviest drinkers to more moderate drinkers. (Moore and Gerstein, 1981:44; emphasis in the original)

Thus far, perhaps, there is nothing here that is counterintuitive. To put it simply, people who drink a lot have many problems, but few people drink a lot. People who only drink a little have fewer problems, but there are a great many people who drink a little. Therefore, the total number of problems experienced by those who drink a little is likely to be greater than the total number experienced by those who drink a lot, simply because more people drink a little than a lot.

What *does* tend to be surprising is the logical implication of this distribution of alcohol problems for intervention. *If the alcohol problems experienced by the population are to be reduced significantly, the distribution of these problems in the population suggests that a principal focus of intervention should be on persons with mild or moderate alcohol problems.* That such a focus may be advisable has been termed "the preventive paradox" (Kreitman, 1986). What seems paradoxical is that the focus of efforts to reduce alcohol problems has characteristically been only on those who manifested many of them, that is, on the heavy drinkers who experience multiple consequences of their drinking. Those often labeled "chronic alcoholics" are commonly seen as the source of the burden of alcohol problems, and it is difficult and somewhat puzzling to be asked to shift one's gaze away from this more troubled population, and to concentrate on a less apparent, albeit more familiar, group.

In health care generally, however, it is not exclusively the major problems that must be dealt with, even though they may be the more immanently hazardous. It has been said of dermatological conditions, for example, that although they may not immediately threaten life, they may make it not worth living. Moreover, there is evidence from a field related to the treatment of alcohol problems, that of smoking cessation, that effective brief interventions can be mounted in a cost-effective manner (Cummings et al., 1989). Reference to the vignettes at the beginning of Chapter 2 may help to illustrate the potential utility of identification, brief intervention, and referral in dealing with alcohol problems of less than the greatest degree of severity or with those which arise from relatively low levels of consumption.

George, a college freshman pledging a fraternity, becomes intoxicated and suffers a broken pelvis as a consequence of an auto accident. Characteristically a low-level consumer of alcohol, he is young (aged 19) and was drinking under the pressure of social conformity; certainly he may "mature out" of his drinking, and it would be difficult to argue that specialized treatment for alcohol problems is indicated. On the other hand, he may not "mature out" of his present drinking pattern. An auto accident and a broken pelvis are matters of no small concern; and even if George's overall level of consumption remains low, another episode of intoxication could produce further serious trauma, especially if it occurred while driving or boating. He is unlikely to be referred for court action with respect to driving while intoxicated, but if this did happen the appropriateness and effectiveness of the intervention could be questioned. Yet some level of attention, albeit short of specialized treatment, would be prudent.

Sally, a young lady with a long-term speech impediment, has begun a pattern of regular drinking because she feels alcohol reduces her disability in some way. Although she initially disliked alcohol, she is beginning to find her drinking gratifying. Being both young and female, she is (on a statistical basis) more likely than George to "mature out." Yet she is already drinking regularly, drinking to cope with a problem, and under the influence of alcohol while working. Again, although specialized treatment for alcohol problems does not seem in order presently, some kind of helpful approach seems to be indicated. Should this initial intervention prove to be ineffective, and should the problems persist or worsen, referral for specialized treatment may indeed be indicated.

Gregory has a very low level of consumption: approximately two drinks in his lifetime. Yet a consequence of his having taken those drinks, as well as other probable factors, is that he is now in jail for murder. Although they may seem excessive, the constellation of symptoms he exhibited has frequently been described (e.g., Banay, 1944; May and Ebaugh, 1953; Marinacci, 1963; Bach-y-Rita et al., 1970; Skelton, 1970; Maletzky, 1976, 1978; Coid, 1979; Wolf, 1980). Little is known of the precise etiology of what has often been referred to as "pathological intoxication" (or, in the current American nomenclature, "alcohol idiosyncratic intoxication") (American Psychiatric Association, 1987:128-129) or of its effective treatment. Perhaps Gregory's experience will prove sufficiently chastening that he will not drink again. In view of the potential consequences, however, it may be better not to leave his treatment entirely to natural processes.

Finally, one may consider Elizabeth. An individual deeply imbedded in the wine-growing culture, and consequently with a high level of alcohol intake, she nevertheless experienced no apparent alcohol problems at all until the very moment of her acute hemorrhage from the gastrointestinal tract. Certainly she would not have sought assistance for problems that, from her point of view, she was not experiencing. Yet there is the hope that someone might have done something to prevent matters from progressing to this point. Excess mortality from cirrhosis of the liver, the presumptive antecedent cause of Elizabeth's acute emergency, is high among those who, like her, are exposed to alcohol in the course of their occupation (Plant, 1988); a program of identification, brief intervention, and referral for this group might be advisable.

None of these four individuals conforms to the stereotypical picture of the alcoholic, nor could any of them be confidently said to exhibit the characteristics of alcohol dependence. All, however, fall within the committee's definition of alcohol problems. Although the level of alcohol consumption in three of these four cases was not high, each individual nevertheless suffered significant consequences in connection with his or her consumption. They are consequences that require address in and of themselves, regardless of whether there may or may not be subsequent progression to more serious alcohol problems. The possibility of progression, although not high, is nevertheless not negligible; furthermore, should brief intervention prove to be ineffective, referral for more extensive intervention may be necessary.

These four cases well illustrate the complex interrelationships, outlined in Figure 9-2, among vulnerability factors, exposure to alcohol, modifying variables, and the consequences of alcohol consumption (Babor et al., 1987b). One important feature of the diagram is that it illustrates the possible independence of the consequences of alcohol consumption from the development of alcohol dependence. Although one pathway illustrates that the development of acute and long-term consequences of alcohol consumption can be preceded or accompanied by the significant symptoms of alcohol use that suggest alcohol dependence, there are other pathways that indicate the occurrence of such consequences in the absence of these symptoms.

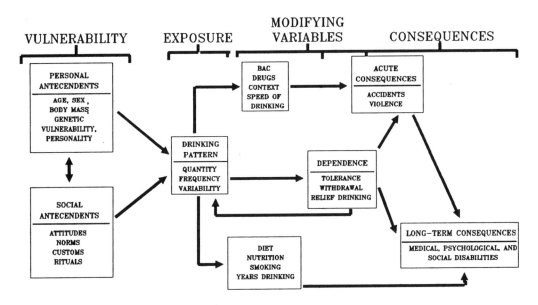

FIGURE 9-2 The complex interrelationships between vulnerability factors, exposure to alcohol, modifying variables, and the consequences of alcohol consumption (Babor et al., 1987:395). The multiple pathways indicate that the acute and long-term consequences of alcohol consumption may or may not be associated with dependence on alcohol.

None of the individuals described in the four case vignettes would be likely to appear in a specialized treatment program for alcohol problems. Rather, George would be seen in the acute medical care inpatient system; Sally might be seen by a speech pathologist or her general practitioner or both; and Gregory would be dealt with primarily by the criminal justice system. If seen at all subsequent to acute treatment for the dramatic event that initiated her difficulties, Elizabeth (absent the implementation of some special program as discussed above) might possibly receive routine attention from occupational health personnel, providing she was employed by a large enough company.

It is unlikely that any of these individuals, with the possible exception of Elizabeth, would have been *referred* as a first order of business to the specialist sector for treatment of their alcohol problems. Because their problems are mild or moderate, such a referral would not be strikingly appropriate. Indeed, the acceptance of an immediate referral to the specialist sector by an individual manifesting mild or moderate problems might be unfortunate, in terms of the potential adverse consequences of mislabeling and the potentially inappropriate use of scarce treatment resources. Moreover, appropriate or not, such a referral might not have been accepted. As a result, under the circumstances that obtain at present, none of these individuals would receive any direct attention for their alcohol problems. Such an outcome would be unfortunate indeed.

The implications of this analysis are clear. *There is a need for a spectrum of interventions that matches the spectrum of alcohol problems.* It may be that, even prior to brief intervention, some work will be required to persuade individuals that even a mild or moderate problem exists; a stepwise progression into treatment interventions of graded levels of intensity should be possible. At present, in the absence of the capability for such a stepwise approach, an individual's denial that entry into, let us say, prolonged inpatient treatment is required is tantamount to a denial that any problem exists.

The specialized treatment sector for alcohol problems cannot be the sole locus of treatment. If significant inroads are to be made into the overall burden of alcohol problems, a widespread, broad-based therapeutic approach must be taken within which gradations of therapeutic attention are possible. For this vision of treatment to be realized, the community and its resources must become a major part of the therapeutic system. How that might be accomplished will be the subject of the balance of this chapter.

Identifying People with Alcohol Problems

The development of an effective role for community agencies in the treatment of alcohol problems depends, first of all, upon the ability to identify persons with such problems. A considerable amount of work has gone into developing methods to accomplish this identification rapidly and effectively (see reviews by Kaplan et al., 1974; Morse and Hurt, 1979; Saunders and Kershaw, 1980; Skinner et al., 1981; Bernadt et al., 1982, 1984; Babor and Kadden, 1985; Babor et al., 1986, 1987a; NIAAA, 1987; Allen et al., 1988; Leigh and Skinner, 1988; J. B. Saunders, 1988). Two major methods of identifying cases in populations have evolved. One is the use of questions or questionnaires. The other is the laboratory examination of body fluids.

There is general agreement in the reviews noted above that currently available laboratory examinations are significantly less useful than questionnaires in identifying new cases. Laboratory examinations have comparatively low levels of sensitivity; that is, they are likely miss a large number of actual cases. They tend to be more costly than are questionnaire methods. They are also difficult to deploy in any but a medical setting, which generally brings with it the necessary skill and the tradition of obtaining samples of body fluids.

Medical care settings do, however, constitute a major potential source of otherwise unrecognized individuals with alcohol problems (see below), and laboratory examinations are often routinely done in such settings. It has been possible to develop methods for using routine laboratory examinations to identify persons with problems (Beresford et al., 1982). Certainly the development of highly sensitive and specific laboratory means of identifying individuals with alcohol problems would do much to enhance physicians' interest in doing so (NIAAA, 1987). Some initially promising new measures such as levels of enzymes in blood platelets, carbohydrate-deficient transferrin, and various acetaldehyde adducts await further investigation (Allen et al., 1988) but may possess more favorable case-finding characteristics than the laboratory methods presently available.

Laboratory examinations may also prove useful for monitoring persons who are receiving brief or other interventions and for providing feedback to treatment personnel and to the individuals being treated regarding the success (or lack thereof) of the treatment effort (Kristenson et al., 1983; Schuckit and Irwin, 1988). Not necessarily a replacement for questionnaires, laboratory examinations may be a useful supplement to them in the case identification process, particularly in instances in which there is reason to suspect a high level of denial of problems. Yet the choice of the appropriate supplementary test may be a rather complex matter (Bernadt et al., 1984). Many laboratory tests involve delays and expense; however, an accurate, inexpensive, and rapid method of measuring alcohol in body fluids that could readily be used outside of medical settings, the alcohol dipstick, has been developed (Kapur and Israel, 1985; Peachey and Kapur, 1986).

The range of available question-based methods for identifying the presence of alcohol problems is impressive. An NIAAA conference achieved consensus that case finding should begin with a single question: "Do you drink now and then?" (NIAAA, 1987). A study in an ambulatory care medical setting came up with two questions: "Have you ever had a drinking problem?" and "When was your last drink?" (the latter question being scored as positive if the drink was within the 24 hours prior to the appointment)(Cyr and Wartman, 1988). The widely used CAGE questionnaire consists of four questions: "Have you ever felt you ought to Cut down on your drinking? Have people Annoyed you by criticizing your drinking? Have you ever felt bad or Guilty about your drinking? Have you ever had a drink first thing in the morning to steady your nerves or get rid of a hangover (Eyeopener)?" (Ewing, 1984).

There are a number of multi-item questionnaires that are useful in case-finding; for example, the Michigan Alcoholism Screening Test (MAST) (Selzer, 1971), the Reich questionnaire (Reich et al., 1975) the Alcohol Dependence Scale (ADS) (Skinner and Allen, 1982), and the Alcohol Use Disorders Identification Test (AUDIT) (J. B. Saunders and Aasland, 1987; Babor et al., 1989). The MacAndrew Scale, which contains no questions having any direct alcohol-related content, was developed on an actuarial basis from the Minnesota Multiphasic Personality Inventory (MMPI) to get around problems of denial (MacAndrew, 1965). Although it has gained some additional notice of late with the development of increased concern about the validity of self-reports (see Chapter 10), a critical review indicates that this particular scale may be fatally flawed (Gottesman and Prescott, 1989). Finally, there are case-finding packages, such as the Alcohol Clinical Index (ACI) (Skinner et al., 1986; Skinner and Holt, 1987) which contain a number of different components used together (clinical, laboratory, and questionnaire data).

Many of the instruments that are currently available for identifying alcohol problems were developed specifically to identify severe alcohol problems. An exception is the AUDIT; items for it were developed from a pool of questionnaires containing no responses from persons with severe alcohol problems (their questionnaires were removed) (J. B. Saunders and Aasland, 1987; Babor et al., 1989). The AUDIT was also developed on a cross-national basis, using large samples from six quite different countries. Its 10 items are simple and readily administered by nontechnical staff, or they can be self-administered. The items cover alcohol consumption, symptoms of alcohol use, and consequences of alcohol use, three areas of content that are desirable for the full description of an alcohol problem (see Chapter 10). Finally, as each of the 10 AUDIT questions is scored on a 0-4 basis, the possible range of scores is 0-40, a potentially useful feature in determining which individuals to retain for brief intervention in a general setting and which to refer directly to specialized treatment settings. Initial indications are that the instrument has highly satisfactory sensitivity and specificity (J. B. Saunders and Aasland, 1987; Babor et al., 1989).

Thus, a range of options is available for the identification of persons with alcohol problems, from single questions to case-finding packages. There is a trade-off between the accuracy of identification desired and the resources available to be expended. Although the more elaborate instruments are generally more precise, their use entails a greater commitment of resources. A possible compromise is to use a staged strategy, with simpler measures deployed first, followed by more elaborate measures for those tentatively identified as possible cases. These issues are discussed further in Chapter 10, which deals at greater length with assessment, of which identification may be considered a subset.

Problem identification in many community settings (see below) might appropriately be undertaken not for alcohol problems alone but for a range of "lifestyle" problems that include those related to alcohol, tobacco, caffeine, medications, nonmedical drugs, diet, sleep, sexual functioning, and exercise (Babor et al., 1987a,b; cf. NIAAA, 1987; J. B. Saunders and Aasland, 1987). Not only is such broadly based inquiry more congruent with the overall mission of many community settings (e.g., physician's offices or social agencies) but "many patients may be willing to discuss their drinking within the broader context of health behaviours, such as smoking, that are less threatening to talk about initially" (Babor et al., 1987a:335).

In one series of studies a lifestyle questionnaire was developed and administered in three different formats while patients were waiting to see their primary care physician. One format was a self-administered computerized version. The level of acceptance of the lifestyle questionnaire in all three formats was very high, and there was evidence that its administration significantly increased the patient's intention to raise questions regarding the target areas in the questionnaire during the subsequent interview with the physician (Skinner et al., 1985a,b).

Brief Intervention

Once persons with alcohol problems have been identified in a community setting, the exercise of a triage function seems advisable. The committee believes that those persons who are identified and who appear to have a substantial or severe alcohol problem (see Chapter 3) should be referred to the specialist sector for treatment. However, those with mild or moderate alcohol problems should be dealt with in the community agency itself by staff who have been trained to deliver brief interventions.

Making the distinction between mild and moderate problems that require only brief intervention on the one hand and substantial and severe problems that require specialized treatment on the other is a function both of the screening instruments used and of the judgment of those who use them. As noted above, some instruments (the AUDIT is an example) provide a wide range of scores that would facilitate the making of such distinctions. Further research and experience will help to sharpen the ability to provide accurate triage of this kind; in particular the continued monitoring of outcomes in individual cases will provide essential information. Irrespective of the triage classification, those who do well following brief intervention need not be referred on, whereas those who do not do well will need additional attention or referral, or both. This type of feedback between intervention and outcome is also important in the specialized treatment sector (see Chapter 13).

Because referral has been an option since the redevelopment of the specialized treatment sector following Prohibition (see Chapter 1), what has facilitated the possibility of an effective community agency role in the treatment of alcohol problems has been the development of effective brief interventions. That anything short of the most heroic efforts might be a reasonable way of dealing with alcohol problems will seem to some quite contrary to experience and common sense. How can such major, serious problems be amenable to a brief and straightforward approach? At first glance, it seems unlikely. However, as has been reviewed in Chapter 6 of this report, a significant proportion of such problems will resolve without any formal treatment (so-called "spontaneous remission"). Given this well-established fact, it is perhaps less surprising that some sort of formal intervention, even a brief one, might add in a significant way to the proportion of positive results.

Not every individual with an alcohol problem, of course, can be helped by a brief intervention. Many persons (as already noted) will require more prolonged and intensive treatment to achieve a good outcome. Yet it seems clear (see below) that some individuals will be helped. Many would otherwise receive no assistance at all for their problems, either refusing a referral outright or, in a pattern that is all too familiar, accepting the referral but failing to see it through. A well-thought-out and effective brief intervention delivered on the spot and immediately following identification of the problem avoids these difficulties. Even if the intervention is ineffective in an individual case, little will have been lost, and possibly the individual may as a consequence of the attempt and its failure be motivated to undertake a more extensive approach to his or her problems.

In recent years a number of controlled studies have demonstrated the efficacy of brief interventions in the treatment of alcohol problems. The committee views this as a highly significant development and will review these studies in some detail below, partly because it senses a high level of ambient skepticism about brief interventions. The review will also serve to describe in some detail the interventions that have been studied. Because the area of smoking cessation is closely related to that of brief intervention for alcohol problems, one of the more important studies in this area will be reviewed as well.

Efficacy of Brief Interventions

The Edwards and Orford study of advice vs. treatment Interest in brief interventions for alcohol problems was stimulated by an important British study (Edwards et al., 1977). A hundred married men who were admitted consecutively to an outpatient clinic for treatment of alcohol problems were randomly assigned, following a careful initial assessment, to one of two treatment conditions. One group was offered a multiplicity of services including an anti-alcohol drug, an introduction to Alcoholics Anonymous, and regular outpatient care, with admission to a 6-week inpatient unit if that seemed advisable. The other group was given a single session of advice, conjointly with their wives, by a professional team that directed them toward abstinence, a good work record for the husband, and mutual effort in improving the marital relationship.

One year later there were no significant differences in outcome between the two groups, and a two-year follow-up (Orford et al., 1976) yielded similar results. That is, for the group as a whole, a single brief session of advice appeared to be as effective as much more extensive treatment. There was evidence of a matching effect, in that those with more severe problems tended to do better with the more extensive treatment program and those with less severe problems tended to do better with the single conjoint session of advice (Orford et al., 1976; see also Glaser, 1980). One of the conclusions of the original paper was that "we should look much more closely at the efficacy of *less* intensive treatment methods than have previously been thought adequate" (Edwards et al., 1977:1027). Following their own advice, the principal authors published a paper on "a plain treatment for alcoholism" (Edwards and Orford, 1977).

The Malmo study Another influential study has been reported from Sweden (Kristenson et al., 1983). As part of an exercise in preventive medicine, all of the male residents of Malmo born between 1926 and 1933 were invited to attend a health screening program at the city's general hospital. Those with high serum levels of gamma glutamyl transferase (GGT), an enzyme often elevated as a consequence of the consumption of alcohol, were offered a second blood test. The study group consisted of all those who had elevated GGT levels on both of these occasions. Systematic evaluation of this group revealed them to be, in general, very heavy drinkers.

These 585 individuals were randomly assigned either to a control group or to the treatment group. The control group was informed by letter that they should be restrictive in their alcohol intake and was asked to return every two years for repeat GGT determinations. The treatment group was provided with continuing follow-up by a consistent physician every three months, together with monthly GGT determinations and contact with a consistent nurse. "The subjects were carefully informed of the GGT level at every [monthly] checkup and stimulated to attain normal levels" (p. 204). The authors comment that "in focusing on the GGT value, which can be completely normalized when alcohol consumption is ceased, the patient perceives a direct advantage of restricting his drinking habits, which cannot be accomplished by the questionnaires" (p. 208). The nurse also offered counseling that was "focused on living habits," and the treatment goal was "moderate drinking rather than abstinence" (p. 204).

In the follow-up period both groups reduced their GGT levels significantly, but there were major differences in favor of the treatment group on absenteeism, hospitalization, and mortality. At four years there was 80 percent more absenteeism in the control group; at five years the control group had 60 percent more hospital days; and at six years there were twice as many deaths in the control group as in the treatment group. "Thus, the intervention program was effective in preventing medico-social consequences of heavy drinking" (Kristenson et al., 1983:203).

The Edinburgh study One hundred fifty-six men who had been admitted to medical wards at the Royal Edinburgh Hospital and the Royal Infirmary and who were identified as problem drinkers by means of a structured interview agreed to participate in this study (Chick et al., 1984). They were randomly assigned to a control and a treatment group. No comments were made about the interview findings to members of the control group, and they received no advice regarding their drinking as a part of the study, though the physician in charge may have advised modification of alcohol consumption "according to his normal practice" (p. 966).

All patients in the treatment group received a counseling session from a nurse. "The session lasted up to 60 minutes, during which the nurse gave the patient a specially prepared booklet and engaged him in a discussion on his lifestyle and health, which helped him to weigh up the drawbacks of his pattern of drinking and to come to a decision about his future consumption. The objective was to help the patient towards problem free drinking, though abstinence was the agreed goal for some" (p. 966).

At the one-year follow-up point, both groups had reduced their consumption of alcohol significantly from what it had been at intake, and there was currently no difference in consumption between them. There had been a 41 percent decline in "problems related to alcohol" for the treatment group, however, as opposed to a 14 percent decline for the controls, a difference achieving statistical significance. The treatment group also experienced a significant decline in mean GGT levels, whereas the control group did not. Finally, there was a significant difference between the two groups in global categories of outcome: 52 percent of the treatment group were categorized as "definitely improved," as opposed to 34 percent of the control group.

The authors describe their results as "encouraging." They further comment that "patients may be especially receptive to counselling when recovering from a medical illness. Screening for alcohol problems should become a routine part of nursing assessment and the medical history so that advice can be given before irreversible physical or psychosocial problems have developed" (Chick et al., 1984:967).

The New Zealand referral study Admissions to three orthopedic and two surgical wards at a general hospital were screened by "two nurses with specific training in alcohol problems" (Elvy et al., 1988), and 198 study subjects were identified using various instruments and criteria. "Most of the patients in this study were non-dependent problem drinkers who did not have medical complications from alcohol abuse, nor were deviant drinking patterns a major feature of their alcohol related problems. Instead they were usually characterized by a number of minor personal and social problems" (p. 87).

These patients were randomly assigned to two groups. One was a control group "where no action was taken." In the "referral group," the patients were "confronted with their self-reported drinking problems . . . and asked if they would accept referral to an alcoholism counsellor for further assessment and possible treatment. In the confrontation, patients were told that their drinking was leading to inappropriate and unacceptable behaviours, and they would need help to overcome their difficulties" (p. 84).

The results of the study were reported principally in terms of those who were referred and those who were not referred to counseling. Only 14 percent of the referral group and 4 percent of the control group were actually admitted to treatment agency programs. Nevertheless, after 12 months the referred group as a whole improved significantly more than the control group "in terms of: time since last drinking; desire to drink less; happiness with the amount drunk; and CAST, the total alcohol problem score" (p. 86).

Interestingly, the control group began to improve after the 12-month research follow-up interview, so that by 18 months the differences between the referral and control groups had diminished; this outcome was interpreted as a reactive effect of the follow-up interview itself. "It seems," observed the authors, "that the 12-month follow-up did act as a form of intervention which still had some beneficial effects at 18 months" (p. 88). But the main effect of the study was, they felt, to show that "there are beneficial effects from screening for problem drinkers and providing brief assessment or counselling" (p. 88).

The British General Practitioner study A large controlled trial of brief intervention (Wallace et al., 1988) has recently been reported from the Medical Research Council's general practice research framework, involving 47 group practices. Most of the practices were in rural or small urban settings. The study recruited 909 patients (641 men and 268 women) whose alcohol consumption exceeded predetermined limits (they were designated as heavy drinkers) and randomly assigned them to a control and a treatment condition. Patients in the control group received no advice from the general practitioner regarding their drinking unless (1) they requested such advice or (2) they had substantially impaired liver function.

The general practitioners who delivered the brief intervention to the treatment group had received a training session in its delivery that featured "a specially recorded video programme to illustrate the elements of the intervention." Patients randomized to the treatment group were then contacted by the practitioners and "asked to attend for a brief interview." After an initial assessment that covered the pattern and amount of their alcohol consumption, evidence of alcohol- related problems, and symptoms of dependence, patients were provided with a histogram "to illustrate how their weekly consumption compared with that of the general population." They were advised about the potential harmful effects of their current level of consumption, which was reinforced by the distribution of an information pamphlet entitled *That's the Limit*. Specific limits for safe drinking were also prescribed, and each patient was given a drinking diary that bore on its cover the likeness of a prescription emblazoned with the words "Cut Down on your Drinking!"

An initial follow-up appointment was routinely offered. Further follow-up appointments at four, seven, and ten months were at the discretion of the individual practitioner. "During these sessions the patient's drinking diary was reviewed and feedback given on the results of blood tests indicating damage due to alcohol." The outcome results were assessed by a research nurse who was blind to whether the patient was in the treatment or the control condition of the study.

The largest changes in reported alcohol consumption took place in the first six months of the trial. Both men and women in the treatment condition showed highly significant reductions in alcohol consumption in comparison with the controls at that point. At one year there were similarly significant differences among men in the treatment and control conditions but some abatement of the differences for women; nevertheless, at that point there was a reduction of nearly one fifth in the proportion of excessive drinkers of both sexes. Reduction in consumption increased significantly with the number of general practitioner interventions. The mean reduction in GGT was significant for men and was significantly associated with the number of general practitioner intervention sessions.

The authors comment that, given the prevalence of heavy drinking in their target population, the frequency with which general practitioners are consulted, and the results of the study, "our findings suggest that if all general practitioners were to participate actively in preventive intervention at least 15% of these patients—that is, around 250,000 men and 67,500 women—would reduce their consumption to moderate levels" (p. 667). Accordingly, they recommend that "general practitioners and other members of the primary health care team should therefore be encouraged to include counselling about alcohol consumption in their preventive activities" (Wallace et al., 1988:663).

The Russell study of smoking cessation As noted earlier, brief interventions have been found to be efficacious in the area of cigarette smoking, which is closely related to alcohol problems and in which similar impressions of intractability exist. It seems reasonable to provide an example of the work that has been done in this area. All adult smokers who attended five London general practices over a one month period (2,138 individuals) were involved in the study. In the intervention group, those whose questionnaire responses indicated a significant level of smoking were advised to stop; given an information leaflet on methods of stopping; "and warned that they would be followed up." This process occupied one to two minutes of the physician's time. At the end of one year, 5.1 percent of the intervention group had stopped smoking, compared with 0.3 percent of the control group, a highly significant result (Russell et al., 1979).

Of course, the corollary of a 5 percent success rate for the two-minute intervention is a 95 percent failure rate. It is the failure rate that often catches the public's attention and is felt to be discouraging. But 5 percent of the original sample in this study amounted to 107 individuals who became smoke-free in one year, and in only five general practices. The authors estimate that, if all British general practitioners adopted this approach, the overall yield would amount to a half million smoke-free individuals in one year. Small, incremental gains of this kind can eventually produce significant cumulative effects.

It is noteworthy that in this study there was no increase in the proportion of individuals who succeeded each time they attempted to stop smoking. That proportion remained constant. However, the effect of the physician's intervention was to increase the number of attempts to stop. Eventually, therefore, the number of persons who succeeded increased. Although not a magical or dramatic approach, it was one that proved effective over the long run.

Further studies of the efficacy of brief intervention for alcohol problems would be most useful. The AMETHYST study, an international collaborative effort mounted by the World Health Organization (see the discussion earlier of its instrument for identifying alcohol problems, the AUDIT), is continuing its efforts with a trial of brief intervention and will provide much in terms of further data. One of the collaborating centers for the project is in the United States, a most welcome development; it is worthy of mention that controlled studies of brief intervention for alcohol problems have yet to be reported from this country.

Taken together, however, the foregoing reports of research already completed are (the committee believes) highly encouraging. *It appears that a variety of techniques can be deployed in different settings by various kinds of personnel without disrupting the usual flow of activities and that such techniques can produce significant and health-relevant effects.* Although they are carefully crafted, the kinds of interventions used in the studies reported in this section are sensible and easily grasped, both by practitioners and by members of the target population. The effects may not be dramatic, but they are palpable. With persistence in their application they could eventually achieve major gains.

Varieties of Brief Intervention

In the foregoing summaries of efficacy studies, particular attention was paid to descriptions by authors of the brief interventions they had actually used. These interventions included many different elements. Some of the more prominent were: persuasion to reduce the consumption of alcohol; information that the level of alcohol consumption was above acceptable, safe, or usual levels for the relevant population; the underscoring of adverse consequences that had already or were likely to accrue to the continued use of alcohol; feedback of laboratory test results; provision for objective and ongoing recordkeeping on alcohol consumption; and ongoing mutual surveillance of the problem. Though relatively straightforward, most of these elements (and this enumeration is hardly exhaustive) have a strong basis in theory (cf. Babor et al., 1987a).

These (and, no doubt, other) elements can be combined in a variety of ways into an intervention package, which can be delivered to the target population by a variety of individuals following a quite modest amount of training. This package is what the committee refers to as a brief intervention. Use of the package is congruent with the normal flow of activities in most settings, because it requires only a few minutes to an hour to deliver, and at most one additional session. An example of brief intervention that is consistent with the foregoing, although not labelled as such, may be found in a pamphlet entitled "The Busy Physician's Five-Minute Guide to the Management of Alcohol Problems" (Kinney, n.d.). In addition to alcohol, the interventions can readily be structured to cover a variety of lifestyle problems. All of these features permit the ready integration of brief interventions into a wide range of settings. Because of these characteristics, as well as a relative or absolute lack of a specialized treatment sector, this kind of brief intervention has become an important element in the therapeutic planning of many developing countries (see Appendix C).

There is another category of interventions that similarly fall short of the complexity of specialized formal treatment for alcohol problems and yet are quite different from brief interventions. They have been referred to collectively as "brief therapy" and are described as follows: "Brief therapy involves instructing clients in specific behavioral methods for reaching abstinence or moderate drinking (i.e. goal-setting, self-monitoring, identification of `high risk´ situations, and instruction in procedures for avoiding drinking or overdrinking). Usually brief therapy is preceded by a comprehensive assessment and does not exceed six sessions of outpatient counselling" (Sanchez-Craig, 1988:3).

Brief therapy may be viewed as an intermediate form of therapeutic approach falling between brief intervention and specialized treatment. It clearly requires much more than does brief intervention in the way of training, and because of its extent is not as readily incorporated into the standard operations of some settings. It might constitute a logical "next step" in the event that brief intervention is not successful and specialized treatment is not acceptable. In settings with a large staff complement and a high proportion of individuals with alcohol problems in the target population, a small number of staff could be trained in a brief therapy and could deliver it on a referral basis to selected individuals. Brief therapy is considerably more complex than brief intervention and probably requires therapists with relatively high levels of professional training. The target population might be those whose problems were somewhat more severe, or who had failed to improve following brief intervention, or who had refused referral for specialized treatment.   Brief therapy is thus a further significant addition to the therapeutic armamentarium.

Mention should also be made of self-help manuals, the use of which for treatment purposes is sometimes referred to as bibliotherapy. Even the most casual bookstore browser knows that self-help manuals are both ubiquitous and popular. There are those who prefer to learn what they need to know and use through the medium of print rather than human interaction. For them the self-help manual may be an excellent way to enter the therapeutic process. They have been widely available for some time (e.g. Miller and Munoz, 1982) and there is evidence for their efficacy (Miller and Taylor, 1980; Heather, 1986; Heather et al., 1986). As noted above in the descriptions of controlled studies, printed materials are sometimes incorporated as an element in brief intervention.

That different kinds of brief interventions exist poses some problems with respect to selection but is on balance a real advantage. As is the case with more complex forms of treatment (see Chapter 11), it is possible that different kinds of brief interventions will prove to be differentially acceptable and effective for different individuals. However, the level of knowledge and, indeed, the level of availability of brief interventions make such sophistication in their use a matter for the future. At present, it is a large enough task for personnel in a given setting to become familiar enough with a single brief intervention package and to deploy it effectively in a generic manner. Once this admittedly limited goal is accomplished, further refinements can be introduced.

Finally, it should be apparent from the foregoing discussion that the committee does not view brief intervention as a one-time activity that is sufficient unto itself. Although there is much evidence for the efficacy of brief interventions, in an individual instance that efficacy cannot be assumed. *Continuity of care is essential to determine whether the brief intervention has sufficed or whether further attention to the alcohol problems of the individual may be required.* Inspection of the efficacy studies summarized above will reveal that continuing contact is an element of most brief interventions and that there is evidence for its efficacy apart from the interventions themselves (see especially the New Zealand referral study).

The provision of such continuity could be viewed as the responsibility of the community provider of brief intervention. Alternatively, the responsibility for this function could be assumed by those who provide it for the specialist sector. A third possibility is to view the responsibility for continuity of care as residing with the individual who manifests the problem. Although there is some evidence linking the provision of continuity of care with favorable outcome in other fields (see the discussion of continuity of care in Chapter 13), little is available in the treatment of alcohol problems. Accordingly, this issue seems to present an important opportunity for future research.

The Target of Brief Intervention

It was emphasized earlier in this chapter that the target of brief intervention is not persons with substantial or severe alcohol problems. However, there is, as has been frequently noted, an important exception. Some proportion of persons with substantial or severe alcohol problems will not accept specialized treatment for them. Under these circumstances, the use of brief interventions (or brief therapies or both) is preferable to no therapeutic action at all. The success rate may not be high, but neither will it be negligible. Moreover, a failure may nevertheless help to persuade the individual to move on to a more rigorous intervention.

As an alternative target of brief interventions, mild or moderate alcohol problems have been put forward. The committee is sympathetic to this formulation but is willing to go somewhat beyond it. Consider the individual whose pattern of alcohol consumption, whether acute or chronic, is *likely* to result in a negative consequence—an alcohol problem, by our definition—but has not done so as yet. (This pattern is consistent with the definition of "hazardous alcohol consumption" proposed by the World Health Organization, namely, "a level of alcohol consumption or a pattern of drinking that is likely to result in harm should present drinking habits persist" [Edwards et al., 1981; J. B. Saunders and Aasland, 1987]). Let us say further that, in some way, this pattern of drinking is identified in a community agency setting. Under these circumstances the committee feels it is reasonable to proceed with a brief intervention.

For example, let us say that, prior to his auto accident and pelvic fracture, George, the fraternity pledge of Chapter 2's vignettes, had developed a severe upper respiratory infection and sought relief from the college infirmary. Because his college infirmary staff had been among those trained to identify alcohol problems and to briefly intervene when they were present, all persons seen there were routinely given a lifestyle questionnaire. The recent change in George's alcohol consumption was detected, and an alert attending physician perceived the potential dangers. No actual problems had occurred as yet, but the physician made the judgment to deploy the brief intervention anyway. As a result, George was sensitized to the problem, took appropriate action to reduce his alcohol consumption and alter its pattern, and the accident and consequent injury did not occur.

It is a possible scenario. Its implication is that brief interventions may also be targeted toward the period slightly prior to the development of actual alcohol problems. Simply put, *the target could be considered to be the consumption of alcohol itself.* To illustrate this concept, the committee has drawn the dotted line in Figure 9-1 that leads to brief intervention very slightly to the left of "mild alcohol problems." As will be seen, this is by no means a plea for any sort of prohibition; but it does involve the recognition, as pointed out in a recent review, that "in effect, any use of alcohol involves risk" (Babor et al., 1987b:392).

In another review the author offers, after meticulous consideration, an alternative approach to the more common preventive plan of reducing alcohol consumption below a specific limit: "an across-the-board reduction for the whole population, eschewing all notions of safe limits" (Kreitman, 1986:261). Anticipating the argument that such an approach will inevitably fail, because people "may see no reason to reduce their consumption for the sake of gains which are more evident to the epidemiologist than to the man in the street," Kreitman draws an analogy to the control of blood cholesterol in the prevention of cardiovascular disease:

> The health message in relation to diet and blood cholesterol is simply to reduce. It seems that the public, at least in the U.S.A., does not pose the question "What is the maximum blood cholesterol that is safe and above which I will take appropriate action?" but rather "What is the minimum level I can reasonably achieve?" The feasibility of promoting a similar strategy for alcohol consumption should at least be debated (pp. 362-363).

The Goal of Brief Intervention

The goal of brief intervention is to reduce or eliminate the alcohol consumption of those individuals to whom it is applied, with the objective of reducing or eliminating their alcohol problems. In the specialized treatment of alcohol problems, which deals with persons who manifest substantial or severe alcohol problems, there has been a prevalent view that the reduction of alcohol consumption to zero should always be the explicit goal. With regard to moderate alcohol problems, a study has been carried out in which individuals manifesting such problems received the same brief therapy but were randomly assigned either to a goal of abstinence or to a goal of reduced drinking. The outcome of treatment at one year was the same in both instances (Sanchez-Craig et al., 1984).

In the review of controlled studies of brief intervention earlier in this chapter, it can be seen that some studies utilized abstinence and some reduced drinking as their goal. The AMETHYST project of the World Health Organization takes a balanced approach with respect to this issue. Subjects in the project are provided with a pamphlet that contains guidelines about whether to choose abstinence or reduced drinking as a goal. The decision is left to the individual (Babor et al., 1987a). In view of the available evidence, the committee considers the approach exemplified by the AMETHYST project, combining guidance and individual choice, to be sound.

Referral

The final element in the community role is referral, which in this instance means referral of individuals to the specialized treatment sector for alcohol problems. One advantage of the committee's vision of a treatment system in the specialized sector (see Chapters 1 and 13) is that it incorporates a pretreatment assessment as an essential element. Referral from the community would logically be to this assessment function, obviating the need for the referring source to make its own determination as to which of many specialized treatments would be most appropriate. Because such a determination is not a simple matter (see Chapter 11), a major advantage of the committee's proposed system is that it lifts a considerable burden from community providers of brief intervention.

There remains, however, a potential problem of continuity of care between the community and the specialized treatment sector for alcohol problems. Some persons may be referred but may not attend. Under such circumstances three options are available: (1) the community provider must assume responsibility for continuity of care; (2) whatever provision is made for continuity of care in the specialized sector must be extended to the community; or (3) continuity of care must become the responsibility of the individual who is manifesting the problem (see Chapter 13).

Implementing the Community Role

Having specified identification, brief intervention, and referral as the principal activities constituting the role of community agencies in treatment, it remains to specify in what settings and by whom this role is to be implemented.

Settings

Health care settings are an obvious and important locus for the activities noted above. There is evidence that persons attending such settings have an increased prevalence of alcohol problems. Although it seems most readily apparent that primary health care settings might yield a large number of cases, the evidence is as compelling in nonprimary as in primary health care venues.

One recent study, for example, found a prevalence of alcohol problems of 20.3 percent among new patients in an ambulatory medical care setting (Cyr and Wartman, 1988). Although there are methodological problems in estimating the prevalence of alcohol problems in the general hospital inpatient population (McIntosh, 1982), an average of 23% has been given; moreover, individual hospitals surveys have resulted in findings of as high as 55 percent (Beresford, 1979). A recent prospective study of all inpatient admissions to the Johns Hopkins Hospital over a 15-month period identified 304 of 2,001 patients, or 19.7 percent, as having substantial or severe alcohol problems. These individuals were to be found in varying proportions on all admitting services and were not identified by the hospital staff in from 44 to 90 percent of instances, depending on the service. The authors noted that a diagnosis related to alcohol "was a primary diagnosis in only 6% of the patients in psychiatry and in none of the patients in the other departments. Therefore, most of these patients had this as a premorbid condition and not as the principal reason for admission" (Moore et al., 1989).

Data from this study and from a related study suggest that there may be a higher prevalence of persons with alcohol problems in the inpatient population of hospitals than in the general population. The lifetime prevalence figure for the Baltimore subset of the Epidemiologic Catchment Area (ECA) study was 15.23 percent (Helzer and Burnham, in press). Although this study was done in 1981-1982 and the Hopkins hospital data were gathered in 1986-1987, per capita consumption of alcohol in Maryland *decreased* during that period (USDHHS, 1987:4, Table 2).

The two studies used different diagnostic instruments: the Hopkins study employed the CAGE questionnaire (Ewing, 1984) and the short version of the Michigan Alcoholism Screening Test (SMAST) (Selzer et al., 1975), and the ECA study used DSM-III criteria with data gathered using the Diagnostic Interview Schedule (DIS) (Robins et al., 1981). Three of the four CAGE questions, however, have close equivalents in the DIS (J. H. Helzer, personal communication, April 29, 1989) and those with a DIS-DSM-III diagnosis for alcohol abuse or dependence tend to achieve very high scores on the full version of the MAST (Ross et al., 1988). Thus the difference between the ECA prevalence for Baltimore of 15.23 percent and the 19.7 percent prevalence found in the recent study at Johns Hopkins Hospital may represent a real difference and may reflect a concentration of alcohol problems in the hospital inpatient population greater than that obtaining in the general population.

The emergency room is another medical setting in which there is extensive contact with alcohol problems. Between 10.8 and 32 percent of casualty case samples seen in emergency departments have had substantial alcohol involvement (Peppiatt et al., 1978; Ward et al., 1982). In another study, 46 percent of 400 casualty cases had positive breathalyzer readings when evening, and particularly weekend evening, admissions were sampled (Holt et al., 1980). A recent study of emergency rooms in San Francisco and the surrounding county area showed a significant and positive association between injuries, high breathalyzer readings, self-reported alcohol consumption, and more frequent heavy drinking (the city sample reported a 21 percent rate of binge drinking in the past year, and the county sample an 8 percent rate, compared with a rate of 1 percent in the general population) (Cherpitel, 1988). Forty-one percent of injured males in the city sample reported alcohol involvement, and more than half of both males and females injured in fights and assaults reported drinking prior to the event (Cherpitel, 1989).

Thus, there is little question that a substantial number of persons with alcohol problems are seen in medical ambulatory care, inpatient, and emergency room settings. The same is true for medical specialty settings. For example, prevalences of 31.9 percent in males and 23.1 percent in females were found among consecutive new admissions for inpatient and outpatient psychiatric service (Davis, 1984). Of all patients admitted to a regional burn center in the Midwest over a six-month period in 1988, 22.9 percent had blood alcohol levels of 100 mg/dl or greater (F. C. Blow, personal communication, February 15, 1989; cf. Howland and Hingson, 1987).

Another example comes from the surgical specialty area of orthopedics. The association between such orthopedic problems as fractures and high alcohol consumption is well known. A prevalence of 30.1 percent was identified among consecutive admissions to an orthopedic service for acute injuries (Beresford et al., 1982). Indeed, the presence of fractures is sufficiently associated with alcohol problems that it has been proposed as a data element in screening for alcohol problems (Skinner et al., 1984; NIAAA, 1987).

In obstetrics, alcohol problems and, indeed, alcohol consumption are of particular importance, and for a reason other than prevalence—the health of the fetus. The full-blown fetal alcohol syndrome (FAS) may develop only in the face of sustained heavy drinking during pregnancy (Rosett and Weiner, 1985). Yet significant adverse consequences, sometimes referred to as fetal alcohol effects (FAE), may occur at lower levels of maternal alcohol consumption (Little, 1977; Hanson et al., 1978; Harlap and Shiono, 1980; Sokol et al., 1980; Streissguth et al., 1980; Rosett et al., 1983). There is evidence that, in this population, an approach such as that recommended here can be effective (Larsson, 1983; Rosett et al., 1983).

Although data are not copious, alcohol problems are likely to be important in other medical care specialty settings as well. Internists, and particularly gastroenterologists, will frequently see patients whose medical problems are directly related to alcohol consumption and would be improved if that consumption decreased (for example, peptic ulcer and hypertension). Given the uncertain state of current treatment for alcohol and other drug problems among adolescents (Blum, 1987; see Chapter 15) adolescent medicine settings may be another area of particular relevance. A further consideration is that, although the general practitioner in some medical care systems is an important gatekeeper and hence an important person in identification and brief intervention (cf. Wallace et al., 1988), the smaller size of the general practitioner pool in the United States and the tendency to take many problems directly to specialists argues against dependence on the general practitioner alone in this country.

In sum, it is possible to conclude from the available data that a significant proportion of persons who seek medical care will either have alcohol problems or will be consuming alcohol in such a way that it contributes substantially to their actual or potential medical problems. *The committee therefore believes that all persons coming for care to medical settings should be screened for alcohol problems. If mild or moderate problems are present, a brief intervention should be provided in situation and observed for its effect; if substantial or severe problems are present, a referral to specialized treatment should be effected.* Put another way, medical settings are a major site in which the role of community agencies in the treatment of alcohol problems should be enacted.

The rationale for this viewpoint should be abundantly clear from the preceding discussion. Absent this kind of approach, alcohol consumption that incurs a risk to the health of the individual or to the health of others, or that incurs a risk of alcohol problems, is likely to go unnoticed or unaddressed. Some persons, in particular those with mild or moderate problems, will not perceive these problems as requiring specialized attention and will not accept a referral to a specialist treatment apparatus. Others who may be willing to grant that alcohol consumption is a problem for them also will not accept referral, for a variety of reasons. For these people the delivery of brief intervention in the medical setting may offer the only opportunity for effective assistance; as noted above, there is considerable evidence that brief interventions can be effective. Even if the intervention is unsuccessful, it is possible that the experience will contribute to an eventual decision to seek more formal help.

These recommendations are consistent with those of the forthcoming *Guide to Clinical Preventive Services*, to be issued by the U.S. Preventive Services Task Force. Section 47 of this report addresses "Screening for Alcohol and Other Drug Abuse. A "clinical intervention" is recommended as follows:

> Clinicians should routinely ask all adults and adolescents to describe their use of alcohol and other drugs . . . Certain questionnaires may be useful to clinicians in assessing important alcohol use patterns . . . All persons who use alcohol should be informed of the health and injury risks associated with consumption and should be encouraged to limit consumption . . . Many patients may benefit from referrals to appropriate consultants and community programs specializing in the treatment of alcohol and other drug dependencies. (U.S. Preventive Services Task Force, 1989:186).

Health care settings are not the only venues to be considered for a community-based program of identification, referral, and brief intervention. *Social assistance agencies* are also a possibility. Less is known about the prevalence of alcohol problems among those seeking social services. However, the ECA study did find that, for black, white, and hispanic women, and for black and white men, the current prevalence of serious alcohol problems was higher for those receiving welfare assistance than for those not receiving welfare assistance (Helzer and Burnham, in press). It has been suggested (Murray, 1977) that vagrants, prisoners, and those cited for legal offenses connected with drinking are other groups likely to be seen in social service settings that may include a high proportion of persons with alcohol problems.

Family service agencies often see individuals whose problems are the result of or are aggravated by alcohol consumption. The same is true of welfare agencies and of agencies that provide assistance for persons with various kinds of handicaps. For example, a survey of all of California's county social services departments found that, on average, 23 percent of individuals on the general assistance caseload were public inebriates (Spieglman and Smith, 1985). Alcohol problems may be manifested by the designated client but also frequently by other members of the family, a traditional focus of family and other social agency concerns.

Alcohol problems are quite significant in the homeless population (IOM, 1988; see also pages 386-388 of this report). Again, referral for formal alcohol treatment will be effective only for a portion of the individuals identified by social agencies, and an onsite identification and intervention capability in social agencies would add an important dimension to overall management. There are exhortations to this effect in the social work literature (Raspa, 1965; Ehline and Tighe, 1977; Deakins, 1983).

Educational settings must also be considered, and are especially important in instances in which students are in residence (e.g., in boarding schools and colleges). In such settings students are away from their parents, and their parents' social support systems, and must depend to a greater degree on the resources and guidance of the institutions they are attending. Recently a number of serious incidents relating to the use of alcohol on college campuses in the United States have risen to general attention, and the time may be propitious for identification and brief intervention efforts in these and other educational settings. Many such settings have health services whose personnel have been trained to help persons with alcohol problems, but other educational personnel may appropriately be involved in such efforts as well (see the discussion on personnel below).

Health and especially alcohol problems have long been a matter of concern in *occupational settings*. Indeed, many such settings have developed employee assistance programs (EAPs) that are designed to deal with a broad spectrum of problems (see Section IV). However, although the identification of persons with alcohol problems has been much stressed in such programs, the therapeutic focus has been primarily on referral rather than on intervention. Referral may, indeed, be appropriate in some instances, but an onsite capability for dealing with at least some proportion of employee alcohol problems would be a logical extension of occupational health and employee assistance programs.

Finally, consideration should be given as well to the *criminal justice system* and the settings it potentially offers for a community agency program. The association between crime and alcohol is complex but significant (cf. Collins, 1981). Alcohol is associated in some way with many activities that come before the courts. Driving while intoxicated (DWI) is an example (see also pages 381-385). Some proportion of persons who drive while intoxicated have severe alcohol problems, but many others do not (Donovan et al., 1983; Vingilis, 1983; Wilson and Jonah, 1985; Perrine, 1986). Yet there is evidence that the specialized treatment sector for alcohol problems is being flooded with DWI and other offenders (Fillmore and Kelso, 1987; State of Connecticut, 1988). In 1986-1987, for example, the state of Connecticut experienced a 400% increase in DWI referrals to alcohol treatment services (State of Connecticut, 1988).

There is scant evidence that an approach such as that recommended in this chapter has been successful in the criminal justice system. On the other hand, there are particular features of the system that would facilitate an approach based on identification, brief intervention, and referral. Persons who enter the criminal justice system are often extensively evaluated in a variety of ways, and it would not be discordant to make the identification of alcohol problems a part of such evaluations. Given the authority of the courts, compliance with intervention and follow-up regimes may prove less of a problem in this system than elsewhere; as noted in Chapter 6, not all persons will respond favorably to such coercion, but some will. Finally, those who enter the correctional system constitute a target population that is at least readily available for interventions of various kinds.

Although the importance of alcohol problems in all of these settings is considerable, it does not follow that the settings will necessarily be receptive to mounting intervention programs. It may be necessary over time to foster a climate of institutional change with respect to alcohol problems. Employee assistance programs have done signal work in industry in this regard, and similar approaches in some school settings (i.e., student assistance programs) have also been effective. Medical settings are not inherently well disposed toward dealing with alcohol problems (Sparks, 1976). The development of specialized consultation teams may be quite helpful in this regard (Lewis and Gordon, 1983; Williams et al., 1985; Glaser, 1988). Institutional change in training settings may be of equal or greater importance in the long run; as noted earlier, one medical school (Johns Hopkins) has made a thorough understanding of alcohol problems the principal goal of its educational efforts (Holden, 1985; Moore et al., 1989). The importance of this example can hardly be overestimated.

To recapitulate: there are a number of settings other than those for the specialized treatment of alcohol problems in which persons with such problems are likely to appear. If these individuals can be effectively identified, a proportion will be appropriate for and will accept referral to specialized treatment programs. But many persons, perhaps most, either will have problems that are not sufficiently severe to require specialized treatment, or, even if their problems are severe, will not accept a referral. For these persons a brief intervention mounted within the setting in which they are identified is probably the only alternative to receiving no assistance at all for their alcohol problems. Even if the brief intervention should be unsuccessful it may serve the purpose of engaging the attention and interest of the individual, who may consequently be more willing to accept referral to the specialist sector. The settings noted in this section as ones in which such a program might be effectively mounted include primary, specialized, and emergency medical services; social agencies; educational institutions; occupational settings; and the criminal justice system. A process of institutional change may be required to foster intervention programs of the kind proposed.

Personnel

Within the settings that have been indicated in the previous discussion, which personnel should be given the responsibility for identification and brief intervention? The simplest answer is that this responsibility should be given to those personnel who already deal with the target populations of the setting. It is a sensible response and leads to a recommendation for an extensive program of on-the-job training.

Yet it is also quite a limited response. The personnel in a given setting are in constant flux. As some leave and others take their places, the new staff will have to be trained, or the capability to perform the community role in treatment will rapidly decline. On-the-job training, however, is a difficult effort to sustain over the long haul.

Alcohol problems have been a part of human history from the beginning. They are not going to go away. Thus, a long-range plan for training various kinds of personnel to identify and deal with alcohol problems must be developed. Such a plan would involve the development of a capability for identification and brief intervention during the training of personnel likely to be active in he target settings. But who are these personnel?

In the medical setting, one thinks immediately of *physicians*. There have been important and effective efforts in recent years to educate physicians about alcohol problems during their period of training (Lewis et al., 1987). Johns Hopkins Medical School in particular has set an important example (see above and Holden, 1985; Moore et al., 1989). Special mention may be made of the career teacher program sponsored jointly by the National Institutes on Drug Abuse and on Alcoholism and Alcohol Abuse, which singled out junior faculty members at medical schools for specialized development in this area. Although the program has now been discontinued, it was felt to be highly effective (Pokorny and Solomon, 1983; see Chapter 4). Certainly, physicians would be a critical target population for training of this kind. The encouragement of physician involvement in a multiplicity of ways in dealing with alcohol problems has come from the highest levels of the government and of the profession (Bowen and Sammons, 1988).

Yet physicians are not the only possible target for such training in the medical setting. *Nurses* represent another important potential resource. There are 220 schools of nursing in the United States, and they admit approximately 14,000 students annually. Enlisting this manpower would constitute a major addition to the personnel pool for treatment based in community agencies. The suitability of nurses for the proposed tasks is attested to by their having implemented them in whole or in part in three of the major trials that have been reported to date: the Malmo study, the Edinburgh study, and the New Zealand referral study (Kristensen et al., 1983; Chick et al., 1984; Elvy et al., 1988).

To take a leaf from past experience, a career teacher program in nursing might be an excellent vehicle through which to achieve the desired competency in this important group. Nurses often work regularly in some settings viewed as important to this effort, such as social agencies, educational and occupational settings, and the criminal justice system. Physicians as well may work in such settings, but unlike nurses they are more often on a consultative or minor part-time basis. Finally, there has been a movement in the United States and elsewhere toward the provision of primary health care by nurse practitioners (Spitzer et al., 1974), making their involvement all the more critical.

Social workers are a significant personnel target group in terms of social agency settings; like nurses, they tend to work in multiple settings and in important, full-time roles in those agencies. Social workers have a long and growing tradition of providing therapeutic services. *Psychologists* are another potential target group; they often play a major evaluative role in educational and criminal justice settings, developing and administering assessment instruments. Theories developed by psychologists have been of particular relevance to the development of brief intervention techniques (cf. Babor et al., 1987a).

Although there are some physicians, nurses, social workers, and psychologists in educational settings, there may be other personnel here to be considered. *Teachers* play a large role in some approaches to primary prevention and might play a role in secondary prevention as well. They spend a great deal of time with students on a regular basis and may be in a good position to identify those who are in difficulty. They are accustomed to imparting large bodies of complex information to their students; brief intervention approaches have a large informational component and may be well within their capabilities. *Guidance and counseling personnel and supervisory personnel* in the systems deployed in large organized living arrangements (e.g., dormitories, and fraternity and sorority houses) may be considered as well.

Occupational services employees in occupational settings—for example, *EAP personnel*—and *parole, probation, and corrections officers* in criminal justice settings may be additional candidates. An increasingly important group that bears consideration, and that is not particularly connected with any one of the target settings but could and perhaps should be, is *alcoholism counselors.* Their training and orientation have traditionally been toward the specialized treatment sector, but this seems more a matter of custom than necessity. Alcoholism counselors might welcome the opportunity to expand their role into this aspect of the field and might bring some unique perspectives and abilities to it.

To recapitulate: on-the-job training will be required in the short run to equip existing personnel within relevant settings to identify and provide brief interventions to persons with alcohol problems. In the long run, however, such capabilities will be most efficiently imparted to relevant personnel during the course of their training. It should be stressed that, to be effective, such training must be broad; it cannot be oriented exclusively toward the more severe problems, as has frequently been the case in the past, but must be oriented toward the entire spectrum of alcohol problems. Among the groups that may be targeted for such training are physicians; nurses; social workers; psychologists; teachers; occupational services employees; parole, probation, and corrections officials; and alcoholism counselors.

Effects and Costs

The successful deployment of a capability for widespread identification of persons with alcohol problems and of brief intervention for those problems, as outlined above, is intended to reduce the overall burden of alcohol problems to the individual and to society at large. There is reason to believe that this desirable result would follow. However, there would be little point in introducing such a major innovation in care unless provisions were made for a careful determination of whether the desired result did in fact occur.

Some may entertain the hope that the costs accruing to the specialized treatment of substantial or severe alcohol problems could be greatly reduced through such a program. This seems a possible but not a necessary consequence. The widespread availability of brief intervention would remove from the specialist treatment pool those individuals who would respond to less extensive kinds of treatment. However, the systematic identification of individuals with alcohol problems in the many settings in which this would take place might result in a significantly increased level of referrals to specialized treatment overall. The net result in this instance would probably be an overall increase in the cost of treatment for alcohol problems. As is discussed further in Chapter 20, the great likelihood is that the overall costs of treatment would continue to be far less than the cost to society of alcohol problems.

An initial financial investment of some magnitude in the development of a comprehensive system of identification and brief intervention would seem to be unavoidable. Further study of these processes, the development and dissemination of appropriate packages of identification and intervention materials, the training of appropriate personnel, and the evaluation of the effort require it. However, once the system is in place, and, one would hope, working well, existing funding mechanisms should be able to cover the provision of services, which will have become part of standard practice. At the same time the overall financial benefits from the reduction of the alcohol problem burden (e.g., reduced collisions, reduced accidents, reduced domestic violence) may begin to be felt. There is evidence that the provision of preventive services of the kind contemplated is at least as cost-effective as many accepted prevention practices (Cummings et al., 1989)

A further comment seems in order regarding the financial implications of brief therapy. Unlike brief intervention (one or two sessions), it is difficult to see how brief therapy (six or eight sessions) can be construed as a part of standard practice, at least for reimbursement purposes. Moreover, although some physicians may be trained in brief therapy, the committee can see no necessary requirement of medical training as a part of its delivery and anticipates that it may be provided for the most part by practitioners other than physicians. In the current climate of health insurance, reimbursement of nonphysicians would very largely not be possible. *The committee urges strongly that a financial mechanism be developed to fund brief therapy outside of, as well as within, the context of funding for medical or medically-supervised services.*

Conclusions and Recommendations

The committee recommends *a broader and more comprehensive nationwide effort to establish a strong community role in dealing with mild to moderate alcohol problems, to complement the efforts of the specialized treatment sector in dealing with substantial and severe alcohol problems.* The goal of this effort is to reduce or eliminate the consumption of alcohol by persons experiencing problems, with the object of reducing the overall burden of problems. The role of community agencies in treatment would involve (1) identifying in a variety of human service settings those persons with alcohol problems, (2) referring those who are appropriate to specialized treatment, and (3) dealing with the rest by providing brief intervention or brief therapy.

To carry out this program, it would be necessary to designate a strong leadership capability in this area. The most appropriate approaches to these activities need to be defined and developed. A major training effort, directed at a variety of human services professionals and their supporting institutions, would need to be mounted, as well as an evaluation effort capable of determining both the outcome of the community role in treatment and its costs. Methods of financing those components of the program not underwritten by existing mechanisms (e.g., planning, materials development, further re-search, feasibility studies, training, and the provision of brief therapy) would also have to be developed.

The committee recognizes that these recommendations constitute a major and (at least initially) a costly proposal, but it also recognizes the appalling magnitude of the cost of alcohol problems to society. For the reasons developed in this chapter, the committee believes that the further development of the community component of treatment offers a significant possibility of ultimately containing these costs.

REFERENCES

Allen, J. P., M. J. Eckhardt, and J. Wallen. 1988. Screening for alcoholism: Techniques and issues. Public Health Reports 103:586-592.

American Psychiatric Association. 1987. Diagnostic and Statistical Manual of Mental Disorders, 3rd Edition, Revised. Washington, D.C.: American Psychiatric Association.

Babor, T. F., and R. Kadden. 1985. Screening for alcohol problems: Conceptual issues and practical considerations. Pp. 1-30 in Early Identification of Alcohol Abuse, N. C. Chang and H. M. Chao, eds. Washington, D.C.: U.S. Government Printing Office.

Babor, T. F., E. B. Ritson, and R. J. Hodgson. 1986. Alcohol-related problems in the primary health care setting: A review of early intervention strategies. British Journal of Addiction 81:23-46.

Babor, T. F., P. Korner, C. Wilber, and S. P. Good. 1987a. Screening and early intervention strategies for harmful drinkers: Initial lessons from the Amethyst Project. Australian Drug and Alcohol Review 6:325-339.

Babor, T. F., H. R. Kranzler, and R. J. Lauerman. 1987b. Social drinking as a health and psychosocial risk factor: Anstie's limit revisited. Pp. 373-402 in Recent Developments in Alcoholism, vol. 5, M. Galanter, ed. New York: Plenum Press.

Babor, T. F., R. de la Fuente, J. Saunders, and M. Grant. 1989. Manual for the Alcohol Use Disorders Identification Test (AUDIT). Geneva: World Health Organization.

Bach-y-Rita, G., J. R. Lion, and F. R. Ervin. 1970. Pathological intoxication: Clinical and electroencephalographic studies. American Journal of Psychiatry 127:698-703.

Baekeland, F., and L. K. Lundwall. 1977. Engaging the alcoholic in treatment and keeping him there. Pp. 161-195 in Treatment and Rehabilitation of the Chronic Alcoholic, Vol. 5 of The Biology of Alcoholism, B. Kissin and H. Begleiter, eds. New York: Plenum Press.

Banay, R. S. 1944. Pathologic reaction to alcohol. I. Review of the literature and original case reports. Quarterly Journal of Studies on Alcohol 4:580-605.

Beresford, T. P. 1979. Alcoholism consultation and general hospital psychiatry. General Hospital Psychiatry 1:293-300.

Beresford, T. P., R. Adduci, D. Low, F. Goggans, and R. C. W. Hall. 1982. A computerized biochemical profile for detection of alcoholism. Psychosomatics 23:713-720.

Bernadt, M. W., J. Mumford, C. Taylor, B. Smith, and R. M. Murray. 1982. Comparison of questionnaire and laboratory tests in the detection of excessive drinking and alcoholism. Lancet 1:325-328.

Bernadt, M. W., J. Mumford, and R. M. Murray. 1984. A discriminant-function analysis of screening tests for excessive drinking and alcoholism. Journal of Studies on Alcohol 45:81-86.

Blum, R. W. 1987. Adolescent substance abuse: Diagnostic and treatment issues. Pediatric Clinics of North America 34:523-537.

Bowen, O. R., and J. H. Sammons. 1988. The alcohol-abusing patient: A challenge to the profession. Journal of the American Medical Association 260:2267-2270.

Cahalan, D. 1970. Problem Drinkers: A National Survey. San Francisco: Jossey-Bass.

Cherpitel, C. J. S. 1988. Alcohol consumption and casualties: A comparison of two emergency room populations. British Journal of Addiction 83:1299-1307.

Cherpitel, C. J. S. 1989. Breath analysis and self-reports as measures of alcohol-related emergency room admissions. Journal of Studies on Alcohol 50:155-161.

Chick, J., G. Lloyd, and E. Crombie. 1984. Counselling problem drinkers in medical wards: A controlled study. British Medical Journal 290:965-967.

Coid, J. 1979. Mania a potu: A critical review of pathological intoxication. Psychological Medicine 9:709-719.

Collins, J. J., Jr., ed. 1981. Drinking and Crime: Perspectives on the Relationships Between Alcohol Consumption and Criminal Behavior. New York: Guilford Press.

Cummings, S. R., S. M. Rubin, and G. Oster. 1989. The cost-effectiveness of counseling smokers to quit. Journal of the American Medical Association 261:75-79.

Cyr, M. G., and S. A. Wartman. 1988. The effectiveness of routine screening questions in the detection of alcoholism. Journal of the American Medical Association 259:51-54.

Davis, D. I. 1984. Differences in the use of substances of abuse by psychiatric patients compared with medical and surgical patients. Journal of Nervous and Mental Diseases 172:654-657.

Deakins, S. M. 1983. In support of routine screening for alcoholism. Pp. 16-22 in Social Work Treatment of Alcohol Problems, D. Cook, C. Fewell, and J. Riolo, eds. New Brunswick, N. J.: Rutgers Center for Alcohol Studies.

Donovan, D. M., G. A. Marlatt, and P. M. Salzberg. 1983. Drinking behavior, personality factors, and high-risk driving: A review and theoretical formulations. Journal of Studies on Alcohol 44:395-428.

Edwards, G., J. Orford, S. Egert, S. Guthrie, A. Hawker, C. Hensman, M. Mitcheson, E. Oppenheimer, and C. Taylor. 1977. Alcoholism: A controlled trial of "treatment" and "advice." Journal of Studies on Alcohol 38:1004-1031.

Edwards, G., and J. Orford. 1977. A plain treatment for alcoholism. Proceedings of the Royal Society of Medicine 70:344-348.

Edwards, G., A. Arif, and R. Hodgson. 1981. Nomenclature and classification of drug- and alcohol-related problems: A WHO memorandum. Bulletin of the World Health Organization 59:225-242.

Ehline, D., and P. O. Tighe. 1977. Alcoholism: Early identification and intervention in the social service agency. Child Welfare 56:584-592.

Elvy, G. A., J. E. Wells, and K. A. Baird. 1988. Attempted referral as intervention for problem drinking in the general hospital. British Journal of Addiction 83:83-89.

Ewing, J. A. 1984. Detecting alcoholism: The CAGE questionnaire. Journal of the American Medical Association 252:1905-1907.

Fillmore, K. M., and D. Kelso. 1987. Coercion into alcoholism treatment: Meanings for the disease concept of alcoholism. Journal of Drug Issues 17:301-319.

Glaser, F. B. 1980. Anybody got a match? Treatment research and the matching hypothesis. Pp. 178-196 in Alcoholism Treatment in Transition, G. Edwards and M. Grant, eds. London: Croom Helm.

Glaser, F. B. 1988. Alcohol and drug problems: A challenge to consultation-liaison psychiatry. Canadian Journal of Psychiatry 33:259-263.

Gottesman, I. I., and C. A. Prescott. 1989. Abuses of the MacAndrew MMPI alcoholism scale: A critical review. Clinical Psychology Reviews 9:223-242.

Hanson, J. W., A. P. Streissguth, and D. W. Smith. 1978. The effects of moderate alcohol consumption during pregnancy on fetal growth and morphogenesis. Journal of Pediatrics 92:457-460.

Harlap, S., and P. H. Shiono. 1980. Alcohol, smoking, and incidence of spontaneous abortions in the first and second trimester. Lancet 2:173-176.

Heather, N. 1986. Change without therapists: The use of self-help manuals by problem drinkers. Pp. 331-359 in Treating Addictive Behaviors: Processes of Change, W. R. Miller and N. Heather, eds. New York: Plenum Press.

Heather, N., B. Whitton, and I. Robinson. 1986. Evaluation of a self-help manual for media-recruited problem drinkers: Six-month follow-up results. British Journal of Clinical Psychology 25:19-34.

Helzer, J. E., and A. Burnham. In press. Alcohol abuse and dependence. In Psychiatric Disorders in America, L. Robins and D. A. Regier, eds. New York: The Free Press.

Hilton, M. E. 1987. Drinking patterns and drinking problems in 1984: Results from a general population survey. Alcoholism: Clinical and Experimental Research 11:167-175.

Hingson, R., T. Mangione, A. Meyers, and N. Scotch. 1982. Seeking help for drinking problems: A study in the Boston metropolitan area. Journal of Studies on Alcohol 43:273-288.

Holden, C. 1985. The neglected disease in medical education. Science 229:741-742.

Holt, S. I., I. Stuart, J. Dixon, R. Elton, T. Taylor, and K. Little. 1980. Alcohol and the emergency service patient. British Medical Journal 281:638-640.

Howland, J., and R. Hingson. 1987. Alcohol as a risk factor for injuries or death due to fires and burns: A review of the literature. Public Health Reports 102:475-483.

Institute of Medicine (IOM). 1988. Homelessness, Health, and Human Needs. Washington, D.C.: National Academy Press.

Institute of Medicine (IOM). 1989. Prevention and Treatment of Alcohol Problems: Research Opportunities. Washington, D.C.: National Academy Press.

Kaplan, H. B., A. D. Pokorny, T. Kanas, and G. Lively. 1974. Screening tests and self-identification in the detection of alcoholism. Journal of Health and Social Behavior 15:51-56.

Kapur, B. M., and Y. Israel. 1985. Alcohol dipstick—a rapid method for analysis of ethanol in body fluids. Pp. 310-20 in Early Identification of Alcohol Abuse, N. C. Chang and H. M. Chao, eds. Washington, D.C.: U.S. Government Printing Office.

Kinney, J. N.d. (ca. 1988). The Busy Physician's Five-Minute Guide to the Management of Alcohol Problems. Produced through a grant from the American Medical Association Department of Substance Abuse.

Kreitman, N. 1986. Alcohol consumption and the preventive paradox. British Journal of Addiction 81:353-363.

Kristenson, H., H. Ohlin, M. B. Hulten-Nosslin, E. Trell, and B. Hood. 1983. Identification and intervention of heavy drinking in middle-aged men: Results and follow-up of 24-60 months of long-term study with randomized controls. Alcoholism: Clinical and Experimental Research 7:203-209.

Larsson, G. 1983. Prevention of fetal alcohol effects: An antenatal program for early detection of pregnancies at risk. Acta Obstetrica and Gynecologica Scandinavica 62:171-178.

Leigh, G., and H. A. Skinner. 1988. Physiological assessment. Pp. 112-136 in Assessment of Addictive Behaviors, G. A. Marlatt and D. M. Donovan, eds. New York: Guilford Press.

Lewis, D. C., and A. J. Gordon. 1983. Alcoholism and the general hospital: The Roger Williams intervention program. Bulletin of the New York Academy of Medicine 59:181-197.

Lewis, D. C., R. G. Niven, D. Czechowicz, and J. G. Trumble. 1987. A review of medical education in alcohol and other drug abuse. Journal of the American Medical Association 257:2945-2948.

Little, R. E. 1977. Moderate alcohol use during pregnancy and decreased infant birth weight. American Journal of Public Health 67:1154-1156.

MacAndrew, C. 1965. The differentiation of male alcoholic outpatients from non-alcoholic psychiatric outpatients by means of the MMPI. Quarterly Journal of Studies on Alcohol 26:238-246.

Maletzky, B. M. 1976. The diagnosis of pathological intoxication. Journal of Studies on Alcohol 37:1215-1228.

Maletzky, B. M. 1978. The alcohol provocation test. Journal of Clinical Psychiatry 39:403, 407-411.

Marinacci, A. A. 1963. A special type of temporal lobe (psychomotor) seizures following ingestion of alcohol. Bulletin of the Los Angeles Neurological Society 28:241-250.

May, P. R. A., and F. G. Ebaugh. 1953. Pathological intoxication, alcoholic hallucinosis, and other reactions to alcohol: A clinical study. Quarterly Journal of Studies on Alcohol 14:200-227.

McEvoy, L., L. N. Robins, J. E. Helzer, and E. L. Spitznagel. 1987. Alcoholism and mental health services: Who comes to treatment? Washington University School of Medicine, Department of Psychiatry, St. Lewis, Mo.

McIntosh, I. D. 1982. Alcohol-related disabilities in general hospital patients: A critical assessment of the evidence. International Journal of the Addictions 17:609-639.

Miller, W. R., and R. F. Munoz. 1982. How to Control Your Drinking, rev. ed. Albuquerque: University of New Mexico Press.

Miller, W. R., and C. A. Taylor. 1980. Relative effectiveness of bibliotherapy, individual and group self-control training in the treatment of problem drinkers. Addictive Behaviors 5:13-24.

Moore, M. H., and D. R. Gerstein. 1981. Alcohol and Public Policy: Beyond the Shadow of Prohibition. Washington, D.C.: National Academy Press.

Moore, R. D., L. R. Bone, G. Geller, J. A. Mamon, E. J. Stokes, and D. M. Levine. 1989. Prevalence, detection, and treatment of alcoholism in hospitalized patients. Journal of the American Medical Association 261:403-407.

Morse, R. M., and R. D. Hurt. 1979. Screening for alcoholism. Journal of the American Medical Association 242:2688-2690.

Moskowitz, J. M. 1989. The primary prevention of alcohol problems: A critical review of the research literature. Journal of Studies on Alcohol 50:54-88.

Murray, R. M. 1977. Screening and early detection instruments for disabilities related to alcohol consumption. Pp. 89-105 in Alcohol Related Disabilities, G. Edwards, M. M. Gross, M. Keller, J. Moser, and R. Room, eds. Geneva: World Health Organization.

National Institute on Alcohol Abuse and Alcoholism (NIAAA). 1987. Screening for Alcoholism in Primary Care Settings: Report of A Workshop Held in Bethesda, Maryland, May 27, 1987. Rockville, Md: NIAAA.

Orford, J., E. Oppenheimer, and G. Edwards. 1976. Abstinence or control: The outcome for excessive drinkers two years after consultation. Behavior Research and Therapy 14:409-418.

Peachey, J. E., and B. M. Kapur. 1986. Monitoring drinking behavior with the alcohol dipstick during treatment. Alcoholism: Clinical and Experimental Research 10:663-666.

Peppiatt, R., R. Evans, and P. Jordan. 1978. Blood alcohol concentrations of patients attending an accident and emergency department. Resuscitation 6:37-43.

Perrine, B. 1986. Varieties of drunken and drinking drivers: A review, a research program, and a model. In Alcohol, Drugs, and Traffic Safety. Proceedings of the 10th International Conference on Alcohol, Drugs, and Traffic Safety, Amsterdam, September.

Plant, M. 1988. Good news for doctors? Alcohol and Alcoholism 23:5-6.

Pokorny, A. D., and J. Solomon. 1983. A follow-up survey of drug abuse and alcoholism teaching in medical schools. Journal of Medical Education 58:316-321.

Popham, R. E., W. Schmidt, and J. de Lint 1975. The prevention of alcoholism: Epidemiological studies of the effects of government control measures. British Journal of Addiction 70:125-144.

Raspa, G. 1965. Public welfare and problem drinkers: Providing financial assistance, therapeutic facilities, and case work help. Pp. 55-62 in Treatment Methods and Milieus in Social Work with Alcoholics. Proceedings of a conference held by the University of California Extension Division, Berkeley, Calif., December 3-5.

Reich, T., L. N. Robins, R. A. Woodruff, Jr., M. Taibelson, C. Rich, and L. Cunningham. 1975. Computer-assisted derivation of a screening interview for alcoholism. Archives of General Psychiatry 32:847-852.

Robins, L. N., J. H. Helzer, J. Croughan, and K. S. Ratcliff. 1981. National Institute of Mental Health Diagnostic Interview Schedule: Its history, characteristics, and validity. Archives of General Psychiatry 38:381-389.

Rosett, H. L., and L. Weiner. 1985. Alcohol and pregnancy: A clinical perspective. Annual Review of Medicine 36:73-80.

Rosett, H. L., L. Weiner, A. Lee, B. Zuckerman, E. Dooling, and E. Oppenheimer. 1983. Patterns of alcohol consumption and fetal development. Obstetrics and Gynecology 61:539-546.

Ross, H. E., F. B. Glaser, and T. Germanson. 1988. The prevalence of psychiatric disorders in patients with alcohol and other drug problems. Archives of General Psychiatry 45:1023-1031.

Russell, M. A. H., C. Wilson, C. Taylor, and C. D. Baker. 1979. Effect of general practitioners' advice against smoking. British Medical Journal 2:231-235.

Sanchez-Craig, M. 1988. Executive summary: Secondary prevention of alcohol problems by brief intervention. Prepared for the IOM Committee for the Study of Treatment and Rehabilitation Services for Alcoholism and Alcohol Abuse.

Sanchez-Craig, M., H. M. Annis, A. R. Bornet, and K. R. MacDonald. 1984. Random assignment to abstinence and controlled drinking: Evaluation of a cognitive-behavioral program for problem drinkers. Journal of Consulting and Clinical Psychology 52:390-403.

Saunders, J. B. 1988. Executive summary: Screening techniques for alcohol problems. Prepared for the IOM Committee for the Study of Treatment and Rehabilitation Services for Alcoholism and Alcohol Abuse.

Saunders, J. B., and O. G. Aasland. 1987. WHO Collaborative Project on Identification and Treatment of Persons with Harmful Alcohol Consumption: Report on Phase I Development of a Screening Instrument. Geneva: World Health Organization, Division of Mental Health.

Saunders, W. M., and P. W. Kershaw. 1980. Screening tests for alcoholism--findings from a community study. British Journal of Addiction 75:37-41.

Schuckit, M. A., and M. Irwin. 1988. Diagnosis of alcoholism. Medical Clinics of North America 72:1133-1153.

Selzer, M. L. 1971. The Michigan Alcoholism Screening Test: The quest for a new diagnostic instrument. American Journal of Psychiatry 127:1653-1658.

Selzer, M. L., A. Vinokur, and L. van Rooijen. 1975. Self-administered Short Michigan Alcoholism Screening Test (SMAST). Journal of Studies on Alcohol 36:117-126.

Skelton, W. D. 1970. Alcohol, violent behavior, and the electroencephalogram. Southern Medical Journal 63:465-466.

Skinner, H. A. 1988. Executive summary: Spectrum of drinkers and intervention responses. Prepared for the IOM Committee for the Study of Treatment and Rehabilitation Services for Alcoholism and Alcohol Abuse.

Skinner, H. A., and B. Allen. 1982. Alcohol dependence syndrome: Measurement and validation. Journal of Abnormal Psychology 91:199-209.

Skinner, H. A., and S. Holt. 1987. The Alcohol Clinical Index: Strategies for Identifying Patients with Alcohol Problems. Toronto: Addiction Research Foundation.

Skinner, H. A., S. Holt, and Y. Israel. 1981. Early identification of alcohol abuse. I. Critical issues and psychosocial indicators for a composite index. Canadian Medical Association Journal 124:1141-1152.

Skinner, H. A., S. Holt, R. Schuller, J. Roy, and Y. Israel. 1984. Identification of alcohol abuse using laboratory tests and a history of trauma. Annals of Internal Medicine 101:847-51.

Skinner, H. A., B. A. Allen, M. C. McIntosh, and W. H. Palmer. 1985a. Lifestyle assessment: Applying microcomputers in family practice. British Medical Journal 290:212-214.

Skinner, H. A., B. A. Allen, M. C. McIntosh, and W. H. Palmer. 1985b. Lifestyle assessment: Just asking makes a difference. British Medical Journal 290:214-16.

Skinner, H. A., S. Holt, W.-J. Sheu, and Y. Israel. 1986. Clinical versus laboratory detection of alcohol abuse: The alcohol clinical index. British Medical Journal 2:1703-1708.

Smart, R. G., M. Gillies, G. Brown, and N. L. Blair. 1980. A survey of alcohol-related problems and their treatment. Canadian Journal of Psychiatry 25:220-227.

Sokol, R. J., S. I. Miller, and G. Reed. 1980. Alcohol abuse in pregnancy: An epidemiological study. Alcoholism: Clinical and Experimental Research 4:135-145.

Sparks, R. D. 1976. Attitudes in medicine toward alcoholism. Man and Medicine 1:173-180.

Speiglman, R., and M. Smith. 1985. California's Services for Public Inebriates: An Inventory and Report to the Department of Alcohol and Drug Programs. Berkeley, Calif.: Alcohol Research Group.

Spitzer, W. O., D. L. Sackett, J. C. Sibley, R. S. Roberts, M. Gent, D. J. Kergin, B. C. Hackett, and A. Olynich. 1974. The Burlington randomized trial of the nurse practitioner. New England Journal of Medicine 290:251-256.

State of Connecticut Drug and Alcohol Abuse Criminal Justice Commission. 1988. The Drug and Alcohol Abuse Crisis within the Connecticut Criminal Justice System. State of Connecticut Drug and Alcohol Abuse Criminal Justice Commission, Hartford, Conn.

Streissguth, A. P., S. Landesman-Dwyer, J. C. Martin, and D. W. Smith. 1980. Teratogenic effects of alcohol in humans and laboratory animals. Science 209:353-361.

U.S. Department of Health and Human Services (USDHHS). 1987. Sixth Special Report to the U.S. Congress on Alcohol and Health. Rockville, Md.: National Institute on Alcohol Abuse and Alcoholism.

U.S. Preventive Services Task Force. 1989. Section 47: Screening for alcohol and other drug abuse. Pp. 182-189 in Guide to Clinical Preventive Services (prepublication copy). U.S. Department of Health and Human Services, Washington, D.C.

Vingilis, E. 1983. Drinking drivers and alcoholics: Are they from the same population? Pp. 299-342 in Research Advances in Alcohol and Drug Problems, vol. 7, R. G. Smart, F. B. Glaser, Y. Israel, H. Kalant, R. E. Popham, and W. Schmidt, eds. New York: Plenum Press.

Wallace, P., S. Cutler, and A. Haines. 1988. Randomized controlled trial of general practitioner intervention in patients with excessive alcohol consumption. British Medical Journal 297:633-638.

Ward, R. E., T. C. Flynn, P. W. Miller, and W. F. Blaisdell. 1982. Effects of ethanol ingestion on the severity and outcome of trauma. American Journal of Surgery 144:153-157.

Williams, C. N., D. C. Lewis, J. Femino, L. Hall, K. Blackburn-Kilduff, R. Rosen, and C. Samella. 1985. Overcoming barriers to identification and referral of alcoholics in a general hospital setting: One approach. Rhode Island Medical Journal 68:131-138.

Wilson, J., and B. Jonah. 1985. Identifying impaired drivers among the general driving population. Journal of Studies on Alcohol 46:531-536.

Wolf, A. S. 1980. Homicide and blackout in Alaskan natives: a report and reproduction of five cases. Journal of Studies on Alcohol 41:456-462.

10 Assessment

In Chapter 9 the committee proposed a broadening of the base of treatment through a wide dissemination of the capability to identify and briefly intervene with persons manifesting mild or moderate alcohol problems. This strategy is intended for implementation in settings other than specialized treatment programs for alcohol problems to which persons identified as having substantial or severe alcohol problems would be referred. In the next three chapters of this section of the report the committee discusses strategies for enhancing the specialized treatment of alcohol problems. Three areas are emphasized: (1) assessment prior to treatment, (2) matching to optimal treatment, and (3) determining treatment outcome.

Considering assessment, matching, and outcome determination in separate chapters is an arbitrary division of material for the purposes of discussion. In practice, each function is related to the others, and all are parts of a unified whole. For example, the treatment modalities that are available influence the content of assessment, and to match individuals to the most appropriate treatments requires pretreatment assessment. Treatment outcomes become increasingly meaningful with assessment and can be utilized to increase the accuracy of matching. How accurate matching has been is, in turn, evaluated by determining treatment outcome. Because the committee wishes to emphasize the importance of a close integration of assessment, matching, and outcome determination, it has elected to discuss how they might be fitted together both at the outset of this report (Chapter 1) and at the close of Section II, "Aspects of Treatment" (Chapter 13). However, because all three of these processes raise particular issues that need to be discussed, the committee has devoted a separate chapter to each.

A key purpose of assessment is to determine which of the available treatment options is likely to be most appropriate for the individual being assessed. Hence, assessment must occur prior to any commitment of the individual to a particular kind of treatment, and its utility is contingent upon the availability of multiple treatment options. "When clinicians apply the same general [treatment] approach to most clients, assessment data can have few treatment implications. With the arrival of more specific interventions, however, the need for guidance by assessment data becomes more obvious" (Hayes et al., 1987:964).

This general principle is particularly pertinent to the treatment of alcohol problems. A major conclusion from the substantial body of research on treatment outcome in this field is that there is no single treatment approach that is effective for all persons with alcohol problems (see Chapter 5). This being so, for optimal treatment matching is not optional but is required (see Chapter 11). Assessment provides the basis for matching.

What Is Assessment?

Assessment is the systematic process of interaction with an individual to observe, elicit, and subsequently assemble the relevant information required to deal with his or her case, both immediately and for the foreseeable future. In general, the collection of detailed initial information is a feature of all human service settings. In particular, alcohol problems are known to affect, and to be affected by, multiple aspects of an individual's life; they frequently manifest themselves as physical problems, psychological problems, social problems, and vocational problems simultaneously. Thus, the initial effort to collect information might be expected to be at least as extended—if not more extended—than in other service settings.

Yet despite the logic and the pervasiveness of this approach, a comprehensive assessment of each individual entering specialized treatment for alcohol problems is a principle honored more in the breach than in the observance. Many specialized treatment settings offer only a single modality of treatment (Glaser et al., 1978). Thus, there is no reason (from the program's standpoint) to develop information that might suggest alternatives, and there may be strong financial incentives not to do so, a point discussed later in this chapter. Although a certain amount of data is usually gathered, it is often simply demographic information and, increasingly these days, information regarding available reimbursement mechanisms. The data are gathered after admission to the treatment program and therefore after a commitment has been made to a particular form of treatment; hence, they have little or no bearing on treatment selection.

A sample statement from the literature documenting the general lack of comprehensive assessment is that "patients were assigned to treatment methods without a thorough evaluation of their problems and without a recorded assessment of severity and were allowed to progress without follow-up or reassessment" (S. Miller et al., 1974:213). In the province of Ontario, where the Addiction Research Foundation has advocated pretreatment assessment for almost a decade, a 1986 survey of 181 programs found that "although there was a very high endorsement of the *systematic assessment* of clients, only about 20-25% of programs include state-of-the-art diagnostic instruments in their assessment protocol. Assessment typically involved a structured or unstructured questioning of the client, without the use of further diagnostic aids" (Rush, 1987:3).

Even if one looks only at the treatment outcome research literature, in which knowledge of pretreatment status is essential to determine whether treatment has affected outcome, what one sees is less than satisfactory. "The failure to provide more comprehensive pretreatment data," reports one group of investigators, ". . . is distressing and is a problem that has not lessened with passage of time . . . Pretreatment data for variables such as severity of dependence, chronicity of drinking problems, and quantitative assessment of pretreatment drinking were reported in only about one-half of the studies" (L. C. Sobell et al., 1988:117).

The committee's general charge was to study the process of treatment and make recommendations for its improvement, and it considers a comprehensive pretreatment assessment to be crucial to such improvement. The "basic justification for assessment is that it provides information of value to the planning, execution, and evaluation of treatment" (Korchin and Schuldberg, 1981). Yet assessment can serve multiple purposes, and an appreciation of the need for assessment should arise from an understanding of all of them.

The Purposes of Assessment for Alcohol Problems

Characterizing the Problem

If alcohol problems differ from one person to another, whether in degree or in kind, it is crucial to document the differences. Otherwise, any changes subsequent to treatment cannot be compared with the individual's pretreatment status. Some persons coming for treatment, for example, will have high alcohol consumption levels, and others will not. Some will be binge drinkers, and others will be steady drinkers. Some will have experienced many symptoms in connection with their use of alcohol, and others will have experienced few symptoms. Some will have accrued a great many adverse consequences of alcohol consumption, and others will have accrued few consequences. As with other drugs, those who have lower levels of consumption will probably exhibit more variety in the problems they manifest than will individuals with higher levels of consumption (Edwards, 1974).

But even among those with many signs and symptoms, the specific manifestations will differ from one person to the next. For example, DSM-III-R lists nine signs and symptoms of "psychoactive substance use disorders," of which any combination of three will qualify for a diagnosis (American Psychiatric Association, 1987). Thus, among those qualifying for this diagnosis on the basis of their alcohol use, many alternative combinations of manifestations will occur. In this spirit physicians have been cautioned to "be aware that not every patient that drinks too much (for whatever reason) will be dependent on alcohol, and different patients need different help and treatment" (Edwards and Gross, 1976:1061).

As this warning suggests, the correspondence between level of consumption, pattern of consumption, signs and symptoms, and consequences is not invariably a close one. Some people with high consumption levels will drink steadily, have many signs and symptoms, and experience many consequences, but others will not. The evidence for the relative independence of these dimensions of alcohol problems will be discussed later in this chapter. That they are not necessarily highly correlated with each other, particularly in younger persons (Fillmore and Midanik, 1984; Fillmore, 1987), introduces still more variance into the clinical picture of alcohol problems.

What should emerge from a comprehensive assessment is a detailed picture of the particular kind of alcohol problem manifested by a particular individual at a particular point in time. Of major importance is to describe the person and the problem in terms that are clear and unambiguous. Not only is precision valuable in itself but, if assessment is to be maximally useful, its terms must be clearly understandable to a variety of individuals. The evolving treatment system is complex. Particularly in cases in which the problem is a chronic one (and many alcohol problems will be), a large number of different treatment personnel will encounter particular persons with alcohol problems over time.

In the absence of a clear and unambiguous picture at initial contact it may not prove possible to understand the evolution of an individual's alcohol problem over time, or to make appropriate decisions regarding care for the present and the future. Let us consider a common clinical situation: a patient reports that he "had a problem before, but it got better; now he has developed a problem again, only this time it is a little different." What sort of problem did he have before? In what sense and to what degree did it improve? In what way is the problem he has now different from the problem he had previously? Skillful interviewing can help to clarify some of these issues, but a comprehensive, understandable, quantitative, recorded account of the patient's earlier status and of his course would be invaluable in providing solid answers.

Precise information regarding the parameters of an alcohol problem is of interest not only to therapists but also to those who manifest the problems. The feedback of assessment data in an understandable form to those from whom it has been obtained is a common and useful practice. Not only does it seem a reasonable courtesy, but there is evidence that feedback can contribute significantly to treatment-seeking behavior.

Thus, in one study, half again as many individuals seeking help for alcohol problems appeared in treatment after receiving a comprehensive assessment compared with those who were not assessed (Annis and Skinner, 1984). In another study, 95 percent of a random sample of such individuals who were given an assessment battery returned for their second appointment, compared with only 56 percent of those who were not given the assessment (Sutherland et al., 1985). General practice patients who completed a brief assessment of their use of alcohol, tobacco, caffeine, medication, and nonmedical drugs during which "feedback was given on how the patient's consumption levels compared with others of the same sex and age" were significantly more likely than those who were not so assessed to query their doctors regarding all of these substances (H. A. Skinner et al., 1985b).

"Taking these [assessment] tests," commented one group of observers, "could have predisposed patients to attend a second session either because they may have expected to obtain some information about the test's results . . . or because they may have been impressed by the amount of care devoted to them" (Sutherland et al., 1985:212). In confirmation, one patient in an assessment program commented that "it helps you to get a hold of yourself and use your mind to sort out what makes you feel [the way you do] about life" (Segal, 1984). Another said that "it slowed down my thinking process and allowed me to have a good, long look at myself. I now know what I am and what I have to do to improve myself."

Characterizing the Individual

Alcohol problems do not occur in a vacuum. The individuals who manifest them are at least as different from one another as are ordinary people (Chapter 2). Or perhaps, more different: Keller's law is that "the investigation of any trait in alcoholics will show that they have either more or less of it" (Keller, 1972). A precise and systematic knowledge of the differing characteristics that each *individual* exhibits at the time he or she is seen for an alcohol problem, as well as a characterization of the problem, is another purpose of assessment.

Eventually, such information will help to unravel which individual characteristics may predispose people to alcohol problems and which are the result of alcohol problems. Beyond these benefits for future research, however, lies the immediate therapeutic utility of such information. Individual characteristics have much to do with a person's acceptance (and, in consequence, the eventual outcome) of various forms of treatment (see the review by Ogborne, 1978). Thus, detailed knowledge of these characteristics is extremely useful in selecting an appropriate treatment.

For example, persons who are well organized and of quite decided opinions may tend to prefer relatively unstructured forms of therapy, whereas those who are disorganized and at a loss may prefer more structured approaches (McLachlan, 1972; McLachlan, 1974; Witkin and Goodenough, 1977; Hartman et al., 1988). Those who prefer structure are more likely to affiliate with programs that provide it, such as Alcoholics Anonymous (Canter, 1966; Reilly and Sugerman, 1967). Those who prefer unstructured settings, on the other hand, may prefer an approach like client-centered or insight-oriented counseling, in which the patient takes the lead and the therapist is relatively inactive. Persons with positive views of themselves may be able to tolerate and benefit from therapeutic approaches that are highly confrontational; those who view themselves negatively may be harmed by such approaches (Annis and Chan, 1983). Persons whose views of the locus of responsibility for alcohol problems (both for developing and for dealing with them) are congruent with the views of program staff may be more likely to sustain treatment (Brickman et al., 1982).

Another aspect of characterizing individuals has to do with their medical and psychiatric status. People with alcohol problems often have medical and psychiatric problems as well (Wilkinson and Carlen, 1981; Ashley, 1982; Popham et al., 1984; Mendelson et al., 1986; Ross et al., 1988). Some of these problems may be the result of alcohol consumption; some may result in drinking (for example, for symptomatic relief); still others may be independent problems. Yet all are important in themselves, requiring clarification and, often, therapeutic attention. To concentrate solely on an individual's alcohol problem and fail to recognize or to deal with a significant medical or psychiatric problem in the same individual is not only poor therapeutic practice but a potential cause for legal action.

There is also evidence that the coexistence of particular problems (e.g., depression, anxiety or panic states, schizophrenia, antisocial personality, drug dependence) may directly affect the outcome of treatment for alcohol problems (Woody et al., 1984; Strayvinski et al., 1986; Rounsaville et al., 1987; Kadden et al., 1990). The effective management of alcohol problems, in other words, may in some instances be contingent upon the effective management of intercurrent problems. Thus, an assessment of medical and psychiatric status should be a standard element of comprehensive assessment. When one considers that alcohol affects both the body and the mind directly, this is hardly a surprising conclusion.

The point that alcohol problems do not occur in a vacuum is paralleled by the point that "no man is an island." It is important during the assessment process to characterize the person's social context as well as the person. A turbulent social context may entirely negate any attempts at individual treatment and may need to be directly addressed as the initial order of business. Individuals with problematic family or home situations or both are unlikely to sustain participation in outpatient treatment programs (H. A. Skinner, 1981c). If there is a history of marital troubles, some attention may be required in this area. If there have been job-related difficulties, vocational evaluation and training may be prudent. If there has been difficulty in allocating leisure time, or a social support network is lacking, social or recreational counseling may be in order. Thus, obtaining an adequate picture of the social context of the individual who has the alcohol problem is an important purpose of assessment.

Characterizing the manifold aspects of individuality is a highly complex matter, and an exhaustive discussion of all of the parameters that may require address during assessment is not possible here. The committee envisions such a discussion as more appropriately part of a consensus exercise that would consider both the relevance of various parameters and the means whereby they can be effectively measured (see below). What the committee hopes will arise from the foregoing discussion is an appreciation of the necessity to characterize individuals as part of a comprehensive assessment process.

Characterizing the Treatment Population

If each individual in the treatment population were characterized in a similar manner, individual data could be aggregated; with aggregation it becomes possible to characterize the treatment population as a whole. As will be discussed further below, accomplishing such a characterization does not mean that the assessment of each individual must be identical in every particular, a practice that would fail to give due recognition to the diversity of individuals and of the problems for which they are seeking treatment. It does suggest, however, that *there should be common data elements in the assessment of all individuals.* Common data would permit not only the characterization of the population of a given program but the comparison of one program population with another.

While it is easy to see that the population characteristics of programs especially targeted for particular population groups—women, youth, or ethnic minorities, for example—are likely to differ, it is less apparent that the populations of treatment programs with a more general orientation may differ as well (Pattison et al., 1969; Pattison et al., 1973; Bromet et al., 1976; Bromet et al., 1977; H. A. Skinner and Shoffner, 1978; Kern et al., 1978; Finney and Moos, 1979; H. A. Skinner, 1981c). Location, history, reputation, publicity, accessibility, treatment orientation, cost, staff composition, funding, and other factors undoubtedly enter into the determination of such differences. They are not stable determinants, and so the characteristics of a treatment program population may change over time. For this reason the occasional assessment of program population characteristics is less useful than their ongoing assessment.

If the characteristics of a program population are known, and the characteristics of the general population from which it is drawn are also known, it is possible to estimate the effectiveness of the program in recruiting its target population. For example, a community assessment service in London, Ontario, saw 14.1 percent of the persons with serious alcohol problems in its catchment area over a three-year period (Malla et al., 1985). A household survey in that area of the province had found that only 3.2 percent of individuals classified as problem or dependent drinkers during the past year had ever received treatment for alcohol problems in their lifetimes (Smart et al., 1980). The authors concluded that "the assessment centre may, over a period of time, increase the penetration rate of a treatment system into the local alcoholic population" (Malla et al., 1985:41).

If comparable data exist for more than one treatment program, between-program comparisons are possible. Two programs may have similar proportions of positive outcomes, but if it is known that the two populations differ on such pretreatment characteristics as, for example, severity of alcohol problems or level of employment, a more exact understanding of the two programs and their relative efficacy is possible. The assessment center noted above (Malla et al., 1985) had a high rate of referral from physicians and employers, while other area programs had high rates of self-referrals and referrals from family and friends; this pattern speaks to differential, and possibly complementary, recruiting from the overall population. Comparable data from all treatment programs would be invaluable in revealing which segments of the community were being served and in planning further services for those who are not entering existing programs.

Planning Treatment for the Individual

Full characterization of a given individual, combined with knowledge of available treatment options, facilitates appropriate, prompt, and effective management of the individual's problem. For example, there is evidence (cf. reviews by Annis, 1986a; W. R. Miller and Hester, 1986) that the results from inpatient and outpatient treatment do not differ for heterogeneous groups of patients. Some (W. R. Miller and Hester, 1986; Saxe et al., 1983) accordingly have advocated that outpatient treatment should be tried first because it is less expensive and that inpatient treatment should be undertaken only if outpatient treatment fails.

But it is well known that individuals with low social stability (as well as other characteristics) are unlikely to sustain participation in outpatient treatment (e.g., H. A. Skinner, 1981c). Thus, rather than a wholesale embargo on inpatient programs for all persons seeking treatment, the more discriminating use of inpatient programs might be envisioned. Those with low social stability, as well as a profile of other indicative features (severe withdrawal symptoms, major medical or psychiatric complications, a markedly noxious environment, crucially aversive temporary circumstances, etc.), might be referred initially to inpatient or residential programs. Others, in more favorable circumstances and with less severe problems, might be referred to outpatient programs (cf. Hoffmann et al., 1987).

To provide another example of the potential utility of pretreatment assessment in assigning individuals to treatment, let us consider a controlled trial in which no advantage was found in the use of a particular treatment (highly confrontational group therapy, or so-called "attack" therapy) in a heterogeneous correctional population (Annis, 1979). Retrospective reanalysis of the data extended these findings. Although there had been no net benefit in the treatment group, in fact some individuals had benefitted and others (in approximately equal numbers) had not. Moreover, data were available to show that these two groups were systematically different.

Those who had benefitted were characterized on initial assessment by positive self-images (determined objectively with appropriate psychometric instruments). Those who failed to benefit—indeed, who appeared to have been harmed by the treatment—were characterized by negative self-images (Annis and Chan, 1983). In future, it is to be hoped that the self-image of persons seeking treatment could be determined in advance, and that only those with positive self-images would be assigned to "attack" therapy.

In other words, *assessment prior to treatment forms the basis on which individual patients are matched to particular treatment programs.* This point was stressed earlier, but is repeated here for emphasis. Matching is the subject of the next chapter in this report (Chapter 11); the implications of assessment for matching are more fully discussed there.

It is worthwhile to point out that additional information on the individual will need to be gathered by program staff following the selection of treatment in order to plan the individual's ongoing treatment course. In some respects, indeed, treatment involves a continual and ongoing gathering of information on the individual. Pretreatment assessment initiates this aspect of treatment, but information gathering continues throughout treatment.

Guiding Treatment for the Population

Assessment provides information that can be used to develop a clinical data base. "A clinical data base is created when well-defined, discrete, and continuous data elements concerning patients are routinely recorded and coupled with outcome descriptors" (Pryor et al., 1985:623). Given knowledge of pretreatment characteristics and knowledge of the outcome of treatment, a comprehensive picture of individual responses to treatment can be elaborated. This information can then be used to estimate the probable responses of future patients to particular treatments. Their characteristics can be documented during the assessment process, and treatment can be selected on the basis of information about how individuals with similar characteristics have previously responded to the available alternatives.

Such a system has been recommended as the basis for medical care generally (Ellwood, 1988). To manage the large amount of information involved and to provide rapid access to that information, computerization of the clinical data base is logical. Yet it is worth noting that the fundamental model is the human clinician. "The ability of a practitioner to couple the process of patient care to the outcome of a disease is the underlying principle enabling physicians to learn from their previous experience" (Pryor et al., 1985:623). Computerized data bases seem foreign or even outlandish to many. Yet they simply imitate and extend a familiar model, formalizing what is done by good clinicians in the management of patients but doing it with greater scope, capacity, accuracy, and speed.

Such data bases are already in existence for many particular kinds of problems. Tumor registries are perhaps the most familiar example (Laszlo, 1985), but clinical data bases exist for such prevalent problems as cardiovascular disease (Hlatky et al., 1984) and such uncommon problems as systemic lupus erythematosus (Fries, 1976), a severe disease that involves the destruction of connective tissue throughout the body. There is at least one extensive clinical data base for alcohol problems that includes outcome information, that of the Chemical Abuse/Addiction Treatment Outcome Registry (CATOR) (Belille, n.d. [ca.1987]; Harrison and Belille, 1987; Harrison and Hoffmann, 1987).

At present, existing data bases are for the most part not used to guide treatment for populations (but see Fries, 1976). Given the increasing availability of computers there is every prospect that they could be so used. In fact, treatment programs offering different treatments could assemble around a shared clinical data base and use the information contained in it to guide the selection of treatment for all individuals presenting to the programs collectively (see Chapter 13). For this proposal to be feasible, however, a comprehensive pretreatment assessment must be an integral part of the clinical process.

To summarize: assessment is a comprehensive gathering of information about each individual who is being considered for specialized treatment for alcohol problems. Its purposes include the characterization of the presenting alcohol problem, the individual who has the problem, and the population seeking treatment, and the facilitation of appropriate treatment for all. Although widely advocated, comprehensive assessment prior to treatment is the exception rather than the rule. To facilitate its more general use, the committee in the next three sections discusses its structure, its content, and its administration.

The Structure of Comprehensive Assessment

There are two important guidelines for structuring comprehensive assessment in the alcohol treatment field. Both are consequences of the heterogeneity of alcohol problems (see Chapter 2). One is that assessment should be *sequential*; the other is that assessment should be *multidimensional.*

Sequential Assessment

Gathering information, and the attendant processes of recording, storing, and retrieving it for various uses, should not be lightly undertaken. Such activities are costly in terms of time, money, and effort. One wants to be certain, therefore, that all of the information gathered is necessary and that no more information is gathered than is required for the purposes at hand. Accordingly, it is advisable to divide the process of assessment into a series of stages, each of which may or may not lead into the next stage (H. A. Skinner, 1981a; 1981b). This approach, which is called sequential assessment, is graphically portrayed in Figure 10-1.

The initial stage in the assessment sequence for those seeking specialized treatment for alcohol problems is *screening*. In common with the process of identification in the community sector of treatment (see Chapter 9), the basic questions asked here are (1) whether an alcohol problem is present and (2) whether it requires specialized treatment. This duplication of what may occur in the community is necessary in a specialized assessment setting for alcohol problems because some individuals—those who did not first attend a primary care physician, social agency, or another community setting in which the identification process is available—will seek specialized treatment directly. Of those who do present for treatment, many will prove to have alcohol problems, but some will not. Hence, screening as the first order of business makes practical sense and, in at least some instances, will suggest that the remainder of the comprehensive assessment process is not necessary.

Even if a problem is present, it may prove to be one that can readily be dealt with through brief intervention. Referral to a community setting rather than to specialized treatment can in such instances be made on the basis of screening alone. Although the yield again will be small, the saving of time and effort devoted to subsequent assessment stages even in a small number of cases will be worthwhile.

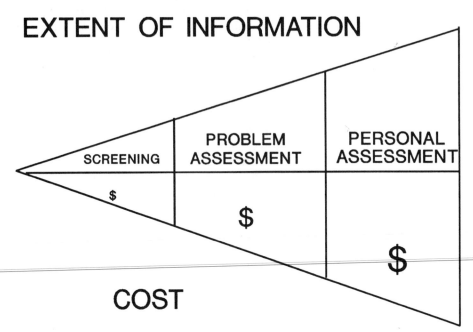

FIGURE 10-1 Sequential Assessment.   As one moves from screening to problem assessment to personal assessment, the extent of information developed is greater but the costs of assessment are also greater.   Performing an assessment sequentially ensures that further information is necessary and justifies its increased cost (adapted from Skinner, 1981a:30; 1981b:330).

If screening suggests that the individual probably does have a problem that is likely to require specialized treatment, the next step in the sequence may be thought of as the *problem assessment*.   This stage of assessment represents a major increment over screening in the extent and variety of the information it yields (as well as in the effort and time required to implement it).   Because screening has indicated the likelihood that an alcohol problem is present, this next stage of assessment both tests and extends that observation.

Many instruments have been developed which may be utilized for problem assessment (cf. Lettieri et al., 1985b).   As discussed in the previous chapter, a single scale instrument is often used for screening purposes.   It may be appropriate in the next stage of assessment to utilize a multiscale instrument, such as the Alcohol Use Inventory (AUI) (Wanberg et al., 1977; H. A. Skinner and Allen, 1983a; Horn, Wanberg & Foster, 1987).   With its extensive item pool and multiple scales, the AUI, together with other elements of the problem assessment, can provide confirmation or disconfirmation of the screening finding that an alcohol problem exists; moreover, it can help to determine what *kind* of alcohol problem it might be.   Additional effort is expended, but additional information is gained.   As is discussed later in the chapter, other measures at this stage of assessment can also be used to provide similarly extensive data on other aspects of the presenting alcohol problem.

Ideally, both the screening stage and the problem assessment stage are uniform in their content for all persons seeking treatment.   Such uniformity is desirable because all such persons may or may not have alcohol problems.   If no alcohol problem is present, or the problem that is present is appropriate for brief intervention rather than specialized treatment, the assessment process can end.

Alternatively, once the presence of a problem appropriate for specialized treatment has been confirmed, and the nature of that problem has been fully characterized during the problem assessment stage, it is appropriate to move on to the next stage of assessment. As discussed earlier, to determine the most appropriate treatment one must take into consideration not only the characteristics of the problem but those of the individual manifesting the problem. Thus, the third stage of a comprehensive assessment, following screening and the problem assessment, is the *personal assessment*.

Before beginning this stage of the assessment, however, it is advisable to undertake a specific screening process as the first order of business. Some of the procedures that must be implemented to gather a full complement of data during the course of a personal assessment are among the most extensive and time-consuming in the assessment repertoire. They therefore should not be deployed unless there is preliminary evidence that it is necessary to do so.

For example, confirmation of the presence of a psychiatric disorder may involve the administration of a structured instrument such as the Diagnostic Interview Schedule (DIS) (Robins et al., 1981), or a psychiatric consultation, or both. Before engaging in these complex procedures, it would be appropriate first to screen as quickly and as accurately as possible for the presence or absence of psychiatric problems. The screening could be accomplished by the use of a brief instrument such as the General Health Questionnaire (GHQ) (Goldberg, 1972, 1978; Ross and Glaser, 1989) or the psychiatric scale of the Addiction Severity Index (ASI) (McLellan et al., 1980; McLellan et al., 1985).

Screening for this and the many other substantive areas one might wish to explore during the personal assessment is essential to ensure that the assessment process is parsimonious; that is, that only those dimensions of the individual that require an extensive assessment receive it. There should be variability in the procedures of the personal assessments of specific individuals because there will be variability in the personal areas in which they have problems. With the exception of certain individual attributes that are sufficiently relevant in all cases to merit routine assessment (e.g., personality), the highly specialized measures would only be utilized if screening indicated a reasonable probability that treatment-relevant information would be gained.

To summarize, *the committee views comprehensive assessment as a sequential process that proceeds from one stage to the next if such a progression is indicated.* Three stages are proposed. The first is a *screening stage*, in which the presence or absence of a problem and the likelihood that specialized treatment may be required are determined; this stage is similar to the identification process in the community setting discussed in Chapter 9. The second stage comprises the *problem assessment*, that is, the characterization of the alcohol problem that screening has indicated is present. The third stage is the *personal assessment stage*, in which the nature of the individual who is experiencing the problem is fully and uniquely characterized; the emphasis in this stage is on areas in which personal problems are being experienced. The overall goal of the assessment is to produce sufficient information to make treatment-relevant decisions.

Multidimensional Assessment

In the previous section of this chapter, it was suggested that assessment be divided into stages. Each of these stages, however, ideally involves the eliciting of information along several important dimensions rather than along a single dimension. Alcohol problems are complex; the people who manifest them are complex; and these complexities defy simple characterization.   Thus, *the assessment of alcohol problems should be multidimensional.*

To illustrate the principle of multidimensional assessment, let us concentrate for the moment on the problem assessment. The task of problem assessment is to describe as fully (and yet as parsimoniously) as possible the problem or problems with alcohol that an individual may have. From the standpoint of multidimensionality, the relevant question is the following: how many different dimensions are required to provide a reasonable description of a given alcohol problem?

There has been a tendency to rely on only a single dimension, a measure of the individual's use of alcohol, to characterize his or her alcohol problem. This measure can be taken, for example, by a tally of the average number of standard drinks the individual consumes per day. Certainly, this is important information, but such a measure of a person's level of use does not even fully characterize alcohol use. Of additional importance is the pattern of use. If an individual consumes four drinks per day on average, it will make a considerable difference (at least in the clinical picture) whether he consumes them in an hour or two or whether they are spaced out over the course of the entire day. With the former pattern, the individual is likely to become intoxicated; with the latter pattern, intoxication is unlikely.

The pattern of alcohol use in turn can make a difference in the consequences the individual experiences. In a recent study (Kranzler et al., 1990) it was found that both an increased level of consumption and a pattern of consumption likely to result in intoxication independently increased the risk of consequences. Interestingly, it was found that an increased level of consumption was more likely to contribute to consequences in males, while an intoxication pattern of consumption was more likely to contribute to consequences in females.   The authors concluded that "these variables, though related, require independent consideration."

Beyond the daily pattern of use, it is important to have information about the pattern of use over longer periods of time. Some persons do drink at the same level and in the same daily pattern over prolonged periods of time. Others, however, vary both their level and their daily pattern of use quite considerably. Binge drinking is a well-known long-term pattern of alcohol use. It is likely that such long-term patterns have important implications for consequences as well as prognosis; hence what can be termed a history of use is an important element in the characterization of an individual's use of alcohol. Such a history would include information as to the time in life the individual began to drink and the length and circumstances of periods of nonuse, as well as the pattern of use over the last few years prior to seeking treatment.

Thus, an adequate assessment of an individual's use of alcohol would include information on the level of use, the pattern of use, and the history of use. It might be felt that such a comprehensive consideration of alcohol use might suffice to characterize an alcohol problem because there is a general and positive correlation between the use of alcohol, signs and symptoms, and consequences, a correlation that becomes most evident when aggregate data from large groups of individuals are explored and when the problems themselves are longstanding and severe. But *treatment is a clinical process that deals with single individuals, one at a time; among individuals, wide variations may be found in the relationship between use, signs and symptoms, and consequences.* The vignettes at the beginning of Chapter 2 of this report include individuals (George, Gregory) with low levels of consumption and serious consequences, as well as one individual (Elizabeth) in whom a high level of consumption was associated for a long period of time with no apparent consequences at all.

Disparities between the level of alcohol consumption and the effects of alcohol are also matters of common experience. Some individuals "can't hold their liquor" and become thoroughly intoxicated on small amounts of alcohol which would not faze most social drinkers. Other individuals drink constantly throughout the day, consuming remarkable quantities of alcohol but without exhibiting the least sign of intoxication (so-called "hollow legs").

That these phenomena are not mere folklore is well substantiated by research that, for example, documents that similar doses of alcohol differ widely in their effects on different individuals, or that even trained observers are unable to identify individuals with elevated blood alcohol levels in from more than a fifth to more than a half of all cases without the aid of such instruments as breathalyzers (Hartocollis, 1962; M. B. Sobell et al., 1979). A study in adolescents found that use-related problems and intensity of drinking were to some degree correlated in the study population but that they were not sufficiently correlated to constitute a single dimension. Rather, they were most accurately viewed as separate dimensions (White, 1987). There have been similar findings in adults (Sadava, 1985). Indeed, a RAND Corporation study found that consequences from drinking were only weakly related either to the amount of alcohol consumed or to the symptomatology of alcohol use (Polich et al., 1981).

All three dimensions appear to contribute useful and independent information to the overall characterization of an alcohol problem. Taken together, they may be seen as illuminating the important question of the severity of the alcohol problem or problems experienced by a given individual. Therefore *in assessing alcohol problems, the committee recommends that information be sought along three specific dimensions*: (1) the *use of alcohol*; (2) the *signs and symptoms of alcohol use; and* (3) the *consequences of alcohol use*. This multidimensional classification is outlined in Table 10-1.

One of the principal advantages of a multidimensional classification system of this type is that, by providing a more fine-grained, specific characterization of individuals with alcohol problems, it facilitates communication among workers in the field. To know where an individual stands on any one of these three proposed dimensions provides significant information. To know where an individual stands on all three provides a significantly greater degree of information. A more detailed example of a multidimensional classification system has been given elsewhere (H. A. Skinner, 1985, 1988).

If all patients entering treatment were characterized according to a common multidimensional basis, enormous advantages would be realized. For example, the equivalence (or lack thereof) of patients in different treatment programs could readily be established. If the treatment provided then proved to be effective, it would be much more securely known for whom the treatment was effective. Should a program for whatever reason tend to deal exclusively with individuals manifesting only the most severe kinds of alcohol problems, its treatment outcomes would necessarily be viewed differently from those of a program that dealt largely with individuals manifesting problems that were not severe.

An analogous multidimensional classification system has been in place in another field for some time. The tumor-node-metastasis (TNM) system, which was first proposed by P. F. Denoix in 1944, subsequently refined and accepted by the Union Internationale Centre de la Cancer (UICC), and widely implemented from about 1968 on, has been of great utility in dealing with cancer (Harmer, 1977), particularly in evaluating prognosis, planning therapy, and reporting results. It considers three significant events in the life history of a cancer: (1) tumor growth (T), (2) spread to primary lymph nodes (N), and (3) distant metastases (M). Cancers occurring in various regions of the body can be classified according to this system, and the effectiveness of differing modalities of treatment (e.g., surgery, radiation, chemotherapy) can be examined using the classification. Such examinations are predicated on the notion that the effects of treatment will vary depending on the classification of the cancer in the TNM system.

Because of the widespread use of the TNM system, treatment results from multiple tumor registries can be aggregated to provide a vast body of information on which to base

Table 10-1 Multidimensional Classification of Alcohol Problems

Dimension	Type of Information
I	Use of alcohol
II	Signs and symptoms of alcohol use
III	Consequences of alcohol use

judgments regarding optimal intervention. The National Cancer Institute offers a Physician Data Query (PDQ) system in which the TNM classification scheme is used to provide physicians with information on prognosis and with treatment protocols for different cancer sites and stages. The TNM system illustrates how a relatively simple but widely utilized multiaxial assessment scheme can greatly facilitate progress in research and treatment. The potential advantages of developing and using a similar scheme in the treatment of alcohol problems are substantial. Potentially, the enormous fund of clinical experience built up from the multitudes of cases seen every year can be directly brought to bear in a systematic manner upon the disposition of future cases (cf. the earlier discussion of clinical data bases).

To some it will come as a surprise that the characterization of the alcohol problems of individuals seeking treatment is not regularly carried out along multiple dimensions. As has already been indicated, however, assessment itself is not commonly carried out in treatment programs. Even in research studies, which explicitly aim at widespread generalizability, characterization of the alcohol problem is often incomplete.

For example, the much-publicized collaborative studies by Swedish and American investigators that have examined the contribution of genetic factors to alcohol problems (Bohman et al., 1981; Cloninger et al., 1981) have been criticized on these grounds: "[T]he data reflect only obvious and reportable instances of the consequences of insobriety. There are no measures of the quantity or frequency of drinking or of the social and personal consequences of private or unreported drunkenness . . . [I]t is quite likely that the obtained results are an artifact of the criteria of abuse" (Searles, 1988:159-160). Further, in a review of 48 alcohol treatment outcome studies published in the period 1980-1984, it was found that reporting on all three dimensions was deficient: only 56.3 percent quantified pretreatment drinking levels; none reported whether the symptom of physical dependence was present or absent; only 18.8 percent reported on alcohol-related arrests; and only 33.3 percent reported on whether or not there had been prior treatment for alcohol problems (M. B. Sobell et al., 1987).

Although the need for a multidimensional approach has been discussed here largely in terms of the characterization of alcohol problems, multidimensionality is a broad structural principle that ideally should be applied to all stages of assessment. For example, a screening instrument such as the AUDIT, although brief, contains questions that cover all three of the axes suggested above for the problem assessment (Saunders and Aasland, 1987; Babor et al., 1989). In like manner the personal stage of assessment requires that multiple aspects of the individual with the alcohol problem be assessed. Agreement on and consequent uniform adoption of a standard multidimensional problem assessment and personal assessment seem essential to progress in clinical services and in research.

To review briefly, more than a single kind of information is required for adequate assessment at each stage of the assessment process. The dimensions along which problem assessments, for example, should proceed include aspects of the individual's use of alcohol, the signs and symptoms of alcohol use, and the consequences alcohol use. This is the principle of *multidimensional assessment*.

The Content of Comprehensive Assessment

An assessment process is comprehensive if it is designed to cover all stages and all dimensions as required. (Depending on the problem and the individual, the full assessment process may not be required.) In what follows the possible content of a comprehensive assessment for alcohol problems is described. The description is intended to be illustrative rather than definitive.

Content of Screening

Screening is by design a brief process (Saunders, 1988). As noted earlier, it must answer two questions: (1) whether an alcohol problem is present and (2) if so, whether it is likely to require brief intervention or specialized treatment. Examples of instruments that accomplish these purposes are the Alcohol Clinical Index (ACI) (H. A. Skinner et al., 1986; H. A. Skinner and Holt, 1987), the CAGE questionnaire (Ewing, 1984), and the AUDIT (Saunders and Aasland, 1987; Babor et al., 1989). Many alternative screening methods are available (Babor and Kadden, 1985; Babor et al., 1986). The reader is referred to Chapter 9 for a more extensive discussion of screening and brief intervention.

Content of the Problem Assessment

In the problem assessment stage, content must address the three dimensions of the multidimensional characterization of alcohol problems. With respect to specifying the prospective client's *use of alcohol*, care must be taken to look broadly at a variety of aspects, including especially the level of use, the pattern of use, and the history of use. Various techniques have been developed for taking a drinking history. These techniques may be divided into three broad classes: (1) retrospective methods that gather information about drinking over a specified time interval in the past, using a self-report questionnaire or a structured interview; (2) prospective methods in which the individual is asked to monitor alcohol use and record it in a daily diary; and (3) laboratory determinations such as various tests performed on body fluids (blood, urine, saliva, sweat) and breath tests. Extensive reviews of these methods have been published (Babor et al., 1987; O'Farrell and Maisto, 1987; L. C. Sobell et al., 1987); they will be discussed further below.

Multiple methods are also available to survey the *signs and symptoms of alcohol use*. Signs and symptoms form the basis of both the 10th edition of the diagnostic manual of the International Classification of Diseases (ICD-10) and DSM-III-R. Methods of making diagnoses within the contexts of these systems, such as the DIS (Robins et al., 1981) or its computerized version (Blouin, 1986), may be useful.

A number of self-report questionnaires have also been developed (Edwards, 1986; Davidson, 1987) that systematically review symptoms of alcohol use. The Severity of Alcohol Dependence Questionnaire (SADQ) (Hodgson et al., 1978; Stockwell et al., 1983) has been extensively used outside of North America, and a considerable amount of data on its measurement properties has been generated. The Alcohol Dependence Scale (ADS) has been widely used in North America (H. A. Skinner and Allen, 1982; Horn et al., 1984). Many treatment outcome studies and almost all epidemiological studies have included alternative scales of this kind.

With respect to the third axis, *consequences of alcohol use,* options abound in this arena as well. The Michigan Alcoholism Screening Test (MAST) (Selzer, 1971; Skinner, 1979), the Alcohol Use Inventory (AUI) (Wanberg et al., 1977; Skinner and Allen, 1983a; Horn et al., 1987) and the Addiction Severity Index (ASI) (McLellan et al., 1980; 1985) are largely concerned with the assessment of this axis. The ASI produces information in the areas of drug abuse, medical problems, psychiatric problems, legal problems, family and social problems, and employment and support problems. Beyond this, there are multiple direct ways of assessing all of these dimensions (e.g., routine medical and psychiatric examinations), as well as scores of psychometric instruments (cf. Lettieri et al., 1985b).

Content of Personal Assessment

Both the screening and problem assessment stages of the comprehensive assessment process may lead to the determination that a problem is present, that it requires a specialized intervention, and that it is of a particular kind. What remains to be specified in order to select the optimum treatment approach is the individual who presents the problem. Some of this information is needed to permit description of the individual and, through the aggregation of individual data, description of the program population. Additional information may be needed to gauge the prognosis, to assist in matching individuals to appropriate treatment, to determine whether prevalent comorbidities are present, to help plan living and working circumstances, to understand certain etiologic possibilities, and for other purposes.

There may be some overlap between information gathered as part of the personal assessment and information gathered as part of the problem assessment when the consequences of alcohol use are being considered. For example, alcohol problems are often manifested in the vocational area. On the other hand, a person with alcohol problems may quite independently have vocational problems, which it may be important from a therapeutic perspective to know about. Fundamentally, *the problem assessment looks at those problems that are reasonably attributable to alcohol consumption, while the personal assessment looks at those problems the individual has whether or not they are attributable to alcohol consumption.* Whatever area of overlap exists is tolerable and ensures that all existing problems will come to light.

Contingent dimensions in personal assessment As has been noted, personal assessment is a particularly complex area. Multiple dimensions that are descriptive of various aspects of the individual might be relevant. Unfortunately, the assessment of any one of these dimensions is often complex and time-consuming. Therefore (in keeping with the principle of sequential assessment), screening should be an important part of the personal assessment process. The purpose of such a screening is to identify which of the many potential dimensions of personal assessment require a more thorough investigation. For example, are there family problems, marital problems, vocational problems, sexual problems, personal problems (problems with assertiveness, with social skills, with particular situations), medical problems, or psychiatric problems? If screening indicates the presence of these problems, a more intensive assessment can be undertaken; if the problems are absent or minimal, no further evaluation may be necessary (and there is a considerable saving of time and effort over the routine administration of intensive assessment in all of these areas). An example was given earlier of screening for psychiatric problems with the GHQ or the ASI and administering the full DIS only when screening is positive.

Noncontingent dimensions in personal assessment With regard to other dimensions of personal assessment, detailed examination should *not* be contingent on screening. For example, the collection of *demographic information* is important both to identify the

ASSESSMENT

individual and to help understand prognosis; age, marital status, and social class are examples of such data. Demographics are also among the principal descriptors of populations; hence, there is a particular need for completeness and uniformity in their compilation.

Yet experience suggests that the collection of demographic data is not as simple a matter as it may seem. Many programs collect age by category, and the categories may not be consistent from one program to another (e.g. persons aged 35-45 vs. persons aged 30-40). Where there is an option to designate that a person is unmarried but living with someone in a stable relationship, this information will be recorded; if the option does not exist, however, the person will probably be designated as single. If data categories vary from program to program, data cannot be aggregated among different programs, nor can different programs be compared.

The *use of tobacco and other drugs* by persons seeking help for alcohol problems is another area of personal assessment that should be surveyed as a matter of routine rather than on the basis of contingent screening. Available data suggest that the correlations between use of alcohol and use of tobacco and other drugs are regularly impressive. With regard to tobacco, one study found that 80 percent of patients in an addiction treatment setting were daily cigarette smokers (Kozlowski et al., 1986); another study of the same population by different means found that 78.3 percent of patients presenting for new episodes of service qualified for the DSM-III diagnosis of tobacco use disorder (Ross et al., 1988). An earlier inpatient study on an alcohol and drug unit found a correlation of 0.74 between amount of alcohol drunk and number of cigarettes smoked for males and females diagnosed as "alcoholics"; the correlation did not hold for individuals not so diagnosed (Maletzky and Klotter, 1974). In an ambulatory medical care setting, 85.1 percent of new patients who answered five or more of the MAST questions affirmatively were smokers, whereas only 47 percent below this cutoff point were smokers (Cyr and Wartman, 1988).

In the large Epidemiologic Catchment Area survey, in which approximately 3,000 persons were diagnostically interviewed in each of five sites, almost one in every five persons (18 percent) who met criteria for alcohol problems also met diagnostic criteria for some type of drug problem (Helzer and Burnham, in press). In aggregate data from three of the five sites, the proportion was much higher (28 percent) among young men (Robins et al., 1984). A study of all persons seeking help from a large alcohol and drug treatment center in Toronto found that exactly the same proportion as in the ECA study (18 percent) of individuals qualified for diagnoses of both alcohol and drug dependence (Ross et al., 1988). A study of a large number of adult women admitted to inpatient treatment for alcohol and drug problems in the United States (N = 1,776) found that, although 61.1 percent of women over the age of 30 reported using only alcohol, the corresponding proportion for women under 30 was 31.2 percent (Harrison and Belille, 1987).

Thus, there is a great deal of evidence that *persons with alcohol problems are highly likely to have problems with tobacco use and quite likely to have problems with drug use.* It also appears, from the data cited here and from the observations of clinicians in the field, that the concurrent use of alcohol and drugs is a more prevalent phenomenon among younger persons entering treatment. These findings suggest that the use of tobacco and of other drugs should be assessed routinely in those seeking treatment for alcohol problems.

The personal stage of assessment should also examine data that are relevant to matching. For example, knowing what *goals* are seen as important by each individual entering treatment can be quite useful in the matching process. In one program that made consistent attempts to match, a treatment goals inventory was extensively utilized (Glaser and Skinner, 1984:76-77, see page 291). Demographics are another dimension that have utility for matching purposes; information collected by AA, for example, suggests that it is a less attractive option for the young and for women (Ogborne and Glaser, 1981; J. K. Jackson, 1988; but see Emrick, 1987). Matching individuals to appropriate treatments is discussed in some detail in Chapter 11.

Personality may be another area that should be routinely assessed. The intent is not to search for evidence of an "addictive personality" (i.e., the one personality pattern that characterizes persons with alcohol problems) because this population is heterogeneous in its personality characteristics (Syme, 1957; Mogar et al., 1970; Partington, 1970; H. A. Skinner et al., 1974; Stein et al., 1977; Barnes, 1979; Cloninger, 1987). Rather, in keeping with the assessment goal of obtaining treatment-relevant information, the intent is to identify personality factors or patterns that may affect in a significant way which treatment programs individuals are likely to find suitable and which they are likely to reject.

Certain pathological personality types, especially antisocial personality but also borderline personality, have been found to have prognostic value in this regard (Schuckit, 1973; Vaillant, 1983; Nace et al., 1986; Cloninger, 1987). Normative factors or traits of personality may also have value in predicting appropriate matches and outcome (see the discussion earlier in this chapter and also Beutler [1979]). It is difficult to assess personality efficiently as a general construct, simply because the scope of the concept is extremely broad. However, potentially suitable structured instruments of reasonable length are available—for example, the Personality Research Form (PRF) (Jackson, 1974), and the Sixteen Personality Factors Inventory (16PF) (Institute for Personality and Ability Testing, 1986).

Intelligence has some influence both on matching and on outcome (Gibbs, 1980). Fortunately, there is a high correlation between intelligence and some measures that can be efficiently administered, such as vocabulary tests. Full-scale intelligence testing with such standard instruments as the Wechsler Adult Intelligence Scales (WAIS) (Wechsler, 1981) is quite exacting, however, and if used at all should be used sparingly.

Cognitive functioning is a related and important area to be assessed, because many kinds of treatment require the ability to process information at a high level of abstraction. Some persons with alcohol problems prove to be cognitively impaired (Wilkinson and Carlen, 1981; Wilkinson, 1987), and this information should enter into the process of treatment selection (Wilkinson and Sanchez-Craig, 1981). The precise evaluation of cognitive functioning is complex and time-consuming, but it is possible to screen briefly for cognitive deficit before embarking on a full-scale evaluation (Barrett and Gleser, 1987; Kiernan et al., 1987; Wilkinson, 1988).

Some aspects of the assessment of the individual may be partly contingent and partly noncontingent. The area of the family is an example. Family circumstances may be an important determinant of alcohol problems and, even in instances in which they do not figure in the etiology of alcohol problems, they may nevertheless affect the outcome of treatment (Cronkhite and Moos, 1978, 1980; Moos et al., 1979). Family history is also important. A significant minority of individuals with serious alcohol problems come from families in which a parent has a similar problem (Cotton, 1979). In some samples potentially treatment-relevant differences have been found between individuals whose families do and do not have a history of alcohol problems (Penick et al., 1987). Recent work in the genetics of alcohol problems (Cloninger, 1987) has enhanced interest in familial factors.

Consequently, data on the family are relevant to the assessment of individuals with alcohol problems. It seems reasonable to recommend that a *family history* of alcohol problems be taken on all persons entering treatment. A full-scale family assessment process, on the other hand, is sufficiently complex (Jacob, 1988) that it should probably be contingent on the results of screening. Although it is often confidently asserted that, in cases in which a member of a family has an alcohol problem, the family itself has a problem, the assertion lacks strong empirical support.

That drinking, and perhaps especially episodes of heavy drinking, may be related to specific life events (deaths, births, marriages, job losses, new jobs, etc.) is a matter of

TABLE 10-2 Comprehensive Assessment of Persons Seeking Treatment for Alcohol Problems

Stage of Assessment	Dimension	Dimension Label	Content of the Dimension	Sample Methods and Instruments
Screening	I	Problem identification	Is an alcohol problem present?	Alcohol Clinical Index CAGE AUDIT Others
	II	Indicated response	Is specialist treatment required?	Alcohol Clinical Index Others
Problem Assessment	I	Use of alcohol	Level of use Pattern of use History of use Other factors	Quantity-frequencyindices Time-line follow- back Lifetime drinking history Diaries Laboratory tests (body fluids; markers)
	II	Signs and symptoms of alcohol use	Narrowing of drinking repertoire Tolerance Withdrawal symptoms Neglect of alternative activities Subjective sense of impaired control Continuation despite consequences Relief drinking Reinstatement liability Sense of compulsion to drink Other signs and symptoms	SADQ ADS Relevant sections of the ICD-10 and DSM-III-R Others
	III	Consequences of alcohol use	Medical Psychiatric Family Employment/ educational Legal (incl. DWI) Financial Other consequences	MAST ASI AUI Others
Personal Assessment	I	Screening for contingent content	Key questions on problem areas	

TABLE 10-2 *continues*

Table 10-2 (continued)

Stage of Assessment	Dimension	Dimension Label	Content of the Dimension	Sample Methods and Instruments
	II	Contingent content	Medical status Psychiatric status Vocational issues Personal problems Sexual problems Social support Family structure Use of leisure time Others	Multiphasic screening, medical consultation DIS; psychiatric consultation Vocational assessment Specific instruments (social skills inventories, assertiveness scales, etc.) Others
	III	Noncontingent content	Demographics Other drug and tobacco use history Family history Prior treatment history Intelligence Cognitive functioning Personality Treatment goals Social stability Situational factors Others	Appropriate forms Vocabulary screen; WAIS Cognitive status Examination; the Reitan battery PRF, 16PF, or other Appropriate inventories Appropriate scale IDS Others

common knowledge. Yet individuals may not report these events unless they are specifically questioned about them. Moreover, it may be the combined weight of such events, whether positive or negative, rather than a specific event that acts as the trigger to particular coping behaviors, including the consumption of alcohol (Holmes and Rahe, 1967; Paykel et al., 1971; Holmes and Masuda, 1973). A systematic attempt to assess the number and kinds of life events may therefore be useful, and a number of instruments have been developed for this purpose.

Related to but different from life events are *situational factors*. These tend to be more complex constellations of individuals, feelings, and circumstances than are life events, but may also be closely related to individual variations in alcohol consumption. Recent studies (Marlatt and Gordon, 1985; Annis, 1986b; Annis and Davis, 1989) have provided both a theoretical and an empirical basis for understanding and dealing with situational factors, including the development of specific assessment devices. The ubiquity of situational stress suggests that careful consideration should be given to the inclusion of such instruments as the Inventory of Drinking Situations (IDS) (Annis, 1982; Annis, Graham, and Davis, 1987) as a noncontingent element of personal assessment.

The preceding review of the potential content of assessment, which is intended to be more heuristic than exhaustive, nevertheless suggests an embarrassment of riches: many instruments are available to assess the relevant dimensions. The development of reliable and valid new instruments should in no way be discouraged, as the development of assessment must be an evolving process. *But a pressing need already exists for shaping what is now available into a reasonable and practical assessment procedure.* To facilitate this development, an outline of the assessment discussed above may be helpful (Table 10-2).

The translation of such an outline into concrete reality—a fully specified comprehensive assessment battery in use across the universe of treatment programs—has both scientific and political aspects. The publication of two monographs on assessment research (Lettieri et al., 1985a, 1985b) which summarize much of the literature to date and provide examples of instruments is a step in the right direction, and every effort should be made to secure the widespread distribution and serial updating of these useful compendia. A caution should be mentioned, however, that the standard means of conveying information (publication in journals and presentation at scientific conferences) will not suffice to bring about the development of comprehensive assessment batteries. Advantage should be taken in this effort of all that is known regarding the dissemination of innovations (cf. Backer et al., 1986).

Leadership of a high order will also be required to produce the desired result of comprehensive and at least partly uniform assessment across all programs. Widely subscribed consensus conferences devoted to the issue are a possible mechanism. The example of large and prestigious programs and of leaders in the field undoubtedly would have a positive influence. Ultimately, the financing of treatment could be made contingent upon the appropriate classification of individuals who are accepted for treatment; a reasonable aspect of accountability is to require a detailed documentation that a type of problem requiring treatment is being dealt with. The present practice of utilization management operations is directed in part toward this end. Surely it would be advisable for the alcohol treatment field itself to assume responsibility for such accountability.

Desirable Qualities of Assessment Content

To be as useful as possible, the information gathered on individuals seeking treatment for alcohol problems should possess certain qualities. These qualities markedly enhance the value of assessment information and also facilitate the aggregation of individual information so that group information can be generated. Most of the data currently gathered on people seeking treatment have never been systematically evaluated to determine whether they possesses these qualities. Published research studies are deficient in this regard to a surprising degree, often making use, for example, of instruments for which reliability and validity have not been established or for which no standardized norms exist.

Ideally, information gathered during an assessment will be quantitative, reliable, valid, standardized, and recordable. Numerical data are precise, easy to record, and amenable to statistical use. That information be reliable (reproducible) and that it measure what it purports to measure (valid) are obvious requirements, but they demand much in the way of effort to establish and certainly cannot be assumed. Information is much more useful if it can be compared to a previously established baseline (standardized); by itself, its meaningfulness may be unclear. In an era in which population mobility is so great, the importance of recordable data is considerable; the likelihood that multiple therapeutic personnel will encounter any given individual seeking treatment is much greater than ever before.

The Administration of Assessment

Obtaining Valid Assessment Data: Problems in Providing Information

Validity, as discussed above, is a desirable property of information. Most of the information obtained during the assessment of an individual seeking assistance for an alcohol problem comes from the individual himself. Although self-reports are a standard procedure in all human therapeutics, they take on a special coloring in the alcohol field. The use of alcohol may negatively affect the validity of self-reported information, especially regarding alcohol consumption.

Contemporary research provides some reason for concern about this issue. Persons with elevated blood alcohol levels tend characteristically to underreport their alcohol consumption (M. B. Sobell et al., 1979). Significant discrepancies have been noted in some recent studies between self-reports of alcohol consumption and alternative lines of evidence, such as laboratory tests or information obtained from collateral informants (spouses, relatives, and close friends) (Orrego et al., 1979; Watson et al., 1984; Peachey and Kapur, 1986; Fuller et al., 1988). These findings have given additional impetus to efforts to find alternative or supplementary methods to self-reports for determining an individual's alcohol consumption.

Methods of obtaining data on alcohol consumption were reviewed in Chapter 9 in relation to their potential use in screening. To recapitulate briefly, there is general agreement that in many circumstances screening questionnaires are significantly more accurate than physical examination findings and currently available laboratory measures (including body fluid examinations and biological markers). Questionnaires also have numerous practical advantages. On the other hand, the validity of the self-reports involved in questionnaire methods remains a matter of concern, and there is some indication that more recently proposed biological markers may possess significant advantages over those that are currently available.

There are particular aspects of assessment that favor the use of laboratory methods in conjunction with other methods. One is the need for a validity check on the assessment process itself. Assessment is lengthy and complex, and its validity might be adversely affected by a high blood level of alcohol. For example, the validity of tests of cognitive functions could be confounded by alcohol intoxication. The use of a breathalyzer test as a preliminary to assessment, in recognition of the fact that high blood alcohol levels are not clinically apparent in a significant proportion of cases (M. B. Sobell et al., 1979), may be advisable.

Because tolerance, physiological parameters (e.g., lean body mass), pharmaco-dynamic parameters (e.g., whether the blood alcohol curve is rising or falling) and other factors make the exact equation of a particular blood alcohol level with actual impairment in a particular individual quite difficult, an arbitrary level—often the legal limit for impaired driving in the jurisdiction of the assessment program—is generally used. Those achieving a level above the legal limit are not assessed but given a return appointment. If, as a matter of usual practice, persons given an assessment appointment are cautioned that they will be tested and that elevated blood alcohol levels will require a postponement, few individuals will need to be turned down. Breathalyzers are well suited for this role, as they are generally quite accurate and easy to use, do not require body fluid collection, are inexpensive to operate (although an initial investment is required), and provide immediate results.

A second consideration is that, although their generally low sensitivity makes biological markers less useful than questionnaires for screening, they may be very useful for monitoring (Kristensen et al., 1983; Schuckit and Irwin, 1988). Thus, establishing a baseline level for one or more markers may be a reasonable assessment procedure, although it should be entertained primarily if there is a specific intent to repeat the measure subsequently. Under these circumstances the time delay involved in a laboratory determination is not a significant problem, and the expense of the test may be quite justifiable.

A sensitive, specific, responsive marker would be a most welcome supplement in assessing individuals with alcohol problems. Some of the newly proposed markers (desialated transferrin, hemoglobin adducts, etc.) are promising, and work continues. At present, however, there is no viable alternative to reliance on verbal self-report for the assessment of alcohol consumption in clinical settings. Fortunately, current research has shed some light on how the validity of self-reports may be enhanced.

Such research (H. A. Skinner, 1984; Babor et al., 1987; O'Farrell and Maisto, 1987; L. C. Sobell et al., 1987) suggests that the concern over whether verbal reports are either valid or invalid has been somewhat misleading. *Verbal reports are inherently neither valid nor invalid; rather, their validity varies, depending on circumstances.* Table 10-3 contrasts those circumstances in which valid and invalid self-reports are likely to be forthcoming.

Attention to the matter of accuracy is clearly of the greatest importance. Not only is an inaccurate assessment not worth doing but, insofar as treatment planning may be based on it, it is potentially harmful. A considerable amount of effort must be expended to ensure that assessment information is accurate and remains so over time. In many clinical settings minimal effort is currently expended toward this end, either because the information the patient gives is presumed to be completely accurate or because the opposite presumption is made. Neither of these presumptions is correct. Programs must come to see themselves as active collaborators with individuals seeking their services to produce the most accurate information possible.

Obtaining Valid Assessment Data: Problems in Gathering Information

Problems with the validity of assessment information can arise not only from those who provide the information but also from those who gather it. Two kinds of factors that operate on assessors, ideological factors and financial factors, have been identified as posing particular threats to the validity of assessment data. They arise from the circumstance, common because it is practically convenient, in which assessment data are obtained by therapists who also provide treatment in a given treatment program.

Those who provide treatment often are, and perhaps ideally ought to be, enthusiastic about the services they provide. It is likely that their enthusiasm will both sustain them in the arduous task of providing treatment and will contribute to positive treatment outcomes. But their enthusiasm may at the same time adversely affect their ability to perceive other aspects of treatment objectively. One such aspect is treatment outcome. Therapists' perceptions of the results of their own efforts are traditionally considered suspect, and it is felt that obtaining objective data on outcome requires that such judgments be made by others. In technical language, this is referred to as the necessity for those who determine outcome to be "blind" to the treatment received by each individual.

The enthusiasm that colors perceptions of treatment outcome may also color perceptions of the suitability of a given patient for a given treatment. Invested in their work, therapists may tend to perceive more individuals as suitable candidates for the treatments they provide than is actually the case. Thus they may not conduct valid assessments.

In a pertinent study (Savitz et al., 1973), hypothetical patient profiles were constructed from actual patient data and were submitted to three groups of staff for disposition. One staff group was not connected with any particular treatment program but ordinarily made dispositional decisions on court-referred cases to a variety of treatment programs. This group assigned 45 percent of the hypothetical patients to treatment A and 35 percent to treatment B. But staff from treatment A assigned 93.8 percent of patients to treatment A, and staff from treatment B assigned 55 percent of patients to treatment B. That is, staff committed to a particular treatment program were significantly more likely to refer patients to that program than staff who were not so committed.

TABLE 10-3 Factors Influencing The Validity Of Self-Reports

Situations Likely to Produce Invalid Self-Reports	Situations Likely to Produce Valid Self-Reports
Patient has positive blood alcohol concentration at time of assessment	Patient is alcohol free at the time of assessment
Patient is experiencing withdrawal symptoms or other acute distress	Patient is stable and has no major symptoms
Unstructured, general, or vague items are used to obtain information	Structured, carefully developed items are used
Patient is not aware that self-reports will be checked against other data	Patient knows that self-reports will be checked against other sources of data (e.g., lab tests, collaterals, records)
Interaction with the patient is brief or minimal	Good rapport is established with the patient
Patient shows poor compliance with the treatment regimen	Patient complies with other aspects of treatment
Patient has clear motive to distort information (e.g., abstinence is a condition of parole or continued employment)	Patient has no obvious reason for distorting self-reports
Patient doubts the confidentiality of the information provided to treatment personnel	Patient can be validly reassured about confidentiality
Staff has obvious expectations that certain behaviors (e.g., abstinence) will be reported	Staff and the information-gathering process are obviously neutral and nonpunitive

Another potential source of bias is the prospect of financial gain. Programs are often reimbursed on a fee-for-service basis. Under this arrangement the more service that is provided, the greater the profits of the provider. To refer a potential patient elsewhere under this type of reimbursement schedule is to turn away income. Financial incentives operating in the opposite direction may influence treatment provided under fixed-price prepayment schemes; here, the more service provided, the smaller the profits of the provider. Although many individuals involved in providing treatment do not deliberately base their treatment dispositions on financial considerations, it may be that such considerations influence them in subtle ways. An exception is the utilization management company, in which the influence of financial considerations upon the provision of services is explicit and paramount. Contracted to ensure that effective services are provided at the least cost, such companies are of increasing importance in alcohol treatment (Korcok, 1988; Lewis, 1988).

In a pertinent study of possible financial influences on assessment (Hansen and Emrick, 1983), five individuals were carefully trained to give histories about their use of alcohol and their concerns about that use; the levels of use and concern chosen by the investigators, although not negligible, did not objectively indicate either the presence of serious alcohol problems or a need for inpatient treatment. Each of these individuals then presented himself or herself to six local agencies that were selected on the basis of their aggressive recruitment practices.

In 59 percent of the ensuing assessments, a diagnosis of "alcoholism" was made. In 100 percent of the diagnosed cases, total lifetime abstinence from alcohol was recommended, and in 53 percent inpatient treatment was recommended. The only agency that made consistently correct dispositional decisions was also the only not-for-profit agency of the six. The researchers concluded that "people who seek out someone to evaluate their drinking behavior may be told they are 'alcoholic' when they are not and are subsequently influenced to receive very expensive, unnecessary, and perhaps harmful treatment" (Hansen and Emrick, 1983:177).

Other data corroborate the potential effect of financial considerations on the provision of treatment. A Citizens League study in Minnesota found that treatment selection was closely related to reimbursement arrangements. Even though inpatient treatment was more than 3.5 times more expensive than outpatient treatment, programs that were reimbursed on a fee-for-service basis treated the great majority of their patients in inpatient treatment programs. The one program that was reimbursed on a fixed prepayment basis treated the majority of its patients in its outpatient treatment program. The Citizens League concluded that "treatment funding is an important factor affecting where people are referred to for treatment, and what services are provided them" (Boss, 1980:15).

That financial or ideological biases may be reasonably widespread is suggested by data on the level of cross-referral among alcohol treatment programs. In two studies that looked at cross-referral in large numbers of persons seeking treatment, no instances could be documented among 600 persons in treatment (Pattison, 1974:640) nor among 6,805 persons in treatment (Glaser et al., 1978:209-210). The reasons for the lack of cross-referral were not explored in either study on a systematic basis. Further studies are needed. Cross-referral probably does exist, but the rate of cross-referral may not be high.

If the purpose of assessment is to provide objective data to serve as a basis for the appropriate referral of those seeking treatment to the variety of treatment programs that are available, the foregoing information is not encouraging. An obvious remedy for ideological and financial biases would be to follow the lead proposed by the common practice in outcome determination and to ensure that assessment and treatment selection were not in the hands of therapists who might be ideologically or financially tied (or both) to particular treatment programs. In other words, perhaps the assessment (and consequent referral) process should be functionally independent of the treatment process.

Experience with independent assessment has been limited but positive. Following its recommendation by Ontario's Addiction Research Foundation in 1978 (Marshman et al., 1978), the establishment of independent assessment/referral centers has been a policy of the province of Ontario in Canada. As of November 1987, 35 such centers were in operation. In comparison with treatment programs in which assessment is *not* independent of treatment, such centers:

- attract a younger population with less serious problems;
- attract clients from a wider array of referral sources;
- are more likely to attract persons with serious alcohol problems;
- are more likely to provide continuity of care; and
- are more likely to involve family members in the therapeutic process (Malla et al., 1985; Rush, 1987).

In the state of Minnesota, the financial independence of assessment from treatment is mandated by law. Partly as a result of the Citizens League report quoted earlier (Boss, 1980), Minnesota Statute 254B was enacted by the state legislature and went into effect on January 1, 1988. This law created a consolidated treatment fund for public assistance recipients, the monies of which were exempted from various federal and state entitlement provisions. As a consequence these funds could follow the patient to whatever treatment was indicated, rather than their availability determining where and how treatment would be provided. From an assessment standpoint the law required that the county shall provide a chemical use assessment ". . . for all clients who seek treatment or for whom treatment is sought for chemical abuse or dependency. The assessor shall complete an assessment summary . . . for each client assessed for chemical dependency treatment services. The form shall be maintained in the client's case record . . . *An assessor under contract with the county shall have no direct financial interest or referral relationship resulting in shared financial gain with a treatment provider*" [emphasis supplied].

Although Minnesota's approach is of recent origin, the preliminary results are encouraging. There is already evidence that individuals seeking treatment are being directed more frequently to low-cost alternatives and that more treatment is being provided at less overall cost (Minnesota Chemical Dependency Program Division, 1989). These findings are consistent with experience elsewhere in the provision of medical care (Feldstein et al., 1988). In neither instance has it been determined that equivalent effectiveness necessarily accompanies a lower overall cost of treatment, but Minnesota has also mandated a uniform evaluation system and plans to address this question as well. Another state, Michigan, is moving toward a similar approach to treatment, involving independent pretreatment assessment and outcome monitoring (Allo et al., 1988).

The problems of financial and ideological bias are well known and at the very least require attention. At issue is whether the independence of the assessment process from the treatment process is required to prevent these biases from operating in a significant manner. The broadly accepted model of complete independence of outcome determination in efficacy studies suggests that such independence may be important, particularly if reassessment is used to determine outcome. On the other hand, objections have been raised on such practical grounds as the delays that may occur in entering treatment and the imposition of an additional structure (independent assessment) between the individual and the treatment he or she is seeking. Rather than settling the issue on a *prima facie* basis, a pilot study involving comparisons of referral patterns and of the results of treatment between independent and nonindependent assessment would be instructive.

In the interim it seems possible that an administratively distinct assessment unit within an overall treatment program could provide some level of assurance that due protection is available from the effects of ideological and financial biases. This assurance would be more credible if the treatment program provided a multiplicity of treatments that were diverse in their treatment philosophies and costs. The arrangement could also provide built-in safeguards such as the regular and independent monitoring of disposition patterns and structural provision for cross-referral to other treatment programs.

Methods of Obtaining Assessment Information

In providing assessment information, individuals seeking treatment may interact with an interviewer, with a questionnaire or other assessment instrument, or with a suitably programmed computer. To some extent these methods represent alternatives; for example, computers are often used to obtain information that would otherwise have been obtained by interview or by questionnaire. The methods are not mutually exclusive: various mixtures of all three can be utilized and ideally should be available because some individuals are quite uncomfortable with particular methods (H. A. Skinner and Allen, 1983b; H. A. Skinner et al., 1985a, 1985b; Lucas et al., 1976; Lucas et al., 1977). In addition, the assessment of sight- and hearing-impaired individuals or of persons not fluent in English poses problems for particular assessment methods.

Face-to-face interviewing is probably the most common method of obtaining assessment information. Its principal advantage lies in the direct person-to-person interaction involved; as noted in Table 10-3, good rapport generally enhances the validity of self-reported data. Such interaction with a member of the staff of a treatment facility may be a prime factor in sustaining participation in treatment; conversely, a program that did not allow such interaction to occur would probably have a high drop-out rate.

On the other hand, interpersonal interaction is not necessarily an unqualified good. Individuals vary widely in their comfort in interpersonal situations. Some of those seeking treatment may prefer a more distant method of interaction. Much of the information gathered during an assessment is of a sensitive nature, and the neutrality of test instruments or of computers may be advantageous in obtaining it. In one study, patients with alcohol problems reported higher levels of alcohol consumption to a computer, lower levels to a psychiatrist, and still lower levels to a higher status psychiatrist (Lucas et al., 1977); both medical status and senior status apparently were intimidating. If assessment and treatment are carried out by different personnel, fostering a close personal relationship with assessment staff could become problematic (W. Skinner and Becks, 1988).

But (as noted) assessment is not an either/or situation with respect to method. Given a sufficiently flexible staff, combinations of interviewing, instruments, and computers can be utilized—perhaps even a different mix of methods for different individuals, depending on preferences and circumstances (e.g., assessment should not have to cease when the computers are "down"). Nevertheless, some degree of face-to-face personal contact is clearly essential and should be part of any assessment process.

To be effective, however, interpersonal interaction must be effectively carried out, and therein lies a possible problem. Potential assessors cannot automatically be assumed to possess the requisite interpersonal skills to conduct a comprehensive assessment. No attribute of an individual, including the possession of a particular academic qualification or the experience of dealing successfully with one's own alcohol problem, in itself guarantees such skills—or, for that matter, guarantees their absence. Even if assessment personnel do possess the requisite skills, it cannot be presumed they will use them consistently. In short, there is no substitute for the careful selection, thorough training, and close supervision of assessment staff.

It should also be noted that, as commonly practiced even by individuals with abundant interpersonal skills, face-to-face interviewing as a method of obtaining assessment information often leaves much to be desired. Such interviewing is most frequently conducted in an unstructured way; that is to say, the content of the questions and the order in which they are asked are left to the interviewer to determine. The result of free-form assessment interviewing is all too frequently spotty and inconsistent data collection. One such interviewer might learn a great deal, for example, about the family history of one individual and nothing about that of the next.

Moreover, the recording of data derived from unstructured interviews presents unusual challenges. Experience suggests that, even if the interview itself has been comprehensive, not everything that is discussed is recorded. Pressed as they often are for time, interviewers are sometimes content with summary statements. Yet the statement that a person has "a moderately severe alcohol problem" could mean just about anything. Finally, the legibility of notes recorded from unstructured interviewing is often a problem; because of the great variability in the structure and content of such interviews the notes are often written out in longhand.

The structured face-to-face interview is another matter entirely. If carefully developed, it can be highly effective even in relatively inexperienced hands. It retains the interpersonal elements of the unstructured interview but substitutes predetermined for spontaneous content. Structure permits the interview to possess (at least potentially) the desired qualities of quantifiability, reliability, validity, standardization, and recordability (see above).

An example of a structured interview from the alcohol field is the time-line (TL) interview, which measures past lifetime alcohol consumption. Its reliability has been examined (L. C. Sobell et al., 1988) and it has been found that individuals given the instrument at different times will come up with consistent estimates of levels of alcohol consumption in past periods of their lives. Whether it is valid, however—whether these estimates are correct—cannot be established because there is no adequate criterion, that is, a certain and alternative method of determining past consumption. Research on biological markers may one day provide the needed criterion. Meanwhile, a reliable means of determining retrospective consumption is to be preferred to one that lacks demonstrated reliability.

The chief disadvantage of structured interviewing as a means of gathering assessment information has to do with personnel time and training. The constant attendance of extensively trained personnel is required to administer a structured interview. In a time of resource constraints on the one hand and increased demand for services on the other, this disadvantage can be considerable. Attention has accordingly been given to the self-administration of assessment. The savings from self-administration can be considerable, even if small amounts of information are concerned. The MAST takes approximately 10 minutes to administer; if 20 patients a day are assessed, the total saving is more than three hours of personnel time.

A common form of self-administration is the use of paper-and- pencil tests. The use of such tests does involve personnel time but of another sort. More than a single test is usually given. Tests must be selected from storage; then each test must be presented to the individual with the appropriate instructions, proofed for completeness, scored, standardized, and recorded. Because different individuals are given different tests and work at different speeds, a one-on-one assessment staffing pattern may be required. In short, although there are resource advantages to self-administration, resource requirements are still apparent.

Computers can be utilized effectively to limit further the resource requirements of assessment. An initial capital investment is needed, but the ultimate saving on resources through the reduced cost of each assessment performed thereafter more than compensates for the original expenditure (Klingler et al., 1977). Although computers can be used in a rather peripheral manner to perform such tasks as the automated scoring of self-administered tests, they truly come into their own when they are used as self-administration devices. For staff, this use involves providing the individuals being assessed with adequate instructions, sitting them down in front of a computer and keyboard (often modified for the sake of simplicity), and being available to provide help and answer questions.

The various instruments or interview schedules to be used for the assessment are held in the capacious and accurate memory banks of the computer. An appropriate program presents the instruments in predesignated order. Responses to individual items can be checked for appropriateness and completeness, ensuring that each response given falls within the designated range for each item and that all questions are completed. If the responses are faulty or incomplete, the computer can (given adroit programming) prompt the individual to make appropriate corrections. In a sequential assessment process, the computer can be programmed to indicate automatically whether it is necessary to proceed from one stage to the next, and to select the requisite instruments to provide in-depth assessment on the basis of scores from the screenings of the prior stage, which it has automatically calculated and compared with the standardized norms in its memory. In addition, the computer can be programmed to integrate multiple assessment results into an understandable and comprehensive assessment report (see an example in H. A. Skinner [1981a:359]).

To some readers the prospect of computerized assessment will sound like magic at best and science fiction at worst. But to others it will be commonplace. Interactive computer games were the best-selling gift item during the 1988 holiday season. The use of computers not only has a high level of initial acceptance in assessment situations but an increasing level of enthusiasm following first exposure, as well as equivalent or superior results to paper-and pencil tests and face-to-face interviewing (H. A. Skinner, 1981; H. A. Skinner and Allen, 1983b; H. A. Skinner et al., 1985a, 1985b). Computer technology has advanced rapidly since the introduction of microcomputers, with the result that equipment of great capability is now available at reasonable cost. Although most frequently criticized as impersonal, the computer can instead increase the interpersonal ambience of assessment. By performing many of the tasks that would ordinarily be required of the assessor it frees time for interpersonal interaction (cf. Levitt, 1972).

Nevertheless, even if assessment is largely automated it may be prudent to design an assessment that is a mixture of face-to-face interviewing, self-administered testing, and computerized testing. None of the methods is foolproof, and some may be precluded by the specialized disabilities or preferences of individual patients. Those carrying out the assessment might optimally be trained to administer the entire process in either of the three options. In that way staff would have a more complete understanding of the process, and maximum flexibility would be assured.

Conclusions and Recommendations

This chapter has made the case that *all individuals seeking specialized treatment for alcohol problems should receive a comprehensive assessment prior to treatment.* The assessment should be carried out in a sequential manner, proceeding in a logical and carefully articulated manner from one stage to the next as needed to produce sufficient information for relevant treatment decisions. *The stages of assessment recommended by the committee include a screening stage, a problem assessment stage, and a personal assessment stage.*

Assessment should also be multidimensional; that is, it should include several different kinds of information within each stage of assessment content. For example, *the committee recommends that the problem assessment stage include information on the individual's use of alcohol, on the signs and symptoms of alcohol use, and on the consequences of alcohol use.* In many instances each of these elements should also be multidimensional; for example, with respect to the use of alcohol, it is important to obtain information on the level of use, the pattern of use, and the history of use. The problem assessment stage is highly multidimensional (see Table 10-2). Finally, *assessment should be uniform to a significant degree for all persons seeking treatment,* so that data from different subjects can be pooled and data from different programs can be compared.

Information gathered during the ideal assessment should be of demonstrated reliability and validity; it should be quantitative and standardized; and it should be readily recordable. Appropriate techniques should be employed to ensure that self-reported assessment information is maximally accurate. Assessments should be administered by a carefully selected, specifically trained, and continuously supervised staff that is adept at using a variety of assessment methods. Due precautions should be taken to assure that assessment staff operated independently of any significant biases, including and especially those that can arise from the prospect of financial gain or from commitment to a specific form of treatment.

The principal purpose of gathering assessment information is to provide a basis for the selection of the most appropriate treatment for the individual being assessed. However, the information also serves a number of other purposes. It constitutes a baseline for subsequent outcome determinations; permits the characterization of treatment populations and facilitates their comparison with one another; and (if analyzed together with outcome data) can be used to guide the future treatment of others with similar problems.

Implementation of a program of comprehensive assessment of this kind will require vigorous and polycentric leadership, adequate funding, and a stepwise developmental process. *The committee believes it is of the essence to foster a consensus within the treatment field both on the general notion of assessment and on all aspects of its content and administration.* To this end, *demonstration models of various kinds of comprehensive assessment should be set up and carefully studied;* such a process would be helpful to those who are not fully persuaded of the need for comprehensive assessment. Those who have already been persuaded should provide information on all aspects of their experience to enrich and accelerate the development of a broad response.

REFERENCES

Allo, C. D., B. Mintzes, and R. C. Brook. 1988. What purchasers of treatment services want from evaluation. Alcohol Health and Research World 12:162-167.

American Psychiatric Association (APA). 1987. DSM III-R: Diagnostic and Statistical Manual of Mental Disorders, 3rd edition, revised. Washington, D.C.: American Psychiatric Association.

Annis, H. M. 1979. Group treatment of incarcerated offenders with alcohol and drug problems: A controlled evaluation. Canadian Journal of Criminology 21:3-15.

Annis, H. M. 1982. Inventory of Drinking Situations. Toronto: Addiction Research Foundation.

Annis, H. M. 1986a. Is inpatient rehabilitation of the alcoholic cost effective? Con position. Advances in Alcohol and Substance Abuse 5:175-190.

Annis, H. M. 1986b. A relapse prevention model for treatment of alcoholics. Pp. 407-433 in Treating Addictive Behaviors, W. R. Miller and N. Heather, eds. New York: Plenum Press.

Annis, H. M., and D. Chan. 1983. The differential treatment model: Empirical evidence from a personality typology of adult offenders. Criminal Justice and Behavior 10:159-173.

Annis, H. M., and C. Davis. 1989. Relapse prevention. Pp. 170-182 in Handbook of Alcoholism Treatment Approaches: Effective Alternatives, R. K. Hester and W. R. Miller, eds. New York: Pergamon Press.

Annis, H. M., J. M. Graham, and C. S. Davis. 1987. Inventory of Drinking Situations User's Guide. Toronto: Addiction Research Foundation.

Annis, H. M., and H. A. Skinner. 1984. Early experiences with assessment. Pp. 107-145 in A System of Health Care Delivery, vol. 2, F. B. Glaser, H. M. Annis, H. A. Skinner, S. Pearlman, R. L. Segal, B. Sisson, A. C. Ogborne, E. Bohnen, P. Gazda, and T. Zimmerman. Toronto: The Addiction Research Foundation.

Ashley, M. J. 1982. Alcohol, tobacco, and drugs: An audit of mortality and morbidity. Pp. 350-366 in Man, Drugs, and Society: Current Perspectives, L. R. H. Drew, P. Stolz, and W. A. Barclay, eds. Canberra: Australian Federation on Alcoholism and Drug Dependence.

Babor, T. F., and R. Kadden. 1985. Screening for alcohol problems: Conceptual issues and practical considerations. Pp. 1-30 in Early Identification of Alcohol Abuse, N. C. Chang and H. M. Chao, eds. Washington, D.C.: U. S. Government Printing Office.

Babor, T. F., E. B. Ritson, and R. J. Hodgson. 1986. Alcohol-related problems in the primary health care setting: A review of early intervention strategies. British Journal of Addiction 81:23-46.

Babor, T. F., R. S. Stephens, and G. A. Marlatt. 1987. Verbal report methods in clinical research on alcoholism: Response bias and its minimization. Journal of Studies on Alcohol 48:410-24.

Babor, T. F., R. de la Fuente, J. Saunders, and M. Grant. 1989. Manual for the Alcohol Use Disorders Identification Test (AUDIT). Geneva: World Health Organization.

Backer, T. E., R. P. Liberman, and T. G. Kuehnel. 1986. Dissemination and adoption of innovative psychosocial interventions. Journal of Consulting and Clinical Psychology 54:111-118.

Barnes, G. E. 1979. The alcoholic personality: A reanalysis of the literature. Journal of Studies on Alcohol 40:571-634.

Barrett, E. T., and G. C. Gleser. 1987. Development and validation of the Cognitive Status Examination. Journal of Consulting and Clinical Psychology 55:877-882.

Belille, C. N.d. (ca. 1987). Bringing Definition to a Soft Science. Saint Paul, Minn.: Chemical Abuse/Addiction Treatment Outcome Registry (CATOR), Ramsey Clinic.

Beutler, L. E. 1979. Toward specific psychological therapies for specific conditions. Journal of Consulting and Clinical Psychology 47:882-897.

Blouin, A. G. 1986. The computerized Diagnostic Interview Schedule. DIS Newsletter 3(Fall):4-8.

Bohman, M., S. Sigvardsson, and C. R. Cloninger. 1981. Cross fostering analysis of adopted women. Archives of General Psychiatry 38:965-969.

Boss, W. A. 1980. Next Steps in the Evolution of Chemical Dependency Care in Minnesota. Minneapolis: The Citizens League.

Brickman, P., V. C. Rabinowitz, J. Karuza, Jr., D. Coates, E. Cohen, and L. Kidder. 1982. Models of helping and coping. American Psychologist 37:368-384.

Bromet, E., R. H. Moos, and F. Bliss. 1976. The social climate of alcoholism treatment programs. Archives of General Psychiatry 33:910-916.

Bromet, E., R. Moos, F. Bliss, and C. Wuthmann. 1977. Posttreatment functioning of alcoholic patients: Its relationship to program participation. Journal of Consulting and Clinical Psychology 45:829-842.

Canter, F. M. 1966. Personality factors related to participation in treatment by hospitalized male alcoholics. Journal of Clinical Psychology 22:114-116.

Cloninger, C. R. 1987. Neurogenetic adaptive mechanisms in alcoholism. Science 236:410-416.

Cloninger, C. R., M. Bohman, and S. Sigvardsson. 1981. Inheritance of alcohol abuse: Cross fostering analysis of adopted men. Archives of General Psychiatry 38:861-868.

Cotton, N. S. 1979. The familial incidence of alcoholism: A review. Journal of Studies on Alcohol 40:89-116.

Cronkite, R. C., and R. H. Moos. 1978. Evaluating alcoholism treatment programs: An integrated approach. Journal of Consulting and Clinical Psychology 46:1105-1119.

Cronkite, R. C., and R. H. Moos. 1980. Determinants of the posttreatment functioning of alcoholic patients: A conceptual framework. Journal of Consulting and Clinical Psychology 48:305-316.

Cyr, M. G., and S. A. Wartman. 1988. The effectiveness of routine screening questions in the detection of alcoholism. Journal of the American Medical Association 259:51-54.

Davidson, R. 1987. Assessment of the alcohol dependence syndrome: A review of self-report screening questionnaires. British Journal of Clinical Psychology 26:243-255.

Edwards, G. 1974. Drugs, drug dependence, and the concept of plasticity. Quarterly Journal of Studies on Alcohol 35:176-195.

Edwards, G. 1986. The alcohol dependence syndrome: A concept as stimulus to enquiry. British Journal of Addiction 81:171-183.

Edwards, G., and M. M. Gross. 1976. Alcohol dependence: Provisional description of a clinical syndrome. British Medical Journal 1:1058-1061.

Ellwood, P. 1988. Outcomes management: A technology of patient experience. New England Journal of Medicine 318:1549-1556.

Emrick, C. D. 1987. Alcoholics Anonymous: Affiliation processes and effectiveness as treatment. Alcoholism: Clinical and Experimental Research 11:416-423.

Ewing, J. A. 1984. Detecting alcoholism: The CAGE questionnaire. Journal of the American Medical Association 252:1905-1097.

Feldstein, P. J., T. M. Wickizer, and J. R. C. Wheeler. 1988. Private cost containment: The effects of utilization review programs on health care use and expenditures. New England Journal of Medicine 318:1310-1314.

Fillmore, K. M. 1987. Women's drinking across the life course as compared to men's. British Journal of Addiction 82:801-811.

Fillmore, K. M., and L. Midanik. 1984. Chronicity of drinking problems among men: A longitudinal study. Journal of Studies on Alcohol 45:228-236.

Finney, J. W., and R. H. Moos. 1979. Treatment and outcome for empirical subtypes of alcoholic patients. Journal of Consulting and Clinical Psychology 47:25-38.

Fries, J. F. 1976. A data bank for clinicians? New England Journal of Medicine 294:1400-1402.

Fuller, R. K., K. K. Lee, and E. Gordis. 1988. Validity of self report in alcoholism research: Results of a Veterans Administration cooperative study. Alcoholism: Clinical and Experimental Research 12:201-205.

Gibbs, L. E. 1980. A classification of alcoholics relevant to type-specific treatment. International Journal of the Addictions 15:461-488.

Glaser, F. B., and H. A. Skinner. 1984. Matching in the real world. Pp. 61-98 in A System of Health Care Delivery, vol. 3, F. B. Glaser, H. M. Annis, H. A. Skinner, S. Pearlman, R. L. Segal, B. Sisson, A. C. Ogborne, E. Bohnen, P. Gazda, and T. Zimmerman. Toronto: Addiction Research Foundation.

Glaser, F. B., S. W. Greenberg, and M. Barrett. 1978. A Systems Approach to Alcohol Treatment. Toronto: ARF Books.

Goldberg, D. P. 1972. The Detection of Psychiatric Illness by Questionnaire: A Technique for the Identification and Assessment of Nonpsychotic Illness. London: Oxford University Press.

Goldberg, D. P. 1978. Manual of the General Health Questionnaire. Windsor: NFER Publishing Company.

Hansen, J., and C. D. Emrick. 1983. Whom are we calling "alcoholic?" Bulletin of the Society of Psychologists in Addictive Behaviors 2:164-178.

Harmer, M. H. 1977. The case for TNM. Clinical Oncology 3:131-135.

Harrison, P. A., and C. A. Belille. 1987. Women in treatment: Beyond the stereotype. Journal of Studies on Alcohol 48:574-578.

Harrison, P. A., and N. G. Hoffmann. 1987. CATOR 1987 Report: Adolescent Residential Treatment: Intake and Follow-Up Findings. Saint Paul, Minn.: Chemical Abuse/Addiction Treatment Outcome Registry (CATOR), Ramsey Clinic.

Hartman, L., M. Krywonis, and E. Morrison. 1988. Psychological factors and health-related behavior change: Preliminary findings from a controlled clinical trial. Canadian Family Physician 34:1045-1050.

Hartocollis, P. 1962. Drunkenness and suggestion: An experiment with intravenous alcohol. Quarterly Journal of Studies on Alcohol 23:376-389.

Hayes, S. C., R. O. Nelson, and R. B. Jarrett. 1987. The treatment utility of assessment: A functional approach for evaluating assessment quality. American Psychologist 42:963-974.

Helzer, J. E., and A. Burnham. In press. Alcohol abuse and dependence. In Psychiatric Disorders in America, L. N. Robins and D. A. Regier, eds. New York: The Free Press.

Hlatky, M. A., K. L. Lee, F. E. Harrel, Jr., R. M. Califf, D. B. Pryor, D. B. Mark, and R. A. Rosati. 1984. Tying clinical research to patient care by use of an observational data base. Statistics in Medicine 3:375-384.

Hodgson, R., T. Stockwell, H. Rankin, and G. Edwards. 1978. Alcohol dependence: The concept, its utility and measurement. British Journal of Addiction 73:339-342.

Hoffmann, N. G., J. A. Halikas, and D. Mee-Lee. 1987. The Cleveland Admission, Discharge, and Transfer Criteria: Model for Chemical Dependency Treatment Programs. Cleveland, Ohio: The Greater Cleveland Hospital Association.

Holmes, T. H., and M. Masuda. 1973. Psychosomatic syndrome: When mothers-in-law or other disasters visit, a person can develop a bad, bad cold. Psychology Today 5(11):71-72, 106.

Holmes, T. H., and R. H. Rahe. 1967. The Social Readjustment Rating Scale. Journal of Psychosomatic Research 11:213-218.

Horn, J. L., H. A. Skinner, K. Wanberg, and F. M. Foster. 1984. Alcohol Dependence Scale. Toronto: Addiction Research Foundation.

Horn, J. L., K. W. Wanberg, and F. M. Foster. 1987. Guide to the Alcohol Use Inventory (AUI). Minneapolis, Minn.: National Computer Systems, Incorporated.

Institute for Personality and Ability Testing. 1986. 16PF Manual. Savoy, Ill.: Institute for Personality and Ability Testing.

Jackson, D. N. 1974. Personality Research Form Manual. Goshen, N.Y.: Research Psychologists Press.

Jackson, J. K. 1988. Testimony presented before the U.S. Senate Governmental Affairs Committee hearing regarding the causes of and governmental responses to alcohol abuse and alcoholism, Washington, D.C., June 16.

Jacob, T. 1988. Executive summary: Approaches to the assessment of family/marital functioning. Prepared for the IOM Committee for the Study of Treatment and Rehabilitation Services for Alcoholism and Alcohol Abuse.

Kadden, R. M., N. L. Cooney, H. Getter, and M. D. Litt. 1990. Matching alcoholics to coping skills or interactional therapies: Posttreatment results. Journal of Consulting and Clinical Psychology 698-704.

Keller, M. 1972. The oddities of alcoholics. Quarterly Journal of Studies on Alcohol 33:1147-1148.

Kern, J. C., W. Schmelter, and M. Fanelli. 1978. A comparison of three alcoholism treatment populations: Implications for treatment. Journal of Studies on Alcohol 39:785-792.

Kiernan, R. J., J. Mueller, J. W. Langston, and C. van Dyke. 1987. The Neurobehavioral Cognitive Status Examination: A brief but differentiated approach to cognitive assessment. Annals of Internal Medicine 107:481-485.

Klingler, D. E., D. A. Miller, J. H. Johnson, and T. A. Williams. 1977. Process evaluation of an on-line computer assisted unit for intake assessment of mental health patients. Behavioral Research Methods and Instrumentation 9:110-116.

Korchin, S. J., and D. Schuldberg. 1981. The future of clinical assessment. American Psychologist 36:1147-1158.

Korcok, M. 1988. Managed Care and Chemical Dependency: A Troubled Relationship. Providence, R.I.: Manisses Communications Group, Inc.

Kozlowski, L. T., L. C. Jellinek, and M. A. Pope. 1986. Cigarette smoking among alcohol abusers: A continuing and neglected problem. Canadian Journal of Public Health 77:205-207.

Kranzler, H. R., T. F. Babor, and R. J. Lauerman. 1990. Problems associated with average alcohol consumption and frequency of intoxication in a medical population. Alcoholism Experimental and Clinical Research 14(1):119-126.

Kristensen, H., H. Ohlin, M.-B. Hulten-Nosslin, E. Trell, and B. Hood. 1983. Identification and intervention of heavy drinking in middle-aged men: Results and follow-up of 24-60 months of long-term study with randomized controls. Alcoholism: Clinical and Experimental Research 7:203-209.

Laszlo, J. 1985. Health registry and clinical data base technology: With special emphasis on cancer registries. Journal of Chronic Disease 38:67-78.

Lettieri, D. J., M. A. Sayers, and J. E. Nelson, eds. 1985a. Summaries of Alcoholism Treatment Assessment Research. Washington, D.C.: U.S. Government Printing Office.

Lettieri, D. J., M. A. Sayers, and J. E. Nelson, eds. 1985b. Alcoholism Treatment Assessment Research Instruments. Washington, D.C.: U.S. Government Printing Office.

Levitt, T. 1972. Production-line approach to service. Harvard Business Review 50:41-52.

Lewis, J. 1988. Growth in managed care forcing providers to adjust. Alcoholism Report 16(24):1.

Lucas, R. W., W. I. Card, R. P. Knill-Jones, G. Watkinson, and G. P. Crean. 1976. Computer interrogation of patients. British Medical Journal 2:623-625.

Lucas, R. W., P. J. Mullin, C. B. X. Luna, and D. C. McInroy. 1977. Psychiatrists and a computer as interrogators of patients with alcohol-related illness: A comparison. British Journal of Psychiatry 131:160-167.

Maletzky, B. M., and J. Klotter. 1974. Smoking and alcoholism. American Journal of Psychiatry 131:445-447.

Malla, A. K., B. Rush, M. Gavin, and G. Cooper. 1985. A community-centred alcoholism assessment/treatment service: A descriptive study. Canadian Journal of Psychiatry 30:35-43.

Marlatt, G. A., and J. R. Gordon, eds. 1985. Relapse Prevention. New York: Guilford Press.

Marshman, J., R. D. Fraser, C. Lambert, A. C. Ogborne, S. J. Saunders, P. W. Humphries, D. W. Macdonald, J. G. Rankin, and W. Schmidt. 1978. The Treatment of Alcoholics: An Ontario Perspective. Toronto: Addiction Research Foundation.

McLachlan, J. F. C. 1972. Benefit from group therapy as a function of patient-therapist match on conceptual level. Psychotherapy: Theory, Research, and Practice 9:317-323.

McLachlan, J. F. C. 1974. Therapy strategies, personality orientation, and recovery from alcoholism. Canadian Psychiatric Association Journal 19:25-30.

McLellan, A. T., L. Luborsky, G. E. Woody, and C. P. O'Brien. 1980. An improved diagnostic evaluation instrument for substance abuse patients: The Addiction Severity Index. Journal of Nervous and Mental Diseases 168:26-33.

McLellan, A. T., L. Luborsky, J. Cacciola, J. Griffith, P. McGahan, and C. P. O'Brien. 1985. Guide to the Addiction Severity Index. Washington, D.C.: U. S. Government Printing Office.

Mendelson, J. H., T. F. Babor, N. K. Mello, and H. Pratt. 1986. Alcoholism and prevalence of medical and psychiatric disorders. Journal of Studies on Alcohol 47:361-366.

Miller, S., E. Helmick, L. Berg, P. Nutting, and G. Shorr. 1974. Alcoholism: A statewide program evaluation. American Journal of Psychiatry 131:210-214.

Miller, W. R., and R. K. Hester. 1986. Inpatient alcoholism treatment: Who benefits? American Psychologist 41:794-805.

Minnesota Chemical Dependency Program Division. 1989. Report on the Status of the Consolidated Chemical Dependency Treatment Fund. Saint Paul: Minnesota Department of Human Services.

Mogar, R. E., W. W. Wilson, and S. T. Helm. 1970. Personality subtypes of male and female alcoholic patients. International Journal of the Addictions 5:99-113.

Moos, R. H., E. Bromet, V. Tsu, and B. Moos. 1979. Family characteristics and the outcome of treatment for alcoholism. Journal of Studies on Alcohol 40:78-88.

Nace, E. P., J. J. Saxon, Jr., and N. Shore. 1986. Borderline personality disorder and alcoholism treatment: A one-year follow-up study. Journal of Studies on Alcohol 47:196-200.

O'Farrell, T. J., and S. A. Maisto. 1987. The utility of self-report and biological measures of alcohol consumption in alcoholism treatment outcome studies. Advances in Behavioral Research and Therapy 9:91-125.

Ogborne, A. C. 1978. Patient characteristics as predictors of treatment outcomes for alcohol and drug abusers. Pp. 177-223 in Research Advances in Alcohol and Drug Problems, vol. 4, Y. Israel, F. B. Glaser, H. Kalant, R. E. Popham, W. Schmidt, and R. G. Smart, eds. New York: Plenum Press.

Ogborne, A. C., and F. B. Glaser. 1981. Characteristics of affiliates of Alcoholics Anonymous: A review of the literature. Journal of Studies on Alcohol 42:661-675.

Orrego, H., L. M. Blendis, J. E. Blake, B. M. Kapur, and Y. Israel. 1979. Reliability of assessment of alcohol intake based on personal interviews in a liver clinic. Lancet 2:1354-1356.

Partington, J. T. 1970. Dr. Jekyll and Mr. High: Multidimensional scaling of alcoholics' self-evaluations. Journal of Abnormal Psychology 75:131-138.

Pattison, E. M. 1974. Rehabilitation of the chronic alcoholic. Pp. 587-658 in Clinical Pathology, Vol. 3 of The Biology of Alcoholism, B. Kissin and H. Begleiter, eds. New York: Plenum Press.

Pattison, E. M., R. Coe, and R. J. Rhodes. 1969. Evaluation of alcoholism treatment: A comparison of three facilities. Archives of General Psychiatry 20:478-488.

Pattison, E. M., R. Coe, and H. O. Doerr. 1973. Population variation among alcoholism treatment facilities. International Journal of the Addictions 8:199-229.

Paykel, E. S., B. S. Prusoff, and E. H. Uhlenhuth. 1971. Scaling of life events. Archives of General Psychiatry 25:340-347.

Peachey, J. E., and B. M. Kapur. 1986. Monitoring drinking behavior with the alcohol dipstick during treatment. Alcoholism: Clinical and Experimental Research 10:663-666.

Penick, E. C., B. J. Powell, S. F. Bingham, B. I. Liskow, N. S. Miller, and M. R. Read. 1987. A comparative study of familial alcoholism. Journal of Studies on Alcohol 48:136-146.

Polich, J. M., D. J. Armor, and H. B. Braiker. 1981. The Course of Alcoholism: Four Years After Treatment. New York: John Wiley and Sons.

Popham, R. E., W. Schmidt, and S. Israelstam. 1984. Heavy alcohol consumption and physical health problems: A review of the epidemiologic evidence. Pp. 148-182 in Research Advances in Alcohol and Drug Problems, vol. 8, R. G. Smart, H. D. Cappell, F. B. Glaser, Y. Israel, H. Kalant, R. E. Popham, W. Schmidt, and E. M. Sellers, eds. New York: Plenum Press.

Pryor, D. B., R. M. Califf, F. E. Harrell, Jr., M. A. Hlatky, K. L. Lee, D. B. Mark, and R. A. Rosati. 1985. Clinical data bases: Accomplishments and unrealized potential. Medical Care 23:623-647.

Reilly, D. H., and A. A. Sugerman. 1967. Conceptual complexity and psychological differentiation in alcoholics. Journal of Nervous and Mental Disease 144:14-17.

Robins, L. N., J. E. Helzer, J. Croughan, and K. S. Ratcliff. 1981. National Institute of Mental Health Diagnostic Interview Schedule: Its history, characteristics, and validity. Archives of General Psychiatry 38:381-389.

Robins, L. N., J. E. Helzer, M. M. Weissman, H. Orvaschel, E. Gruenberg, J. D. Burke, Jr., and D. A. Regier. 1984. Lifetime prevalence of specific psychiatric disorders in three sites. Archives of General Psychiatry 41:949-958.

Ross, H. E., and F. B. Glaser. 1989. Psychiatric screening of alcohol and drug patients: The validity of the GHQ-60. American Journal of Drug and Alcohol Abuse. 15:429-442.

Ross, H. E., F. B. Glaser, and T. Germanson. 1988. The prevalence of psychiatric disorders in patients with alcohol and other drug problems. Archives of General Psychiatry 45:1023-1031.

Rounsaville, B. J., Z. S. Dolinsky, T. F. Babor, and R. E. Meyer. 1987. Psychopathology as a predictor of treatment outcome in alcoholics. Archives of General Psychiatry 44:505-513.

Rush, B. 1987. Executive summary: Assessment procedures and specialized assessment in Ontario. Prepared for the IOM Committee for the Study of Treatment and Rehabilitation Services for Alcoholism and Alcohol Abuse.

Sadava, S. 1985. Problem behavior theory and consumption and consequences of alcohol use. Journal of Studies on Alcohol 46:392-397.

Saunders, J. B. 1988. Executive summary: Screening techniques for alcohol and drug problems. Prepared for the IOM Committee for the Study of Treatment and Rehabilitation Services for Alcoholism and Alcohol Abuse.

Saunders, J. B., and O. G. Aasland. 1987. World Health Organization Collaborative Project on Identification and Treatment of Persons with Harmful Alcohol Consumption: Report on Phase I Development of a Screening Instrument. Geneva: World Health Organization, Division of Mental Health.

Savitz, L. D., K. File, and T. W. McCahill. 1973. Referral decision-making in a multi-modality system. Pp. 158-168 in Proceedings of the Fifth National Conference on Methadone Treatment. New York: NAPAN.

Saxe, L., D. Dougherty, K. Esty, and M. Fine. 1983. The Effectiveness and Costs of Alcoholism Treatment. Washington, D.C.: U. S. Congress, Office of Technology Assessment.

Schuckit, M. A. 1973. Alcoholism and sociopathy—diagnostic confusion. Quarterly Journal of Studies on Alcohol 34:157-164.

Schuckit, M. A., and M. Irwin. 1988. Diagnosis of alcoholism. Medical Clinics of North America 72:1133-1153.

Searles, J. S. 1988. The role of genetics in the pathogenesis of alcoholism. Journal of Abnormal Psychology 97:153-167.

Segal, R. L. 1984. The administration of the Assessment Unit. Pp. 198-214 in A System of Health Care Delivery, vol. 2, F. B. Glaser, H. M. Annis, H. A. Skinner, S. Pearlman, R. L. Segal, B. Sisson, A. C. Ogborne, E. Bohnen, P. Gazda, and T. Zimmerman. Toronto: Addiction Research Foundation.

Selzer, M. L. 1971. The Michigan Alcoholism Screening Test: The quest for a new diagnostic instrument. American Journal of Psychiatry 127:1653-1658.

Skinner, H. A. 1979. A multivariate evaluation of the MAST. Journal of Studies on Alcohol 40:831-834.

Skinner, H. A. 1981a. Assessment of alcohol problems: Basic principles, critical issues, and future trends. Pp. 316-369 in Research Advances in Alcohol and Drug Problems, vol. 6., Y. Israel, F. B. Glaser, H. Kalant, R. E. Popham, W. Schmidt, and R. G. Smart, eds. New York: Plenum Press.

Skinner, H. A. 1981b. Benefits of sequential assessment. Social Work Research and Abstracts 17:21-28.

Skinner, H. A. 1981c. Comparison of clients assigned to in-patient and out-patient treatment for alcoholism and drug addiction. British Journal of Psychiatry 138:312-320.

Skinner, H. A. 1984. Instruments for assessing alcohol and drug problems. Bulletin of the Society of Psychologists in Addictive Behaviors 3:21-33.

Skinner, H. A. 1985. The clinical spectrum of alcoholism: Implications for new drug therapies. Pp. 123-135 in Research Advances in New Psychopharmacological Treatments for Alcoholism, C. A. Naranjo and E. M. Sellers, eds. Amsterdam: Elsevier.

Skinner, H. A. 1988. Executive summary: Toward a multiaxial framework for the classification of alcohol problems. Prepared for the IOM Committee for the Study of Treatment and Rehabilitation Services for Alcoholism and Alcohol Abuse.

Skinner, H. A., and B. A. Allen. 1982. Alcohol dependence syndrome: Measurement and validation. Journal of Abnormal Psychology 91:199-209.

Skinner, H. A., and B. A. Allen. 1983a. Differential assessment of alcoholism. Journal of Studies on Alcohol 44:852-862.

Skinner, H. A., and B. A. Allen. 1983b. Does the computer make a difference? Computerized versus face-to-face versus self-report assessment of alcohol, drug, and tobacco use. Journal of Consulting and Clinical Psychology 51:267-275.

Skinner, H. A., and S. Holt. 1987. The Alcohol Clinical Index: Strategies for Identifying Patients with Alcohol Problems. Toronto: Addiction Research Foundation.

Skinner, H. A., and H. Lei. 1980. The multidimensional assessment of stressful life events. Journal of Nervous and Mental Disease 168:535-541.

Skinner, H. A., and K. R. Shoffner. 1978. Sex differences and addiction: A comparison of male and female clients at the Clinical Institute. Substudy No. 983. Toronto: Addiction Research Foundation.

Skinner, H. A., D. N. Jackson, and H. Hoffmann. 1974. Alcoholic personality types: Identification and correlates. Journal of Abnormal Psychology 83:658-666, 1974.

Skinner, H. A., B. A. Allen, M. C. McIntosh, and W. H. Palmer. 1985a. Lifestyle assessment: Applying microcomputers in family practice. British Medical Journal 290:212-14.

Skinner, H. A., B. A. Allen, M. C. McIntosh, and W. H. Palmer. 1985b. Lifestyle assessment: Just asking makes a difference. British Medical Journal 290:214-216.

Skinner, H. A., S. Holt, W.-J. Sheu, and Y. Israel. 1986. Clinical versus laboratory detection of alcohol abuse: The alcohol clinical index. British Medical Journal 292:1703-1708.

Skinner, W., and W. Becks. 1988. Executive summary: The assessment setting: Should assessment/referral centers be independent of treatment programs? Prepared for the IOM Committee for the Study of Treatment and Rehabilitation Services for Alcoholism and Alcohol Abuse.

Smart, R. G., M. Gillies, G. Brown, and N. L. Blair. 1980. A survey of alcohol-related problems and their treatment. Canadian Journal of Psychiatry 25:220-227.

Sobell, L. C., M. B. Sobell, and T. D. Nirenberg. 1987. Behavioral assessment and treatment planning with alcohol and drug abusers: A review with emphasis on clinical application. Clinical Psychology Review 8:19-54.

Sobell, L. C., M. B. Sobell, G. Leo, and A. Cancilla. 1988. Reliability of a timeline method: assessing normal drinkers' reports of recent drinking and comparative evaluation across several populations. British Journal of Addiction 83:393-402.

Sobell, M. B., L. C. Sobell, and R. VanderSpek. 1979. Relationships among clinical judgment, self-report, and breath-analysis measures of intoxication in alcoholics. Journal of Consulting and Clinical Psychology 47:204-206.

Sobell, M. B., S. Brochu, L. C. Sobell, J. Roy, and J. A. Stevens. 1987. Alcohol treatment outcome evaluation methodology: State of the art 1980-84. Addictive Behaviors 12:113-128.

Stein, K. B., V. Rozynko, and L. A. Pugh. 1977. The heterogeneity of personality among alcoholics. British Journal of Social and Clinical Psychology 10:253-259.

Stockwell, T., D. Murphy, and R. Hodgson. 1983. The Severity of Alcohol Dependence Questionnaire: Its use, reliability, and validity. British Journal of Addiction 78:145-155.

Strayvinski, A., Y. Lamontagne, and Y.-J. Lavallee. 1986. Clinical phobias and avoidant personality disorder among alcoholics admitted to an alcoholism rehabilitation setting. Canadian Journal of Psychiatry 31:714-719.

Sutherland, G., T. Stockwell, and G. Edwards. 1985. The impact of a research interview on clinical re-attendance: A happy finding. British Journal of Addiction 80:211-212.

Syme, L. 1957. Personality characteristics and the alcoholic: A critique of current studies. Quarterly Journal of Studies on Alcohol 18:288-302.

Vaillant, G. E. 1983. The Natural History of Alcoholism: Causes, Patterns, and Paths to Recovery. Cambridge, Mass.: Harvard University Press.

Wanberg, K. W., J. L. Horn, and F. M. Foster. 1977. A differential assessment model for alcoholism: The scales of the Alcohol Use Inventory. Journal of Studies on Alcohol 38:512-543.

Watson, C. G., C. Tilleskjor, E. A. Hoodecheck-Schow, J. Pucel, and L. Jacobs. 1984. Do alcoholics give valid self-reports? Journal of Studies on Alcohol 45:344-348.

Wechsler, D. 1981. Wechsler Adult Intelligence Scale. New York: Psychological Corporation.

White, H. R. 1987. Longitudinal stability and dimensional structure of problem drinking in adolescents. Journal of Studies on Alcohol 48:541-50.

Wilkinson, D. A. 1987. C. T. scan and neuropsychological assessments of alcoholism. Pp. 76-102 in Neuropsychology of Alcoholism, O. A. Parsons, N. Butters, and P. E. Nathan, eds. New York: Guilford Press.

Wilkinson, D. A. 1988. Executive summary: Neuropsychological screening. Prepared for the IOM Committee for the Study of Treatment and Rehabilitation Services for Alcoholism and Alcohol Abuse.

Wilkinson, D. A., and P. L. Carlen. 1981. Chronic organic brain syndromes associated with alcoholism: Neuropsychological and other aspects. Pp. 107-145 in Research Advances in Alcohol and Drug Problems, vol. 6, Y. Israel, F. B. Glaser, H. Kalant, R. E. Popham, and R. G. Smart, eds. New York: Plenum Press.

Wilkinson, D. A., and M. Sanchez-Craig. 1981. Relevance of brain dysfunction to treatment objectives: Should alcohol-related cognitive deficits influence the way we think about treatment? Addictive Behaviors 6:253-260.

Witkin, H. A., and D. R. Goodenough. 1977. Field dependence and interpersonal behavior. Psychological Bulletin 84:661-689.

Woody, G. E., A. T. McLellan, L. Luborsky, C. P. O'Brien, J. Blaine, S. Fox, I. Herman, and A. T. Beck. 1984. Severity of psychiatric symptoms as a predictor of benefits from psychotherapy: The Veterans Administration-Penn Study. American Journal of Psychiatry 141:1172-1177.

11 Matching

Selecting patients properly
Is one of treatment's tricks;
For whether one does well or not
Depends on whom one picks.
—Anonymous

In Chapter 5 of this report the principal conclusion drawn from a review of the available evidence on the efficacy of treatment was that there was no single treatment approach that was effective for all persons with alcohol problems. The chapter went on to state that "reason for optimism in the treatment of alcohol problems lies in the range of promising alternatives that are available, each of which may be optimal for different types of individuals." Research data corroborating these conclusions are extensively reviewed in Appendix B. Matching—that is, selecting from among available alternatives the treatment or treatments that are most likely to facilitate a positive outcome in a particular individual—is a necessary consequence of these conclusions.

Because it has recently received much attention (cf. Annis, 1987; Gordis, 1987; Holden, 1987), matching in the treatment of alcohol problems may appear to be a new concern. *In fact, it has been an object of attention for some time.* The first major review of the treatment of alcohol problems (Bowman and Jellinek, 1941) stressed the need for matching. The first major experimental study of matching in the treatment of alcohol problems, the Winter VA Hospital study, was initiated in 1950 (Wallerstein, 1956, 1957). Matching was advocated in the December 1971 *First Special Report to the U.S. Congress on Alcohol and Health* (USDHEW, 1971), and has also been endorsed in subsequent reports in this series.

However, there *has* been a recent acceleration of interest in matching. Perhaps (as was suggested in the introduction) the passage of time has been required to appreciate the varieties of individuals and problems involved and to develop differing forms of treatment. In recent years there have been multiple reviews of matching in the treatment of alcohol problems (Gibbs and Flanagan, 1977; Pattison, 1978, 1979; Gibbs, 1980; Glaser, 1980; McLellan et al., 1980; Gottheil et al., 1981; Skinner, 1981; Solomon, 1981; Finney and Moos, 1986; Longabaugh, 1986; Miller and Hester, 1986; Annis, 1987, 1988; IOM, 1989). Nor has interest been restricted to the United States and Canada (cf. Matakas et al., 1978; Lindstrom, 1986; Anokhina et al., 1987).

Developments in the treatment of alcohol problems do not occur in a vacuum. As is suggested by the bit of medical student doggerel collected some three decades ago that is the epigraph to this chapter, matching has long been an integral part of medical practice. Differential diagnosis followed by specific treatment is a pattern of clinical activity that dates back to the Hippocratic corpus (Veith, 1964), and remains the hallmark of contemporary medical therapeutics. Consider, for example, the selection of the appropriate varieties, the appropriate sequences, and the appropriate intensities of surgery, radiation, and chemotherapy in the contemporary management of cancers or the careful selection of particular antibiotics to deal with specific infections.

Yet medicine is hardly alone in its use of matching. In education it has become important to recognize "the differential effectiveness of [educational] approaches on different kinds of students" (Hunt, 1971:1). In corrections (in fulfillment of the "object all sublime" of Gilbert and Sullivan's *Mikado*—"to make the punishment fit the crime") it has

279

been recognized that "treatment methods will relate specifically to the goals for the various offender subgroups" (Warren, 1969:48). Psychology has a long history of appreciation of the therapeutic significance of individual differences (Kiesler, 1966; Paul, 1967; Abramowitz et al., 1974; Berzins, 1977; Beutler, 1979), and a growing interest has been developing in psychiatry (Frances et al., 1984; Clarkin and Perry, 1987). Thus, *matching in the treatment of alcohol problems is appropriately viewed not as a unique and idiosyncratic development but as a particular application of a general strategy in human therapeutics.*

Studies of Matching in the Treatment of Alcohol Problems

A brief description of two studies will demonstrate the effect of matching on the outcome of treatment for alcohol problems. One study involved incarcerated offenders with a history of alcohol problems treated with a highly confrontational type of group therapy (Annis, 1979). A retrospective analysis of outcome results from this randomized controlled trial indicated a significant difference in the effect of treatment depending on the self-image of the individual. Persons who entered treatment with a positive self-image achieved outcomes that were significantly better than those of control subjects who were not treated; however, those who entered treatment with a negative self-image did significantly worse than controls. For example, they were reconvicted of crimes more frequently than those who were not treated at all to a significant degree (Annis and Chan, 1983).

The implications of such a study for the future conduct of treatment are straightforward, assuming further validation of the findings. Pursuing them briefly will provide an example of how results from matching studies might influence subsequent clinical practice. The therapy under consideration cannot reasonably be given to all individuals because it will harm some of them (cf. Chapter 6). Rather, individuals should be carefully assessed on the relevant variable(s)—in this case, self-image—prior to a decision regarding treatment. Those who have a positive self-image can be treated by this method with a reasonable expectation of good results; those who do not should be provided with alternative treatments.

In another study the relevant individual variable was "conceptual level," a complex construct derived from educational theory (cf. Hunt, 1971). It was hypothesized that individuals with alcohol problems who operated at a high conceptual level (i.e., were independent, empathic, and cognitively complex) would do better in relatively unstructured therapeutic situations, whereas those who operated at a low conceptual level (i.e., were impulsive, poorly socialized, and cognitively simple) would respond more favorably to directive therapists and structured therapies. The hypothesis was tested simultaneously with respect to initial treatment and aftercare. Those who were correctly matched to either treatment or aftercare did better than those who were mismatched; however, those who were matched to both did strikingly better than those who were matched to neither (77 percent positive results as compared with 38 percent) (McLachlan, 1972, 1974).

Again, the application in practice is quite straightforward, but it involves an extension of the prior example that is instructive. Implementing the findings from this study in practice would involve assessing not only potential clients but also potential therapists and therapies; the properties of both need to be determined to create the appropriate match. This was true as well of the prior example, but there only a single therapeutic approach was considered. Here, multiple approaches as well as multiple therapists would need to be evaluated. In addition, the importance of matching to "aftercare," as well as to initial treatment, is stressed.

The results of these and other studies of matching in the treatment of alcohol problems are summarized in Table 11-1 (slightly modified from Annis, 1988). All of the studies listed involve (a) a reliable matching variable that can distinguish between at least two types of individuals with alcohol problems; (b) at least two well-defined treatment conditions; (c) assignment (preferably random) of each type of individual to each treatment condition; (d) an adequate post-treatment follow-up period; and (e) objective, reliable measure(s) of treatment impact. These elements are considered desirable methodological criteria for the investigation of matching phenomena (Annis, 1988; cf. Hayes et al., 1987).

The studies indicate that *matching individuals to specific treatments on a variety of variables* including demographic factors, psychiatric diagnoses, personality factors, severity of alcohol problems, and antecedents to drinking *has the potential to improve treatment outcome significantly*. These are not the only variables that may be useful but simply those that have been studied to date utilizing an adequate methodology. Nor are these studies the only kind that are capable of shedding light on possible matching effects. Rather, there are a variety of methodologies that can be used to illuminate such effects.

For example, simple outcome monitoring often demonstrates a close association between some particular variable and successful outcome. Of course, this method does not definitively prove that a matching effect has occurred, but it is certainly suggestive. As a next step, the variable (or variables) identified from outcome monitoring as associated with positive outcome can be used as a guide to the matching of a subsequent group of individuals to treatment. The outcomes from the subsequent group can then be compared with those of the previous group. A higher proportion of positive outcomes suggests that (other factors being equal between the two trials) an effective match has been identified.

This "bootstrapping" strategy has been used effectively in the treatment of persons with alcohol and drug problems (McLellan et al., 1980, 1983a). It does not involve the random assignment of individuals to treatments (although such a finding could be tested in a randomized controlled trial as well) but instead is a methodology that is more readily implemented in clinical treatment settings (cf. Chapter 5). It does involve obtaining systematic knowledge of treatment outcomes. Although this practice is not a common one at present, it is rapidly becoming a major requirement for the certification of treatment programs (Schroeder, 1987; Commission on Accreditation of Rehabilitation Facilities, 1988; see also Chapter 12).

Beyond studies that investigate ways in which researchers and treatment personnel may attempt to match patients to treatment programs are studies suggesting that patients may be attempting to match themselves to the most appropriate treatments. For example, there is evidence that patients entering treatment expect to be matched. A careful study of informed consent (Appelbaum et al., 1983), in which elaborate explanations of random assignment to treatment were provided, found that prospective patients persisted in believing, despite what they had been told, that they would in fact be assigned to what-ever treatment the experimenters had concluded was most suitable for them. The implication of the study is that the selection of treatment according to the principle of matching is generally assumed to be an integral element of therapeutics. This view is also held by some therapists (Angell, 1984; Taylor et al., 1984; Imber et al., 1986) and some ethicists (Marquis, 1983).

It has been shown repeatedly that the populations of different treatment programs for alcohol differ significantly from one another (Pattison et al., 1969, 1973; Bromet et al., 1976, 1977; Kern et al., 1978; Skinner and Shoffner, 1978; Finney and Moos, 1979; Skinner, 1981). To some extent, the differences may be due to such factors as eligibility requirements (it is hardly surprising to find more males and more veterans in a Veterans Administration treatment program than in other programs).

Yet differential eligibility requirements and other administrative and practical factors do not appear to provide a complete explanation for the population differences that have been observed among various treatment programs. A belief on the part of individuals that certain programs may serve them better than others—a belief in matching—may contribute importantly to these consistent findings. In programs that are targeted specif-

TABLE 11-1 Findings from Selected Studies on Matching

Study	Matching Variable(s)	Description of Match
Demographic variables		
Azrin et al. (1982)	Marital status	Single persons required behavior therapy in addition to disulfiram for favorable outcome, whereas married persons did well on disulfiram alone.
Mayer and Myerson (1971)	Social stability	Disfulfiram was associated with successful outcomes in persons with low social stability but not in those with high social stability.
Kissin et al. (1970)	Social and psychological stability	Persons with both social and psychological stability did best in psychotherapy; those with social stability only did better in drug therapy; those with neither did best in an inpatient program.
Psychiatric diagnosis (plus alcohol problems)		
Wallerstein (1957)	Various diagnoses	Those diagnosed as compulsive characters did better on disulfiram; those who were passive dependent did better in group hypnotherapy; those who were less aggressive did better in conditioned reflex therapy; those with a "positive attachment factor" did better in milieu therapy.
Tomsovic and Edwards (1970)	Schizophrenia	Persons with alcohol problems but without schizophrenia did better than controls who did not receive lysergic acid diethylamide (LSD); persons with both alcohol problems and schizophrenia who were given LSD did worse than controls.
Merry et al. (1976) Reynolds et al. (1977)	Depression	Depressed persons with alcohol problems had successful outcomes on lithium compared with controls, whereas nondepressed persons with alcohol problems given lithium did worse than controls.
McLellan et al. (1980, 1983)	Psychiatric severity	Persons with high severity did poorly in both inpatient and outpatient treatment; those with low severity did well in both; and those with intermediate severity had outcomes that were sensitive to careful matching to either setting.
Kadden et al. (1990)	Global psychopathology, sociopathy, and neuropsychological impairment	Following inpatient treatment, those high in global psychopathology and sociopathy did better in a relapse prevention group; those high in neuropsychological impairment did better in interactional group psychotherapy.

TABLE 11-1 (continued)

Study	Matching Variable(s)	Description of Match
Personality factors		
McLachlan (1972, 1974)	Conceptual level	High conceptual level individuals did best with nondirective therapists and unstructured aftercare; low conceptual level individuals did best with directive therapists and structured aftercare.
Annis and Chan (1983)	Self-image	Persons with a positive self-image benefited from a highly confrontational form of group therapy, whereas those with a negative self-image did worse than no-treatment controls.
Hartman et al. (1988)	Locus of control	Persons with an internal locus of control did better in brief, unstructured therapy; those with an external locus of control did better in more structured and intensive treatment conditions.
Severity of alcohol problem(s)		
Edwards et al. (1977) Orford et al. (1976)	Jellinek classification	Gamma alcoholics (severe, dependent) did best in intensive treatment; nongamma alcoholics did best with simple advice.
Sokolow et al. (1980) Lyons et al. (1982)	Sex and severity	Females did better in treatment programs that had a medical orientation; males with less severe problems did best in programs with a rehabilitation orientation.
Polich et al. (1981)	Alcohol dependence, age, and marital status	Older (over 40) married individuals with high levels of physical and psychological dependence were less likely to relapse if abstinent; younger unmarried individuals with low levels of dependence were less likely to relapse with nonproblem drinking.
Antecedents to drinking		
Rosenberg (1979)	Anxiety related to drinking	Those with high levels of anxiety related to drinking were markedly improved with relaxation training; those with low levels of anxiety were not improved.
Annis and Davis (1989)	Situational factors	Those who could relate their risk of drinking to specific stressful situations were highly successful with relapse prevention; those who perceived a generalized risk of drinking across all stressful situations had much less favorable outcomes with relapse prevention.

SOURCE: Modified from Annis (1988).

ically at special populations (e.g., women, blacks, Indians), the belief that these programs may serve them better is likely to be responsible for the presence of most of the individuals in the program. Programs for special populations are further discussed in Section IV of this report.

Examples of Matching Programs

There are alternatives to defining matching as the sole responsibility of those seeking treatment. Matching can be carried out by treatment programs themselves. Indeed, this practice may be advisable because matches elected by individuals seeking treatment may speak more to the attractiveness of the treatment than to its probable efficacy and because their judgment may be constrained by the pressures of the problems for which they are seeking relief. It is also highly unlikely that individuals seeking treatment will be fully conversant with all of the available therapeutic alternatives. The foregoing is not to say, however, that individual preferences should not be consulted, a matter that will be discussed in more detail later in this chapter.

When queried, many programs will state that they engage in matching on a regular basis (cf. Maisto and Nirenberg, 1986). However, what is often meant by this response is (a) that they screen potential admissions to their program and do not accept all applicants, and (b) that although they provide the same principal treatment to all persons whom they accept, they also provide supplementary or ancillary services on an individualized basis. Although such practices are commendable they do not, in the committee's view, constitute matching. Matching involves varying the principal treatment approach utilized from one individual to another in accord with a preconceived and explicit plan. For example, the Winter VA Hospital study involved four completely different therapeutic approaches (disulfiram, conditioned reflex therapy, group hypnosis, or milieu therapy) (Wallerstein, 1956, 1957).

The frequency with which programs match to different primary therapies is currently unknown because few studies have examined the question. From an impressionistic standpoint it is not done frequently. Some data suggest a reason may be that few programs offer more than a single major therapeutic option. In a study of all treatment programs for alcohol problems in one state, it was found that only 5 percent of all programs offered two or more such options. These were large programs and serviced approximately 15 percent of all of the individuals in treatment in the state at that time. However, this meant that 85 percent of all individuals in treatment could not have been offered alternative options because there was also evidence that cross-referral between programs was nonexistent (Glaser et al., 1978).

There are programs that have made matching a fundamental part of their clinical operations. As of January 1, 1988, pretreatment assessment and matching to the appropriate level of care are mandated by law in the state of Minnesota for all individuals whose treatment involves the expenditure of public funds (the relevant portions of the law are quoted in Chapter 10). Based on an advisory report issued in 1978 (Marshman et al., 1978), the province of Ontario in Canada has fostered the development of assessment centers that were independent of treatment operations and thus were necessarily engaged in matching. There is evidence that these centers have achieved high levels of community acceptance (Ogborne, Dwyer, and Ekdahl, 1984) and are evaluated as producing positive results (Malla, Rush, Gavin et al., 1985). By 1987 there were some 35 such centers throughout the province (Rush, 1988).

The Brookfield Clinics, a private treatment program for alcohol and drug problems that operates at several sites in the state of Michigan, has for some time based its operations on matching (MacDonnell, 1981; O'Dwyer, 1984, 1988). Another development in the private sector may signal the arrival there of matching on a wholesale basis: the phenomenal rise of utilization management (Lewis, 1988; Korcok, 1988).   At least as currently practiced, utilization management is primarily a mechanism to control costs, but it may also serve to direct individuals to programs that are more effective for them as well as being less expensive. To date, there is some evidence that utilization management is an effective cost-containment strategy (Feldstein et al., 1988); evidence that superior or even equivalent therapeutic results have been produced is not available.

A program tested in the Clinical Institute of Ontario's Addiction Research Foundation, the Core-Shell Treatment Program, attempted to match all individuals seeking treatment for alcohol and drug problems to the most appropriate treatment (cf. Glaser et al., 1984). The central position of matching in the program is illustrated in Figure 11-1. At its center, splayed arrows indicate the multiple matching options that were utilized (Skinner, 1984).

To recapitulate: the matching of particular individuals to specific treatments that are more likely than others to produce positive results has had wide therapeutic application. It has also been a matter of interest in the treatment of alcohol problems for some time. In a large number of studies conforming to specific methodological standards, a variety of variables have been shown to have value in the matching of individuals to more effective treatments for their alcohol problems.

Reviews of these and other studies cited earlier have identified many additional variables that might be useful in matching. Persons entering treatment may expect to be matched to the most appropriate intervention and may engage in efforts at matching on their own. Several clinical treatment programs have been developed recently that use the process of matching as their basis for providing services; in addition, the rapid growth of utilization management may herald the arrival of matching on a very broad basis, indeed (although nothing is currently known about the outcome as opposed to the cost containment effects of utilization management).

Nevertheless, matching can be a complex matter (cf. Finney and Moos, 1986). Few studies are beyond criticism; some of the treatments dealt with in the matching literature are no longer in use, and none of the existing studies has been replicated to date. Further research on matching is indicated and in fact is being actively pursued.   In September 1989 the participants in a multisite collaborative study of matching were selected from a peer-reviewed competition implemented by NIAAA.

Clinical application, however, is not in all instances and under all circumstances necessarily contingent on further research.   Research often performs the function of corroborating the validity of clinical practice. Two illustrative examples can be provided from the history of medicine. Dr. Edward Jenner (1749-1823), who paid attention to the local belief that dairymaids who contracted cowpox were immune to smallpox, introduced the practice of inoculation in 1796. Dr. William Withering (1741-1799) paid attention to the local belief that foxglove was effective against dropsy and introduced it into clinical medicine in 1785. Both proved to be major advances in therapeutics that were adopted and widely used, to good effect, long before the introduction of controlled trials into medicine. Both were based on attentiveness to therapeutic possibilities and empirical observation.

Two caveats must, of course, be posted. The first is that not everything that is claimed to be therapeutic is in fact therapeutic.   Another outcome of research is to demonstrate that treatments believed to be therapeutic are not; regrettably, this seems to be a more frequent outcome than the success that followed Jenner's and Withering's innovations. The second caveat, which follows from the first, is that the need for and the results of research cannot simply be dismissed. The foregoing discussion should not be read as advocating an "anything goes" philosophy in treatment. Rather, the committee ad-

286

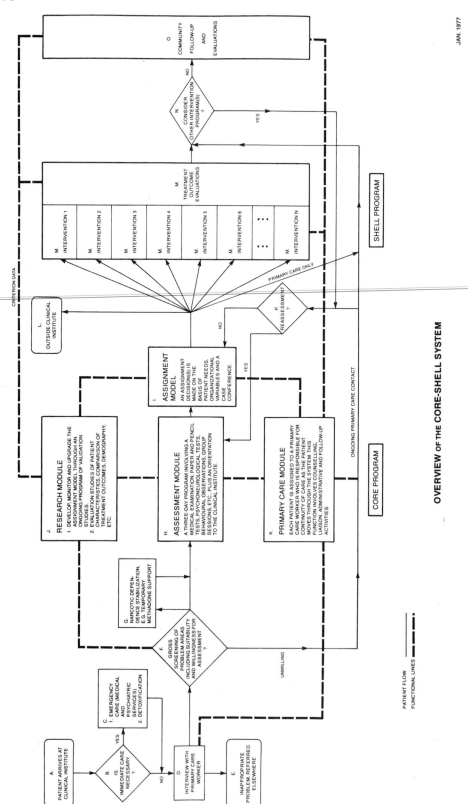

OVERVIEW OF THE CORE-SHELL SYSTEM

JAN 1977

FIGURE 11-1 Flow diagram for the Core-Shell Treatment Program (Skinner, 1984, p. 18). The multiple arrows in the center of the diagram illustrate the matching

vocates a balanced approach in which both practical experience and research findings are carefully weighed to find a reasonable compromise course for the present, always subject to review and reconsideration in the face of additional evidence. At the same time the obligation to provide the best possible treatment in the light of current knowledge must also be recognized. Given that no existing treatment for alcohol problems is universally effective, attempts to match individuals to treatments that are optimal for their particular needs seems to be a practical necessity even at the present time.

How may matching be carried out in a responsible manner prior to the completion of the major research efforts that are only now beginning to get under way? In much the same way as clinical medicine has always proceeded: cautiously, empirically, and collectively. Matching is an issue of central importance around which researchers and clinicians can come together to determine what might best be done given the current state of knowledge.

An appropriate model is the expert committee mechanism that has been employed to good effect by the World Health Organization. Where steps must be taken in an area that has been less than fully illuminated by research, a convening authority brings together a group of persons that is highly knowledgeable to share their information and to put forward, often in writing, their best advice on a particular subject. The committee considers matching to be an ideal focus for such an expert committee because it is the central process in the committee's vision and implies both a need for pretreatment assessment and for the determination of outcome.

One matter that such a committee might consider is the further specification of additional elements of treatment. In Chapter 10 the committee discussed the specification of problems and individuals through the process of assessment. To match individuals to treatment, however, additional kinds of specification are required: a specification of treatments; a specification of matching guidelines; and a specification of outcomes.

If fully specified individuals with fully specified alcohol problems are matched by fully specified matching criteria to fully specified treatment programs, and if the results of these treatment matches are fully specified, sufficient information will be at hand to refine the process so that during the next iteration better results are produced. As noted above, this "bootstrapping" strategy has already been shown to be effective for persons with alcohol and drug problems (McLellan et al., 1980, 1983a). A long-range advantage of adopting this strategy is that, when the results of matching research do become available, just such specifications of the relevant components of treatment will be required for their implementation. Hence, the committee discusses the remaining kinds of specifications in the following pages: those of treatments and of matching guidelines in this chapter and that of outcome in the next.

Specification of Treatment

If individuals seeking treatment are to be matched to particular treatments, there must be detailed knowledge of the treatments that are to be provided. Otherwise, how can a choice be made among them? This requirement is familiar from the practice of referral, for which similar knowledge is required. Often, such knowledge is gained by visiting a program and observing it in action before making referrals. Although this is an excellent strategy, it is problematic in several ways. The time and expense involved may be considerable, and sampling problems may exist; that is, it is sometimes difficult to know whether what one observes under such circumstances is representative of the program's activities.

Moreover, although most programs offer only a single kind of treatment, some programs offer many potentially effective interventions in what has sometimes been referred to as a "smorgasbord approach." As also occurs at table, there is a strong impression that individuals obtaining treatment in these programs often sample a small amount of each intervention, to a degree known only to themselves and not documented in the written record of treatment. Under these circumstances the treatments provided are often not well characterized, and it is not possible to determine what their individual contributions might be to the outcome of treatment.

Reading the written descriptions of the treatment provided is a more efficient alternative than site-visiting all treatment programs, and many such descriptions exist. Often, however, they are neither fully explicit nor consistent with one another. For example, they will indicate that individual psychotherapy is provided but neglect to specify what kind (according to one estimate, there are more than 140 varieties [Karasu, 1977]). Alternatively, one description will contain an explicit statement of the goals of the treatment, whereas another will assume that the goals are understood and omit them.

It would be a happy circumstance if the capability to describe programs was as advanced as the capability to describe individuals and their problems—if, in a word, the assessment of treatment programs was well understood. Unfortunately, this is not the case (see, however, Moos and Daniels, 1967; Moos, 1968; Moos et al., 1973; Moos, 1974). Research studies often involve the development of treatment manuals that fully embody all aspects of the therapeutic interventions that are being tested, so as to be able to specify exactly what the treatment was that did or did not produce positive results. Sometimes these manuals are retranscribed into a form appropriate for clinical application (cf. Sanchez-Craig, 1984). Embodying what is done in treatment in a well-specified treatment manual is a practice that treatment programs might well emulate.

To be maximally useful, the content of such treatment descriptions should be reasonably uniform. That is, it would be important to achieve consensus on those critical dimensions along which programs need to be characterized and on the methods for specifying those dimensions. Following the achievement of consensus the resultant descriptive paradigm could be generally applied to all treatment programs.

In Chapter 3, four dimensions are discussed as general descriptors of treatment programs: the philosophy and orientation of the program (e.g., medical model, social model); the stage of the alcohol problem at which the treatment is directed (e.g., acute intervention, rehabilitation, maintenance); the setting of the program (e.g., inpatient, outpatient, residential), and the modality (e.g., disulfiram, cognitive behavior therapy). All of these descriptors may be important in achieving an appropriate match. Other dimensions that may need to be considered both for matching purposes and to achieve a comprehensive description include an explicit statement of the objectives or goals of the treatment; the criteria for assignment to the treatment and the target population or kind of problem at which the treatment is directed; its length; its intensity; its cost; and a reasonably detailed description of what is expected to occur during the course of treatment.

The general application of a set of uniform descriptive dimensions would create a gazetteer of available treatments that would be of considerable value. For example, if most treatment programs offer only a small complement of interventions, and if they engage in careful matching, they are likely to find it necessary to refer a large number of persons to programs that provide alternative interventions. But how are they to know whether these other programs constitute a better match in terms of the treatments they offer? Only if there is a relatively detailed and uniform method of program description is it likely that an appropriate referral can be made. Conversely, such descriptions make it possible to utilize effectively the full complement of interventions that may be available on a local or regional basis.

Descriptions of treatments constructed along the lines of common dimensions are at present not plentiful, but they do exist. The appendix to this chapter reproduces the so-called Cleveland criteria as an example (Hoffmann et al., 1987). The criteria were developed on the basis of a comprehensive review of both the relevant literature and of "clinical criteria developed by various treatment providers, state agencies, and professional groups" (p. 2). The criteria in the appendix are for the admission of adults to what are termed "levels of care." For each such level (e.g., mutual/self-help, low intensity outpatient treatment, intensive outpatient treatment, etc.) a "programmatic description" is provided along six dimensions—(1) setting, (2) support systems, (3) staff, (4) therapies, (5) assessments/treatment plan review, and (6) documentation.

Although the committee has some problems with the concept of "levels of care," the specification of each component of the treatment system along the same set of descriptive dimensions is an important contribution to the specification of treatment. Another example of treatment specifications are those of the Brookfield Clinics, which were mentioned earlier. They provide an intervention rationale, general objectives, criteria for assignment, and a detailed outline of each session for all interventions provided by the program (P. O'Dwyer, Brookfield Clinics, personal communication, January, 1988).

The potential utility of uniform descriptions goes well beyond matching. Those seeking treatment, for example, might well wish to know the content of the proposed treatment; with rising consumer consciousness in therapeutics, this is increasingly likely. Third-party payers providing reimbursement for treatment might wish to know for what they are paying. For these and other reasons, such explicit descriptions may soon be required.

Specification of Matching Guidelines

Even assuming that adequate specification of individuals, problems, and treatments might be accomplished, there is an additional need to specify how to connect them in the most appropriate manner—that is, for specifying matching guidelines. Several methods can be used to guide the selection of optimal treatment for a particular individual. Far from being mutually exclusive, they are potentially complementary, even if occasionally contradictory. Ideal matching guidelines would take them all into account. The methods include therapist selection of the optimal intervention; patient selection; selection on the basis of the most prominent problem or problems; selection on the basis of theory; selection on the basis of research; and selection on the basis of empirical data about outcome.

Therapist Selection

It seems likely that many therapists select treatments for individuals differentially on the basis of their experience and knowledge. The committee does not doubt that this is in many respects a valid procedure and believes that the knowledge of therapists ought to be tapped systematically in creating guidelines for matching. Unfortunately, there are no data that establish the validity of therapist selection of treatment; the committee could identify no studies of treatment for alcohol problems that compare outcomes from reatments selected by therapists with outcomes from treatments selected in other ways. The lack of data does not necessarily mean that the method lacks validity but only that it has not been studied.

Even though therapists may select treatments for their patients, experience suggests that they do not commonly make explicit the reasons why one treatment was selected in preference to another. However, matching guidelines can be examined carefully only if they are made completely explicit. As well, only if they are explicit can they be shared and ap-

Matching Patient Needs and Treatment Methods

Listed are a series of statements related to specific treatment needs and goals. Read each statement carefully and decide how important this treatment goal is for you. Circle the appropriate response on the accompanying answer sheet.

1. I need a structured inpatient program to learn how to live without taking drugs.
2. I want to make changes in my life-style that I can continue back in the community.
3. I want to learn how to cope more effectively with my urges to drink.
4. I need someone who will know me and help in sorting out my situation.
5. I need to learn better ways of coping with my problems.
6. I want to argue less frequently with my family.
7. I want to learn how to communicate more honestly with my husband/wife.
8. I want to learn better ways of talking with others in a group.
9. I want to learn how to be tense less often.
10. I need help in organizing a more effective job search.
11. I want to learn how to enjoy my free time without using drugs or alcohol.
12. I want to learn how to manage my financial affairs.
13. I want to learn how to improve my physical fitness.
14. I want to take Antabuse or Temposil and stop drinking completely.
15. I would like to learn more about attending Alcoholics Anonymous (A.A.) meetings.
16. I want to stop my illegal use of narcotics.
17. I want to become free of narcotics within six months.
18. I want to stop drinking completely.
19. I want to stop my nonmedical use of drugs.
20. I want to work on my drug problems in an inpatient program with people my own age.
21. I want to understand the conditions under which I tend to drink.
22. I need a half-way house where I can learn how to handle my drinking problems.
23. I would like to have one counsellor I can count on to discuss my problems and concerns.

24. I want an inpatient program that will help me deal with my drinking problems at work.
25. I want a therapist to help me develop a greater awareness of my alcohol (drug) dependence.
26. I want family counselling to help us deal with problems around my drinking or drug use.
27. I want a residential program where I can learn how to get along with others.
28. I need counselling with my husband/wife regarding problems related to my alcohol or drug use.
29. I want to learn how to feel at ease with other people.
30. I want to be able to improve my sleeping patterns.
31. I want to explore new career-educational possibilities.
32. I want to learn how to enjoy my free time along with other responsibilities.
33. I need long-term (six months or more) methadone support.
34. I want a program where I can gradually decrease my dependence on narcotics.
35. I want to stay in a half-way house and develop new interests outside of drinking.
36. I need someone to help me with day-to-day problems like finding a place to stay.
37. I want an inpatient program that will involve my employer.
38. I want a therapist to help me look beneath the surface and find better ways of handling my problems.
39. I need a temporary change (inpatient program) to start working on my alcohol-drug problems.
40. I want to learn how to relax in everyday situations.
41. I want to learn ways of making my work more satisfying.
42. I want to learn how to spend free time out of my home in the community.

FIGURE 11-2 Treatment Goals Inventory for the Core-Shell Treatment Program (Glaser and Skinner, 1981:312-313). Each goal related to a particular treatment offered as part of the program. By indicating which of these goals were theirs, individuals indicated which of the available treatments was a potential match for themselves.

plied in other program settings. This requirement applies not only to guidelines used by therapists, but to matching guidelines derived from any source.

Patient Selection

Some of the problems involved in exclusive dependence on patient selection of major treatment interventions have been noted already. Those seeking treatment may select programs on the grounds of their attractiveness rather than their probable efficacy, may make their choice under the constraint of their problems, and may be unaware of possible alternatives. Nevertheless, reliance upon self-selection—the so-called "cafeteria plan"—has been recommended (Ewing, 1977).

It would certainly be unwise as well as unnecessary to exclude personal preference from the treatment selection process. Attrition from treatment programs characteristically has been high (cf. Baekeland and Lundwall, 1977; Silberfeld and Glaser, 1978; Brandsma et al., 1980). Obviously this will continue to be the case unless a very considerable degree of customer satisfaction can be generated. Involving the person who is to undergo treatment in the treatment selection process may contribute importantly to customer satisfaction and to involvement in treatment. Treatment seekers have been known to make shrewd and interesting choices of therapy (Obitz, 1975). What seems to be required, then, are methods to elicit individual therapeutic preferences on a systematic basis and to combine them with other methods of selecting treatment.

Many possible ways of doing this are available. For example, persons seeking treatment may be most comfortable in treatment programs whose fundamental beliefs about alcohol problems they share. Treatment programs differ on these beliefs; some assign the responsibility for developing alcohol problems and for dealing with them to the person seeking treatment, and others do not (Brickman et al., 1982). Accordingly, one can systematically assess such beliefs in both potential clients and potential treatment programs prior to treatment and take them into account in the matching process.

Another method that has been used is the construction of a treatment goals inventory (Glaser and Skinner, 1981). Each of the therapeutic programs in one system of care was asked to provide three statements in simple terms of what its goals might be. These goals were then organized into a checklist. Individuals being considered for treatment were asked, first, to check off all goals they felt were personally relevant and, second, to select their top five goals in rank order. Since each goal statement was tied to a specific treatment program, the goal choices could be used as an important guideline for matching. Figure 11-2 of this chapter reproduces this goal inventory.

These examples do not exhaust the possible methods for tapping patient preference. Educational programs are another possibility that has been utilized (Bohnen, 1984). Prospective patients have been shown audiovisual presentations of different therapists providing treatment and have been asked to make their selection on this basis (Obitz, 1975). With some ingenuity, it should be quite possible to develop a broad repertory of methods for involving the individual significantly in the selection of treatment, with the hope thereby of assisting him or her to "buy into" the treatment process.

Problem-Oriented Selection

When persons with alcohol problems are assessed, they may be found to have a variety of other problems that may contribute in a crucial manner to their alcohol problems. For some of these problems, specific therapeutic measures are available. For example, if it were felt that an individual's drinking was closely related to his or her marital problems, marital therapy might be indicated. A sample decision sequence of this kind is provided in Figure 11-3 (Skinner, 1981).

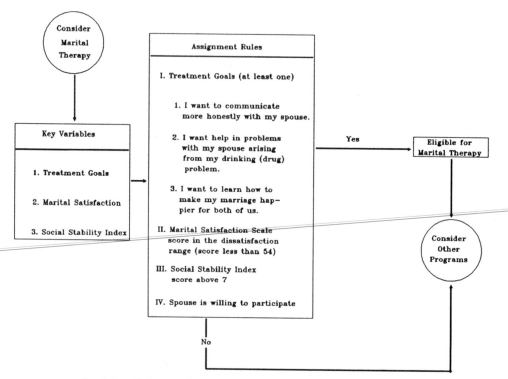

Decision Schema for the OPD Marital Therapy Program.

FIGURE 11-3 An example of problem-oriented selection of treatment (Glaser and Skinner, 1981:319). The selection of the treatment goals of marital therapy and a low score on a marital satisfaction scale were key elements in eligibility for marital therapy on an outpatient basis. Willingness of the spouse to participate and a high social stability score, the latter indicating a reasonable likelihood of sustaining attendance in outpatient treatment, also contributed to eligibility.

In addition, the figure demonstrates the contribution of several kinds of selection guidelines to an ultimate decision regarding treatment selection. The key assessment variables are a treatment goals inventory, a marital satisfaction scale, and a social stability index. To be eligible for outpatient marital therapy, four assignment rules must be satisfied. The person seeking treatment must have selected a marital therapy goal statement as one of their top five goals on the treatment goals inventory; must have scored within the dissatisfaction range on the marital satisfaction scale; must have a reasonable level of social support on the social stability scale to support an outpatient intervention; and must have a spouse who is willing to participate. Exclusion criteria include the presence of a major medical or psychiatric disorder.

A series of similar problem-oriented decision rules may be developed for a whole range of problem-oriented interventions. In our present state of knowledge, rules of this kind are in large measure arbitrary and lack research validation. Still, they are fully explicit and unambiguous; were they to be used, there could be little question about why a particular individual was provided with a particular treatment. They constitute a reasonable point of departure in matching. Because they have been made explicit, they can be tested and modified by subsequent experience.

Theory-driven Selection

Theories of human behavior can be utilized as guidelines for the selection of treatment. Conceptual-level theory, for example, has been used to construct a matching paradigm that subsequently proved to have validity (McLachlan 1972, 1974; see also the description above). Another example is the use of Bandura's self-efficacy theory to derive both a therapeutic approach and a method of matching (Annis, 1986a; Annis et al., 1987; Annis and Davis, 1988; Annis and Davis, 1989).

Theories have the advantage not only of making disparate facts meaningful but of transcending them by leaping from the particular to the universal. Whether such a leap is justified, however, may be problematic; and, in view of the diversity of individuals and problems in the treatment of alcohol problems, universal approaches can only be viewed with some skepticism. A claim that theory-based methods of matching are superior to others is difficult to sustain. Nevertheless, as one among several approaches to the construction of matching guidelines, theory has an important place and one of demonstrated utility.

Research-driven Selection

As is noted earlier, the committee favors the conduct of further research on matching. What has been learned to date is summarized in Table 11-1. Further research is under way, and no doubt it will make an important contribution.

The committee has nevertheless given its reasons for wishing to proceed cautiously and empirically with matching without awaiting the results of further research. As discussed, the principal reason is that, because research carried out to date suggests there is no single treatment method that is effective for all persons seeking assistance, matching is a current necessity. But there are other reasons as well. Many of the limitations of randomized controlled trials that are discussed in Chapter 5 may apply to the resultant research and particularly to the problem of its generalizability. Research conducted primarily or exclusively in academic settings on highly selected subjects treated with comparatively exotic interventions may not be immediately translatable into routine clinical settings. The probable generalizability of research results could be greatly enhanced through careful study design.

Matching research, as it is presently conceptualized, seems to be directed at the elucidation of universal matching guidelines. It may be questioned, however, whether matching guidelines are likely to prove to be universal. Even robust guidelines are likely to be affected by local program conditions (e.g., staffing patterns, unavoidable local variations in the delivery of treatments, specific local traditions and other circumstances; and most guidelines are not likely to be robust. For these and other reasons, research should perhaps be viewed as an important but not an exclusive source of matching guidelines, and the need to evaluate and possibly modify research guidelines when they are applied to particular programs should be accepted as a fact of clinical life.

Data-driven Selection

In Chapter 10 the development of a clinical data base was discussed as a way to provide guidelines for matching to various interventions. To recapitulate that discussion briefly, such a data base contains information on individuals, on their problems, on the treatments they have been provided, and on the outcomes that have ensued. When a subsequent individual approaches treatment, those in the data base having similar characteristics can be readily identified. The known responses of these similar individuals to treatment can then guide the selection of treatment for other individuals.

It was pointed out that this process mimics one of the ways in which an experienced clinician operates. A facet of experience is knowledge about response to various therapeutic approaches and the prediction of future success based on that experience. Thus, in a certain sense this discussion has come full circle and is again addressing selection on the basis of clinical experience. However, the computers that are now commonly the vehicle for clinical data bases can retain and access a larger amount of specific information than can most individuals and (through modern communications techniques) are potentially more widely available for consultation.

Tumor registries are perhaps the most familiar of clinical data bases, although they have not been widely used in the manner described above (Laszlo, 1985). Data bases in other areas have been used in this way (Fries, 1976), and a recommendation has been made (Ellwood, 1988) that, in future, the selection of treatment in medical practice should be largely based on this method. To date, there are no examples of the use of a clinical data base to select treatment for individuals with alcohol problems, but there is no reason in theory why this could not be done.

Such a tactic would have many advantages. One is that it would potentially take into account the uniqueness of local circumstances. However desirable it may be to standardize treatment interventions, and however close it may be possible to come in achieving such standardization, the goal will never be fully achieved. Each program will retain some unique characteristics that will differentiate it from other programs, even of the same kind. For one thing, different people will staff the program. For another, different people will seek treatment there. For yet another, each program will develop its own history, ambience, procedural methods, and so forth.

Other methods of matching (e.g., theory-driven, problem-driven, and research-driven methods) tacitly assume that all programs of a given type are the same; accordingly, they develop assignment rules that are assumed to be universally applicable. An empirically based selection strategy does not necessarily make such an assumption. Rather, by deriving its guidelines from actual outcome experience on a reiterative basis, it takes account of individual program, staff, population, and other differences insofar as they are affecting outcome. In the time-honored phrase, an empirically derived matching strategy deals with treatment "in our hands," and not with all treatment. It is not possible to be certain at this point, in the absence of actual experience, how decisive an advantage this gives to guidelines constructed in this manner. But it may be a substantial advantage.

In summary, there are several approaches to the construction of guidelines for the matching of individuals to treatment programs. Therapist experience, individual preference, the demands of particular problems, theories, research information, and accumulations of empirical outcome data can all be consulted. None of these approaches needs to be viewed as having exclusive validity in comparison with the others, although each has its potential particular advantages. All can be combined to create an explicit and reasonable set of initial guidelines that can then be continuously reappraised and modified. Eventually, the committee believes, a highly effective set of matching guidelines can evolve.

Some Treatment Controversies as Matching Problems

In addition to being a method for the potential improvement of treatment outcomes, matching is a perspective that may help to resolve controversies that arise from time to time in the treatment of alcohol problems. Such controversies sometimes arise from sharply polarized thinking about a given issue. Thinking of this kind has been aptly parodied and paraphrased in the statement that "There are two ways of approaching this problem: my way and the wrong way" (cf. Cook, 1985).

If approaches of this kind can accurately be characterized as either/or approaches, matching can be said to constitute a both/and approach. A simple analogy to the giving of directions may be instructive. One way of giving directions is to assume that there is only one way to get from point A to point B. An alternative is to assume that there are many ways to get to point B—"all roads eventually lead to Rome"—and that what is required is to choose the route best suited to the needs of the individual traveler. Some will wish to get where they are going as directly as possible, while others will prefer the scenic route. Neither group will embark if they cannot take their preferred route.

Two recent areas of discussion may be cited which may benefit from being viewed as problems in matching. One is the issue of inpatient versus outpatient treatment, discussed in the previous chapter. Rather than thinking of either form of treatment as having exclusive validity, one can instead suppose that each is especially valid for some persons with some kinds of problems (cf. Annis, 1986b). The issue then becomes one of developing appropriate matching guidelines that can successfully discriminate who should go where. The so-called Cleveland criteria, noted earlier in the chapter, are a recent example of such guidelines (Hoffmann et al., 1987). At present, they lack empirical validation. But they seem a reasonable place to start and embody the view that no one setting or "level of care" is appropriate for all, while at the same time there may be specific indications for each.

Another active area of discussion has been centered on the appropriate goals of treatment for alcohol problems with respect to the acceptable level of consumption. All are agreed that a reduction in the consumption of alcohol is a principal goal of the treatment of persons with alcohol problems. Some, however, feel that only a reduction to zero consumption is acceptable, whereas others are willing to accept a lesser degree of reduction, depending on individual circumstances.

A matching perspective would suggest that zero consumption is an appropriate goal for some individuals with some kinds of problems but is not necessarily appropriate for others. There is evidence (see Table 11-1) that zero consumption may be a more appropriate, if not always realizable, goal for most persons with substantial or severe alcohol problems; something short of zero consumption, however, may be acceptable for most persons with mild or moderate alcohol problems. (It is likely that appropriate matching here, as elsewhere, will require the use of other information in addition to that regarding severity of the problem—for example, age, sex, cultural background, previous history, and so forth.)

Whatever turns out to be the case—and at this point it is a matter that requires further investigation—the goal must always be to achieve for the individual the optimum possible outcome for him or her, whether or not that outcome happens to be an ideal outcome. For example, one recent set of guidelines stated (in part) the following:

> The [Addiction Research] Foundation strongly advocates that total abstinence is the appropriate treatment goal for persons with severe alcohol or drug problems . . . Irrespective of the Foundation's position in this matter, those with serious alcohol problems who refuse to accept abstinence, despite the consequences and our advice, still require treatment. In these circumstances, the role of the Foundation's therapists is to negotiate treatment plans that will reduce the severity of damage. The Foundation will not refuse treatment or care to a client because he or she is either unwilling or incapable of accepting the Foundation's advice related to abstinence as a treatment goal. (Addiction Research Foundation, 1988:2)

The committee commends the position of the Addiction Research Foundation. Its implementation may require a high degree of flexibility. Uniform goals for all individuals may be a simpler approach, but the notion of different goals for different individuals seems more consistent with the heterogeneity of alcohol problems and the individuals who manifest them. Consistent with its approach on other issues, the committee is prepared to accept differential goals for treatment.

To summarize, matching is not only a useful technique for enhancing the effectiveness of treatment but casts new light on at least some treatment controversies. Two such controversies are those that have been presented as "inpatient versus outpatient treatment" and "controlled drinking versus abstinence." A matching perspective, considered in the context of the broad spectrum of alcohol problems and of those who manifest such problems, moots the adversarial nature of these controversies.

Conclusions and Recommendations

Because the accumulated evidence from treatment outcome studies to date indicates that no single treatment approach is effective for all persons with alcohol problems, the effort to match each person seeking help with that treatment that is most likely to facilitate a positive outcome is now a practical necessity. Some research has been carried out that substantiates the value of matching and provides an indication of how to proceed in this regard. More research, however, would be helpful and is in fact going forward.

However, the committee believes that matching can be carried out at the present time if care is taken to specify the multiple parameters and components of the treatment situation. Individuals and their problems must be specified through a process of comprehensive assessment (see Chapter 10). The treatments to which they are being matched must be specified through the development of explicit and detailed written descriptions, such as those embodied in the treatment manuals that are a feature of some research endeavors; one cannot match to treatments of unspecified content, any more than one can determine the outcome of such treatments when provided in unspecified amounts. The guidelines used to make the match must be specified both in order to be examined and, should they prove effective, in order to be used by others. The outcomes of treatments must be specified for a variety of reasons (see Chapter 12), among them the need to test critically the matching guidelines.

Under these circumstances it is possible to learn whether a positive match has been effected and to proceed accordingly, either utilizing the proposed guidelines if results have been satisfactory or modifying them if they have not been satisfactory. Ideally, this approach would be undertaken as a cooperative effort among many treatment programs so that each could learn from the other. Such an undertaking would facilitate the research effort, and would also enable the results of research to be incorporated into clinical practice without undue delay once they are available.

To facilitate the development and application of matching, it is recommended that an expert committee be convened on a regular basis (perhaps once every two years) to focus on what is currently known about matching individuals with alcohol problems to appropriate treatments. The committee should consist of representatives of major organizations and disciplines involved in the treatment of alcohol problems, and should include both researchers and clinicians. A written report advising the field on how best to proceed with matching, based both on available research and current clinical experience, should be the expected product of each meeting.

REFERENCES

Abramowitz, C. V., S. I. Abramowitz, H. B. Roback, and C. Jackson. 1974. Differential effectiveness of directive and nondirective group therapies as a function of client internal-external control. Journal of Consulting and Clinical Psychology 42:849-853.

Addiction Research Foundation. 1988. The position of the Addiction Research Foundation on reduced substance use as a treatment goal. Approved by Program Policy Committee August 3. Toronto, Ontario, Canada.

Angell, M. 1984. Patients' preference in randomized clinical trials. New England Journal of Medicine 310:1385-1387.

Annis, H. M. 1979. Group treatment of incarcerated offenders with alcohol and drug problems: a controlled evaluation. Canadian Journal of Criminology 21:3-15.

Annis, H. M. 1986a. A relapse prevention model for treatment of alcoholics. Pp. 407-433 in Treating Addictive Behaviors: Processes of Change, W. R. Miller and N. Heather, eds. New York: Plenum Press.

Annis, H. M. 1986b. Is inpatient rehabilitation of the alcoholic cost effective? Con position. Advances in Alcohol and Substance Abuse 5:175-190.

Annis, H. M. 1987. Effective treatment for drug and alcohol problems: What do we know? Presented at the Annual Meeting of the Institute of Medicine, Washington, D.C., October 21.

Annis, H. M. 1988. Optimal treatment for alcoholism and drug dependencies. Presented to Kaiser Permanente, Southern Permanente Medical Group, Los Angeles, California, March 30.

Annis, H. M., and D. Chan. 1983. The differential treatment model: Empirical evidence from a personality typology of adult offenders. Criminal Justice and Behavior 10:159-173.

Annis, H. M., and C. M. Davis. 1988. Assessment of expectancies. Pp. 84-111 in Assessment of Addictive Behaviors, D. M. Donovan and G. A. Marlatt, eds. New York: The Guilford Press.

Annis, H. M., and C. M. Davis. 1989. Relapse prevention. Pp. 170-182 in Handbook of Alcoholism Treatment Approaches: Effective Alternatives, R. K. Hester and W. R. Miller, eds. New York: Pergamon Press.

Annis, H. M., J. M. Graham, and C. S. Davis. 1987. Inventory of Drinking Situations Users Guide. Toronto: Addiction Research Foundation.

Anokhina, I. P., N. N. Ivanets, Y. V. Burov, and B. M. Kogan. 1987. Alcohol and alcohol problems research 13. U.S.S.R. British Journal of Addiction 82:23-30.

Appelbaum, P. S., L. H. Roth, and C. Lidz. 1983. The therapeutic misconception: Informed consent in psychiatric research. International Journal of Law and Psychiatry 5:319-329.

Azrin, N. H., R. W. Sisson, R. Meyers, and N. Godley. 1982. Alcoholism treatment by disulfiram and community reinforcement therapy. Journal of Behavior Therapy and Experimental Psychiatry 13:105-112.

Baekeland, F., and L. K. Lundwall. 1977. Engaging the alcoholic in treatment and keeping him there. Pp. 161-195 in Treatment and Rehabilitation of the Chronic Alcoholic. Vol. 5 of the Biology of Alcoholism. B. Kissin and H. Begleiter, eds. New York: Plenum Press.

Berzins, J. I. 1977. Therapist-patient matching. Pp. 222-251 in Effective Psychotherapy: A Handbook of Research, A. S. Gurman and A. M. Razin, eds. New York: Pergamon Press.

Beutler, L. E. 1979. Toward specific psychological therapies for specific conditions. Journal of Consulting and Clinical Psychology 47:882-897.

Bohnen, E. 1984. Background to the Core-Shell client education programme. Pp. 154-168 in A System of Health Care Delivery, vol. 1, F. B. Glaser, H. M. Annis, H. A. Skinner, S. Pearlman, R. L. Segal, B. Sisson, A. C. Ogborne, E. Bohnen, P. Gazda, and T. Zimmerman. Toronto: Addiction Research Foundation.

Bowman, K. M., and E. M. Jellinek. 1941. Alcohol addiction and its treatment. Quarterly Journal of Studies on Alcohol 2:98-176.

Brandsma, J. M., M. C. Maultsby, Jr., and R. J. Welch. 1980. Outpatient Treatment of Alcoholism: A Review and Comparative Study. Baltimore, Md.: University Park Press.

Brickman, P., V. C. Rabinowitz, J. Karuza, Jr., D. Coates, E. Cohn, and L. Kidder. 1982. Models of helping and coping. American Psychologist 37:368-384.

Bromet, E., R. H. Moos, and F. Bliss. 1976. The social climate of alcoholism treatment programs. Archives of General Psychiatry 33:910-916.

Bromet, E., R. H. Moos, F. Bliss, and C. Wuthmann. 1977. Posttreatment functioning of alcoholic patients: its relation to program participation. Journal of Consulting and Clinical Psychology 45:829-842.

Clarkin, J. F., and S. W. Perry. 1987. Differential therapeutics. Pp. 327-441 in American Psychiatric Association Annual Review, vol. 6, R. E. Hales and A. J. Frances, eds. Washington, D.C.: American Psychiatric Press, Inc.

Commission on Accreditation of Rehabilitation Facilities. 1988. Program Evaluation in Alcoholism and Drug Abuse Treatment Programs. Tucson, Ariz.: Commission on Accreditation of Rehabilitation Facilities.

Cook, D. R. 1985. Craftsman vs. professional: Analysis of the controlled drinking controversy. Journal of Studies on Alcohol 46:433-442.

Edwards, G., J. Orford, S. Egert, S. Guthrie, A. Hawker, C. Hensman, M. Mitcheson, E. Oppenheimer, and C. Taylor. 1977. Alcoholism: A controlled trial of "treatment" and "advice." Journal of Studies on Alcohol 38:1004-1031.

Ellwood, P. M. 1988. Outcomes management: A technology of patient experience. New England Journal of Medicine 318:1549-1556.

Ewing, J. A. 1977. Matching therapy and patients: The cafeteria plan. British Journal of Addiction 72:13-18.

Feldstein, P. J., T. M. Wickizer, and J. R. C. Wheeler. 1988. Private cost containment: The effects of utilization review programs on health care use and expenditures. New England Journal of Medicine 318:1310-1314.

Finney, J. W., and R. H. Moos. 1979. Treatment and outcome for empirical subtypes of alcoholic patients. Journal of Consulting and Clinical Psychology 47:25-38.

Finney, J. W., and R. H. Moos. 1986. Matching patients to treatments: Conceptual and methodological issues. Journal of Studies on Alcohol 47:122-134.

Frances, A., J. Clarkin, and S. Perry. 1984. Differential Therapeutics in Psychiatry: The Art and Science of Treatment Selection. New York: Brunner/Mazel.

Fries, J. F. 1976. A data bank for the clinician? New England Journal of Medicine 294:1400-1402.

Gibbs, L. E. 1980. A classification of alcoholics relevant to type-specific treatment. International Journal of the Addictions 15:461-488.

Gibbs, L. E., and J. Flanagan. 1977. Prognostic indicators of alcoholism treatment outcome. International Journal of the Addictions 12:1097-1141.

Glaser, F. B. 1980. Anybody got a match? Treatment research and the matching hypothesis. Pp. 178-196 in Alcoholism Treatment in Transition, G. Edwards and M. Grant, eds. London: Croom Helm.

Glaser, F. B., and H. A. Skinner. 1981. Matching in the real world: A practical approach. Pp. 295-324 in Matching Patient Needs and Treatment Methods in Alcoholism and Drug Abuse, E. A. Gottheil, A. T. McLellan, and K. A. Druley, eds. Springfield, Ill.: Charles C. Thomas.

Glaser, F. B., S. W. Greenberg, and M. Barrett. 1978. A Systems Approach to Alcohol Treatment. Toronto: ARF Books.

Glaser, F. B., H. M. Annis, H. A. Skinner, S. Pearlman, R. L. Segal, B. Sisson, A. C. Ogborne, E. Bohnen, P. Gazda, and T. Zimmerman. 1984. A System of Health Care Delivery, 3 vol. Toronto: Addiction Research Foundation.

Gordis, E. 1987. Accessible and affordable health care for alcoholism and related problems: Strategy for cost containment. Journal of Studies on Alcohol 48:579-585.

Gottheil, E. A., A. T. McLellan, and K. A. Druley, eds. 1981. Matching Patient Needs and Treatment Methods in Alcoholism and Drug Abuse. Springfield, Ill.: Charles C. Thomas.

Hartman, L., M. Krywonis, and E. Morrison. 1988. Psychological factors and health-related behavior change: Preliminary findings from a controlled clinical trial. Canadian Family Physician 34:1045-1050.

Hayes, S. C., R. O. Nelson, and R. B. Jarrett. 1987. The treatment utility of assessment: A functional approach to evaluating assessment quality. American Psychologist 42:963-974.

Hoffmann, N. G., J. A. Halikas, and D. Mee-Lee. 1987. The Cleveland Admission, Discharge, and Transfer Criteria: Model for Chemical Dependency Treatment Programs. Cleveland, Ohio: The Greater Cleveland Hospital Association.

Holden, C. 1987. Alcoholism and the medical cost crunch. Science 235:1132-1133.

Hunt, D. E. 1971. Matching Models in Education: The Coordination of Teaching Methods with Student Characteristics. Toronto: Ontario Institute for Studies in Education.

Imber, S. D., L. M. Glanz, I. Elkin, S. M. Sotsky, J. L. Boyer, and W. R. Leber. 1986. Ethical issues in psychotherapy research: problems in a collaborative clinical trials study. American Psychologist 41:137-146.

Institute of Medicine (IOM). 1989. Prevention and Treatment of Alcohol Problems: Research Opportunities. Washington, D.C.: National Academy Press.

Kadden, R. M., N. L. Cooney, H. Getter, and M. D. Litt. 1990. Matching alcoholics to coping skills or interactional therapies: post treatment results. Journal of Consulting and Clinical Psychology 57:698-704.

Karasu, T. B. 1977. Psychotherapies: An overview. American Journal of Psychiatry 134:851-863.

Kern, J. C., W. Schmelter, and M. Fanelli. 1978. A comparison of three alcoholism treatment populations: Implications for treatment. Journal of Studies on Alcohol 39:785-792.

Kiesler, D. J. 1966. Some myths of psychotherapy research and the search for a paradigm. Psychological Bulletin 65:110-136.

Kissin, B., A. Platz, and W. H. Su. 1970. Social and psychological factors in the treatment of chronic alcoholism. Journal of Psychiatric Research 8:13-27.

Korcok, M. 1988. Managed Care and Chemical Dependency: A Troubled Relationship. Providence, R.I.: Manisses Communications Group, Inc.

Laszlo, J. 1985. Health registry and clinical data base technology: With special emphasis on cancer registries. Journal of Chronic Diseases 38:67-78.

Lewis, J. S. 1988. Growth in managed care forcing providers to adjust. The Alcoholism Report 16(24):1.

Lindstrom, L. 1986. Val av Behandlung for Alkoholism. Malmo: Liber Forlag.

Longabaugh, R. 1986. The matching hypothesis: Theoretical and empirical status. Presented at the Annual Meeting of the American Psychological Association, Washington, D.C., August 24.

Lyons, J. P., J. Welte, J. Brown, L. Sokolow, and G. Hynes. 1982. Variation in alcoholism treatment orientation: Differential impact upon specific subpopulations. Alcoholism: Clinical and Experimental Research 6:333-343.

MacDonnell, F. J. 1981. How effective are our current methodologies for the treatment of alcoholism? EAP Digest 2(1):32-35.

Maisto, S. A., and T. D. Nirenberg. 1986. The relationship between assessment and alcohol treatment. Presented at the Annual Meeting of the American Psychological Association, Washington, D.C., August 24.

Malla, A. K., B. Rush, M. Gavin, and G. Cooper. 1985. A community-centred alcoholism assessment/treatment service: A descriptive study. Canadian Journal of Psychiatry 30:35-43.

Marquis, D. 1983. Leaving therapy to chance. Hastings Center Report 13(4):40-47.

Marshman, J., R. D. Fraser, C. Lambert, A. C. Ogborne, S. J. Saunders, P. W. Humphries, D. W. Macdonald, J. G. Rankin, and W. Schmidt. 1978. The Treatment of Alcoholics: An Ontario Perspective. Toronto: Addiction Research Foundation.

Matakas, F., H. Koester, and B. Leidner. 1978. Welche Behandlung fur welche Alkoholiker. Psychiatrische Praxis 5:143-152.

Mayer, J., and D. J. Myerson. 1971. Outpatient treatment of alcoholics: Effects of status, stability, and nature of treatment. Quarterly Journal of Studies on Alcohol 32:620-627.

McLachlan, J. F. C. 1972. Benefit from group therapy as a function of patient-therapist match on conceptual level. Psychotherapy: Theory, Research, and Practice 9:317-323.

McLachlan, J. F. C. 1974. Therapy strategies, personality orientation, and recovery from alcoholism. Canadian Psychiatric Association Journal 19:25-30.

McLellan, A. T., C. P. O'Brien, R. Kron, A. I. Alterman, and K. A. Druley. 1980. Matching substance abuse patients to appropriate treatment methods: A conceptual and methodological approach. Drug and Alcohol Dependence 5:189-195.

McLellan, A. T., G. E. Woody, L. Luborsky, C. P. O'Brien, and K. A. Druley. 1983a. Increased effectiveness of substance abuse treatment: A prospective study of patient-treatment "matching." Journal of Nervous and Mental Diseases 171:597-605.

McLellan, A. T., L. Luborsky, G. E. Woody, C. P. O'Brien, and K. A. Druley. 1983b. Predicting response to alcohol and drug abuse treatments: Role of psychiatric severity. Archives of General Psychiatry 40:620-25.

Merry, J., C. M. Reynolds, J. Bailey, and A. Coppen. 1976. Prophylactic treatment of alcoholism by lithium carbonate: A controlled study. Lancet 2:481-482.

Miller, W. R., and R. K. Hester. 1986. Matching problem drinkers with optimal treatments. Pp. 175-203 in Treating Addictive Behaviors: Processes of Change, W. R. Miller and N. Heather, eds. New York: Plenum Press.

Moos, R. H. 1968. Differential effects of ward settings on psychiatric patients: A replication and extension. Journal of Nervous and Mental Diseases 147:386-393.

Moos, R. H. 1974. Evaluating Treatment Environments: A Social Ecological Approach. New York: John Wiley and Sons.

Moos, R. H., and D. N. Daniels. 1967. Differential effects of ward settings on psychiatric staff. Archives of General Psychiatry 17:75-82.

Moos, R. H., R. Shelton, and C. Petty. 1973. Perceived ward climate and treatment outcome. Journal of Abnormal Psychology 82:291-298.

Obitz, F. W. 1975. Alcoholics' perceptions of selected counseling techniques. British Journal of Addiction 70:187-191.

O'Dwyer, P. 1984. Cost effective rehabilitation: A process of matching. EAP Digest 4(2):33-34.

O'Dwyer, P. 1988. Executive summary: Assessment procedures currently used by alcohol treatment programs. Prepared for the IOM Committee for the Study of Treatment and Rehabilitation Services for Alcoholism and Alcohol Abuse.

Ogborne, A. C., D. Dwyer, and A. Ekdahl. 1984. The Niagara Alcohol and Drug Assessment Service: Referral Patterns, Client Characteristics, and Community Reactions. Toronto: Addiction Research Foundation.

Orford, J., E. Oppenheimer, and G. Edwards. 1976. Abstinence or control: The outcome for excessive drinkers two years after consultation. Behavior Research and Therapy 14:409-418.

Pattison, E. M. 1978. Differential approaches to multiple problems associated with alcoholism. Contemporary Drug Problems 7:265-309.

Pattison, E. M. 1979. The selection of treatment modalities for the alcoholic patient. Pp. 126-227 in The Diagnosis and Treatment of Alcoholism, J. H. Mendelson and N. K. Mello, eds. New York: McGraw-Hill Book Company.

Pattison, E. M., R. Coe, and R. J. Rhodes. 1969. Evaluation of alcoholism treatment: A comparison of three facilities. Archives of General Psychiatry 20:478-488.

Pattison, E. M., R. Coe, and H. O. Doerr. 1973. Population variation among alcoholism treatment facilities. International Journal of the Addictions 8:199-229.

Paul, G. L. 1967. Strategy of outcome research in psychotherapy. Journal of Consulting Psychology 31:109-118.

Polich, J. M., D. J. Armor, and H. B. Braiker. 1981. The Course of Alcoholism: Four Years After Treatment. New York: John Wiley and Sons.

Reynolds, C. M., J. Merry, and A. Coppen. 1977. Prophylactic treatment of alcoholism by lithium carbonate: An initial report. Alcoholism: Clinical and Experimental Research 1:109-111.

Rosenberg, S. D. 1979. Relaxation Training and a Differential Assessment of Alcoholism. Ann Arbor, Mich.: Dissertation Abstracts International (University Microfilms No. 8004362).

Rush, B. 1988. Executive summary: Assessment procedures and specialized assessment in Ontario. Prepared for the IOM Committee for the Study of Treatment and Rehabilitation Programs for Alcoholism and Alcohol Abuse.

Sanchez-Craig, M. 1984. Therapist's Manual for Secondary Prevention of Alcohol Problems: Procedures for Teaching Moderate Drinking and Abstinence. Toronto: Addiction Research Foundation.

Schroeder, S. A. 1987. Outcome assessment 70 years later: Are we ready? New England Journal of Medicine 316:160-162.

Silberfeld, M., and F. B. Glaser. 1978. Use of the life table method in determining attrition from treatment. Journal of Studies on Alcohol 39:1582-1590.

Skinner, H. A. 1981. "Different strokes for different folks": Differential treatment for alcohol abuse. Pp. 349-367 in Evaluation of the Alcoholic: Implications for Research, Theory, and Treatment, R. E. Meyer, T. F. Babor, B. C. Glueck, J. H. Jaffe, J. E. O'Brien, and J. R. Stabenau, eds. Washington, D.C.: U. S. Government Printing Office.

Skinner, H. A. 1984. An overview of the Core-Shell Treatment System. Pp. 17-26 in A System of Health Care Delivery, vol. 1, F. B. Glaser, H. M. Annis, H. A. Skinner, S. Pearlman, R. L. Segal, B. Sisson, A. C. Ogborne, E. Bohnen, P. Gazda, and T. Zimmerman. Toronto: Addiction Research Foundation.

Skinner, H. A., and K. R. Shoffner. 1978. Sex differences and addiction: A comparison of male and female clients at the Clinical Institute. Toronto: Addiction Research Foundation.

Sokolow, L., J. Welte, G. Hynes, and J. Lyons. 1980. Treatment-related differences between female and male alcoholics. Focus on Women—Journal of Addictions and Health 1:42-56.

Solomon, S. D. 1981. Tailoring Alcoholism Therapy to Client Needs. Washington, D.C.: U. S. Government Printing Office.

Taylor, K. M., R. Margolese, and C. L. Soskolne. 1984. Physicians' reasons for not entering eligible patients in a randomized clinical trial of surgery for breast cancer. New England Journal of Medicine 310:1363-1367.

Tomsovic, M., and R. V. Edwards. 1970. Lysergide treatment of schizophrenic and nonschizophrenic alcoholics: A controlled evaluation. Quarterly Journal of Studies on Alcohol 31:932-949.

U.S. Department of Health, Education, and Welfare. 1971. First Special Report to the U. S. Congress on Alcohol and Health. Rockville, Md.: National Institute on Alcohol Abuse and Alcoholism.

Veith, I. 1964. The infancy of psychiatry. Bulletin of the Menninger Clinic 28:186-197.

Wallerstein, R. S. 1956. Comparative study of treatment methods for chronic alcoholism: The alcoholism research project at Winter VA Hospital. American Journal of Psychiatry 113:228-233.

Wallerstein, R. S. 1957. Hospital Treatment of Alcoholism: A Comparative, Experimental Study. New York: Basic Books.

Warren, M. Q. 1969. The case for differential treatment of delinquents. Annals of the American Academy of Political and Social Science 381:47-59.

Appendix: Excerpts From The Cleveland Admission, Discharge and Transfer Criteria

The *Cleveland Admission, Discharge and Transfer Criteria* are guidelines for use by treatment providers in documenting placement decisions, by third party payors in monitoring placement, and by researchers in evaluating treatment. The guidelines were prepared for the Northern Ohio Chemical Dependency Treatment Directors Association by the CATOR/Ramsey Clinic and published by the Greater Cleveland Hospital Association (Hoffman et al., 1987:3-33). In their original form the *Cleveland Criteria* include criteria for both adults and adolescents. Only portions of the adult criteria are reproduced in this appendix. The criteria are presented as guidelines to be used carefully with consideration of both individual and combinations of symptoms when making placement decisions. Exceptions based on extenuating circumstances (e.g., admission to a higher level than that specified in the guidelines) require presentation of further justification.

Overview of Adult Admission Criteria

Diagnosis

In general all individuals accepted for the treatment of chemical dependency in these levels of care are expected to have met diagnostic criteria for a psychoactive substance use disorder as defined by DSM-III, DSM-III-R or other standardized and widely accepted criteria. Exceptions to this would be individuals who have experienced only a few problems or adverse consequences as a result of their use and who would benefit from further assessment or low levels of therapeutic involvement.

It is assumed that diagnostic assessment typically can be accomplished in two to four hours of contact time with adult patients. This may need to be extended in some unusual cases or where the collection of collateral information is necessary.

Levels of Care

Levels of care have been identified which reflect the general consensus of a wide range of previously developed criteria available to this project. The type and extent of treatment services necessary define each level, not the specific site of the services. Staffing and local factors also contribute more to costs and charges than simply the site of the program.

These criteria assume not only that the levels of care are available, but also that they are reimbursed at an adequate rate. Numerous illustrations can be found where reimbursement policies or logistical and economic factors effectively preclude provision of services at a given level of care. It is assumed that clinical parameters and standards of care, *not* economic policies, are the driving force for the appropriate treatment placement.

The criteria are designed to place individuals into an appropriately intensive treatment level in accordance with appropriate standards of clinical practice. Movement between levels typically is expected to be from a higher, or more intense, level to a lower level as the patient's treatment progress warrants.

Any clinical criteria should be considered as guidelines which must evolve with advances in clinical procedures and with accumulating empirical evidence.

Placement Criteria Consideration

Two factors must be considered in making treatment placement decisions which override the patient-treatment match determined by these criteria: (1) prior treatment failure and (2) availability of the criteria-selected level of care.

A treatment failure at any given level of care indicates the need for treatment at a *higher* level of care, unless the patient is uncooperative or would not benefit from such a treatment placement. These criteria attempt to minimize the occurrence of failures by initially placing individuals into an appropriately intense level of care. However, the explicit incorporation of documented prior treatment failures provides for a correction mechanism when a failure occurs.

The second consideration is the availability of the optimal level of care indicated by the criteria. If that level is not available, the next higher level of care available should be utilized rather than a less adequate lower level of treatment.

Both of these considerations should be relatively automatic and not require extensive justification for utilization review or reimbursement.

While these criteria are intended to be as inclusive as possible, unique clinical presentation or extenuating circumstances may require some flexibility in the application of the criteria to insure the safety and welfare of the patient.

Dimensions for Making Placement Decisions

The following seven dimensions have been identified as the general assessment dimensions used nationally in treatment placement criteria and guidelines. These dimensions are analogous to the categories in the routine medical "Review of Systems."

1. Acute alcohol and/or drug intoxication and/or withdrawal potential;
2. Physical complications;
3. Psychiatric complications;
4. Life areas impairments;
5. Treatment acceptance/resistance;
6. Loss of control/relapse crisis;
7. Recovery environment.

LEVEL I: MUTUAL/SELF-HELP

A. Brief Description of Treatment Level

This level of care encompasses services provided by organizations such as Alcoholics Anonymous, Narcotics Anonymous, Cocaine Anonymous, Alateen, Emotions Anonymous and other mutual self-help groups. It may also include other formal social support or peer groups that do not rely on other recovering persons to provide mutual/self-help support and therapeutic milieu.

The principal criterion for admission to mutual/self help groups is that the individual wishes to stop using alcohol and/or other mood altering substances. There is no role for formal diagnostic determinations at this level; however, individuals may seek to reflect on their substance use and its consequences (a self-assessment).

B. Programmatic Description

1. *Setting*
Any appropriate setting for group meetings and peer counseling.

2. *Support systems*
No direct support required, but a referral list or mechanism for referral to treatment and other services is highly recommended.

3. *Staff*
No professional staff required. Volunteers typically provide administrative services.

4. *Therapies*
Peer interaction/mutual help.

5. *Assessments/treatment plan review*
Self/peer assessment.

6.   *Documentation*
        None required.

C. Brief Description of Typical Patient

Individuals who feel they may have an alcohol/drug use problem may seek the advice and counsel of peers based on trust, respect, and privacy in a mutual self-help setting. Patients who require professional assessment or treatment services would not be appropriate for Level I care alone.

D. Dimensional Admission Criteria

No formal admission criteria are required for this level; however, the following specifications are suggested.

1.   *Acute alcohol and/or drug intoxication and/or potential withdrawal*
        a.   History of recent or current drinking and/or drug use may be evident;
        b.   No indication of serious physical complications due to current intoxication or withdrawal.

2.   *Physical conditions and complications*
        a.   Physical state is sufficiently stable to permit participation in mutual help treatment.

3.   *Psychiatric conditions or complications*
        a.   Any anxiety, guilt, and/or depression present is (are) related to chemical use rather than another psychiatric condition;
        b.   Mental state sufficiently stable to permit participation in mutual self help;
        c.   Sufficient cognitive functioning to understand the requirements of mutual help.

4.   *Life areas impairment*
        a.   Subjective report of problems related to use;
        b.   Evidence of adverse consequences (vocational, social, or legal) related to use may be evident.

5.   *Treatment acceptance/resistance*
        a.   Willingness to cooperate and attend activities;
        b.   Feels that life areas impairment is associated with alcohol/drug use or wishes to use mutual self help to self-evaluate status of use.

6.   *Loss of control/relapse crises*
        a.   Acknowledges personal problem with use.

7.   *Recovery environment*
        a.   Sufficient environmental stability to indicate safe and adequate living conditions and support of recovery goals.

* * *

LEVEL II: LOW INTENSITY OUTPATIENT TREATMENT

A.   **Brief Description of Treatment Level**

Low Intensity Outpatient Treatment is the provision of outpatient services by appropriately trained professionals. This level of care involves weekly sessions usually supplemented by involvement in Mutual/Self Help. As in primary treatment, intensity typically does not exceed 10 contact hours per week over a period of one to three months. This level of care may be utilized in maintenance services for persons who have recently completed a more intensive level of care. Such maintenance treatment typically involves no more than four hours per week for a period of up to one year. This level of care also may be appropriate for protracted evaluation of patients who require some additional time to make a commitment to a more intensive recovery effort.

B.   **Programmatic Description**

1.   *Setting*
Any appropriate professional setting.

2.   *Support systems*
Contractual availability of specialized professional consultation and supervision.

3.   *Staff*
Any appropriately trained personnel, e.g., certified chemical dependency counselors, licensed mental health professionals, etc.

4.   *Therapies*
Focused counseling and/or medical monitoring.

5.   *Assessment/treatment plan review*
Documented initial treatment plan with update at least every 30 days.

6.   *Documentation*
Problem oriented progress notes at each visit.

C.   **Brief Description of Typical Patient**

For admission to this level of care the patient should have few or no continuing symptoms of withdrawal or intoxication; manifest only stable (if any) physical or psychiatric conditions; demonstrate sufficient motivation and supportive environmental factors to participate in a low intensity, low control treatment program. A typical patient at this level may have completed a more intensive program but still requires maintenance services.

Patients inappropriate for Level II include those who are at risk for imminent relapse without more intensive services and/or those who cannot stay focused on recovery efforts and goals because the severity of any of the criteria dimensions distracts them from following through with a low intensity plan.

D.   **Dimensional Admission Criteria**

Admission to this level of care requires meeting the specifications in all of the following seven dimensions:

1.   *Acute alcohol and/or drug intoxication and/or potential withdrawal*
a.   Discharge referral from a higher level of care or;
b.   One of the following:
(1)   History of recent or current drinking and/or drug use;
(2)   Mild symptoms related to withdrawal such as: headaches, insomnia, vague somatic complaints;
(3)   History of withdrawal syndrome with withdrawal symptoms that can safely be managed without medical intervention.

2.   *Physical conditions or complications*
a.   Any physical conditions, if present, are sufficiently stable to permit participation in outpatient treatment.

3.   *Psychiatric conditions or complications-all of the following:*
a.   Significant anxiety, guilt, and/or depression, if present, are related to chemical dependency problems rather than another psychiatric condition;
b.   Mental state is sufficiently stable to permit participation in the outpatient treatment program;
c.   Sufficient comprehension to understand the materials presented.

4.   *Life areas impairment-one of the following:*
a.   Absence from work as a consequence of substance use;
b.   Occupational difficulties as a consequence of substance use;
c.   Legal difficulties as a consequence of substance use;

d.   Deteriorating job performance as a consequence of substance use;

e.   Damage of personal relationships as a consequence of substance use;

f.   Documentation of substance use great enough to damage social functioning as a consequence of substance use;

g.   Patient has completed a more intensive program but still requires services until recovery efforts result in additional stability.

5.   *Treatment acceptance/resistance-all of the following*:

        a.   Willingness to participate in the treatment program and attend all scheduled activities;

        b.   Evidence that the patient has restorative potential (e.g., accepts treatment; absence of organic mental disorder that would prevent improvement);

        c.   Willing to work toward recovery goals with minimal supervision.

6.   *Loss of Control/Relapse Crises-either of the following*:

        a.   Recent history of use despite commitment not to use;

        b.   Patient is able to maintain short term abstinence goals with support and therapeutic contact.

7.   *Recovery environment-all of the following:*

        a.   Sufficiently supportive psychosocial environment for low intensity outpatient treatment (e.g., significant others in agreement with recovery efforts; supportive work or legal coercion);

        b.   Lack of environmental impediments to recovery (e.g., adequate transportation to program, accessibility of support meeting locations);

        c.   Adequate environmental stability to indicate safe adequate living conditions and support of recovery goals (e.g., spouse is not active alcoholic).

* * *

LEVEL V: MEDICALLY SUPERVISED INTENSIVE INPATIENT TREATMENT

A.   **Brief Description of Treatment Level**

This level of care utilizes a multidisciplinary staff for patients whose physical, psychiatric, and/or psychosocial problems are severe enough to require inpatient services. Twenty-four hour observation, monitoring, and treatment should be available; however, the full resources of an acute care general hospital system are not necessary. The treatment is specific to chemical dependency, but the multidisciplinary team and availability of support services allows for the conjoint treatment of coexisting physical and/or psychiatric condition(s) which could jeopardize recovery.

B.   **Programmatic Description**

1.   *Setting*
A free-standing residential facility or specialty hospital with a chemical dependency treatment unit. General hospitals may also have units at this level of care, but the full resources of such a medical system are not essential for this level of care.

2.   *Support systems*
Availability of specialized professional consultation and supervision; direct affiliation with more intensive levels of care.

3.   *Staff*
Multidisciplinary team of appropriately trained professionals; 24 hour availability of physician with direct patient management as necessary; 24 hour skilled nursing care and observation (16 hours of nursing coverage if based in a JCAH approved general or psychiatric hospital where supplemental nursing coverage is available); counseling services are available on site 16 hours per day.

4.   *Therapies*
A multidisciplinary team will be available to meet the individual needs of each patient; at least four skilled treatment services will be provided per day for at least five days per week. Skilled treatment services include but are not limited to: psychotherapy, family

therapy, individual and groups counseling, educational groups, occupational and recreational therapy.

5.   *Assessments/treatment plan review*
Documented initial treatment plan; ongoing reassessment; weekly update of treatment plan by multidisciplinary treatment team.

6.   **Documentation**
Daily problem orientation progress notes.

C.   **Brief Description of Typical Patient**

Admission to this level of care requires at least one of the following: a significant likelihood of the development of a withdrawal syndrome; previous history of having failed at attempts at outpatient withdrawal; the presence of a medical condition serious enough to warrant inpatient management; the presence of isolated medical symptoms of concern; external mandates for inpatient treatment; a recent history of inability to function without some externally applied behavioral controls; and significant denial of the severity of his/her own addiction. In addition, high motivation for a multifaceted intensive inpatient treatment program does not preclude admission to an inpatient setting provided other criteria are met. In addition, loss of control or impending relapse crises is suitable for the level of care. Detrimental recovery environmental factors likely to prevent a patient from maintaining treatment progress merits admission to this level of treatment.

D.   **Dimensional Admission Criteria**

Admission to this level of care requires the presence of one or more symptoms from at least one of the following seven dimensions.

1.   *Acute alcohol and/or drug intoxication and/or potential withdrawal-at least one of the following:*

a.   Patient is in need of 24 hour observation and/or skilled nursing care;
b.   History of significant multiple alcohol/drug ingestion during present episode;
c.   Failure of ambulatory detoxification;
d.   Inability to continue in, or lack of availability of, ambulatory alcohol/drug detoxification program;
e.   Motor and/or gait incoordination;
f.   For opioid withdrawal-the presence of two or more withdrawal symptoms warrants admission: Rhinorrhea; lacrimation; mydriasis; piloerection; bone pain; diarrhea.

2.   *Physical conditions or complications-at least one of the following:*
a.   Physical conditions related to the excessive use of alcohol and/or drugs (e.g., metabolic abnormalities, which are not life threatening but impair physiological functioning, severe enough to warrant inpatient treatment, such as unstable diabetes);
b.   Documentation of alcohol/drug use great enough to damage physical health.

3.   *Psychiatric conditions or complications-at least one of the following:*
a.   Significant depression but no active suicidal ideation;
b.   Recent death or other significant personal loss causing daily distress and distraction from recovery efforts;
c.   Overly complaint and pathologically dependent personality disorders that interfere with recovery without direct intervention e.g., individual who needs intensive therapy interventions to improve recovery chance);
d.   Histrionic display of emotions or hostile dependency with attempts to have others take responsibility.

4.   *Life areas impairment-at least one of the following:*
a.   Violent behavior while intoxicated;
b.   The patient has demonstrated an inability to sustain independent functioning without a controlled environment;
c.   Legal system (e.g., probation officer, courts, etc.) mandates the patient to participate in an inpatient treatment program.

[Note: a court order or legal mandate resulting from criminal behavior or civil commitment should not require a treatment program to accept a patient that the staff feels is inappropriate for that program or facility. Likewise, adequate reimbursement for treatment dictated by such mandate should be the responsibility of the court.];

d. Treatment mandated by employee assistance referral program.

5. *Treatment acceptance/resistance-at least one of the following:*

   a. Absence from three or more scheduled outpatient treatment sessions without adequate explanation, arrangement, or documentation;
   b. Significant denial and minimization of the effects of chemical dependency which would prevent the patient from following through with rehabilitative care in a lesser setting;

6. *Loss of control/relapse crisis-at least one of the following:*

   a. Currently unable to effectively control chemical use at the time of evaluation;
   b. Requires the continuous use of alcohol and/or other drugs in order to function adequately;
   c. If abstinent, the patient is experiencing an acute crisis and feels himself going out of control and possibly reactivating his/her addiction and outpatient services have failed to improve the crisis;
   d. Demonstrated inability to remain substance free for at least five days;
   e. Failure to maintain abstinence while engaged in an outpatient program.

7. *Recovery environment-at least one of the following*:

   a. Actual or threatened major losses (e.g., death, divorce, job change);
   b. Severe isolation or withdrawal from social contacts;
   c. Lives in an environment (social and interpersonal network) in which treatment is unlikely to succeed (e.g., a chaotic family, rife with interpersonal conflict, which undermines patient's efforts to change);
   d. Seriously impaired social, family or occupational observation/care in a structured inpatient treatment program (i.e., patient is unable to abstain from the use of chemicals, and this condition and associated behaviors result in the patient's inability to function on the job or in the home, in even a limited capacity);
   e. Patient's family and/or significant others are opposed to his/her treatment efforts and not willing to participate in recovery program;
   f. Family members and/or significant others living with the patient manifest current substance use disorders, and are likely to undermine the patient's recovery;
   g. Living situation not conducive to life style change necessary for recovery;
   h. Logistic impediments (e.g., distance from treatment facility, mobility limitations, lack of drivers license, etc.) preclude participation in outpatient treatment services;
   i. Danger of physical, sexual, and /or severe emotional attack or victimization in his/her current environment will make recovery unlikely without removing the individual from the environment;
   j. The patient is employed in an occupation where his/her continued employment could jeopardize public or personal safety in the event that he/she resumed use as a consequence of treatment failure.

* * *

ADULT DISCHARGE & TRANSFER CRITERIA

Introduction

These Discharge & Transfer Criteria are measured along several dimensions of patient participation in treatment:

Dimension 1 (Acceptance/Awareness) is predicated on the patient's ability to accept treatment and his or her awareness of the need for treatment.

Dimension 2 (Cooperation) assesses the patient's ability to cooperate with treatment.

Dimension 3 (Follow-Through) assesses the patient's ability to follow the designed treatment plan.

Dimension 4 (Medical Stability) assesses the stability and control of any existing biomedical problems.

Dimension 5 (Psychological Stability) assesses the stability and control of any existing psychiatric or psychological problems.

Dimension 6 (Environmental Support) assesses the extent to which the patient's external environment is supportive of treatment goals.

These Discharge & Transfer Criteria dimensions are compatible with but not identical to the Admission dimensions. The Admission Criteria dimensions also involve historical information which is less relevant to the status evaluation for discharge or transfer.

In this conceptualization of treatment the traditional discharge may be considered as a transfer to mutual/self-help networks (Level I) and/or aftercare, or maintenance, services (Level II). While Level I or Level II care may also be primary treatment for select cases, these levels would typically provide additional assistance after a more intensive treatment experience. The current conceptualization explicitly deals with these less intensive services on their own merit rather than as adjuncts to more intensive programs.

Exceptions to Transfer Criteria

In some cases a patient's conditions may have improved so as to warrant transfer to a lower level of care, but a transfer which preserves the appropriate continuity of care is not available. In other cases it may be more efficient to retain the patient on the higher level of care for an additional brief period and effect a full discharge (or transfer to Level I or II) earlier than would be possible with a transfer to an intermediate level of care. Under these conditions the transfer guidelines appropriately may be overridden.

Transfer to a Higher Level of Care

Transfer to a higher level of care is warranted if any of the following apply:

1. There is deterioration in any of the transfer criteria dimensions.
2. There is lack of progress in any of the transfer criteria dimensions.
3. There is identification of additional chemical dependency related problems.

and all of the following apply:

1. There is evidence of restorative potential in the areas involved.
2. Greater intensity and/or range of services would positively impact the problem areas involved.
3. The required service(s) is (are) not available at the current level of care.

Transfer to a Lower Level of Care

In general, transfer to a lower level of care is warranted if all of the following apply:

1. There is sufficient improvement across all the transfer criteria dimensions;
2. There is sufficient progress in all appropriate dimensions;
3. There is sufficient resolution of problems;
4. Lower intensity services will continue to positively impact remaining problem areas;
5. Such services are available and can be provided while maintaining the continuity of care.

A more detailed and explicit set of guidelines for transfer and discharge are provided in the following section. A discharge could be viewed as a transfer from the current level to either Level I or Level II without any intermediate level services. Levels are presented from the highest to the lowest.

* * *

LEVEL V: MEDICALLY SUPERVISED INTENSIVE INPATIENT TREATMENT

All of the following must be present for a patient to be transferred from intensive inpatient treatment to a lesser level of care.

1.   **Acceptance/Awareness**
      Patient's awareness and acceptance of an addiction problem and commitment to definitive treatment is sufficient to expect treatment compliance in a less structured setting.

2.   **Cooperation**
      Patient's cooperation and acceptance of treatment is high enough that the need for motivating strategies has diminished sufficiently to reduce counseling observation, and availability of outpatient services to at least five hours of contact time per day for at least five hours of contact time per day for at least four days all week.

3.   **Follow-Through**
      Patient is capable of following a specific and complete post-inpatient recovery treatment plan. The patient's integration of therapeutic gains is established enough that transfer to a lesser level of care does not substantially risk reactivating the patient's addiction.

4.   **Medical Stability**
      Patient's biomedical problems, if any, have diminished or stabilized to the extent that daily availability of skilled medical/nursing care is no longer necessary.

5.   **Psychological Stability**
      Patient's psychological/psychiatric problems have diminished in acuity to the extend that daily availability of skilled psychiatric care is no longer necessary.

6.   **Environmental Support**
      Patient's social system and significant others are supportive of recovery to the extent that the patient can adhere to a post-inpatient treatment plan without substantial risk or reactivating his/her addiction.

* * *

LEVEL II: LOW INTENSITY OUTPATIENT TREATMENT

All of the following must be present for a patient to be transferred from Outpatient Treatment to a lesser level of care.

1.   **Acceptance/Awareness**
Patient's awareness and acceptance of an addiction problem and commitment to recovery is sufficient to expect maintenance of a self-directed recovery plan.

2.   **Cooperation**
Patient's cooperation and acceptance of treatment is high enough that the need for motivating strategies has diminished sufficiently to allow contact to be at the patient's discretion and experienced need.

3.   **Follow-Through**
Patient is capable of following a self-motivating recovery plan involving mutual/self-help support groups. The patient's integration of therapeutic gains is established enough that transition to a lesser level of care does not substantially risk reactivating the patient's addiction.

4.   **Medical Stability**
Patient's biomedical problems, if any, have diminished or stabilized to the extent that they can be managed through outpatient appointments at the patient's discretion as the need arises.

5.   **Psychological Stability**

Patient's psychological/psychiatric problems have diminished or stabilized to the extent that they can be managed through outpatient appointments at the patient's discretion as the need arises.

6.   **Environmental Support**

Patient's social system and significant others are supportive of recovery to the extent that the patient can adhere to a self-directed treatment plan without substantial risk or reactivating his/her addiction.

* * *

12 Determining Outcome

We can no longer afford to provide health care without knowing more about its successes and failures. The Era of Assessment and Accountability is dawning at last; it is the . . . latest—but probably not the last—phase of our efforts to achieve an equitable health care system, of satisfactory quality, at a price we can afford.
—Arnold Relman

The Rationale for Outcome Determination

This report focuses primarily on ways to improve the outcome of treatment for alcohol problems. In previous chapters it was suggested that the clarification of basic concepts, comprehensive pretreatment assessment, more precise characterizations of the treatments provided, and careful matching of individuals to treatment by means of explicitly stated and modifiable guidelines would enhance the proportion of positive outcomes. In this chapter the committee examines issues involved in understanding the target of all of this activity, the outcome of treatment.

For purposes of orientation, a distinction may be drawn between the short-term goals of treatment and its outcome. The goals of treatment include detoxification (where required); the reduction or elimination of alcohol use; the concomitant reduction of the signs and symptoms and of the consequences of alcohol use; the resolution of intercurrent medical, psychiatric, and social problems; and a modification in attitude toward drinking behavior leading to a commitment to its amelioration in future. The attainment of these goals is a major therapeutic achievement, a fact that should not be obscured by what follows. Goals will not be extensively discussed in this chapter, although it should be emphasized that, as with outcomes, there is a great need for their more frequent and detailed documentation.

The outcome of treatment has to do with the maintenance of these goals over the longer term; that is, with whether the commitment to the amelioration of drinking behavior has been realized. Although achievement of the short-term goals of treatment is laudable, it does not ensure a favorable outcome. And as the epigraph suggests, outcome is the bottom line. A health economist put it with characteristic directness in discussing the issue of quality of care: "Quality means: did the patients get better?" (McClure, 1985a:43). Organizations that accredit treatment facilities have increasingly stressed the evaluation of treatment outcome as a prerequisite for accreditation (Schroeder, 1987). One such organization recently advised as follows:

> The Commission now has an entire subsection of standards specifically focused on program evaluation and the importance of program results. This reflects a blending of technical requirements and the Commission's long-term emphasis on utilization of outcome measurements . . . organizations should keep in mind that an important focus of accreditation site surveys will be on the extent that evaluation reports are actually assisting them to accomplish their goals. (Commission on Accreditation of Rehabilitation Facilities, 1988:10-11)

Current interest in treatment outcome is fueled in large measure by concern over the growth of health care expenditures. There is an understandable desire to be certain that a return on such expenditures is being realized. Yet clinicians have long been concerned about treatment outcomes—and for other reasons.

The provision of treatment in the absence of knowledge of results has been likened to playing golf in the fog (Ziskin, 1970). One can stand at the tee, drive balls into the distance with impeccable form, fantasize about what good drives they were, and congratulate oneself on being a surpassingly good golfer. Yet what does this avail if one does not know where the balls are landing? Golfing under these circumstances becomes an exercise in unreality; no reasonable feedback can be provided that will be useful in improving one's game.

In addition to its potentially improving effect on clinical practice, there are ethical and legal reasons for promoting a systematic knowledge of treatment outcome. Because an effective treatment may nevertheless prove harmful to some individuals (see Chapter 6), an ethical obligation exists to monitor outcome so that deleterious effects can be detected and countered. Such an obligation is consistent with the principle of *primum non nocere*—the first duty of the treater is to do no harm. Should the detection of adverse effects of treatment be overlooked or ignored by treaters, remedies may be sought at law.

Wishing to practice in the most effective and ethical manner possible, clinicians commonly take steps to assure positive outcomes. In the regular follow-up of individuals after treatment, they observe them closely and often modify their therapeutic approaches accordingly. They are also at increased pains to utilize those treatments that sophisticated research studies have indicated are efficacious.

Unfortunately, accumulated experience now suggests that such strategies, while laudable, are not sufficient. Following patients clinically is an appropriate and useful practice, but one that is directed primarily at a determination of whether the goals of treatment were achieved rather than at treatment outcome. It is likely to provide an incomplete picture of outcome results: attrition is considerable, and those who fail to improve are less likely to return for follow-up appointments. If a follow-up visit is not carefully structured, it may not systematically and quantitatively explore the multiple aspects of outcome that are now felt to be important. If follow-up is carried out by those who administered treatment, there is a tendency to perceive more favorable outcomes than may actually exist, and treatment recipients will be reluctant to bring forth evidence that the treatment they have been given has not been effective.

Being guided by research studies in the provision of treatment may enhance the probability of positive results, but it does not guarantee them. The results of a treatment outcome study are considered positive if, in the aggregate, the outcomes are significantly better than those following either no treatment or a comparison treatment. But it is rare that all treated subjects have positive outcomes, and the relevant clinical question is whether a particular individual had a positive outcome.

Moreover, there are factors that may constrain the more general applicability of research findings to clinical practice. The subjects of research studies frequently differ in important ways from persons seen in clinical settings (Seiden, 1961; Hlatky et al., 1984; Longabaugh and Lewis, 1988). Although a treatment may be effective for research subjects, it is not necessarily effective for a very different clinical population.

Apart from subject differences, there may also be differences in the treatment as delivered. It used to be common for discussions of treatment outcome to be graced by a modest qualifying phrase: "Treatment X had the following results *in our hands*." Although now used only infrequently, the phrase is still highly meaningful, especially in the case of complex nonbiological interventions, such as those that are often utilized in the treatment of alcohol problems. Even with adequate quality assurance mechanisms in place (see Chapter 5) there are likely to be differences between a treatment as studied in a research setting and the same treatment as delivered in a treatment setting. This state of affairs is not necessarily unfortunate—variations on a basic treatment theme may be advantageous in dealing with an extremely variable target population—but it does mean that results obtained in a research setting cannot automatically be extrapolated beyond it.

Thus, although the carefully controlled research study may be an important method for exploring treatment efficacy, its clinical applicability is limited by numerous factors. From the standpoint of an individual seeking treatment, controlled studies have commonly been carried out in other programs, at other times, by different staff. What the prospective consumer of treatment services wants to know, however, is whether, given *his* problem, *his* characteristics, and *his* circumstances, he can reasonably expect to achieve a positive result from *this* program, at *this* time, and with *these* staff (cf. Paul, 1967; Pattison et al., 1977). The desire for such knowledge is shared by prospective third-party reimbursers. Knowledge of outcome results is a cornerstone of the "buy right" strategy advocated for all purchasers of health care (McClure, 1985a,b). According to this strategy, third party reimbursers can improve the quality of treatment by systematically shifting their economic support to providers who produce the best results at the most reasonable cost. In the past the limited number of treatment providers constrained such a strategy, but the growth of the treatment enterprise has now made it feasible.

What may be concluded from the foregoing considerations of clinical practice, research design, accreditation, ethics, legal considerations, marketing, and financing is relatively straightforward. Knowledge of the achievement of treatment goals is important, and very much to be encouraged, but it is not sufficient. Individual treatment programs must develop systematic and detailed knowledge of the outcomes experienced by those to whom they deliver services. Because of constant flux in critical dimensions of the treatment scene over time (changes in the patient population, in the treatment staff, in the available alternatives, in funding policy, etc.), such knowledge cannot be occasional but must be ongoing.

Although information regarding the achievement of short-term treatment goals is sometimes sought, the development of a comprehensive understanding of outcome is not common in the treatment of alcohol problems. Why this should be the case when multiple considerations favor knowledge of outcome is uncertain, and (as will be seen in the next section) there are some important exceptions. The reasons for the relative neglect of outcome determination may not be specific to the treatment of alcohol problems, since it is also a feature of the treatment of medical problems (Schroeder, 1987; Bunker, 1988; Relman, 1988; Lohr et al., 1988; Wennberg, 1988).

Some Examples of Systematic Outcome Determination

In some instances, concerted attempts have been made to determine the outcome of treatment for alcohol problems. The state of Oklahoma operates a mental health information system that generates data on the performance of all psychosocial treatment programs. An addition to this system has been made by the state agency responsible for the treatment of alcohol problems:

[W]e require the alcoholism programs to submit follow-up data on a random sample of all the clients taken in. This information is collected in a standardized form, and the service is reimbursed [for the collection of this data] in the amount designated by the schedule of payments. The random sample is generated every month by the computer from the pool of patients intaken [sic] by the program 6 months earlier. The level of completion of the follow-up quota is an important criterion in the decision of our department to renew or deny renewal funding by each program. (Paredes et al., 1981:384).

More recently (as of January 1, 1988), the state of Minnesota has instituted a requirement that all alcohol treatment programs receiving public monies must participate in a similar sort of management information system that includes regular follow-up of treated individuals. The development of systems of outcome monitoring is not a feature of the public sector of service delivery exclusively, however. With the rise of utilization management in the treatment of alcohol problems (Korcok, 1988; Lewis, 1988) a concern with outcome has surfaced in the private sector. Given increasing competition among providers of treatment for alcohol problems, documentation of positive outcomes may become a critical element in marketing. Commercial organizations that retail such documentation in the alcohol field, for example, the Chemical Abuse/Addiction Treatment Outcome Registry (CATOR), already include this inducement in their promotional materials.

Some details of the CATOR operation may be cited to illustrate how such an organization operates. A private corporation located in Saint Paul, Minnesota, CATOR contracts with individual treatment programs on a per capita basis (currently $98 per client per year) to provide treatment outcome data. Program staff are trained by CATOR staff working onsite to administer client data forms and forms documenting the details of treatment. These forms are then submitted to CATOR, which conducts posttreatment follow-up of individual clients by telephone from its main office.

The data that have been gathered are analyzed by CATOR staff, and feedback is provided to the individual programs that subscribe to the service, not only in terms of aggregate outcome for the program itself but in terms of how the program is doing in comparison with similar programs in the same registry. Such comparisons are possible because uniform data are obtained from all subscribing programs. The CATOR registry is quite large; its most recent version contains individual data on approximately 31,000 persons, with completed follow-up data on approximately 17,000 (N. G. Hoffmann, CATOR, personal communication, March 2, 1989). Although it is used primarily to prepare reports for its subscribers, the registry can also be employed to explore general issues in the treatment of alcohol and drug problems.

Thus reports have been prepared on 1,776 women in treatment (Harrison and Belille, 1987), on 1,824 adolescents in treatment (Harrison and Hoffmann, 1987), on 569 adults who completed outpatient treatment and were successfully followed for four consecutive six-month intervals after treatment (Harrison and Hoffmann, 1988), and on 2,303 adults discharged from inpatient treatment who were successfully followed in the same manner (Hoffmann and Harrison, 1988).

In summary, there are multiple reasons for favoring the systematic monitoring of the outcome of treatment, both in health care generally and in treatment for alcohol problems specifically. Many treatment programs attempt to develop information on the achievement of short-term treatment goals; although this is praiseworthy, it is not sufficient. The systematic determination of the status of individuals at the end of treatment is not common, and determination of outcome during the postdischarge period is even less common. Several examples can be cited in which monitoring of the outcome of treatment for alcohol problems has been and is currently being carried out. In view of the fundamental importance of knowledge of outcome, however, much more needs to be done.

A Major Caveat

For all of the reasons discussed above, the monitoring of outcome results is of central importance to the treatment of persons with alcohol problems. In addition to its many advantages, however, outcome monitoring has an important limitation. It does not prove that the outcomes observed following treatment are the result of the treatment provided.

From the manner in which outcome information is often used in marketing treatment programs, this limitation seems not to be well understood. Imputations of treatment efficacy based on outcome monitoring are a regular feature of mass media advertising. The committee believes that outcome monitoring should be used only with an understanding of its limitations; it also considers an examination of its limitations to be a necessary counterbalance to the foregoing discussion.

If a given result occurs following a given event, there is an understandable tendency to believe that the event caused the result. The belief is particularly compelling if the event was *intended* to cause the result. Treatment is intended to produce positive results; when a positive outcome is observed after treatment, the tendency is to conclude that it is due to the treatment provided. Certainly, that is one possibility. Yet a little reflection will indicate that there are alternative possibilities and that this sequence—treatment followed by a positive result—does *not necessarily* mean that the positive result was caused by the treatment.

As an example, let us take the familiar sequence of the alarm clock going off, followed by the rising of the sun. That this sequence occurs is readily and repeatedly verifiable. But the alarm clock does not cause the sun to rise, as may also be readily verified by not setting the clock. The two events happen to occur in a time sequence identical to the one that would be observed if the second event in the sequence were the result of the first, that is, if there were a causal relationship between them. But there is not. The temporal sequence is consistent with causality but does not demonstrate causality. So frequent and ancient is the logical fallacy of the assumption that a temporal sequence demonstrates causality that there is a Latin tag for it: *post hoc ergo propter hoc*, or (roughly) "after this, therefore because of this."

It follows that improvement subsequent to treatment is not necessarily the result of the treatment provided. Of what might it be the result, then, if not of the treatment itself? There are many possible alternative explanations. Alcohol problems, like other problems, have a natural course—or, more accurately, several natural courses (see Chapter 2). They may come and go. Treatment may have happened to occur in the middle of this process but may not have affected it (much as the alarm clock happened to ring while the sun was in the process of rising but did not cause it to rise). Life goes on while people are in treatment, and such life events as the threatened loss of a job or an important relationship may be the crucial determinants of outcome rather than treatment. That alcohol problems can improve in the absence of any formal treatment is well known (see Chapter 6).

None of these considerations negates the value or importance of treatment. There is ample evidence (see Chapter 5) that treatment can be crucial to positive outcome in many persons. Moreover, treatment can be carried out with certainty; nontreatment events or processes that might favor positive outcomes may, indeed, exist, but their occurrence is far from certain. Some alcohol problems come and go, but others do not. Even if improvement were eventually to occur without formal treatment, formal treatment may still be indicated because it might accelerate the process. Thus, treatment is very important; but the point here is that, because positive outcomes can occur that are related to factors other than treatment, proof that treatment has produced a positive outcome is not a simple matter.

To establish with certainty in a given instance that there was a causal relationship between treatment and improvement requires a more elaborate procedure. Basically, the results obtained in a group of persons who receive treatment must be compared with the results obtained in an essentially similar group who do not receive treatment. If there are differences in outcome between these two groups beyond what can be expected on the basis of chance, the results can be attributed to the treatment with confidence.

The randomized controlled trial (RCT) is this kind of procedure (see the discussion in Chapter 5). Randomization is the method commonly used to ensure the essential comparability of the treated and untreated groups on factors affecting outcome. The term *controlled,* used in this context, means that the presence of treatment has been controlled for by having a comparison group that was not treated (or, in a common variant, received a different kind of treatment). Outcome studies characteristically look only at people who have been treated; they do not look at randomly selected, untreated controls drawn from the same admission population. Hence the RCT, aided by a suitably selected comparison group, is better able to test the effect of treatment.

Yet the RCT has its disadvantages (see Chapter 5), and outcome monitoring has corresponding (and in many respects complementary) advantages. In a recent editorial in the *New England Journal of Medicine,* the disadvantages of the RCT in medicine generally were summarized as being of a practical nature: "We cannot afford to conduct randomized controlled trials for every test, procedure, or medication in use. To do so would require far too many research resources and would not produce results soon enough" (Greenfield, 1989:1142). In contrast,

> The scope of observational studies can be expanded much more easily than that of randomized controlled trials to include large numbers of patients and providers, maximizing the opportunity to gauge the effectiveness of routine medical care practices in various clinical settings, by various clinicians, and for various patient groups. Answers to questions about the effectiveness of care for important subgroups of patients (including those with specific coexisting morbid conditions), which would not be supplied by randomized controlled trials, can therefore be provided . . . . Longitudinal observational studies permit both the examination of a complex set of decisions, including the decision not to perform a procedure, and the assessment of the supportive care that follows. (Greenfield, 1989:1142)

The editorial goes on to caution that "care must be taken in interpreting the results of longitudinal observational studies, even though they are intuitively appealing and offer a quick solution to the information needs of policy makers." (p. 1143) It speaks of the capability of such studies to "reduce our dependence on randomized controlled trials" (p. 1143) rather than eliminating the need for such trials. A similar note is struck in a recent Institute of Medicine background paper on the assessment of technological innovation in medical practice (Gelijns, 1989). The virtues of observational methods, which are felt to have been enhanced by recent methodological developments, are enumerated (pp. iii, 51-52), but the recommendation is for a mixture of methods: "Evaluation of the risks and benefits of new technologies during their development will have to rely not only on experimental methods (including randomized controlled clinical trials) but also on improved observational methods of clinical conditions" (p. 51).

As these sources suggest, there is an important and highly complementary relationship between the RCT and the treatment outcome study. The RCT furnishes evidence that improvements in outcome are due to the treatment provided but only under the conditions of the experiment; it does not demonstrate, as indicated above, that the same results will consistently be produced in "the real world." On the other hand, the treatment outcome study does not prove that positive outcomes are due to the treatment provided. But it does demonstrate that improvements have occurred "in the real world" following the delivery of the treatment.

Let us suppose that there has been (a) ample demonstration from controlled trials that a particular treatment can be efficacious and (b) ample demonstration from treatment outcome monitoring that the same treatment, concretely embodied in a specific treatment program, is consistently associated with positive results. If these two circumstances coexist, one can entertain a reasonable certainty that effective treatment is being provided. If either element (a) or (b) is absent, one cannot be as certain. Thus, an important goal for the immediate future is the increased implementation of both randomized controlled trials and routine monitoring of treatment outcome.

Implementing Outcome Monitoring

Setting the Stage for Outcome Monitoring

Imagine a situation in which the following statement is made: "Sixty percent of the people who pass through our treatment program achieve a positive outcome." Let us assume that the statement is valid. How meaningful is it?

"A cautious response to the presentation of any treatment outcome rate," it has been noted, "requires that we ask several questions" (Emrick and Hansen, 1983:1086). One question that immediately comes to mind is "What sorts of alcohol problems do the people who come to your program exhibit?" A second question might be "What are the characteristics of the people that are treated in your program?" A third question might be "What sort of treatment is provided by your program?" In the absence of answers to these and other questions, a simple statement about the proportion of positive outcomes is not highly meaningful.

Specifying the Problem and the Individual A 60 percent positive outcome rate in a program seeing persons with mild alcohol problems of brief duration has a different meaning than the same rate in a program seeing persons with severe problems of long duration. A 60 percent positive outcome rate in a program seeing socially stable individuals has a different meaning than the same rate in a program seeing socially unstable individuals. The specification of problems and of individuals being considered for treatment has been discussed earlier in Chapter 10. In a very real sense the determination of outcome is a process of reassessment, in which the individual's status following treatment is compared with his status prior to treatment. As has been noted, "pretreatment functioning needs to be assessed for comparison with posttreatment adjustment, using parallel pre-post data-gathering procedures" (Emrick and Hansen, 1983:1082). Assessment thus helps to set the stage for outcome determination.

Specifying the Treatment A 60 percent positive outcome rate in an elaborate, time-consuming, and expensive form of treatment has a different meaning than the same rate in a simple, brief, and inexpensive form of treatment. The relevant question here is "Outcome of what?" The specification of treatment is also important for the classification of treatment programs and for matching to particular treatments (see Chapters 3 and 11). Briefly, there is a need to specify the treatments that are provided along multiple dimensions including treatment orientation or philosophy, the stage of the problem at which the treatment is directed, the setting of the program, the treatment modality utilized, its goals or objectives, the criteria for selecting individuals for treatment, its length, its intensity, its content, and other factors.

For purposes of outcome determination it is not enough to know what treatment was provided; one should also know what treatment the individual *received*.   Many treatment programs offer several treatment options simultaneously (e.g. group therapy, individual counselling, and educational lectures), and it is assumed that all persons in the program receive all of them in similar proportions; in fact, this may not be the case (W. J. Filstead, Parkside Medical Services, personal communication, March, 1988).   If a medication such as disulfiram (Antabuse) is dispensed, it is important to know whether it is being taken. Experience suggests that compliance with a prescribed regime of medication does not always occur, and a monitoring mechanism may be advisable to ensure that the medication is actually being used (cf. Peachey and Annis, 1984; Peachey and Kapur, 1986).

Perhaps it is only stating the obvious to emphasize that, in order to understand treatment outcome data, one must be clear about the nature of the problems being treated, the nature of the individuals undergoing treatment, and the nature of the treatment. Unfortunately, clarity about these matters is too frequently lacking at the present time. It has long been a goal of research on the treatment of alcohol problems that all of these critical dimensions should be explicitly accounted for (but the goal is not always realized; see Sobell et al., 1987). What is being urged, in a sense, is that the distinction between treatment and research practice be reduced to the point that they approximate each other.

The Content of Outcome Monitoring

Knowledge of an individual's status after completing treatment is much more meaningful if it can be compared closely with his or her status prior to treatment. Accordingly, *there should be a parallelism between the content of assessment and the content of outcome determination*. A comparison of the "core indices [of outcome] to be used for all treatment-evaluation studies" noted in a recent review (Emrick and Hansen, 1983:1084-1085) and the content of assessment suggested in Table 10-2 of this report demonstrates such parallelism. Among the shared content domains are physical health, including morbidity and mortality; drinking behavior; other substance use; legal problems; vocational functioning; family and social functioning; emotional functioning; cognitive functioning; and the operation of situational variables and life events.

Some aspects of a comprehensive pretreatment assessment might not be directly relevant posttreatment—for example, a specification of the individual's treatment goals. On the other hand, it would be of great importance to determine at the follow-up point or points whether the goals initially viewed as appropriate had been achieved, or whether there had been a shift of goals during the course of treatment. A thorough posttreatment assessment of customer satisfaction might be valuable in several ways. Guidance about modifications in program content and process could be obtained, but a more positive and participatory feeling toward the program and toward treatment generally might also be engendered by the fact of soliciting such feedback. In addition, regular reports of customer satisfaction may serve as an incentive and reward to the staff.

Prior treatment history would not be reassessed in outcome monitoring, but it would be essential to document any further treatment received in the interim between treatment and follow-up. Certain individual characteristics that might remain relatively unchanged (e.g., intelligence, personality, and family history) might not be reassessed, although specific reasons for doing so in individual cases come to mind. Because full testing of cognitive functioning is an expensive and time-consuming procedure, it might be repeated only if initial impairment had been detected. However, it is a common experience that marked improvement in cognitive functioning within the normal range can be characteristic of a positive treatment outcome, and the documentation of this improvement may have a salutary effect on the individual's outlook.

There has been a tendency in the field to rely primarily on changes in the level of use of alcohol to determine the outcome of treatment. Certainly, level of use is a critical focus for both treatment and outcome, and its status will bear a strong relationship to other outcome parameters (Babor et al., 1988). But the relationship is not invariable and may be quite discordant in some individuals, particularly those with lower levels of alcohol use (cf. Edwards, 1974). A case can therefore be made, as with assessment, for the use of multiple dimensions in the determination of outcome. "Because of the non-orthogonal relationships among treatment outcome domains," one authoritative paper states succinctly, "use of multiple outcome measures is essential" (Emrick and Hansen, 1983:1084).

Brief mention should be made here of a problem in selecting individuals for treatment that was touched upon earlier in this chapter. It has long been clear that certain population characteristics are associated *in general* with favorable outcomes. Those with less severe problems accompanied by fewer symptoms and consequences and of shorter duration, as well as such personal and situational characteristics as affluence, high intelligence, high educational levels, social stability, a high level of verbal skills and personal attractiveness are likely to do well in treatment and are more attractive to work with (cf. the "YAVIS syndrome" of Schofield [1964]). A program could substantially improve its proportion of positive outcomes, and the ease of its staff, by choosing to deal only with problems and individuals of this kind. Although it is true that some such individuals do not do well and that persons in this group may have as profound a need for treatment as any others, a high proportion of positive outcome results in a population of this kind carries a rather different meaning than would be the case in other populations (e.g., a population of skid row inhabitants). Less substantial gains in a more impaired and less advantaged group may represent an equal or superior therapeutic achievement. Thus, in the understanding of outcome results, relative rather than absolute standards are best employed.

At present, there is great variability in the measures that are used when outcomes are examined (Emrick and Hansen, 1983; Sobell et al., 1987). The use of a uniform set of treatment outcome criteria would be an enormous advantage because it would permit the aggregation of data and the comparison of treatment outcomes across programs. For example, with uniform outcome criteria it would be possible to compare the outcomes of individuals treated with pharmacotherapy and those treated with counseling. At present, data cannot be aggregated in this way because different and often incompatible outcome measures are used. The argument that particular programs need to present their data in particular ways to satisfy various data and funding requirements does not preclude the use of uniform criteria as well. If unique information is required, it can be collected in addition to shared uniform measures.

As with the development of a uniform assessment process, agreement on uniform outcome criteria needs to be forged through a series of consensus exercises involving all segments of the treatment community. Indeed, if the determination of outcome is conceptualized in large measure as reassessment, consensus on the content of both assessment and outcome determination could be sought simultaneously. The increment in useful information that would result from uniformity in assessment and outcome data would be considerable and would contribute importantly to the further enhancement of positive treatment outcomes.

The Process of Outcome Monitoring

Training A quite practical aspect of viewing outcome monitoring as reassessment is that only one set of staff, rather than two, is required. The measures being parallel, training to use them for assessment is also training to use them for follow-up. In many instances, staff will be reassessing individuals that they assessed initially; such familiarity may contribute to a greater likelihood that reassessment will be accepted and provides valuable feedback directly to relevant staff.

Timing How long after treatment should outcome be determined? In practice the range has been very wide indeed, ranging from a few weeks to as many as five years (Ogborne, 1984). What period might be optimal is a knotty question. Outcome results tend to be unstable—that is, individuals who are evaluated at time A tend to have different outcomes than when evaluated at time B (Annis and Ogborne, 1980)—and it is questionable whether time A or time B represents the "real" outcome.

There is also the issue that "although a lengthy period of follow-up may cast important light on the course of patients' drinking and related problems posttreatment, as the period of evaluation is lengthened less of what is observed can be attributed directly to treatment" (Emrick and Hansen, 1983:1082). What one may be observing over lengthy periods of time is the effect of nontreatment factors (e.g., loss of jobs, promotions, marriages, divorces, etc.) rather than the effect of treatment (Cronkite and Moos, 1980). Accordingly, there may be a progressive decline in treatment effect from the point of treatment termination. Such a progressive decay curve is often seen in medical treatments, in which the active ingredient in therapy is what the treater does. It has also been seen in treatment for alcohol problems, as well as for similar problems (Hunt et al., 1971). Individuals pursuing such a posttreatment course have been termed "faders" (Moos et al., 1982).

But there are other patterns of response over time. For example, in some treatments for alcohol problems, individuals are taught skills that they then apply to their life situations. With increased practice, they may apply the skills more effectively. In these circumstances the treatment effect may increase rather than decrease from the point of formal treatment termination. Such a pattern has been observed (Annis and Ogborne, 1980); in this case the individuals have been called "sleepers" (Moos et al., 1982). If different forms of treatment have variable effectiveness curves over time after treatment, how can one specific point in time be chosen as the "gold standard" for determination of outcome?

The answer probably is that it cannot be. A compromise would be to assess outcome at regular intervals following treatment and to continue to do so for a reasonable period of time. A schedule of reassessment, then, at 6 months, 12 months, and 18 months seems defensible, especially if the reassessment serves clinical as well as outcome determination purposes. For clinical reasons alone one would wish to evaluate individuals posttreatment on a schedule of at least this stringency. It would be possible, with such a pattern, to identify both "faders" and "sleepers."

Sampling Outcome monitoring can be carried out for all persons who enter treatment. As an alternative the determination can be made on selected samples (e.g., every third admission) as in the Oklahoma system. Using a sample is an effective procedure if a *generalized* knowledge of outcome is what is required. However, if the purposes of outcome monitoring are also in part clinical, it is more reasonable to opt for the monitoring of outcome for all persons who have entered treatment. For clinical purposes, one must know the outcome of treatment in every case, not excluding those who have failed to complete the prescribed course of treatment. The effectiveness of sampling in meeting the ethical obligations of *primum non nocere* and in preventing the potential legal consequences of failure to identify harmful effects of treatment upon particular individuals is unclear.

Setting In research studies, follow-up interviews are commonly carried out by means of a face-to-face interview, often in the patient's home. As an alternative, patients may be asked to return to the scene of their treatment for follow-up interviews. Because either of these options involves direct personal contact, additional direct observations can be made, and such procedures as breathalyzer testing or the use of biological markers can be deployed.

CATOR, as noted earlier, has conducted its follow-up interviews by telephone; others have used mailed questionnaires. These techniques, although less costly and time-consuming, do not permit the observations and methods available with direct contact and are thought to be less likely to produce valid responses, particularly from those who have not been satisfied with the treatment they have received. There is little in the way of empirical data to substantiate this impression. It may be that, to achieve a satisfactory response level—the higher, the better—a combination of methods will need to be used.

Corroboration The issue of the reliability of self-reports was discussed in Chapter 10. Self-reports seem inherently to be neither reliable nor unreliable; rather, they are markedly affected by the circumstances in which they are elicited. Under favorable circumstances, self-reports achieve a satisfactory level of reliability.

On the other hand, it is undoubtedly useful to obtain corroborating data from various external sources, and, at least in research studies, there has been an increasing tendency to do so (Sobell et al., 1987). The usual sources include family and other informants, public records, and the use of various biochemical tests to measure alcohol consumption either directly (e.g., breathalyzers, urinalyses) or indirectly (e.g., such markers as gamma glutamyl transpeptidase and high-density lipoprotein). These measures increase the validity of outcome information but at a cost of time, money, and effort.

Utility Outcome information may be principally useful in persuading third-party payers to purchase services from a particular treatment program, in persuading prospective clients to enter the program, and in qualifying for accreditation. In a larger sense, however, outcome data provide an ethical justification for purveying treatment and a means of improving its effectiveness. From an ethical standpoint the provision of treatment in the absence of knowledge of results is a questionable procedure. (Of course, if the results are not favorable, the ethical problems in continuing to provide treatment may be insuperable.) In most instances, outcome information is likely to indicate that admission to a given treatment program is followed by positive outcomes in a significant proportion of the people who seek its services; at the same time, however, it is followed by no significant change or by a worsening of problems in another but also significant proportion. A number of responses are possible in the face of such information: (a) improvements to the treatment being currently provided may be introduced, after which outcome may be examined again; (b) additional treatments that seem likely to help those who are not being helped may be introduced, and their outcomes may be examined; and (c) those who are not being helped by the treatment provided may be preferentially referred to programs whose outcome information indicates a higher probability of a positive outcome for individuals with their characteristics and types of problems. These alternatives are more extensively discussed in Chapters 11 and 13. All of them may substantially improve treatment outcomes, both for the individual programs and for the persons seeking treatment.

The Locus of Responsibility for Outcome Monitoring

The monitoring of treatment outcomes can be carried out under differing auspices. Responsibility for determining outcome can be taken (a) by individuals external to the program, (b) by the program itself, or (c) by some combination of the two. Theoretical and practical advantages may be advanced for all three approaches.

The principal advantage of external evaluation is greater objectivity. Programs themselves may be presumed to have an interest in demonstrating that their treatment is associated with a high level of positive outcomes; external evaluators presumably would not share such an interest. The principal disadvantages of external evaluation include lack of understanding of the program being evaluated, lack of availability, and cost. In Chapter 10, some of the advantages of an assessment process that was functionally independent of treatment were discussed. Similar advantages would accrue to functionally independent determination of treatment outcome; and, because outcome determination and reassessment are substantially the same process, both could be performed by the same functional unit. Because this option has already been discussed, the focus here will be on options (b) and (c).

Programs themselves may conduct treatment outcome monitoring. Indeed, when clinical as opposed to research treatment programs are being evaluated, this method is probably the most common. Program personnel are at least geographically available and presumably sympathetic to and knowledgeable about their own programs. In this case, information on treatment outcomes would be directly useful to the very personnel who carried out the evaluation and hence would tend to ensure its pertinence and perhaps also narrow the notorious treatment-research gap (cf. Garfield, 1978; Miller, 1987). Mounting research projects within treatment programs may also foster a more observing and objective attitude among staff toward their program than would otherwise be the case.

As an example of a within-program evaluation, half of a group of 100 patients who were seen for initial assessment of alcohol problems were randomly sent "a personal letter expressing concern for the patient's well-being and repeating our invitation for further assistance." Fifty percent of those sent the letter returned for additional contact, as compared with 31 percent of those not sent the letter; 76 percent returned the same day the letter was received, as compared with 12.5 percent; and 80 percent returned sober, as compared with 31 percent. All results were significantly beyond what would have been expected on the basis of chance (Koumans and Muller, 1965). A second and similar study demonstrated the effectiveness of a telephone call versus no call (Koumans et al., 1967).

A large residential treatment program visited by staff and committee members of this study conducted an evaluation of the effects of their program on persons who had alcohol or drug problems (or both) and eating disorders. The evaluation was carried out by an internal research group, which designed the study in close collaboration with clinical staff. Records were reviewed to establish the prevalence of eating disorders, and special questionnaires to be used both at admission and at follow-up were devised. The key finding was that individuals with eating disorders were found to have outcome results with respect to alcohol or drug problems that were similar to those of individuals without eating disorders. After much discussion, the program decided to continue to admit individuals with both alcohol or drug problems and eating disorders (J. Spicer, Hazelden Foundation, personal communication, 1988).

If programs conduct their own evaluations, problems arise in terms of validity, allocation of resources, and the uniformity of the data gathered. How objective program personnel would be in evaluating the results of their own work is an important issue. If the research were in the hands of program but nonclinical personnel, as in the example immediately above, the effects of bias might be somewhat attenuated. Even if the results were in fact not biased, their persuasiveness to others might be less than with an external evaluation. Finally, when individual programs gather data on their own clients they tend to gather them in an idiosyncratic manner. This lack of uniformity makes comparisons across programs, even on such seemingly straightforward items as demographic variables, difficult or impossible. Consensus on outcome measures, as recommended above, could be helpful in reducing this problem.

At present, most programs do not possess staff devoted to outcome monitoring. One approach would be to reallocate staff assignments so that some proportion of clinical time (and thus some proportion of the program budget, depending upon the intensity of follow-up to be done and the methods to be employed) was used for this purpose.

Alternatively, individual programs could be enriched by providing them with additional personnel to design and carry out outcome monitoring.

Programs may collaborate with external organizations to monitor their outcomes. CATOR is an example of this approach. It relies upon program personnel (after training) to produce descriptive data on patients and treatments but does its own follow-up and data analysis. In its promotional material, CATOR stresses the value of its externality: "Perhaps most importantly, potential patients and referral sources know you care about treatment outcomes by your willingness to have them audited by an objective, respected outside source" (Belille, n.d. [ca. 1987]:4).

The state systems in Oklahoma and Minnesota that were described earlier are similar in their approach, in that they involve collaborations between programs and external agencies. However, they differ in that treatment program personnel, rather than personnel of the collaborating agency, are responsible for conducting the outcome determinations. This practice also changes the financing pattern; in Oklahoma, for example, programs are paid for conducting outcome determinations on a prearranged per capita basis. Also, of course, the basis of participation differs; participation in CATOR is optional, but participation in the state systems is obligatory for programs receiving public funds.

It would appear from this brief consideration of the locus of responsibility for outcome monitoring that all of the options described have both advantages and disadvantages. If validity is the bottom line with respect to outcome determination (and it is for most of the purposes that outcome information is asked to serve) then the maximum feasible degree of externality in outcome determination is desirable. If outcome determination for practical reasons cannot be wholly external, some combination of internal and external loci of responsibility would be the next most desirable option. Examples would be a commercial organization such as CATOR in the private sector or the state systems in Oklahoma and Minnesota in the public sector. Providing that steps were taken to ensure functional independence, the use of an assessment or research group within a program might be yet another option.

Wholly internalized outcome monitoring may be useful for various local purposes but will tend not to be persuasive beyond the confines of the program. Nevertheless, as indicated above, such internal program research can be of great value in making sound decisions about the future course of the program. In addition, a program that has become accustomed to such internal research may well develop a capacity for objective self-scrutiny that will eventually result in an openness to external evaluation. Although not a fully satisfactory method of determining treatment outcome, internal monitoring is much to be preferred to an absence of effort toward this end.

The Funding of Outcome Determination

It is generally assumed that the introduction of widespread, comprehensive, and ongoing outcome monitoring, whether in the alcohol treatment field or in the medical treatment field generally, will raise the costs of providing treatment. At the least it is assumed that outcome monitoring will require an initial investment until a payoff of improved treatment efficiency is realized. Thus a medical periodical has editorialized that "To achieve these objectives will require much new financial support and unprecedented cooperation among physicians, government, private insurers, and employers" (Relman, 1988:1222).

Some are uncertain whether a financial payoff will in fact be realized. In calling for a national system of "outcomes management," Ellwood (1988) says that such a program "will not automatically favor a decrease or increase in health care expenditures" (p. 1556).

This is especially the case if any increase in the efficiency of treatment makes it more attractive so that demand for treatment is also increased.

As will be discussed in Chapter 21, the cost of treatment for alcohol problems is great, but is dwarfed by the cost of the consequences of alcohol problems. Systematic knowledge of outcome and its application to treatment may increase effectiveness and efficiency by improving treatment matching. The committee considers it likely that the overall costs of treatment may rise as a result of its recommendations because savings owing to improved effectiveness and efficiency will be more than offset by additional costs arising from the treatment of greater numbers of persons who are newly attracted to an expanded and improved system. Even though the costs increase, however, they will continue to represent only a fraction of the cost of the consequences of alcohol problems. The effort involved in determining treatment outcome and utilizing that knowledge to improve treatment is thus likely to prove worthwhile. More people will be treated, and they will be treated more appropriately; these constitute important benefits.

Conclusions and Recommendations

There is much to be said for determining whether the short-term goals of treatment for alcohol problems, such as reduction in the level of use of alcohol, have been achieved. More needs to be done in this regard. But a more pressing (although related) need is the determination of the longer-term outcome of treatment. Not a substitute for more rigorous controlled techniques that can demonstrate treatment efficacy, outcome monitoring nevertheless offers benefits in that it addresses many important issues, is more readily implemented on a broad basis, and complements significantly what can be learned in other ways.

Ideally, the outcome of treatment for all individuals entering specialized treatment programs for alcohol problems should be determined. There are a multiplicity of reasons for such a course, including ethical reasons, but the principal purpose would be to improve the ability to provide the most effective treatment to each individual by serving as a guide to matching. To reach this goal, *consensus must be achieved on the need for outcome determination, on the parameters to be used in determining outcome, and on the optimal way(s) to go about making outcome determinations.* Many variant approaches to all of these matters are possible. The committee believes, however, that *a quantum increment in attention to outcome determination is crucial to the future of the effort to treat alcohol problems.*

REFERENCES

Annis, H. M., and A. C. Ogborne. 1980. The temporal stability of alcoholism treatment outcome results. Addiction Research Foundation, Toronto.

Babor, T. F., Z. Dolinsky, B. Rounsaville, and J. H. Jaffe. 1988. Unitary versus multidimensional models of alcoholism treatment outcome: An empirical study. Journal of Studies on Alcohol 49:167-177.

Belille, C. n.d. (ca. 1987). Bringing definition to a soft science. Saint Paul, Minn.: Chemical Abuse/Addiction Treatment Outcome Registry (CATOR), Ramsey Clinic.

Bunker, J. P. 1988. Is efficacy the gold standard for quality assessment? Inquiry 25:51-58.

Commission on Accreditation of Rehabilitation Facilities (CARF). 1988. Program Evaluation in Alcoholism and Drug Abuse Treatment Programs. Tucson, Arizona: Commission on Accreditation of Rehabilitation Facilities.

Cronkite, R. C., and R. H. Moos. 1980. Determinants of the posttreatment functioning of alcoholic patients: A conceptual framework. Journal of Consulting and Clinical Psychology 48:305-316.

Edwards, G. 1974. Drugs, drug dependence, and the concept of plasticity. Quarterly Journal of Studies on Alcohol 35:176-195.

Ellwood, P. M. 1988. Outcomes management: A technology of patient experience. New England Journal of Medicine 318:1549-1556.

Emrick, C. D., and J. Hansen. 1983. Assertions regarding effectiveness of treatment for alcoholism: Fact or fantasy? American Psychologist 38:1078-1088.

Garfield, S. L. 1978. Research on client variables in psychotherapy. Pp. 191-232 in Handbook of Psychotherapy and Behavior Change: An Empirical Analysis, 2nd ed., S. L. Garfield and A. E. Bergin, eds. New York: John Wiley and Sons.

Gelijns, A. C. 1989. Technological Innovation: Comparing Development of Drugs, Devices, and Procedures in Medicine. Washington, D.C.: National Academy Press.

Greenfield, S. 1989. The state of outcome research: Are we on target? New England Journal of Medicine 320:1142-1143.

Harrison, P. A., and C. A. Belille. 1987. Women in treatment: Beyond the stereotype. Journal of Studies on Alcohol 48:574-78.

Harrison, P. A., and N. G. Hoffmann. 1987. CATOR 1987 Report: Adolescent Residential Treatment: Intake and Follow-Up Findings. Saint Paul, Minn.: Chemical Abuse/Addiction Treatment Outcome Registry (CATOR), Ramsey Clinic.

Harrison, P. A., and N. G. Hoffmann. 1988. Adult Outpatient Treatment: Perspectives on Admission and Outcome. Saint Paul, Minn.: Chemical Abuse/Addiction Treatment Outcome Registry (CATOR), Ramsey Clinic.

Hlatky, M. A., K. L. Lee, F. E. Harrell, Jr., R. M. Califf, D. B. Pryor, D. B. Mark, and R. A. Rosati. 1984. Tying clinical research to patient care by use of an observational data base. Statistics in Medicine 3:375-384.

Hoffmann, N. G., and P. A. Harrison. 1988. Treatment Outcome: Adult Inpatients Two Years Later. Saint Paul, Minn.: Chemical Abuse/Addiction Treatment Outcome Registry (CATOR), Ramsey Clinic.

Hunt, W. A., L. W. Barnett, and L. G. Branch. 1971. Relapse rates in addiction programs. Journal of Clinical Psychology 27:455-456.

Korcok, M. 1988. Managed Care and Chemical Dependency: A Troubled Relationship. Providence, R.I.: Manisses Communications Group, Inc.

Koumans, A. J. R., and J. J. Muller. 1965. Use of letters to increase motivation for treatment in alcoholics. Psychological Reports 16:1152.

Koumans, A. J. R., J. J. Muller, and C. F. Miller. 1967. Use of telephone calls to increase motivation for treatment in alcoholics. Psychological Reports 21:327-328.

Lewis, J. S. 1988. Growth in managed care forcing providers to adjust. Alcoholism Report 16(24):1.

Lohr, K. N., K. D. Yordy, and S. O. Thier. 1988. Current issues in quality of care. Health Affairs 7:5-18.

Longabaugh, R., and D. C. Lewis. 1988. Key issues in treatment outcome studies. Alcohol Health and Research World 12:168-175.

McClure, W. 1985a. Buying right: The consequences of glut. Business and Health 2(9):43-46.

McClure, W. 1985b. Buying right: How to do it. Business and Health 2(10):41-44.

Miller, W. R. 1987. Behavioral alcohol treatment research advances: Barriers to utilization. Advances in Behavior Research and Therapy 9:145-164.

Moos, R. H., R. C. Cronkite, and J. W. Finney. 1982. A conceptual framework for alcoholism treatment evaluation. Pp. 1120-1139 in Encyclopedic Handbook of Alcoholism, E. M. Pattison and E. Kaufman, eds. New York: Gardner Press.

Ogborne, A. C. 1984. Issues in follow-up. Pp. 173-215 in A System of Health Care Delivery, vol. 3, F. B. Glaser, H. M. Annis, H. A. Skinner, S. Pearlman, R. L. Segal, B. Sisson, A. C. Ogborne, E. Bohnen, P. Gazda, and T. Zimmerman. Toronto: Addiction Research Foundation.

Paredes, A., D. Gregory, and O. H. Rundell. 1981. Empirical analysis of the alcoholism services delivery system. Pp. 371-404 in Research Advances in Alcohol and Drug Problems, vol. 6, Y. Israel, F. B. Glaser, H. Kalant, R. E. Popham, W. Schmidt, and R. G. Smart, eds. New York: Plenum Press.

Pattison, E. M., M. B. Sobell, and L. C. Sobell. 1977. Emerging Concepts of Alcohol Dependence. New York: Springer Publishing Company.

Paul, G. L. 1967. Strategy of outcome research in psychotherapy. Journal of Consulting Psychology 31:109-118.

Peachey, J. E., and H. M. Annis. 1984. Pharmacologic treatment of chronic alcoholism. Psychiatric Clinics of North America 7:745-756.

Peachey, J. E., and B. M. Kapur. 1986. Monitoring drinking behavior with the alcohol dipstick during treatment. Alcoholism: Clinical and Experimental Research 10:663-666.

Relman, A. S. 1988. Assessment and accountability: The third revolution in medical care. New England Journal of Medicine 319:1220-1222.

Schofield, W. 1964. Psychotherapy: the Purchase of Friendship. Englewood Cliffs, N.J.: Prentice-Hall.

Schroeder, S. A. 1987. Outcome assessment 70 years later: Are we ready? New England Journal of Medicine 316:160-162.

Seiden, R. H. 1961. The use of Alcoholics Anonymous members in research on alcoholism. Quarterly Journal of Studies on Alcohol 21:506-509.

Sobell, M. B., S. Brochu, L. C. Sobell, J. Roy, and J. A. Stevens. 1987. Alcohol treatment outcome evaluation methodology: State of the art 1980-84. Addictive Behaviors 12:113-128.

Wennberg, J. E. 1988. Improving the medical decision-making process. Health Affairs 7:99-106.

Ziskin, J. 1970. Coping with Psychiatric and Psychological Testimony. Beverly Hills, Calif.: The Law and Psychiatry Press.

13 Implementing the Vision: Toward Treatment Systems

To provide the reader with an overview of its conclusions on the treatment of alcohol problems, in the first chapter of this report the committee presented its perceptions about the probable form toward which the treatment effort is evolving. The preceding four chapters in this section of the report have discussed some important components of this proposed treatment system: the community share of treatment, which involves the identification of alcohol problems by community agencies, as well as dealing with them either by brief intervention and referral for specialized treatment; and the specialized treatment of alcohol problems, which involves the processes of comprehensive assessment, matching of individuals to the most appropriate treatment options, and determining the outcomes of the treatments provided. It is now time to revisit the structure that ensues when these components and others are combined into an integrated whole (Figure 13-1).

In this system, which was previously discussed in Chapter 1, a concerted effort is made by community agencies to identify all persons with alcohol problems by evaluating those individuals who come to their attention. (Some proportion of persons with alcohol problems will, of course, enter the treatment process after identifying themselves as having alcohol problems.) Those persons who are identified are dealt with through brief interventions provided by the various community agencies if their problems are mild or moderate or are referred for specialized treatment if their problems are substantial or severe.

Those referred for specialized treatment are first provided with a comprehensive assessment that specifies in detail both their alcohol problems and those of their individual needs and characteristics that are treatment relevant. This information is then used to select the treatment that is most likely to facilitate a positive outcome. In moving between the elements of the specialized treatment sector, which is sometimes a difficult process for some individuals, provision is made for the assurance of continuity of care. Following the completion of treatment, the outcome achieved is monitored at regular intervals to determine whether it has been positive. This information is used both to reach a decision regarding future treatment of the individual and to provide guidance for the more precise matching of other individuals seeking treatment.

What is outlined in Figure 13-1 and the accompanying text is simply an example of one possible systems approach. Systems designs often differ greatly in form, but they serve similar purposes. Fundamentally, they are carefully planned approaches for the efficient and cooperative solution of various problems. *It is this generic approach that the committee finds compelling,* rather than any specific design, although the presence of certain elements is viewed as critical. Most of the elements have been developed at length in their own chapters; the system is simply a way of linking the elements together into a coherent whole. There are parallels in the development of the computer chip, also by definition a system, in which the principal innovation was the inclusion of the links between elements as an integral element (Reid, 1984).

Two components of the committee's proposed system for treating alcohol problems still require consideration here: the assurance of continuity of care and the feedback of outcome information. They are discussed below as a preface to an audit of the implementation and evaluation of such systems.

Assuring Continuity of Care

Care is appropriately provided for those who require it because they have problems of various kinds. On account of these problems, as well as for other reasons (for example,

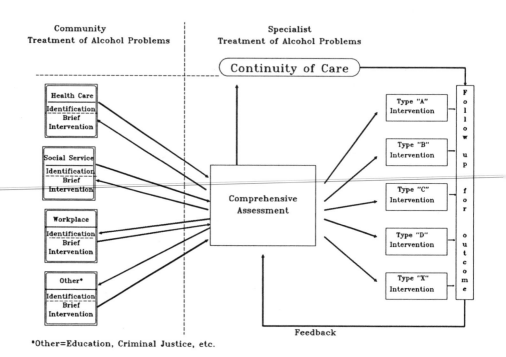

*Other=Education, Criminal Justice, etc.

FIGURE 13-1   The committee's view of the evolving treatment system. All persons seeking services from community agencies are screened for alcohol problems. A brief intervention is provided by agency personnel for persons with mild or moderate problems. Persons with substantial or severe problems are referred for a specialized comprehensive assessment. Where treatment is indicated, they are matched to the most appropriate specialized type of intervention. The outcome of treatment is determined and feedback of outcome information is used to improve the matching guidelines. Continuity of care is provided as required to guide individuals through the treatment system.

because of personal characteristics and attributes such as diminished capacity to understand, impaired sensory functioning, and so forth), some persons will require guidance through the process of care in order to engage it effectively. The need for such guidance is neither a new concept nor one uniquely related to alcohol problems; it has been claimed that all societies have created functionaries "who can listen, clarify needs, provide responses, and who will bear the responsibility for the continuity of care" (Parker, 1974:16).

Terminology has flourished in the area of continuity assurance, which creates some difficulties for the present discussion. "Case manager" has been most frequently used to refer to those who provide continuity assurance. Other terms enjoying some frequency of use include primary care worker, indigenous paraprofessional, mental health expediter, integrator, broker, ombudsman, advocate, patient representative, personal program coordinator, systems agent, continuity agent, clinical secretary, and (in one extremely large individual program offering multiple services) personal services shopper (cf. Intagliata,

1982). These differing terms may be understood to designate the same individual perform-ing similar functions, but the various terms give particular emphasis to one among the many possible functions that may accrue to the role.

What makes "case manager" problematic for the committee in the current discussion is the association of that term with managed care in the treatment of alcohol problems (Korcok, 1988; Lewis, 1988). The committee believes that the term has become linked to the notion of making decisions regarding care with a principal regard to cost savings. It is aware that distinctions have been made between "financial case management" and "clinical case management," but it prefers in this discussion to avoid the use of the term altogether. The committee's concept of continuity assurance is not tied to notions of cost containment, although savings may, indeed, be effected. In what follows, then, reference will simply be made to "the person who assures continuity of care," except in cases in which direct quotation of other sources involves alternative designations.

Discussions of continuity assurance in the literature are characteristically framed in terms of the individuals designated to fulfill this function. Although the discussion in this chapter will follow suit, it is worth noting that alternative strategies are available. One is to design the treatment system in such a way that the system itself, rather than specific individuals within it, provides for the assurance of continuity. For example, highly structured interrelationships among components of the system could serve this purpose. Another approach is to make the individual seeking treatment responsible for the continuity of care. The committee considers any or all of these to be effective strategies in particular circumstances. *The crucial matter is that continuity of care be assured; how this is accomplished is of secondary importance.* However, because the most prevalent approach is to assign the role of continuity assurance to an individual or individuals, the committee's discussion will continue in this vein.

In recent years the provision of continuity assurance has received increased emphasis because of the growth in size and complexity of treatment services. It is a practice that is more common in areas other than the treatment of alcohol problems—for example, in the treatment of the chronically mentally ill, in which it has attained great importance in the wake of deinstitutionalization initiatives. There are many definitions of the function, but "their common theme suggests that case management is a process or method for ensuring that consumers are provided with whatever services they need in a coordinated, effective, and efficient manner" (Intagliata, 1982:657). The same authority goes on to say that "the specific meaning of case management . . . depends upon the system that is developed to provide it" (p. 657).

There are some examples of continuity assurance in the treatment of alcohol problems. The role of the AA sponsor comes to mind (although this role, as with other examples, tends to serve more than continuity assurance functions). For many years the Donwood Institute in Toronto, a treatment facility for alcohol and drug problems, made use of "clinical secretaries," lay persons who served continuity assurance and other functions for small groups of individuals in treatment; regrettably, there appears to be no published record of this experience. One of the functions of the primary care workers in the Core-Shell Treatment System Project at the Addiction Research Foundation was continuity assurance (Glaser, 1984; Pearlman, 1984a, b). It is likely that there are other examples of personnel who serve the function of continuity assurance in treatment for alcohol problems that have not come to the notice of the committee, but it can probably be said with confidence that the practice has not been widespread.

Other elements of the system, such as assessment, matching, treatment, and the determination of outcome, can be viewed as the vertical components of care; they occur in more or less serial order and are time limited. Continuity assurance is the horizontal element in the system, cutting across the other elements and providing a coherent experience for the individual. The continuity assurance role is usually played by the same person during a given episode of care and ideally thereafter; should a problem develop again after an episode of care has been concluded, the person who provided continuity assurance is the logical point of recontact.

A common example will perhaps help to bring home the importance of designating a specific individual as responsible for continuity of care. Following the completion of a period of inpatient care, it is common to refer many persons to outpatient care. Let us suppose, however, that the referred person does not keep the first outpatient appointment. Under such circumstances, continuity of care can fall victim to a disjuncture in the treatment system. The inpatient service has discharged its responsibility by making the referral and therefore has no sense of responsibility for the individual's care. The outpatient service has not seen the individual and therefore has no sense of responsibility for his or her care. Thus, no one is responsible for continuity assurance, and the individual may be lost to care. If, however, responsibility for continuity of care is a specifically designated function—if some particular staff person is responsible for it—it is that person's job to bridge the gap and reestablish the thread of continuity.

Although many professional persons and such highly trained nonprofessional persons such as counselors could carry out the role well, an additional and perhaps more suitable source of personnel to assume the continuity assurance function may be the lay public. Those with extensive training might more appropriately occupy the formal therapeutic roles in the system. Assigning the continuity assurance function to lay persons does not gainsay the need for careful selection, training, and supervision, as in any role that has responsibility for the care of others. Yet the literature on continuity assurance stresses the importance of the personal qualities of those who assume this function. Consider the following list of attributes that are desirable for a "primary care worker" (slightly modified from Pearlman, 1984a):

1.   perseverance—an ability to follow through;
2.   comfort in working with difficult, marginally motivated patients;
3.   knowledge about and comfort in a supportive counseling role;
4.   knowledge about community resources;
5.   comfort in working in a secondary capacity with other treatment staff;
6.   relative ease in handling crises;
7.   an ability to relate to and cope with many people and problems simultaneously;
8.   thoroughness, organization and responsibility in the area of recordkeeping;
9.   willingness to get involved in a relatively unstructured and evolving work role;
10.   flexibility in terms of relating differentially to patients in a less formal, structured manner than is characteristic of psychotherapy;
11.   patience and a sense of humor;
12.   some knowledge of alcohol and drug dependency and the pharmacology of alcohol and drug abuse;
13.   an ability to formulate and sustain realistic expectations for self and patient; and
14.   ease in shifting among the various roles and functions inherent in the primary care role—counselor, ombudsman, facilitator, problems solver, and coordinator.

These are largely personal characteristics. They tend to be present in a given individual independently of the professional training he or she may have received, or perhaps even in spite of it (Becker et al., 1961; Shem, 1978; LeBaron, 1981). The literature on the effectiveness of nonprofessional therapists supports the presence in lay people of interpersonal characteristics favorable to positive therapeutic outcomes (Carkhuff, 1968; Lynch et al., 1968; Bergin, 1971; Emrick et al., 1978).

The foregoing should not be read as a brief against professional therapists. Continuity assurance is not in itself therapy. It might be said that therapeutic effects *ensue* from the efforts of those who provide continuity assurance, but are not *pursued* by them. That is, they provide continuity of care as an essential component of treatment in its own right and not because it may have a therapeutic effect—which it sometimes does. Those who assure continuity primarily facilitate the therapeutic efforts of the system as a whole, and therefore are a key element in whatever success the system may have.

Research on the impact of continuity assurance has been limited to the study of case management in the aftercare of the chronically mentally ill. One review noted mixed results: some studies had positive outcomes while others showed no significant addition to outcome over customary mental health aftercare services (Anthony et al., 1988). However, a recent study in which individuals who received case management were compared to matched controls found that the case managed individuals exhibited better occupational functioning, improved living conditions, and were less socially isolated (Goering et al., 1988).

Certainly, further research is needed on this important function. Indeed, the whole area of what happens following the initial treatment effort with the individual is one that requires much further investigation (cf. Moos et al., 1988; Moos et al., 1990). For example, two studies have already suggested that matching individuals to the appropriate intervention approach in this phase of their treatment is associated with more positive outcomes (McLachlan, 1972, 1974; Kadden et al., 1989). With the further development of relapse prevention techniques a variety of highly suitable approaches for this crucial phase of treatment are becoming available (Marlatt and Gordon, 1985; Annis, 1986).

Nevertheless, the committee believes that, at least for some persons, continuity assurance is a pressing and immediate requirement that should be acted upon forthwith. As services in general increase in number and complexity, the need will be even greater. There are already a variety of implementation strategies, as has been discussed above. Practical and theoretical advantages may be found for all of these options. That the function be available to those who need it is the crucial consideration.

Feedback of Outcome Information

Feedback may be defined as the use of information to modify the system that gathered the information. Provision for feedback makes a system self-reflecting and greatly increases its options (Hofstadter, 1979). Where it is present in biological systems, it facilitates their ongoing adaptation to current reality (Young, 1957); what has happened is taken into consideration, and future action is directed accordingly.

All too frequently a particular treatment is provided repeatedly without knowledge of its effects. For example, the antialcohol drug disulfiram (Antabuse) has enjoyed widespread general use in the treatment of alcohol problems since its introduction into clinical use more than 40 years ago (Hald and Jacobsen, 1948). Only recently have the results that accrue to its use been definitively examined in a large-scale investigation (Fuller et al., 1986). Those results suggest a much more discriminate and selective use of the drug than has often obtained in the past. It is good to have this information, but it would have been preferable to have it within a shorter time frame. Feedback has eventually occurred but has been much delayed.

The feedback that the committee sees as an integral part of the proposed treatment system is the feedback of outcome results in order to modify guidelines for matching persons to treatments. Simply put, if a particular set of matching guidelines is not productive of a reasonable level of positive outcomes, that information should be available within a reasonable time frame and should lead to a modification and retesting of those guidelines. Nor does the committee foresee a time when this process will not be necessary and when matching guidelines can be permitted to go untested by outcome results. There is too much change in too many of the key parameters of treatment on too regular a basis to assume that the guidelines will remain optimal for a prolonged period (cf. McLellan et al., 1983a). Rather, they must be tested constantly against the realities of outcome and readjusted frequently according to what is learned.

Active feedback of this kind permits the responsible evaluation of matching guidelines within standard clinical settings and within a shorter time frame than is possible using more rigorous methodologies—for example, the randomized controlled trial. RCTs have an important role to play in the evaluation of treatment, but so, too, do observational outcome studies of the kind the committee envisions as informing this sort of feedback (cf. Chapters 5 and 12; Gelijns, 1989; Greenfield, 1989). More of both are required, but outcome monitoring is more congruent with the circumstances of clinical treatment than is the conduct of RCTs. Outcome monitoring is also able to focus much more precisely on particular treatment programs, which is very much to the point.

Over the longer term there is another use to which the feedback of outcome information can be put. It may happen that, however creatively matching guidelines are modified during several iterations of the modification process, some proportion of individuals seeking treatment may persistently fail to achieve positive outcomes. These failures may signify a gap in treatment services; that is, some treatment that is not currently being provided may be necessary for a particular subgroup of the population being served. Given, however, the existence of the feedback loop that facilitated this conclusion, a new treatment can be identified, set in place, and evaluated in the same manner as already described. Thus, the successful closure of potential gaps in treatment services is another possible benefit of feedback.

Finally, it is worth stressing that generating outcome data is one thing, but using it to provide feedback is something else again. The first is a precondition to the second—outcomes that are not known cannot be used to provide feedback—but feedback does not necessarily occur simply because the results of treatment are available. Effort, planning, and vigilance will be required to ensure that outcome information is developed and is actually used to modify the functioning of treatment. Feedback will not happen automatically.

An Audit of the Systems Approach

The committee has now identified and described the key components of its proposed treatment system. To summarize briefly, they include (in addition, of course, to the availability of a reasonable number of alternative treatments) a community component, consisting of identification followed by brief intervention or referral for specialized treatment; and a specialized treatment component, consisting of comprehensive pre-treatment assessment, matching to a variety of treatment options, assurance of continuity of care, determination of outcome, and the effective feedback of outcome information. It now seems in order to audit the degree to which the system has been implemented in practice, and the existing evidence that, taken as a whole, it works.

As a preface to the audit, it is worth noting that there are considerable practical difficulties in implementing a systems approach. Most treatment programs do not offer more than a single treatment option (cf. Glaser et al., 1978). Perhaps because in the absence of treatment alternatives there seems little reason for it, neither do most offer the kind of comprehensive assessment discussed in this report. Even if they did, the assessment could not be carried out prior to a commitment to a particular kind of treatment; where only one treatment option is available, admission to the program entails a commitment to that treatment.

With only a single treatment option, matching cannot be carried out, as it requires the availability of multiple treatment options. Although external referral could serve the purpose of matching, it is rare in practice (Pattison, 1974; Glaser et al., 1978) and in a fee-for-service system there are financial incentives against it. Finally, few treatment programs engage in comprehensive outcome monitoring, and without monitoring there can be no feedback. Reasoning from this perspective, it is unreasonable to expect more than a few examples of the implementation of a systems approach.

On the other hand, the organization of activities into planned systems to achieve particular goals in an efficient and effective manner, as an alternative to independent activity at multiple sites, has a long history. An early example was the rapid re-outfitting of Admiral Nelson's fleet during the Napoleonic wars. Pulley-blocks were the problem. They were traditionally made, very well but very slowly, by individual craftsmen. Under the supervision of the engineers Sir M. I. Brunel (1769-1849) and H. Maudslay (1771-1831), the work was systematically organized, and the blocks were produced very well, very rapidly, and in large numbers. The improved condition of the fleet was a major factor in the victory at Trafalgar in 1805.

The integration of the "assessment devices" of the newly developed radar and ground observers with a central command structure and multiple "interventions" (e.g., antiaircraft defenses and the many fighter squadrons) was essential to victory in the Battle of Britain in September, 1940. Out of this and other wartime experiences evolved operations research, the beginning of the formal study and application of systems approaches (Miser, 1980). To date the adoption of systems approaches has been widespread in health care generally (cf. Van Eimeren and Kopcke, 1979; Tilquin, 1981). From this historical perspective, then, there might be some reason to expect the application of systems approaches in the treatment of alcohol problems.

In searching the literature, the committee has concluded that both of its presumptions are correct. The components of the proposed system are not represented in most treatment that is currently provided for alcohol problems. On the other hand, there are a number of examples in which one or more of the components are represented in programs that have existed, are currently viable, or are planned for the future. It is unlikely that all such programs have come to the committee's attention; and with some that have, the information is less complete than might be hoped. Bearing these cautions in mind, Table 13-1 summarizes this information by indicating those components of the system that are represented in particular treatment efforts.

Description of the Table

To facilitate an understanding of the table, the committee briefly discusses each of the individual examples offered. It should be understood that the designations in the table are often arbitrary because information on a number of the examples is incomplete or dated or both, and that the exercise is intended to be illustrative rather than definitive. The following section discusses the conclusions that arise from the table as a whole.

Oklahoma State System This system is basically for outcome monitoring, and was discussed earlier (see page 315; see also Paredes et al., 1981). The system collects initial data on individuals, but the data are gathered after admission to treatment programs and are not used to determine which treatment is to be delivered. Outcome determinations are made on a systematic sample of individuals admitted to treatment.

TABLE 13-1 An Audit of the Systems Approach to the Treatment of Alcohol Problems in North America

Examples	Components					
	Community Component	Comprehensive Pretreatment Assessment	Matching	Continuity Assurance	Outcome Determination	Feedback
Oklahoma State System					X	
Ontario Assessment and Referral System		X	X			
Brookfield Clinics		X	X	X		
Chemical Abuse/Addiction Treatment Outcome Registry (CATOR)		(X)	(X)		X	?,(X)
Minnesota State System		?	X		X	X
Managed care systems		?	X	X	X	
Penn-VA Project		X	X		X	X
National Collaborative Matching Project		(X)	(X)		(X)	(X)
Core-Shell Project		X	X	X	(X)	(X)
Northern Addictions Centre		(X)	(X)	(X)	(X)	(X)
Regional Youth Substance Abuse Project	(X)	(X)	(X)	(X)	(X)	(X)

NOTE: X = Component present in implemented program; (X) = component and/or program planned; ? = component present but questionable.

Ontario Assessment and Referral System In this system of multiple independent assessment and referral programs, a pretreatment assessment is carried out, and the data are used to match individuals seeking treatment to the most appropriate programs (see pages 265-266; see also Marshman et al., 1978; Ogborne et al., 1984; Malla et al., 1985; Rush, 1988). Other components of the committee's system have not been a planned part of this approach. Although there is an extensive program of prevention activities in the province, they do not appear to be explicitly connected with the assessment and referral system.

Brookfield Clinics A private treatment program operating at multiple sites in Michigan and Ohio, the Brookfield Clinics have adapted practices of the Core-Shell Treatment System Project (see the discussion below) to their operations (MacDonnell, 1981a,b; O'Dwyer, 1984, n.d.). They provide an individualized pretreatment assessment that is used to match individuals to very carefully specified treatments by using explicit guidelines. Continuity assurance is also provided.

Chemical Abuse/Addiction Treatment Outcome Registry (CATOR) CATOR is a private St. Paul-based program that provides outcome monitoring (see page 316; Harrison and Belille, 1987; Harrison and Hoffmann, 1987; Harrison and Hoffmann, 1988). It was also the primary contractor in the development of the so-called Cleveland criteria, which are designed to match individuals to various "levels of care" (see pages 289, 303-312; see also Hoffmann et al., 1987). In addition to outcome determination, CATOR provides feedback on this information to its subscribers, but whether it is used to modify the operations of those subscribers (an integral part of the definition of feedback) is uncertain. Although in the course of its usual operations CATOR, like the Oklahoma State system, obtains staff-generated information on individuals after admission to treatment, the Cleveland criteria are clearly intended to be used prior to treatment and to match individuals to the appropriate "level of care."

Minnesota State System In the state of Minnesota the legislature has mandated a pretreatment assessment to determine the appropriate treatment setting through matching guidelines that are required by law and specified in explicit regulations (see Chapter 10). Yet whether this pretreatment assessment can accurately be described as comprehensive is questionable. Although the gathering of additional information on individuals entering treatment is also mandated (through the state's own Drug and Alcohol Abuse Normative Evaluation System [DAANES] or an acceptable equivalent), this additional information is not at present used in matching. Determining the outcome of treatment is also mandated, and staff of the state program have begun to use this information to examine the state's matching guidelines.

Managed care systems A feature of recent years has been the growth of managed care in the treatment of alcohol problems (Korcok, 1988; Lewis, 1988) as well as in medical treatment generally. The data presented in the table are based on an imaginary composite of such programs and must be considered only approximate, as managed care programs vary a good deal. Almost all provide a pretreatment assessment of some sort and use this information to place individuals seeking treatment; however, the information gathering often cannot be realistically described as comprehensive. Monitoring of the individual's status while in treatment and afterwards is a reasonably consistent features of these programs.

Penn-VA Project Investigators in this research project, conducted jointly at the University of Pennsylvania and the Philadelphia and Coatesville Veterans Administration Hospitals, first described a system of care involving many of the components of the committee's vision (McLellan et al., 1980b). They then conducted a prospective study using the system in which the outcomes of those matched to treatment and those not matched were compared (McLellan et al., 1983a; see also below). A particular feature of this series of exercises was their stress on the use of feedback data to modify matching guidelines. The investigators continue to examine issues related to assessment and matching on a research basis; it is uncertain whether the program is used in either setting as a basis for routine clinical operations.

National Collaborative Matching Project   Recently announced by the Treatment Research Branch of the National Institute on Alcohol Abuse and Alcoholism (RFA AA-89-02A and AA AA-89-02B), this project will set up multiple clinical research units and a coordinating unit to conduct "multisite trials of patient-treatment matching." In these studies, individuals seeking treatment will be assessed on relevant variables, randomly assigned to treatment conditions, and be followed up to determine the outcomes of treatment.   The purpose of these studies is to test matching guidelines that may subsequently be utilized by other treatment programs.   They are expected to be completed in approximately five years, that is, in approximately mid-1994.

The Core-Shell Treatment System Project   During the period 1975-1981 a model treatment system was evaluated in the Clinical Institute of the Addiction Research Foundation in Toronto (Glaser et al., 1984).   Persons seeking treatment were given a lengthy and uniform pretreatment assessment in a discrete assessment unit; they were then assigned to treatment through a detailed set of explicit matching guidelines.   Continuity assurance was the responsibility of the Primary Care Unit.   Determination of treatment outcomes for the clinical population and the use of this information to modify the matching guidelines were a prominent part of the plans for this project but were not implemented.

Northern Addictions Centre   Some years ago the Alberta Alcoholism and Drug Abuse Commission (AADAC) prepared plans for an adaptation of the Core-Shell treatment system model to be located in Grande Prairie, a rural setting (Bazant, n.d.; Glaser and Hubbard, 1985; Skirrow, 1986).   Its original implementation was delayed by an economic recession, but the project was reactivated recently and is expected to receive persons seeking treatment in its specially designed facility within two years.   Pretreatment assessment, matching to a variety of interventions, continuity assurance, outcome determination, and modification of matching guidelines through feedback are planned.   Although prevention activities for the region are to be carried out by an office located in the same facility, no specific connection between the prevention and treatment activities has been articulated.

Regional Youth Substance Abuse Project   A United Way program located in Bridgeport, Connecticut, this project recently received a grant from the Robert Wood Johnson Foundation to set up the Youth Evaluation Service (YES) in cooperation with the Alcohol Research Center at the University of Connecticut (Babor and Del Boca, 1988). Focusing on adolescent problem drinkers and drug abusers, the program includes the following components: (1) a community action component that is concerned with access to treatment, availability of services, integration of services, and identification of high risk youth; (2) comprehensive pretreatment assessment using standardized questionnaires, structured interviews, and laboratory tests; (3) a rational treatment matching strategy that presents the individual with a long-term treatment plan and referral options; (4) continuity assurance guaranteed by a case manager who follows the individual for up to 18 months; (5) outcome monitoring by an independent university research center; and (6) feedback of outcome and process evaluations to improve treatment response.

Although components of the committee's system are not at present to be found in most treatment settings, there are (or have been) a number of settings in which they have been present to a variable degree.   The data in the table represent a conservative estimate; there are probably other relevant programs that are not listed of which the committee is unaware. Also, some that are known are not listed; for example, a system with many of the proposed components has been proposed for the state of Michigan (Allo et al., 1988), but is not included because its implementation at present is uncertain.

Of the proposed components only one program, the Regional Youth Substance Abuse Project, which is planned for the future, embodied all six components (it was the only one to have a community component similar to that envisioned by the committee).

The community component and the continuity assurance component were the two elements least in evidence in the examples discussed. Comprehensive pretreatment assessment, matching, and outcome determination were most frequently present in these examples. Feedback occupied a middle ground, and was more often planned than implemented.

Evaluation of the Systems Approach

It is reasonable to ask for evidence that the approach embodied in the committee's perception of the future is valid, that is, that it will improve outcomes following treatment compared with possible alternative approaches. The comparative effectiveness of most of the implemented programs in Table 13-11 has not at this writing been evaluated. The National Collaborative Matching Project offers the possibility of comparing the outcomes of those who are and are not matched to treatment on relevant variables. The Northern Additions Centre and the Regional Youth Substance Abuse Project will determine outcomes in individual cases; however, a comparison with alternative approaches is not contemplated in either project at present.

Because the Penn-VA project was a prospective study of the effectiveness of an approach resembling that of the committee, a brief summary of it seems in order. Four hundred seventy-six male veterans were assessed prior to treatment using the Addiction Severity Index (ASI) (McLellan et al., 1980a; McLellan et al., 1985); 178 are described as alcohol dependent and 298 as drug dependent. Previous work with the ASI had suggested that its scale for rating the severity of psychiatric symptomatology was predictive of outcome in various kinds of treatment. Together with other data, this information was used to construct explicit "program assignment decision criteria" for the alcohol-dependent and the drug-dependent groups. Because the construction of these criteria was based on the known outcomes of persons fully characterized prior to treatment, the criteria used in the study are a product of feedback.

Although an attempt was made to match all patients to treatment using these criteria, only 62 percent of the alcohol dependent and 48 percent of the drug dependent patients could be so matched, due largely to such practical matters as lack of treatment slots in the appropriate settings. Treatment staff were blinded to whether a given individual had been appropriately matched. Outcome data were collected on all patients six months after their admission to treatment. For the patients who were dependent on alcohol, 17 of the 19 dimensions on which their outcomes were compared showed better outcome status in the matched patients; 8 such comparisons achieved statistical significance. The authors stated their belief that "our ongoing 'matching' strategy will continue to be helpful in optimizing outcome" (McLellan et al., 1983a:604).

Yet a number of methodological shortcomings, pointed out by the authors themselves, constrain the conclusions that can be drawn from this study. Assignment to treatment was not random, although multivariate statistical techniques were employed in an attempt to equate the two comparison groups on initial characteristics. The follow-up period was brief and differed for different individuals. Nevertheless, this was a large-scale, creative study. The results are consistent with the potential effectiveness of treatment conducted along the lines envisioned by the committee.

There have been other prospective studies of matching of persons with alcohol problems to treatment (see Table 11-1) that have produced positive results. Although not in the area of alcohol treatment, a study of a geriatric assessment unit (GEU) in a VA Hospital in California met methodological criteria similar to those used in screening for the table and produced similarly positive results (Rubenstein et al., 1984). Thus, there is some if not an inordinate amount of evidence for the efficacy of the approach envisioned by the committee. Additional evidence is likely to come from at least one of the major projects planned for the future, the National Collaborative Study on Matching.

More evidence would be welcome indeed. Perhaps those responsible for similar projects (e.g., the Northern Treatment Centre and the Regional Youth Substance Abuse Project) will be able to work out ways of including comparative efficacy considerations within their scope of work. Little else is on the horizon. Unfortunately, health services research, the name given to the kind of research aimed at studying questions of this kind, is not currently considered to be of unusual urgency; "at the present time, research on alcohol service systems receives a relatively low priority within the Federal Government and in the alcoholism field generally" (Wallen, 1988:605).

Conclusions and Recommendations

The committee views the treatment of alcohol problems as evolving toward a system in which an active component of care undertaken by community agencies and consisting of identification, brief intervention, and referral is closely coupled with a specialized treatment sector that includes a comprehensive pretreatment assessment, the matching of individuals to a variety of treatment interventions, the assurance of continuity of care, the regular determination of outcome, and the feedback of outcome information. Many of the components of this system have been separately deployed and tested. The results have been documented in this section of the report and have generally been positive.

The committee recognizes the need for a further deployment and evaluation of these individual components of the system. It also recognizes that some work has already been done (Table 13-1) in bringing combinations of these components together. The committee lauds such efforts but believes that they have been too few and far between. It concludes that *what is now most needed is a major initiative to combine these separate components into fully integrated treatment systems of the sort envisioned in this report and to conduct careful and complete process and outcome evaluations of these model systems.* It is likely, and desirable, that alternative versions of such a systems approach should be mounted in a variety of different settings and directed at diverse populations—for example, with medically indigent persons in a public treatment system, with insured persons in a proprietary treatment system, and with particular subgroups such as those discussed in the next section of this report. Ideally, outcomes obtained through the treatment system would be rigorously compared with outcomes obtained through nonsystematic treatment.

A purpose of this series of demonstration projects would be to define effective models that could be transferred to the treatment field in general; they would also provide timely evaluation data to guide the formulation of treatment policy. Funds should be made available through public or private sources, or through a combination of sources, sufficient to support a minimum of four to five such demonstrations. Previous and current efforts, such as those discussed in this chapter, could serve as prototypes for these projects.

The committee recognizes that this is both a major and a novel undertaking, even though its continuity with the current thrust in the field is quite clear. It is a formidable task. But an undertaking of appropriate magnitude is required if the challenge of alcohol problems is to be met. There is also the promise that what is learned may be useful in advancing the ability of our society to cope with the many other health problems with which it is faced.

REFERENCES

Allo, C. D., B. Mintzes, and R. C. Brook. 1988. What purchasers of treatment services want from evaluation. Alcohol Health and Research World 12:162-167.

Annis, H. M. 1986. A relapse prevention model for treatment of alcoholics. Pp. 407-433 in Treating Addictive Behaviors: Processes of Change, W. R. Miller and N. Heather, eds. New York: Plenum Press.

Anthony, W. A., M. Cohen, M. Farkas, and B. F. Cohen. 1988. Case Management—More than a Response to a Dysfunctional System. Boston: Center for Psychiatric Rehabilitation, Boston University.

Babor, T. F., and F. Del Boca. 1988. Evaluation of Regional Youth Substance Abuse Project. Prepared for the Robert Wood Johnson Foundation. Farmington, Connecticut: Alcohol Research Center, University of Connecticut.

Bazant, W. F. N.d. Program Proposal for the Establishment of an A. A. D. A. C. Centre at Grande Prairie, Alberta. Edmonton, Alberta: Alberta Alcohol and Drug Abuse Commission.

Becker, H., B. Geer, E. C. Hughes, and A. L. Strauss. 1961. Boys in White: Student Culture in Medical School. Chicago: University of Chicago Press.

Bergin, A. E. 1971. The evaluation of therapeutic outcomes. Pp. 217-270 in Handbook of Psychotherapy and Behavior Change: An Empirical Analysis, A. E. Bergin and S. L. Garfield, eds. New York: John Wiley and Sons.

Carkhuff, R. R. 1968. Differential functioning of lay and professional helpers. Journal of Consulting Psychology 15:117-126.

Emrick, C. D., C. L. Lassen, and M. T. Edwards. 1978. Nonprofessional peers as therapeutic agents. Pp. 120-161 in Effective Psychotherapy: A Handbook of Research, A. S. Gurman and A. M. Razin, eds. Oxford: Pergamon Press.

Fuller, R. K., L. Branchey, D. R. Brightwell, R. M. Derman, C. D. Emrick, F. L. Iber, K. E. James, R. B. Lacoursiere, K. K. Lee, I. Lowenstam, I. Maany, D. Neiderhiser, J. J. Nocks, and S. Shaw. 1986. Disulfiram treatment of alcoholism: A Veterans Administration cooperative study. Journal of the American Medical Association 256:1449-1455.

Gelijns, A. C. 1989. Technological Innovation: Comparing Development of Drugs, Devices, and Procedures in Medicine. Washington, D.C.: National Academy Press.

Glaser, F. B. 1984. The nature of primary care. Pp. 3-34 in A System of Health Care Delivery, vol. 2, F. B. Glaser, H. M. Annis, H. A. Skinner, S. Pearlman, R. L. Segal, B. Sisson, A. C. Ogborne, E. Bohnen, P. Gazda, and T. Zimmerman. Toronto: Addiction Research Foundation.

Glaser, F. B., and R. N. Hubbard. 1985. Application of a treatment system model in rural Alberta. Presented at the 34th International Congress on Alcoholism and Drug Dependence, Calgary, Alberta.

Glaser, F. B., S. W. Greenberg, and M. Barrett. 1978. A Systems Approach to Alcohol Treatment. Toronto: ARF Books.

Glaser, F. B., H. M. Annis, H. A. Skinner, S. Pearlman, R. L. Segal, B. Sisson, A. C. Ogborne, E. Bohnen, P. Gazda, and T. Zimmerman. 1984. A System of Health Care Delivery, 3 vols. Toronto: Addiction Research Foundation.

Goering, P. N., D. A. Wasylenki, M. Farkas, W. J. Lancee, and R. Ballantyne. 1988. What difference does case management make? Hospital and Community Psychiatry 39:272-276.

Greenfield, S. 1989. The state of outcome research: Are we on target? New England Journal of Medicine 320:1142-1143.

Hald, J., and E. Jacobsen. 1948. A drug sensitising the organism to ethyl alcohol. Lancet 2:1001-1004.

Harrison, P. A., and C. A. Belille. 1987. Women in treatment: Beyond the stereotype. Journal of Studies on Alcohol 48:574-578.

Harrison, P. A., and N. G. Hoffmann. 1987. CATOR 1986 Report: Adolescent Residential Treatment: Intake and Follow-up Findings. Saint Paul, Minn.: Chemical Abuse/Addiction Treatment Outcome Registry (CATOR), Ramsey Clinic.

Harrison, P. A., and N. G. Hoffmann. 1988. CATOR 1987 Report: Adult Outpatient Treatment: Perspectives on Admission and Outcome. Saint Paul, Minn.: Chemical Abuse/Addiction Treatment Outcome Registry (CATOR), Ramsey Clinic.

Hoffmann, N. G., J. A. Halikas, and D. Mee-Lee. 1987. The Cleveland Admission, Discharge, and Transfer Criteria: Model for Chemical Dependency Treatment Programs. Cleveland, Ohio: The Greater Cleveland Hospital Association.

Hofstadter, D. R. 1979. Goedel, Escher, Bach: An Eternal Golden Braid. New York: Basic Books.

Intagliata, J. 1982. Improving the quality of community care for the chronically mentally disabled: The role of case management. Schizophrenia Bulletin 8:655-674.

Kadden, R. M., N. L. Cooney, H. Getter, and M. D. Litt. 1989. Matching alcoholics to coping skills or interactional therapies: Posttreatment results. Journal of Consulting and Clinical Psychology 57:698-704.

Korcok, M. 1988. Managed Care and Chemical Dependency: A Troubled Relationship. Providence, R.I.: Manisses Communications Group, Inc.

LeBaron, C. 1981. Gentle Vengeance: An Account of the First Year at Harvard Medical School. New York: Richard Marek Publishers.

Lewis, J. 1988. Growth in managed care forcing providers to adjust. Alcoholism Report 16(24):n.p.

Lynch, M., E. A. Gardner, and S. B. Felzer. 1968. The role of indigenous personnel as clinical therapists: Training and implications for new careers. Archives of General Psychiatry 19:428-434.

MacDonnell, F. J. 1981a. Alcoholism in the work place: differential diagnosis. Occupational Health Nursing 29:14-16.

MacDonnell, F. J. 1981b. How effective are our current methodologies for the treatment of alcoholism? EAP Digest 2(1):32-35.

Malla, A. K., B. Rush, M. Gavin, and G. Cooper. 1985. A community-centred alcoholism assessment/treatment service: A descriptive study. Canadian Journal of Psychiatry 30:35-43.

Marlatt, G. A., and J. R. Gordon, eds. 1985. Relapse Prevention. New York: The Guilford Press.

Marshman, J. A., R. D. Fraser, C. Lambert, A. C. Ogborne, S. J. Saunders, P. W. Humphries, D. W. Macdonald, J. G. Rankin, and W. Schmidt. 1978. The Treatment of Alcoholics: An Ontario Perspective. Toronto: Addiction Research Foundation.

McLachlan, J. F. C. 1972. Benefit from group therapy as a function of patient-therapist match on conceptual level. Psychotherapy: Theory, Research, and Practice 9:317-323.

McLachlan, J. F. C. 1974. Therapy strategies, personality orientation, and recovery from alcoholism. Canadian Psychiatric Association Journal 19:25-30.

McLellan, A. T., L. Luborsky, G. E. Woody, and C. P. O'Brien. 1980a. An improved diagnostic evaluation instrument for substance abuse patients: The Addiction Severity Index. Journal of Nervous and Mental Disease 168:26-33.

McLellan, A. T., C. P. O'Brien, R. Kron, A. I. Alterman, and K. A. Druley. 1980b. Matching substance abuse patients to appropriate treatments: A conceptual and methodological approach. Drug and Alcohol Dependence 5:189-195.

McLellan, A. T., G. E. Woody, L. Luborsky, C. P. O'Brien, and K. A. Druley. 1983a. Increased effectiveness of substance abuse treatment: A prospective study of patient-treatment "matching." Journal of Nervous and Mental Diseases 171:597-605.

McLellan, A. T., L. Luborsky, G. E. Woody, C. P. O'Brien, and K. A. Druley. 1983b. Predicting response to alcohol and drug abuse treatments: Role of psychiatric severity. Archives of General Psychiatry 40:620-625.

McLellan, A. T., L. Luborsky, J. Cacciola, J. Griffith, P. McGahan, and C. P. O'Brien. 1985. Guide to the Addiction Severity Index. Washington, D.C.: U. S. Government Printing Office.

Miser, H. J. 1980. Operations research and systems analysis. Science 209:139-146.

Moos, R. H., J. W. Finney, and R. C. Cronkite. 1990. Alcoholism Treatment: Context, Process, and Outcome. New York: Oxford University Press.

O'Dwyer, P. 1984. Cost effective rehabilitation: A process of matching. EAP Digest 4(2):33-34.

O'Dwyer, P. N.d. A Systems Approach to Substance Abuse and Mental Health Treatment. Garden City, Mich.: Brookfield Clinics.

Osborne, A. C., D. Dwyer, and A. Ekdahl. 1984. The Niagara Alcohol and Drug Assessment Service: Referral Patterns, Client Characteristics, and Community Reactions. Toronto: Addiction Research Foundation.

Paredes, A., D. Gregory, and O. H. Rundell. 1981. Empirical analysis of the alcoholism services delivery system. Pp. 371-404 in Research Advances in Alcohol and Drug Problems, vol. 6, Y. Israel, F. B. Glaser, H. Malant, R. E. Popham, W. Schmidt, and R. G. Smart, eds. New York: Plenum Press.

Parker, A. W. 1974. The dimensions of primary care: Blueprints for change. Pp. 15-80 in Primary Care: Where Medicine Fails, S. Andreopoulos, ed. New York: John Wiley and Sons.

Pattison, E. M. 1974. Rehabilitation of the chronic alcoholic. Pp. 587-658 in Clinical Pathology Vol. 3 of The Biology of Alcoholism, B. Kissin and H. Begleiter, eds. New York: Plenum Press.

Pearlman, S. 1984a. Early experiences with primary care. Pp. 35-48 in A System of Health Care Delivery, vol. 2, F. B. Glaser, H. M. Annis, H. A. Skinner, S. Pearlman, R. L. Segal, B. Sisson, A. C. Ogborne, E. Bohnen, P. Gazda, and T. Zimmerman. Toronto: Addiction Research Foundation.

Pearlman, S. 1984b. Later experiences with primary care. Pp. 49-66 in A System of Health Care Delivery, vol. 2, F. B. Glaser, H. M. Annis, H. A. Skinner, S. Pearlman, R. L. Segal, B. Sisson, A. C. Ogborne, E. Bohnen, P. Gazda, and T. Zimmerman. Toronto: Addiction Research Foundation.

Reid, T. R. 1984. The Chip: How Two Americans Invented the Microchip and Launched a Revolution. New York: Simon and Schuster.

Rubenstein, L. Z., K. R. Josephson, G. D. Wieland, P. A. English, J. A. Sayre, and R. L. Kane. 1984. Effectiveness of a geriatric evaluation unit: A randomized clinical trial. New England Journal of Medicine 311:1664-1670.

Rush, B. 1988. Executive Summary: Assessment prodedures and specialized assessment in Ontario. Prepared for the IOM Committee for the Study of Treatment and Rehabilitation Services for Alcoholism and Alcohol Abuse.

Shem, S. 1978. The House of God. New York: Richard Marek Publishers.

Skirrow, J. 1986. Waging the war against alcohol abuse. Canadian Medical Association Journal 135:434.

Tilquin, C. 1981. Systems Science in Health Care: Proceedings of the International Conference on Systems Science in Health Care, Montreal, July 1980, 2 vols. Toronto: Pergamon Press.

Van Eimeren, W., and W. Kopcke. 1979. State of the Art Report: Health Systems Research. 2 vols. Munich: Institute for Medical Information Processing, Statistics, and Biomathematics.

Wallen, J. 1988. Alcoholism treatment service systems: A health services research perspective. Public Health Reports 103:605-611.

Young, J. Z. 1957. The control of living systems. Pp. 1-30 in The Life of Mammals, J. Z. Young. New York: Oxford University Press.

14 The Treatment of Special Populations: Overview and Definitions

Over the past 20 years, a number of subgroups have been identified as special populations for the purposes of planning and evaluating the national system of treatment for alcohol problems. Through the years, barriers to accessing and successfully completing treatment were identified for a variety of such groups. Efforts were initiated to provide funding for separate programs or to make sure that generic, or mainstream, programs were structured so as to provide appropriate outreach and treatment (USDHEW, 1974; Gunnerson and Feldman, 1978; USDHHS, 1981, 1983, 1986; Saxe et al., 1983; McGough and Hindman, 1984). Emphasis has been placed on developing treatment strategies that would be delivered through separate treatment programs employing clinical and administrative staff from the affected group whenever possible or with special training for staff of mainstream programs in understanding the normative environment in which the persons that they are treating have functioned and developed alcohol problems.

Throughout the history of its funding of specialty programming for the treatment of alcohol problems, the federal government has emphasized that there are certain populations or subgroups that must receive special attention because of their unique characteristics and their inability to receive appropriate treatment within what might be called "generic" treatment programs (e.g., USDHEW, 1974; USDHHS, 1986). These special populations have been defined in terms of either their apparently greater risk for alcohol-related problems, whether the reasons are primarily biological or sociocultural (e.g., American Indians, children of alcoholics) or legal or political (e.g., public inebriates, drinking drivers, the homeless). From the perspective of general health care, people with alcohol problems are themselves seen as a special population whose needs have not been adequately met within the overall health care system nor within the specialty mental health system (e.g., Plaut, 1967; Heckler, 1985). Just as there is still debate over whether a separate specialty alcohol problems treatment sector is necessary or whether integration and mainstreaming are possible, there is still debate over whether specialty alcohol problems treatment programs are needed for the various special populations that have been identified.

The term *special populations* takes in a wide range of categories, many of which do not truly make up a self-identified group (Diesenhaus, 1982). Yet, the concept is still seen by those in the field as instructive for designing and implementing treatment programs in instances in which there is information on commonly shared characteristics that are thought to have relevance for treatment attraction, retention, and maintenance. The concept has remained important at the state and local service delivery level. The states report that they are continuing to provide services targeted toward a variety of special populations (ADAMHA, 1984, 1986), even though the federal government no longer requires such targeting (other than to women and American Indians) as a condition of receiving federal block grant funds (see Chapter 18).

Legislators, clinicians, and researchers recognize the need not only to define but also to provide culturally relevant treatment of alcohol problems for individuals who belong to special populations. Yet there is little consensus about what such treatment entails, for whom it is specifically designed, and what the term *special populations* actually means. The purpose of Section IV is to review some of the history and issues involved in the delineation of treatment programming for special populations, to review selected research and practice, and to make recommendations regarding future research and programming needs.

344

Defining Special Populations: A Historical Perspective

Alcoholic beverages have been a part of the heritage and culture of the United States since the first Spanish colonists arrived in this country in 1565. All of the European groups that established colonies imported alcoholic beverages and rapidly developed local production as an early priority. Each group of settlers brought over its unique views of the positive and negative aspects of alcohol use, as well as its own alcoholic beverage of choice. Early on, this country's ambivalent relationship toward alcohol use led to economic, medical, and social support for drinking on the one hand and to control and prohibition of alcohol use for some population groups on the other. Those leading religious and moral/social movements directed toward all drinkers of alcoholic beverages began to describe subpopulations that they considered to have unique problems associated with alcohol ingestion. These initial efforts at control were directed mainly toward Indians, blacks, and Irish and Scottish immigrants all of whom were singled out as special subgroups that consumed alcohol at levels far above "normal" and had a higher rate of problems associated with drinking. Since those early times, efforts have continued to classify those individuals who misuse alcohol into categories as a way to facilitate assessment and treatment, but it was not until the establishment of NIAAA in the early 1970s that using the concept of special populations as a categorizing strategy (both for funding and for the development of treatment programs) became prominent.

Historical perspective on the changing or progressive definition of what constitutes a special population represents progress in recognizing the complexity of treatment for alcohol problems. Gomberg (1982) notes that the *Third Special Report to Congress on Alcohol and Health* (USDHEW, 1978) refers to special populations as groups defined in terms of demographic variables: age, gender, and race. The groups discussed in that report were young people, women, the elderly, American Indians, Spanish-speaking persons, and blacks. These groupings were seen as very different from those described in the 1940s, when the focus was on grouping by differences in social class and psychiatric symptoms. Gomberg further noted that the fourth report, published in 1981, had added Native Alaskans, Asian Americans, and gays to this list (USDHHS, 1981). Although she questioned why the special populations discussed did not include such white ethnic groups as Irish-Americans or Polish-Americans or those groups at higher risk for alcohol problems by virtue of their socioeconomic status, she concluded that the definition of special populations then current represented real progress in recognizing the complexities of alcohol problems. As Gomberg noted, "[t]he term has come to mean those groups who have special treatment needs and who have been underserved (Gomberg, 1982:351)."

A major arena in which there has been an effort to define special populations for the treatment of alcohol problems has been legislative activity at the federal level. Special populations first began to be identified legislatively in the mid 1960s when the Alcohol Countermeasures program was established within the National Highway Safety Administration; this effort ultimately led to the funding by NIAAA of categorical grants for the treatment of drinking drivers (Diesenhaus, 1982). Public inebriates were singled out for state and federal legislative attention as a result of federal court decisions that the chronic alcoholic could not be held criminally liable for public inebriety. The establishment of the National Center for the Prevention and Control of Alcoholism and of NIAAA, in the early 1970s, also drew attention to special populations (Plaut, 1967; Gunnerson and Feldman, 1978).

Alcohol problems among the poor were seen by many as an area of particular need. Efforts to provide targeted service were initiated through grants made for outreach, advocacy, and outpatient counseling as part of the Model Cities Act and the Antipoverty Act in the late 1960s; in 1972 these so-called poverty grants were transferred from the Office of Economic Opportunity to NIAAA and became its largest special population grant category (Gunnerson and Feldman, 1978; DeVita, 1988). Another piece of legislation targeting special populations was the 1970 Hughes Act (Public Law 91-616). The Hughes Act authorized a formula grant to the states which required them to identify needs and services for women and youth under 18 years of age. These two groups were also included in the legislation authorizing NIAAA to provide categorical grants for community-based services.

Parallel to the federal effort, a number of states had also begun focusing on the need for differentiating treatment to meet the needs of identified subgroups (e.g., Minnesota's programming for American Indians; California's funding of commissions to focus on the needs of women and Hispanic Americans).

Yet despite this apparent interest, the term *special populations* does not appear in the *First Special Report to the U.S. Congress on Alcohol and Health* from the secretary of health, education, and welfare (USDHEW, 1971). The chapter, "Treatment of Alcoholism," in the report was organized around the multiple interacting systems that must be taken into account in developing treatment strategies (biological, biochemical, organ, intrapsychic, interpersonal, social, small group, and large group). However, several population subgroups were singled out in this discussion of treatment as requiring specialized programming: skid row alcoholics, alcoholic employees, persons arrested for driving while intoxicated, and those who have suffered injuries to the central nervous system.

The report also identified six priority areas for the development of research and services programs. Three of these areas were related to special populations: (1) rehabilitating the public inebriate; (2) providing help to alcoholic employees, and (3) identifying and treating drunken drivers. The priorities also served to introduce a fourth subgroup: American Indians. The priority involved was to reduce alcoholism among them. Adolescents were also discussed but as part of prevention programming; the report singled out for attention those adolescents "who exhibit delinquent behavior or personality traits of incipient alcohol abuse."

The term *special population programs* was finally introduced in the *Second Special Report to the U.S. Congress on Alcohol and Health* (USDHEW, 1974) in describing NIAAA's efforts to carry out these priorities:

> Recently the NIAAA has also launched a series of special-population programs in addition to those already functioning for American Indians and Alaskan natives. They include projects to bring aid and rehabilitation to alcoholic people in certain hitherto neglected segments of our society: blacks, Spanish-speaking Americans, migrant farm workers, women, and persons caught up in the criminal justice system. (p. xviii)

> To increase resources to meet the needs of the ethnic groups noted above, the NIAAA has developed separate program guidelines that encourage the recognition and use of each group's unique cultural characteristics in developing treatment services and has supported these services through the award of project grants. (p. 113)

The *Third Special Report* (USDHEW, 1978) continued this emphasis on services to specially designated populations, including both a separate chapter on special populations and a discussion of the research findings and clinical observations in the chapter on treatment. The report included a description of the current status of research on cultural or subgroup drinking practices and on the prevalence and form of problem drinking among subgroup members. The emphasis of the discussion on treatment was the barriers to gaining access to treatment experienced by members of each special population and the design of "culturally specific" or "culturally relevant" treatment interventions to ensure the retention of group members in treatment and a successful outcome of treatment efforts.

The Research Perspective on Special Populations

Diesenhaus (1982) attempted to offer a comprehensive definition of special populations as groups that have common social, psychological, or legal characteristics and that have encountered barriers in obtaining appropriate treatment. He reviewed the status of specialized treatment programming for a number of groups: drinking drivers, incarcerated alcoholics, migrant farm workers, military personnel and other occupational groups, public inebriates and skid row alcoholics, the physically impaired, and those experiencing problems with both alcohol and other drugs. Diesenhaus also described what he considered to be the current research trend to develop a unifying conceptual framework of special population classification schemes to be used in evaluation of treatment for alcohol problems. According to Diesenhaus, this trend had evolved from the need to design specialized and culturally sensitive treatment programs that might better meet the needs of those special population groups whose members shared common psychosocial attributes or social status.

Prior to 1970 scientific research and clinical experience in the treatment of alcohol problems was based predominantly on studies of Caucasian males aged 40 or older in inpatient treatment settings (cf., Gomberg, 1982; Vannicelli, 1984; Lex, 1985; Westermeyer, 1988). The preeminence of the Minnesota model as the most widely used model for treatment has arisen from its success in treating alcohol problems among this same core group of identified men (see Chapter 3). Treatment for special populations was also structured on the increasingly popular model of short-term inpatient primary rehabilitation followed by a variable period of aftercare using a multidisciplinary approach and incorporating the principles of Alcoholics Anonymous; efforts were made, however, to use counselors who were recovering alcoholics from the same socioeconomic and ethnic group as the persons being treated (e.g., Staub and Kent, 1973; Mitnick, 1978; Rosenberg, 1982) (see Chapter 4). In the early 1970s, a consensus developed that using findings of studies of middle-aged white males to understand attitudes, treatment concepts, and prognostic expectations for members of special population groups was not useful. Rather, there was a need to develop treatment approaches tailored to what was known about the relevant culture of each group. This consensus was not limited to the treatment of alcohol problems; it was a major theme in the development of community-based general health and mental health services (Rogler et al., 1987). Lex (1985) summed up this change in perspective:

> It is now recognized that a society as heterogeneous as the United States is best viewed as an aggregation of numerous subgroups. There is considerable variation in patterns of alcohol use and alcohol problems in distinctive subgroups who share common racial or ethnic backgrounds—such as blacks, Hispanics, and American Indians. Persons who share demographic characteristics of sex or age—such as women, youth, and the elderly—similarly constitute discernible subgroups whose alcohol use patterns and problems also have implications for diagnosis and treatment. (p. 90)

By the early 1980s, it became apparent that there had been little evaluation of these efforts to develop treatment programs tailored to the diverse needs of special populations. Saxe and colleagues (1983) reviewed the status of treatment programming for nine special populations: the elderly, youth and adolescents, women, blacks, Hispanics, American Indians, problem drunk drivers, and public inebriates and skid row alcoholics. The Saxe team reviewed a variety of studies for each of these subgroups to try to establish whether their overrepresentation (e.g., blacks, American Indians) or underrepresentation (e.g., women, the elderly) in the treatment population reflected real differences in the incidence and prevalence of alcohol problems among groups or the lack of appropriately designed, culture-specific treatment programs. They concluded that there was insufficient evidence to resolve what had come to be ongoing disagreement between those who advocated culturally specialized treatment programs using staff who share the patients' cultural and experiential background (and language, when appropriate) and those who believed that treatment should focus on the alcohol problem itself rather than on the cultural considerations.

Saxe and coworkers also stressed the heterogeneity of the groups discussed in their review. They particularly noted this quality among the Hispanic American subgroup. Although most research up to that point had focused on Mexican Americans, the Saxe team urged attention also to the alcohol problems of Hispanic Americans whose cultural origin was Puerto Rico, Cuba, or one of the other Central or South American countries. Similarly, Saxe and his group pointed to the socioeconomic heterogeneity that exists among public inebriates who do not all fit the stereotype of the homeless, skid row alcoholic.

The *Fifth Special Report to Congress* (USDHHS, 1983) introduced the concept of *special need populations*, focusing on informal selection of treatments by members of these groups and the matching of needs to specific treatments:

> Despite the increasing variety of programs, settings and treatment modalities, many alcoholics do not have the opportunity to find an informal match between their own specific needs and the type of treatment available. This is especially true of special needs populations, such as women, ethnic minorities, the multidisabled, the elderly, and skid row alcoholics. For these groups access to treatment and successful rehabilitation are often impeded by cultural barriers, financial constraints, and program design characteristics. (p. 108)

The report's listing represents another expansion of the groups identified as special populations. The most important common characteristic of the groups is that they all face barriers to treatment access that the report states are being dealt with in program design: "With the growing recognition that utilization rates may be improved by removing barriers to access, greater attention is now being given to special population groups in the design of treatment programs" (USDHHS, 1983:108). A new emphasis found in this report is the need to evaluate these programs once they have been implemented: "As these programs become available, research will need to move from program descriptions to actual evaluation studies in which programs designed for special population groups are compared with more traditional approaches" (p. 109).

The *Fifth Special Report* identifies specific services that are thought to be needed by some of the special populations if treatment is to be more attractive and retention and outcome is to be improved: (1) for women, child care services and same-sex counselors are needed; (2) minority groups for whom language differences impose a barrier require minority staff who speak the same language and come from the same cultural background; (3) for American Indians and Hispanic Americans, native healing and folk medicine should be included; and (4) those who have problems with alcohol as well as other drugs need combined alcohol/drug treatment programs. Financial restrictions on the availability of treatment are identified as a concern for all these special need populations. The report raises the issue of the unknown impact that the shift from federal categorical grants targeted toward special need populations to the block grant has on the continuing efforts to improve access for these groups.

The review of treatment in the *Sixth Special Report to the U.S. Congress on Alcohol and Health* (USDHHS, 1987) does not contain a discussion of the treatment needs of special populations. The questions about the impact on efforts to improve access identified in the prior report remain largely unstudied. Yet NIAAA's most recent publication on the planning of treatment services does include a section on the consideration of the special needs for members of several special populations which ". . . research suggests may be particularly underserved by alcoholism treatment programs" (McGough and Hindman, 1986:41). The report identifies eight major groups on the basis of sex, age, race, and ethnicity: (1) elderly; (2) youth; (3) multidisabled; (4) American Indians; (5) Black Americans; (6) Hispanic Americans; (7) Asian/Pacific Americans; and (8) women. The report contains a brief chapter for each of these special populations summarizing research findings and actual program experiences. For several, there is further discussion of the differences among subgroups with need be taken into account in planning. For example, the multidisabled individual can be physically or mentally disabled. Specific subgroups identified within this special population are the mobility impaired, hearing impaired, vision impaired, mentally retarded, and developmentally disabled. Similarly, the American Indian special population is further broken down to identify Aleuts and Alaskan Natives as distinct subgroups; the existence of tribal variation on key variables relevant to the treatment process is also stressed. The Hispanic American special population is similarly divided into subgroups that differ in terms of national origin, educational attainment, socioeconomic status, and degree of acculturation. Subgroups that are specifically mentioned include Mexican Americans, Puerto Ricans, Cubans, Caribbean Islanders, and Central and South Americans. Additionally, Hispanic American migrant and seasonal workers are identified as a high-risk occupational group whose mobile lifestyle calls for special efforts to coordinate treatment services.

The planning manual has two key criteria for defining a special population: (1) the group must be identified by research as underserved in current treatment programs and (2) clinical experience and research must demonstrate the necessity for subgroup-specific interventions (e.g., linking the elderly with recreational, medical and social services; dealing with educational and vocational issues for youth; providing employment counseling and job placement within a program targeted at black Americans; and being sensitive to language barriers with Hispanic Americans).

Over the years, Congress has also reviewed the status of alcohol problems treatment for individual special population groups and included specific references to them in legislation and reports. Groups so identified have been drinking drivers, "federal offenders," military personnel, federal employees, the elderly, families of alcoholics, the handicapped, the homeless, victims of domestic violence, public inebriates, Native Americans, poverty groups, veterans, Native Hawaiians, ethnic minority groups, women, underserved populations, and youth (DeVita, 1988).

Legislative actions have covered a wide range of assistance efforts. Legislation has been enacted mandating that treatment for alcohol problems be provided or made available to particular groups (the military, federal employees); it has also been used to require representation of identified underserved or high-risk groups (e.g., the elderly, racial and ethnic minority groups, poverty groups, and women) in the state advisory councils that had to be established for a state to obtain formula grant funds. Legislation has also required that the states conduct surveys to determine needs and ensure services for particular special populations (the elderly, youth, and women); it also required the Department of Health and Human Services (DHHS) and NIAAA to give special consideration to certain applications for treatment funds that were directed to these groups (the elderly, the physically and mentally handicapped, families of alcoholics, underserved populations such as ethnic and racial minorities, Native Americans, public inebriates, victims of domestic violence, women, and youth under age 18).

Legislative activity in regard to federal employees has focused on providing employee assistance programs and on the question of whether treatment for alcohol problems should be mandated in the Federal Employees Health Benefits Plan. Legislative activity in regard to other groups (most notably, the elderly, youth, and women) has been directed toward ensuring that the identified special populations receive the services that they need. At times Congress has been quite directive in its designation of a special population that requires additional consideration in planning and funding treatment services; for example, in 1980, the Congress required DHHS to give special consideration to grants and contracts designed to provide specialist treatment programs for the elderly. Its action was prompted by the belief that older persons are less likely to seek services in centers populated by young alcohol abusers. Also in 1981, Congress instructed DHHS to provide funding for a designated center for research on the effects of alcohol on the elderly.

In the years since the passage of the block grant in 1981, congressional emphasis has been on meeting research needs rather than on directing federal funding to meet service access needs of selected populations. The authorization for services funding efforts was subsumed under the new block grant in 1981, with the expectation that the states would carry on the efforts to meet the service needs of special populations according to their own priorities. The three special population groups which have received some degree of congressional attention in recent years have been women, youth, and the homeless.

In 1984, Congress mandated that at least 5 percent of the block grant funds for alcohol and drug abuse services be used to support new or expanded services for women. Congress also singled out for research attention the problems that are created when pregnant women drink. High risk youth, including those at risk of becoming an alcohol abuser, are the target population for the new services demonstration programs to be carried out by the Office of Substance Abuse Prevention, established in 1986. In 1987, research demonstration projects for the treatment of homeless persons with alcohol problems were authorized along with more broadly defined efforts to provide health care, emergency shelter, and social services to the homeless. In 1988, the new alcohol and drug abuse treatment resources block grant identified desirable services to nationally targeted populations; these groups were most often identified as the homeless, youth and adolescents, and intravenous drug abusers (ADAMHA, 1988).

Given the diversity of special population groups identified as needing culturally sensitive treatment in legislative and program development activity, it becomes necessary to ask: where then has the research and clinical emphases lain? What groups are being defined in clinical and services research efforts as special populations? What special treatments or treatment programs have been developed for them? Does the availability of culturally appropriate treatment increase accessibility, retention, and outcome for special populations?

First, as a means of understanding the historical evolution of the interest in special populations in the alcohol literature, the committee examined the field's research and clinical practice priorities as captured by the National Clearinghouse for Alcohol and Drug Abuse Information (NCADI) since the inception of its data base in 1973. The NCADI database, one of the most complete resources in the field, classifies the materials in its file of abstracts into the 14 special population groups shown in Table 14-1. Catalogued materials include research studies, books, newsletter articles, case studies, program descriptions, journal articles, monographs, communications, and so forth. Table 14-1 shows the frequency distribution of materials in each of the specified areas for three distinct time periods: 1973-1982, 1983-1985, and 1986-1987. The table also contains a summary for the total 15-year period, 1973-1987.

TABLE 14-1 Total Number of Resource Materials on Special Population Groups Included in the National Clearinghouse for Alcohol and Drug Abuse Information (NCADI) Data Base

Special Population Group	1973-1982	1983-1985	1986-1987	Total 1973-1987
Youth	722	1,120	511	2,353
College/university students	8	119	134	261
Elderly	205	186	49	440
Alcoholic females	425	347	208	980
Homosexuals	16	14	22	52
Economically disadvantaged	39	66	47	152
Racial and ethnic groups (general)	301	338	165	804
Blacks	103	131	69	303
Hispanics	48	54	42	144
Asians and Pacific Islanders	54	60	30	144
American Indians	117	85	35	237
Religious groups	79	113	51	243
Public inebriates	2	33	46	81
Handicapped/disabled	0	22	23	45

SOURCE: Committee analysis of data from the National Clearinghouse for Alcohol and Drug Abuse Information data base.

Over the 15 year period the emphasis in catalogued material has been predominantly on youth, women, and racial and ethnic groups. The increase in abstracted materials for all the special populations in the last five years deserves notice; youth and women are the categories for which the most materials are recorded. There is also a marked increase in attention paid to college students, whereas there seems to be a slight tapering off in attention paid to elderly, youth, and American Indians.

It is possible to characterize the literature abstracted in the NCADI data base as containing only a very few controlled trials in which the effectiveness of generic treatment is compared with treatment specifically tailored to the characteristics of the special population under consideration. There is a paucity of adequate studies on treatment outcome for any of the groups identified (Gilbert and Cervantes, 1988; Vannicelli, 1988; Westermeyer, 1988). The comment on treatment outcome made by Braiker (1982) continues to have current general applicability to all special population groups:

> A review of the general literature on alcoholism treatment effectiveness reveals that most studies either fail to distinguish between outcome rates for men and women alcoholics or exclude the latter group from the study samples altogether. Among those studies that distinguish outcome rate by sex, varying and often conflicting results are reported. (p. 127)

Whereas the NCADI data base offers with insight into the research and and clinical practice emphasis on special populations, data from the National Drug and Alcohol Treatment Survey (NDATUS) can help to identify both the trends and the current distribution of treatment programs available for special population groups. These were surveys of alcoholism treatment services provided by all known public and private alcoholism and drug abuse facilities and units in the United States (NIAAA, 1983; Reed and Sanchez, 1986; NIDA/NIAAA 1989) (see Chapters 4 and 7). Table 14-2 presents data on the number of specialized programs offered by alcoholism treatment units by the year

TABLE 14-2 Specialized Programs Offered by Alcoholism Treatment Units by Survey Year[a]

| | Percentage of Total Units Reporting | | |
Specialized Program	1982[b]	1984[c]	1987[d]
Youth	21	27	31
Elderly	9	9	8
Women	23	22	28
Hispanics	9	9	11
Blacks	8	7	6
American Indians/Alaskan natives	—[e]	5	5
Public inebriates	13	9	7
Other	13	9	15
None	51	46	41
Total units reporting	4,233	6,963	5,791

[a]Includes both alcoholism-only units and combined alcoholism and drug abuse units.
[b]Data from the 1982 National Drug and Alcoholism Treatment Utilization Survey (NIAAA, 1983).
[c]Data from the 1984 National Alcoholism and Drug Abuse Program Inventory (Reed and Sanchez, 1986).
[d]Data from the 1987 National Drug and Alcoholism Treatment Unit Survey (NIDA/NIAAA, 1989).
[e]Not included in the 1982 survey.

of the survey. Youth, women, the elderly, Hispanics, public inebriates, and blacks were the only special population groups included in all three of these surveys; American Indians/Alaskan natives were included in the last two surveys.

The inventory asked respondents to identify whether they offered one or more specialized programs to certain population groups. Judging on the basis of the treatment units reporting, it appears that an increasing percentage of units are offering one or more specialized programs. In 1987 the largest number of specialized programs offered in treatment units were for youth (31 percent), followed closely by those for women (28 percent), with a sharp drop to programs for Hispanics (11 percent) and the elderly (8 percent).

Changes in the total number of units reporting and in the number of specialized programs must be interpreted cautiously because there was a more thorough outreach effort in 1984 to locate all units that were either not identified in 1982 or that did not respond; this effort may simply have uncovered existing units that had not responded earlier rather than identifying new units that had only recently been established (cf. Reed and Sanchez, 1986:2).

An examination of these two sources—the NCADI database and the NIAAA surveys of treatment units—shows that women and youth are the special population groups that have received the most attention since the early 1970s. What they do not reveal are the most effective ways to meet the needs of individual problem drinkers or how to identify factors germane to a special population that might affect treatment. The overviews are also unable to provide guidance on when treatment should emphasize an individual's special population membership to facilitate a successful outcome. Indeed, if these overviews tell us anything, it is that women and youth appear to be the special population groups that people are most concerned about.

Given the historical dilemmas, variations, and inconsistencies in defining which groups should be considered as special populations in the planning, funding and evaluation of alcohol problems treatment, Lex (1985:90) has suggested that a special population be defined as any subgroup that is "special in terms of their uniformity on some dimension and their differences from more typical societal patterns and problems." The committee agrees with this definition.   However, the definition does not fully capture the problems encountered in attempting to review existing knowledge on the value of special population programming.

This review of the history of attention to special population groups suggests that their definition is often not only in terms of the unique biological and sociocultural characteristics that define a group with similar risk factors and drinking practices but also in terms of the momentary concern regarding access to appropriate services. Interest in each group has waxed and waned. There has been no systematic follow up to determine whether access has been improved or treatment outcome positively affected by these periods of attention. What is challenging, for both researchers and clinicians, is to determine where and how the emphasis on special population membership can best facilitate effective treatment for alcohol problems.

Given this background, for the purposes of this report, a special population will be viewed as any subgroup that has been identified by the field as needing a specifically tailored "culturally sensitive" treatment program. The committee has chosen to look at developments and issues for only a few of the commonly identified special population groups and the evolution and effectiveness of treatment programs designed for them as portrayed in the research and clinical literature. It is important to note that these groups are by no means inclusive of all special population groups; rather, they have been selected as representatives of special populations as a whole. Chapter 15 considers these groups on the basis of structural characteristics (i.e., demographic characteristics); Chapter 16, adapts the perspectives of functional characteristics (i.e., circumstantial concerns) as a definitional framework. Chapter 17 presents the committee's conclusions and recommendations on the issue of treatment for alcohol problems among special populations.

REFERENCES

Alcohol, Drug Abuse, and Mental Health Administration (ADAMHA). 1984. Alcohol and Drug Abuse and Mental Health Services Data: Report to Congress. Rockville, Md.: ADAMHA.

Alcohol, Drug Abuse, and Mental Health Administration (ADAMHA). 1986. Alcohol and Drug Abuse and Mental Health Services Block Grant: Report to Congress. Rockville, Md.: ADAMHA.

Alcohol, Drug Abuse, and Mental Health Administration (ADAMHA). 1988. Alcohol and Drug Abuse Treatment and Rehabilitation Block Grant: Report to Congress. Rockville, Md.: ADAMHA.

Braiker, H. B. 1982. The diagnosis and treatment of alcoholism in women. Pp. 111-139 in Special Population Issues, J. de Luca, ed. Washington, D.C.: U.S. Government Printing Office.

DeVita, A. 1988. Congressional activity to define and address alcohol-related problems of special populations: Selected provisions, 1970-1987. Compiled for the IOM Committee for the Study of Treatment and Rehabilitation Services for Alcoholism and Alcohol Abuse. Office of Policy Analysis, National Institute on Alcohol Abuse and Alcoholism, Rockville, Md., July.

Diesenhaus, H. I. 1982. Current trends in treatment programming for problem drinkers and alcoholics. Pp. 219-290 in Prevention, Intervention, and Treatment: Concerns and Models, J. de Luca, ed. Washington, D.C.: U.S. Government Printing Office.

Gilbert, M. J., and R. C. Cervantes. 1988. Alcohol treatment for Mexican Americans: A review of utilization patterns and therapeutic approaches. Pp. 199-231 in Alcohol Consumption among Mexicans and Mexican Americans: A Binational Perspective, M. J. Gilbert, ed. Los Angeles: Spanish Speaking Mental Health Research Center, University of California, Los Angeles .

Gomberg, E. L. 1982. Special populations. Pp. 337-354 in Alcohol, Science, and Society Revisited, E. L. Gomberg, H. R. White, and J. A. Carpenter, eds. Ann Arbor, Mich.: University of Michigan Press.

Gunnerson, U., and M. L. Feldman. 1978. Alcohol and Alcoholism Programs: A Technical Assistance Manual for Health Systems Agencies. San Leandro, Calif.: Human Services, Inc..

Heckler, M. M. 1985. Report of the Secretary's Task Force on Black and Minority Health. Washington, D.C.: U.S. Department of Health and Human Services.

Lex, B. W. 1985. Alcohol problems in special populations. Pp. 89-187 in The Diagnosis and Treatment of Alcoholism, J. H. Mendelson and N. K. Mello, eds. New York: McGraw-Hill.

McGough, D. P., and M. Hindman. 1986. A Guide to Planning Alcoholism Treatment Programs. Rockville, Md.: National Institute on Alcohol Abuse and Alcoholism.

Mitnick, L. 1978. Manpower issues in community alcoholism programs. Pp. 159-169 in Report of the ADAMHA Manpower Policy Analysis Task Force. vol. 2, Working Papers and Other Supporting Documents, D. M. Kole, ed. Rockville, Md.: Alcohol, Drug Abuse, and Mental Health Administration.

National Institute on Alcohol Abuse and Alcoholism (NIAAA). 1983. Executive Report: Data from the September 1982 National Drug and Alcoholism Treatment Utilization Survey. Rockville, Md.: National Institute on Alcohol Abuse and Alcoholism.

National Institute on Drug Abuse/National Institute on Alcohol Abuse and Alcoholism (NIDA/NIAAA). 1989. Highlights from the 1987 National Drug and Alcoholism Treatment Unit Survey (NDATUS). Rockville, Md.: NIDA/NIAAA.

Plaut, T. F. A., ed. 1967. Alcohol Problems: A Report to the Nation. New York: Oxford University Press.

Reed, P. G., and D. S. Sanchez. 1986. Characteristics of Alcoholism Services in the United States-1984: Data from the September 1984 National Alcoholism and Drug Abuse Program Inventory. Rockville, Md.: National Institute on Alcohol Abuse and Alcoholism.

Rogler, L. H., R. G. Malgady, G. Costantino, and R. Blumenthal. What do culturally sensitive mental health services mean: The case of Hispanics. American Psychologist 42:565- 570.

Rosenberg, C. M. 1982. The paraprofessionals in alcoholism treatment. Pp. 802-809 in Encyclopedic Handbook of Alcoholism, E. M. Pattison and E. Kaufman, eds. New York: Gardner Press.

Saxe, L., D. Dougherty, K. Esty, and M. Fine. 1983. The Effectiveness and Costs of Alcoholism Treatment. Washington, D.C.: U.S. Congress, Office of Technology Assessment.

Staub, G. E., and L. M. Kent, eds. 1973. The Paraprofessional in the Treatment of Alcoholism. Springfield, Ill.: Charles C. Thomas.

U.S. Department of Health and Human Services (USDHHS). 1981. Fourth Special Report to the U.S. Congress on Alcohol and Health. Rockville, Md.: National Institute on Alcohol Abuse and Alcoholism.

U.S. Department of Health and Human Services (USDHHS). 1983. Fifth Special Report to the U.S. Congress on Alcohol and Health. Rockville, Md.: National Institute on Alcohol Abuse and Alcoholism.

U.S. Department of Health and Human Services (USDHHS). 1986. Toward a National Plan to Combat Alcohol Abuse and Alcoholism. Report submitted to the United States Congress. Rockville, Md.: National Institute on Alcohol Abuse and Alcoholism.

U.S. Department of Health and Human Services (USDHHS). 1987. Sixth Special Report to the U.S. Congress on Alcohol and Health. Rockville, Md.: National Institute on Alcohol Abuse and Alcoholism.

U.S. Department of Health, Education, and Welfare (USDHEW). 1971. First Special Report to the U.S. Congress on Alcohol and Health. Rockville, Md.: National Institute on Alcohol Abuse and Alcoholism.

U.S. Department of Health, Education, and Welfare (USDHEW). 1974. Second Special Report to the U.S. Congress on Alcohol and Health. Rockville, Md.: National Institute on Alcohol Abuse and Alcoholism.

U.S. Department of Health, Education, and Welfare (USDHEW). 1978. Third Special Report to the U.S. Congress on Alcohol and Health. Rockville, Md.: National Institute on Alcohol Abuse and Alcoholism.

Vannicelli, M. 1984. Treatment outcome of alcoholic women: The state of the art in relation to sex bias and expectancy effects. Pp. 369-412 in Alcohol Problems of Women: Antecedents, Consequences, and Interventions, S. C. Wilsnack and L. J. Beckman, eds. New York: Guilford.

Vannicelli, M. 1988. Executive summary: Key issues related to the treatment of alcoholic women. Prepared for the IOM Committee for the Study of Treatment and Rehabilitation Services for Alcoholism and Alcohol Abuse, March.

Westermeyer, J. 1988. Executive summary: Culture, special populations, and alcoholism treatment. Prepared for the IOM Committee for the Study of Treatment and Rehabilitation Services for Alcoholism and Alcohol Abuse, April.

15 Populations Defined by Structural Characteristics

This chapter specifically examines current research and clinical practice emphases for several representative special populations. The discussion is not meant to be a comprehensive review of research and clinical practice but a selective evaluation of the current state of knowledge about these groups in order to suggest what needs to be taken into account in future program development efforts and the studies of treatment organization and outcome that are required for such development. The groups discussed in this chapter are those which are defined by a common structural (demographic) characteristic: women, adolescents, the elderly, American Indians, Asian Americans and Pacific Islanders, blacks and Hispanics. These special populations are defined in terms of a fixed characteristic (gender, race, or ethnicity) or a developmental characteristic (age).

Women

The studies conducted over the last seven years have shown nothing to warrant significant changes in the conclusions reached following a systematic review of the treatment outcome literature from 1972 to 1980 on women with alcohol problems (Vannicelli, 1984, 1988; Blume, 1986, 1987; Roman, 1988). In keeping with earlier reviews, Vannicelli concluded that there are relatively few solidly established facts about the specific interventions that increase the probability of successful outcomes of treatment for women with alcohol problems. A number of treatments have been enthusiastically endorsed for women including family therapy, group therapy, separate rather than combined treatment for men and women, and female rather than male therapists. Yet, there are few scientific studies that examine or support: (a) the superiority of group versus individual therapy for women, (b) the value of family therapy over other modalities, (c) the need for women to be treated separately, and (d) the value of a female over a male therapist. Moreover, there appears to be little evidence supporting the superior efficacy of any particular treatment modality for women.

Blume (1987) and Roman (1988) also note that there has been no systematic research on the differential effectiveness of treatment programs designed for women. In general, in treatment for alcohol problems, males and females with comparable sociodemographic characteristics (marital status, employment, social stability, etc.) and at the same levels of problem severity appear to do equally well in the same treatment settings. Outcome monitoring in a selected set of programs that participate in the Chemical Abuse/Addiction Treatment Outcome Registry (CATOR) showed little difference on the basis of sex, leading Blume to suggest that there is no reason to believe that females are harder to treat than males or are less likely to recover—a common perception. What is not known are the components of treatment that would improve treatment outcome for both males and females (Blume, 1987).

What is known is that there has been a notable increase in the number of women appearing for treatment over the past 10 years, particularly younger women, although they are still seen as seriously underrepresented in treatment when prevalence rates are considered (National Council on Alcoholism, 1987). The male-to-female ratio in national prevalence rates for alcohol problems and dependence appears to be about 2 to 1, while the treated prevalence rate appears to be closer to 4 to 1 (Gomberg, 1981; Beckman and Amaro, 1984; Blume, 1987, Roman, 1988). There is some evidence that these ratios vary for those in treatment in publicly funded programs and those in treatment in private sector programs. The increase in women in treatment is paralleled by an increase in women affiliated with AA: 34 percent of its members are now women. The reasons commonly given for the continued under-representation of women in formal treatment are the greater stigma still associated with a diagnosis of having alcohol problems for women, including the associated stigma of perceived sexual promiscuity (Blume, 1987), and the lack of specialized treatment facilities, particularly the lack of child care facilities (Lex, 1985; Blume, 1987; Vannicelli, 1988). There is also evidence suggesting that age of onset of drinking problems is later for women than for men and is often tied to important life transitions that have implications for the types of treatment needed. Age and marital status are seen as important variables for establishing both risk status and treatment response (Braiker, 1982; Harrison and Belille, 1987; Blume, 1987; Roman, 1988). Research relating prognostic factors to treatment efficacy in females is equally nondefinitive.

Debate continues regarding both how much of what we know about treatment outcome for males with alcohol problems can be applied to women and the extent to which special programs and treatment modalities for females are needed (Blume, 1987; Roman, 1988; Vannicelli, 1988). These issues become especially problematic because the data for males comparing specific treatment modalities within subgroups of males with differential prognoses are also quite sparse. There are those who argue (e.g., Braiker, 1984) that much of what we know about treating males can be meaningfully applied to females as well. However, until the advent of systematic studies examining individual and key subgroup differences in response to various types of treatment, knowledge will continue to be limited regarding the therapeutic modalities differentially suited to females rather than to males and to different types of females with alcohol problems.

It is important to note that there are also many subgroups within the population of women that may have specific needs for differential treatment services in addition to those required by all women. Typologies have been suggested based on personality differences, sexual orientation, age of onset, race/ethnicity, psychopathology, other drug use, childbearing status, and socioeconomic factors (Schuckit and Morrisey, 1976; Braiker, 1982; Dawkins and Harper, 1983; Vannicelli, 1984; Lex, 1985; Amaro et al., 1987; Blume, 1987; Roman, 1988):

> Although an inclination to draw a profile of "the typical alcoholic woman" still exists, it is generally agreed that female alcoholics comprise a heterogeneous group . . . Like male alcoholics, female alcoholics differ from one another on a variety of important dimensions including age, race, ethnicity, religion, psychopathology, occupational status, education and socioeconomic status. Consequently numerous classifications have appeared in recent years. (Lex, 1985:101)

Clinical data supported by several studies (Braiker, 1984; Beckman and Amaro, 1986) suggest a number of areas in which females may differ from males, thereby suggesting differential programming needs. These findings indicate that women are more likely than men to have (a) primary affective disorders (as well as depressed/sad mood states); (b) serious liver disease; (c) marital instability; (d) instability of family of origin; (e) spouses with alcohol problems; (f) lower self-esteem; (g) a pattern of drinking in response to major life crises; (h) a history of sexual abuse; (i) opposition to treatment from family and friends; and (j) more child care responsibilities, which is inferred from data indicating that women in treatment are more likely to be divorced and single heads of households than are men.

These apparent differences between men and women with alcohol problems point to a number of practical considerations in the treatment of women. Until definitive studies are undertaken, it is best to infer that treatment programs that specifically attend to some of the particular issues that are of more frequent concern to women will be most effective with women. For example, it is best in light of current knowledge to assume that more effective outcomes with women will be obtained with treatment programs that offer the following: (a) child care; (b) assessments of psychiatric disorder and treatment for depression, when indicated; (c) methods of building self-esteem, perhaps through skills training; (d) support offered to and education of family and friends; (e) assessments of accompanying medical disorders; (f) availability of staff to work with families; and (g) provisions for teaching coping strategies for dealing with stress. In the absence of outcome monitoring, however, the value of these recommendations remains speculative; providing the services detailed above may be just as significant in improving outcome for men who do not do well in standard treatment.

In general, distinct types of treatment differ in attractiveness for different types of persons, but knowledge is currently limited regarding which women do best in particular treatment modalities. The potential gains in effectiveness of treatment for women with alcohol problems offered by programs that attend specifically to their needs are supported by the work of Beckman and her colleagues (1984). These researchers indicated that environmental, social, and situational circumstances, as well as characteristics of the treatment delivery system, influenced whether women entered treatment in those facilities.

In addition to the research noted thus far, there are studies that suggest useful approaches but that require replication before alternative policy recommendations can be made. Recommendations for gender-specific treatment that are based primarily on clinical experience emphasize providing social support (e.g. Gomberg, 1981; Roman, 1988). Yet a study of structural factors in treatment program utilization in California suggested that women were more likely to choose programs on the basis of their need for alcohol problems treatment, with social support being a lesser consideration (Beckman and Kocel, 1982). What is required to answer the question of whether gender-specific treatment programs for women are more effective than the standard treatment is a battery of adequate clinical and services research studies. The committee suggests that consideration be given to establishing a research demonstration grant program for women, similar to the former NIAAA categorical services demonstration grants but with much more stringent research and evaluation components (perhaps modelled after the current NIAAA homeless research demonstration program [NIAAA, 1987]). Currently there are a sufficient number of specialized women's treatment programs that could be brought together in properly managed research consortia to examine the effect of individual characteristics and treatment program structures and activities, similar to those listed earlier, on the outcome of treatment (Vannicelli, 1988).

At this point controversy persists regarding differences in prognoses for males and females and whether the course or quality of recovery differs for men and women. Although not substantiated by research, the myth prevails that women have a poorer treatment prognosis than men. *The perpetuation of this myth in the face of available outcome monitoring data, combined with the minimal available data regarding the superiority of any particular treatment for women, demonstrates a critical need for more and better treatment outcome research. Such research should clearly specify the treatment process and define the differential ingredients applicable to men and women. The results of treatment outcome studies should be analyzed and reported for both males and females.*

Adolescents

The committee encountered several major problems in attempting to review the current status of treatment programming for youthful problem drinkers that make it difficult to develop a coherent description of the field. Current efforts in treating youthful problem drinkers are marked by the following: (a) a lack of clinical studies comparing the variety of treatment approaches recommended as a result of clinical experience; (b) concerns about the overutilization and cost-efficiency of hospital-based and residential inpatient rehabilitation; (c) the lack of precision in and agreement on the definition of problem drinking and alcohol dependence in adolescents; (d) disagreement over the need for a combined substance abuse approach or an alcohol-focused approach to treatment; and (e) controversy over the need for age-segregated facilities.

There is perhaps no special population about which so much has been written; yet, despite the more than 2,000 published papers, the common feeling among investigators in this area is that very little is known about how best to treat youth with alcohol and other drug problems (Filstead and Anderson, 1983; Blum, 1987, 1988; Winters and Henley, 1988). On the one hand (as is the case with women), there is very little systematic research involving well-designed clinical trials that compare the alternative strategies suggested by clinical experience (e.g., Maloney, 1976; Millman and Khuri, 1982) for providing culturally and developmentally appropriate alcohol problems treatment to adolescents. It is not known, for example, which of the youths who drink heavily during adolescence will continue to do so as adults or and which will "mature out" of a course of heavy drinking without formal intervention or treatment (Fillmore et al., 1988) (see Chapter 6). It is not known whether there are any biologic markers of juvenile addiction. Moreover, to date there has never been a treatment matching study conducted among youthful drinkers.

Given the dramatic increases in the number of programs that purport to offer specialized treatment to youth (see Chapter 14) and given the concerns that have been expresses expressed regarding the overutilization of inpatient and residential treatment (e.g., Rodriguez, 1988), there has been a lamentable paucity of funding for studies to evaluate treatment process, outcome, and matching for youth. There are virtually no experimental studies on the effectiveness of treatment for alcohol problems among adolescent and young adult problem drinkers. Most research efforts with youth have studied the extent of alcohol use and problem drinking; few have investigated treatment effectiveness (Smart, 1979; Filstead and Anderson, 1983; Blum, 1988). The design of treatment services for youth is proceeding primarily on the basis of limited clinical experience and values rather than on solid, generalizable empirical findings.

On the other hand, some advances have been made over the last decade, particularly in understanding the processes by which youth are introduced to alcohol and other drug use. The Johnston team's Monitoring the Future Project has made an important contribution with its finding that although slightly more than 90 percent of high school seniors reported having had an alcoholic beverage, only approximately 5 percent reported drinking on a daily basis, with a male-to-female ratio of almost 2 to 1 (Johnston et al., 1987). In addition, the natural history of alcohol abuse through adolescence into young adulthood has been more clearly elucidated by Kandel and her colleagues (Kandel and Logan, 1984; Yamaguchi and Kandel, 1984). They reported a peak prevalence between 16-18 years of age, with maximal consumption continuing for the subsequent four years, then diminishing significantly. Likewise, in a large longitudinal study in Colorado, Donovan and his colleagues found that 57 percent of male and 73 percent of female subjects originally categorized as "problem drinkers" were either abstinent or moderate drinkers at the time of follow-up seven years later (Donovan, Jessor, and Jessor, 1977). Fillmore and her colleagues (1988) report similar findings in their review of longitudinal studies.

Beyond the demographic trends, there is a spate of social-psychological research that characterizes the heavy juvenile drinker as follows (Blum, 1988): (a) males predominate over females; (b) male drinkers tend to have lower achievement orientation and tend to be more rebellious than nondrinking peers; (c) heavy drinking correlates strongly with other socially deviant juvenile behaviors (e.g., precocious sexual behavior); (d) early onset drinking is the best single predictor of substance abuse; (e) juvenile drinking behavior tends to parallel that of parents; and (f) for youths in treatment programs, significant numbers have other problems concurrent with their drinking (e.g., learning disabilities, major depression).

Yet for neither adults nor adolescents is there any consensus on what constitutes problem drinking or substance abuse. For juveniles, definitions range from the legal perspective that any use of a substance by juveniles is tantamount to abuse (National Council of Juvenile and Family Court Judges (1987) to defining abuse based on the impact which drinking has on adolescent development (Jessor et al., 1980). Without agreement in the field as to what constitutes the disease or condition, the clinician is left to his or her own resources; as a result, adult definitions of alcohol problems tend to be applied to juveniles without the empirical justification to support such applications.

Because there is considerable disagreement about the definition of alcohol dependence and problem drinking among youth, great care must be exercised in making such a diagnosis with youth. Juvenile possession or use of alcohol in most situations outside the home is legally defined as a status offense (Marden and Kolodner, 1978; Morrisey and Schuckit, 1978). Labeling an adolescent a problem drinker as a result of being picked up for drinking or being intoxicated can be an unnecessarily stigmatizing and traumatizing experience. Furthermore, it may be an incorrect diagnosis.

For example, Schuckit and Morrisey (1978) interviewed 693 adolescents (aged 20 and under) who had been referred by the courts to alcohol counseling and education centers (for evaluation and referral for treatment, if needed) as part of a diversion project for those arrested for alcohol-related crimes. The study compared three groups: (1) those who were arrested for some crime but who had never been arrested as a minor in possession (MIP) of alcohol, (2) those who had only one MIP arrest, and those with two or more MIP arrests. The multiple-MIP-arrests group manifested the most serious problems with antisocial behavior, drug and alcohol use, school problems, and other life problems. The no-MIP-arrests group was quite heterogeneous and demonstrated moderate levels of problems. The single-MIP-arrest group did not manifest any severe personal, social, alcohol, or drug problems; referral to treatment was not indicated, and they could have been harmed by being labeled a problem drinker. The authors concluded that the multiple-MIP-arrests group would be the least likely to be harmed by referral to alcoholism treatment, but even they might pass out of the adolescent drinking problem status if left untreated. Morrisey and Schuckit recommended against such mandatory programs in which all youths who had been picked up were referred for treatment.

Thus, definitional issues must be clarified before systematic treatment design and implementation can take place. In addition to questions about what constitutes a youthful problem drinker, there is no agreed-upon standard as to which age groups make up the youth special population. Some define the age group as individuals 25 years of age or younger; others limit it to those in childhood and adolescence, setting the upper age at 18. In its original categorical grant and state plan initiatives, the federal government focused on adolescents aged 18 and under, but in some instances considered those aged from 19 to 24 as "youths". Some practitioners and researchers consider the upper age limit to coincide with the age at which purchase and possession of beverage alcohol becomes legal; formerly, the age limit varied among the states, but it has now been increased to 21 in all states in response to concerns over drinking and driving.

The increase in alcohol use and problem drinking by adolescents and young adults has generated increasing concern in recent years, and much popular attention has been paid to alcohol as the "number one drug" abused by youth. Yet, there is still much disagreement about what constitutes a clinical state requiring formal treatment (Marden and Kolodner, 1978; Filstead and Anderson, 1983; Blum, 1985). The point on which there is agreement is that the use of treatment facilities by young persons is on the increase, and as noted earlier, there has been a dramatic increase in the number of treatment units that either offer a specialized program for youth in a mixed age setting or serve as a specialized program only for youth.

Another area in which little is known either pathophysiologically or psychologically is the comparability between heavy juvenile and adult alcohol ingestion. The lack of consensus as to what constitutes juvenile alcohol dependence weighs against any comparability among treatment center approaches. As Skinner (1981) notes, assessment decisions tend to be guided by the philosophical orientation of the specific treatment center.

These concerns raise the question of whether adolescents and/or young adults should be treated in separate programs, whether existing adult-oriented programs should be modified to serve them more appropriately, or whether both changes are needed. There is a general assumption that those under the age of 18 are still struggling with the developmental tasks of adolescence and need separate programs which include specialized attention to these concerns (Blum, 1988; Filstead and Anderson, 1988). Yet many treatment programs set their upper or lower age limits with no regard for this boundary. The age at which a minor can legally consent to treatment varies from state to state; this and other legal considerations can affect treatment design. There have been no recent studies of the varieties of approaches that are being used and the differential outcome, if any.

Existing youth treatment programs for alcohol problems can be classified as traditional or nontraditional (Maloney, 1976). Traditional treatment programs utilize many of the same techniques and concepts as adult programs and label the young person as an alcoholic or problem drinker. Concerns have been voiced by some in the treatment field that most of the new residential programs being established are based on the adult model of brief inpatient rehabilitation with minimal aftercare (Woltzen et al., 1986; Blum, 1988; Durst, 1988).

Nontraditional treatment facilities tend to use a different approach. They avoid labelling the youth as an alcoholic and try to work within the framework of the youth's culture and developmental tasks. The focus in this kind of treatment is on alcohol use as one of many expressions of the growing up process. Labeling the young person as an alcoholic is seen as potentially harmful, a technique that may restrict the individual's opportunities to grow out of the period of excessive use. Such nontraditional programs are usually conceptualized as youth services agencies and try to offer a wide range of activities—educational, recreational, and vocational as well as those focused on the adolescent's drinking behavior. Nontraditional programs stress outreach and early intervention. Nontraditional agencies are most likely to use peer counseling, a treatment modality in which young people who have recently been through the program are trained to work with newcomers. The premise is that the adolescent peer counselor will be better able to reach the youth new to treatment because of their shared personal and cultural experiences. The use of peer counselors in adolescent programs embodies the same principles as the use of recovered alcoholic counselors in AA-oriented adult programs and of counsels who share a common cultural background in other special population programs.

There have been no recent studies to evaluate the effectiveness of either approach or to determine whether particular youth do better in one type of program or the other. Until recently, for the adolescent, no empirical base existed for the clinical assessment of the juvenile in need of treatment for alcohol problems. Yet many clinicians and researchers deem it essential that treatment of youth begin with such an assessment (Blum, 1988; Winters and Henley, 1988). For example, Filstead and Anderson (1983) stressed the importance of beginning the treatment of adolescents, whether on an inpatient or outpatient basis, with an extended "evaluation-assessment" period. Hoffmann and colleagues (1987) described such a process for evaluation and assignment to the appropriate level of care: they called for either a 3 to 6 hour assessment on an outpatient basis for adolescents who are socially and behaviorally compliant, or an inpatient assessment of approximately one week for noncompliant, nonstable adolescents. The assessment they proposed covered seven dimensions of clinical status that are held to be important for making such a placement decision: (1) acute alcohol or drug intoxication, or both, and potential for withdrawal; (2) physical conditions or complications; (3) psychiatric conditions or complications; (4) life area impairment (behavioral, social, academic, legal); (5) treatment acceptance or rejection (motivation; potential for compliance); (6) loss of control over drinking precipitating a possible relapse crisis; and (7) the recovery environment (supportive and remedial versus pathogenic and destructive). The levels of care which they identify are mutual/self-help, low-intensity outpatient treatment, intensive after-school treatment, structured day treatment, medically supervised intensive inpatient treatment, and medically managed intensive evaluation.

However promising this approach appears, neither its program classification scheme nor its assessment battery has been empirically validated. Indeed, the majority of work on assessment and on matching has been done with adults. Specific research to develop concepts and assessment tools that are appropriate for use with adolescents is required. There continues, however, to be a lack of well-developed, standardized, and validated assessment instruments for use by clinicians in the identification, referral, level of care placement, and treatment planning for youth (Owen and Nyberg, 1983; Filstead and Anderson, 1986; Winters and Henley, 1988). Although there have been some brief screening tools (e.g., the Adolescent Alcohol Involvement Scale; Mayer and Filstead, 1979) or high school survey instruments (e.g., Johnston et al., 1987) that were developed for use with adolescents, most programs tend to use questionnaires that they develop in-house and informal assessment procedures (Owen and Neyberg, 1983).

More recently, a three-dimensional assessment schema exploring the impact of drinking on psychosocial, biomedical, and school functioning was developed (Halikas, et. al., 1984). The model was based on a study of 1,185 adolescents and has been useful in distinguishing problem drinkers from nonproblem drinkers. This work has been used in the development of the placement criteria described above (Hoffmann et al., 1987).

Most importantly, a new adolescent assessment instrument has recently been developed by the Adolescent Assessment Project in St. Paul, Minnesota, and it promises to be the most comprehensive adolescent alcohol assessment tool to date (Winters and Henley, 1988). The assessment employs both a written instrument—the Personal Experience Inventory—and an interview—the Adolescent Diagnostic Interview. It could be validated through cooperative study in the many new programs which have been recently implemented, given a sufficient desire to remedy the lack of investment in studies on youth treatment process and outcome.

For the adolescent, as for the adult with a drinking problem, there is a wide array of treatment alternatives that include: behavioral, operant conditioning, social learning, psychosocial, and self-help approaches. Yet despite the diversity of approaches, there has been little attempt at treatment matching for adolescents' and no controlled studies of treatment outcomes have ever been undertaken for this special population.

The CATOR data base currently provides the most extensive outcome monitoring longitudinal data on juveniles who have been in treatment, conducting 6- and 12-month follow-ups on 493 youths (Harrison and Hoffmann, 1987). The data collected through the registry are self-reported, which always raises methodological problems in interpreting the findings. Keeping this caveat in mind, Harrison and Hoffmann determined the following, using total abstinence of at least 3 months every 6 month posttreatment period as their criterion: (a) females did better than males; (b) for females, a prior history of a suicide attempt correlated poorly with outcome; (c) for males, those who viewed themselves more negatively at treatment initiation have a lower relapse rate; (d) certain factors appeared to be unrelated to outcome including: prior sexual abuse, learning disabilities, a lack of intimate relationships, relationship with parents, or parental substance abuse; (e) treatment completion was positively correlated with outcome; and (e) a strong positive relationship between the duration of posttreatment involvement in AA and abstinence, such that two-thirds of those who remained in AA for the entire follow-up year reported total abstinence, compared with 11 percent of those who never attended.

Although these data provide some clues about the individual characteristics that are most highly correlated with posttreatment abstinence, little is known of the treatment center and treatment modality characteristics that best meet this outcome objective. Most importantly, nothing is known of the treatment match or matches that will optimize outcome for adolescents who are problem drinkers.

Moreover, a single criterion of treatment success (e.g., abstinence) has limited utility, as does a single follow-up evaluation source (e.g., adolescent themselves). Rather, a multiple-factor assessment model, such as that proposed in Chapter 10, is desirable for adolescents as well as adults. It is critical to include measures of school and job performance, as well as measures of interpersonal and social adjustment that are tailored to the adolescent's living situation. Such a multidimensional assessment model has rarely, if ever, been applied to assessing adolescent alcohol treatment programs and those who complete treatment.

Because of the paucity of substantive evaluation or longitudinal data on adolescents in alcohol treatment programs, one is left with only vague impressions: that in the short run (e.g., 6 to 12 months), some kind of treatment is better than no treatment if abstinence is the goal. On the other hand, in the long run, it is uncertain whether the steady improvement which has been reported over a seven-year period is more a function of "maturing out" than of treatment itself (Barr and Antes, 1981; Fillmore et al., 1988).

An important innovation has been the development of the student assistance programs, which are modeled after employee assistance programs, or EAPs (Anderson, 1979; USDHHS, 1987). As in an EAP, a critical feature of student assistance programs is the development of a policy and procedure for how the school will handle the problem drinking student. The policy development procedure is seen as helping school officials and students to confront their own ambivalent attitudes toward alcohol use and yields a consistent rather than erratic response to youth who are identified as needing assistance for alcohol problems. Proponents recommend that students be involved in the policy development process. Proponents also suggest that students be involved in program operations as lecturers, discussion leaders, and peer counselors should the school choose to implement its own alcohol education and intervention program in addition to the providing the identification components.

The four essential ingredients of the student assistance program are (1) a clear policy that establishes expectations and limits; (2) consistent application of the policy; (3) identification, motivation, and referral of problem drinking adolescents; and (4) follow-up monitoring. These activities are generally carried out by a resource coordinator or counselor who acts as a safe, confidential linking agent between the troubled student, the school administration, and treatment personnel.

The identification of students with alcohol problems is often an unforeseen outcome of alcohol education programs whose focus is primary prevention. Teachers ordinarily are ill-prepared to make an appropriate referral if and when a student comes forward. The implication is that didactic prevention programs should be linked with student assistance programs whenever prevention programs are introduced into a school setting. And, whenever these programs are designed as "broad-brush" efforts—that is geared to assisting the student with any type of problem—labeling and stigmatization can be avoided. Appropriate screening and assessment by the counselor to identify the variety and severity of problem drinking manifested can lead to early intervention either through brief intervention delivered on the spot or through referral to the most appropriate treatment setting as well as the definition of realistic goals. Student assistance programs, like employee assistance programs for adults in the workplace, can serve as the independent assessment and referral centers needed to ensure the appropriate use of specialty and primary care treatments. This mode of functioning is the essence of the committee's vision (see Chapter 9).

Again, like many of the recent innovations in treatment for adolescents, the number of student assistance programs has grown significantly, but the drawback is that there have been no systematic evaluations of their effectiveness.

The evaluation of treatment for youth with alcohol problems is complicated by the lack of a single system that can be described and by the heterogeneity of adolescents' drinking problems (e.g., Welte and Barnes, 1987). Indeed, an effort is required to describe in detail the many programs and agencies that are trying to provide such treatment. Assessment, intervention, and treatment are offered in a wide variety of school, social services, primary health care and correctional settings as well as in the specialty mental health and alcohol problems treatment sectors. There are no good available data on who is being treated where, by what modalities, and with what outcome. Although there has been concern expressed regarding the number of youths being admitted to inpatient treatment settings, there is data that suggest that young people are still underrepresented in treatment when publicly funded treatment programs are surveyed (Butynski et al., 1987). Clearly, specific recommendations on how and where to treat adolescents are impossible without a better data base on existing treatment programs and their effectiveness for different individuals.

The Elderly

The prevalence of alcohol problems in the elderly (persons aged 60 and older) is given by the U.S. Department of Health and Human Services (1987) as 2 percent, which is less than the rate for younger age groups. The prevalence rate has been found to be higher for men (5 percent) than for women (1 percent). There are still concerns about the exact rate because of questions about the appropriateness of the methods used to identify elderly persons with alcohol problems (Graham, 1986, 1988; Douglas et al., 1988).

Generally, two different subgroups have been identified—early onset problem drinkers and late onset problem drinkers—with different histories and prognoses. A threefold classification has also been proposed that has a third group with a history of experiencing mild or moderate problems earlier in life and developing a severe problem only in later years (Williams, 1985). The value of these typologies for differential treatment assignment has yet to be established (Atkinson, 1988; Hurt et al., 1988). Early onset problem drinkers are thought to account for two-thirds of elderly persons with alcohol problems; they generally have a history of long-term problem drinking and are likely to have serious physical problems. Late onset drinkers have no history of alcohol problems prior to their identification and typically begin heavy drinking in response to a major life stress (e.g., retirement, death of a spouse or friend, poor health). Early onset problem drinkers are assumed to have a poorer prognosis. It has been assumed by some clinicians that all elderly persons with alcohol problems can benefit more from psychological and sociocultural approaches than to physiological approaches (e.g., Zimberg, 1978, 1983); this assumption remains untested.

As with the other special population groups being discussed in this section, reports of empirical studies that compare treatment tailored to the special needs of the elderly with standard, "generic" treatment for alcohol problems are lacking. Indeed, there are very few studies of treatment effectiveness which focus on the elderly; much of what is currently believed about the assessment and treatment of the elderly remains based on unsystematic clinical observations and indirect evidence (Graham, 1988). There are, however, a number of descriptive studies beginning to appear which do attempt to explore whether mixed-age settings or programs were more or less effective for treating elderly persons with alcohol problems (e.g., Kofoed et al., 1987; Hurt et al., 1888). The results of these studies are conflicting, possibly because of the differing socioeconomic status of the persons studied (Atkinson, 1988). A number of other studies have reviewed retention and outcome rates for younger and older persons treated in the same mixed-age programs. However, these studies were inadequate to establish which approach can lead to more successful outcome, and it is not possible at this time for the committee to suggest specific guidelines.

There have also been a number of attempts to identify those factors that were associated with successful outcome in the elderly regardless of the modality or approach used. Characteristics that have been associated with poorer prognosis are chronic physical problems, psychiatric comorbidity, family drinking practices, and isolation (Williams, 1985). There have been no studies on the long-term impact of treatment in this special population (Mishara, 1985; Hurt et al., 1988).

Another question often raised is whether elderly persons with alcohol problems can and should be treated in special programs within the alcohol problems sector or in special programs within the specialized geriatric services system (Williams, 1985). There does not seem to be a great deal of activity in the development of either type of program at this time, although several states (e.g., New Jersey, Michigan, Connecticut) have made special outreach efforts to bring more elderly persons into standard treatment programs. Elderly persons continue to underrepresented in standard treatment programs (Graham, 1988).

American Indians

According to May (1982), the "drunken Indian" stereotype has been prevalent throughout American society since early colonial days. The literature is replete with descriptions that reinforce negative myths about the Indian and alcohol, and it is only in the last decades that researchers have attempted to consider the complexity and variation among the American Indian peoples and their associations with alcohol. Indeed Westermeyer (1974) maintains that understanding the cultural diversity among American Indians is crucial in avoiding the "drunken Indian" stereotype. Notwithstanding, although "alcoholism" may not be a universal Indian problem, it is a problem for many tribal groups (Mail and McDonald, 1980), and it has been identified by the Indian Health Service as requiring significant federal attention (USDHEW, 1971; Mason et al., 1985; Rhoades et al., 1988).

With the 280 recognized tribes in the United States, alcohol consumption rates, prevalence of alcohol problems, drinking practices, and beliefs about alcohol use are found to vary among tribal groups or communities (Westermeyer, et al., 1981; USDHHS, 1987). There appear to be no common patterns of drinking behavior among the tribes, but instead high rates of both heavy drinking and abstinence are reported (Lemert, 1982; May, 1982; Lex, 1985). Despite the abstinence patterns for some tribal groups, alcohol-related problems remain a major source of difficulty for American Indians. There is a strong correlation between American Indian alcohol problems and economic factors; in addition, alcohol abuse has been cited consistently as a major disruptive factor in the family life of American Indians (Lex, 1985).

American Indians and Alaska Natives constitute less than 1 percent of the total population in the United States (USDHHS, 1987). These 1.5 million people maintain relatively higher rates of alcohol problems than the general population (Lex, 1985; Rhoades et al., 1988). American Indians also rank higher in the proportion of abstainers, many of whom are former heavy drinkers who have given up alcohol (Lemert, 1982). Alcohol consumption is reported to be highest and most problematic for American Indian men between the ages of 25 and 44, with a decline after the age of 40 in total consumption and number of drinkers (Indian Health Service, 1980).

Few studies have specifically focused on alcohol use in American Indian females, although the number of females who drink alcohol reportedly is increasing (Lex, 1985). Although American Indian women drink less than men, they account for nearly half of all deaths among Indians from cirrhosis, and they appear to be at particular risk for giving birth to children with fetal alcohol syndrome. The death rate from cirrhosis for American Indian women is three times higher than the rate for other nonwhite women and almost six times higher than that for the population at large (S. Johnson, 1979).

American Indian adolescents show a high rate of alcohol use in comparison with other adolescent groups. Weibel-Orlando (1984) reported that American Indian adolescents began involvement with alcohol at younger ages than other subcultural groups in the United States. Donovan and Jessor (1978) found that 42 percent of American Indian adolescent male drinkers and 31 percent of Indian adolescent female drinkers reported alcohol problems, compared with 34 percent of white male and 25 percent of white female adolescent groups.

Alcohol-related mortality rates are significantly higher for American Indians than for the general population. Thirty-five percent of all American Indian deaths involve alcohol, and 5 of the 10 most frequent causes of death among Indians are alcohol-related. Such deaths include accidents (the rate of motor vehicle accident deaths is 2.5 to 5.5 times higher than that of the general population), liver cirrhosis (2.6 to 3.5 times higher), clinical alcoholism, including psychosis and alcohol related cirrhosis (5.4 to 5.5 times higher), suicide (1.2 to 2.3 times higher), and homicide (1.7 to 2.3 times higher).

In their review of alcohol problems among American Indians, Westermeyer and Baker (1986) cited six studies relating alcohol use in the group with incidents of pneumonia, burns, accidents, fatalities from freezing, malnutrition among children, and infant mortality. American Indians also have a high rate of arrests related to alcohol use (e.g., driving under the influence, drunkenness, disorderly conduct, and violations of liquor laws), which is 12 times that of the general population (Lemert, 1982).

Despite the knowledge that alcohol use has created widespread problems among American Indians, there are relatively few studies that investigate treatment use and treatment effectiveness in this population group. Basic issues concerning the prevalence of problem drinking and the patterns of treatment for alcohol problems among American Indians remain unresolved (Lewis, 1982; Weibel, 1982).

In 1971 NIAAA adopted the reduction of alcoholism among Indians as a priority goal (USDHEW, 1971). A consistent problem in planning alcohol treatment for this special population has been the differing cultural orientations of American Indians and mainstream society, upon whose values prevention and treatment programs are generally based. In general, treatment for the American Indian has been concluded to fall into one of four areas: (1) "nativistic endeavors"; (2) conversion of Indians to evangelistic religions; (3) individually invented types of aids provided by psychotherapy and AA (i.e., the medical model); and (4) programs oriented specifically toward Indians (Lewis, 1982). While the literature is inconclusive about which type of treatment focus is most effective, it is widely believed that few Indians with alcohol problems have been helped by the traditional medical approach to rehabilitation or through non-Indian chapters of AA. Indeed, Westermeyer and Baker (1986) state that "[t]o be effective, programs for Indians must consider cultural, historical, psychological, and social forces. It is also crucial that the treatment staff include positive Indian role models with whom the recovering Indian alcoholic can identify."

There has been relatively rapid growth in the development of Indian treatment programs for alcohol problems, growth that began in the late 1960s and has continued until the present (Rhoades et al., 1988). These programs have had a rather short and frustrating history coupled with an active political life (Levy and Kunitz, 1981). In general, these initial efforts were low-budget programs that provided client-oriented counseling staffed by recovered Indian alcoholics (Towle, 1975). Today, there are over 190 reservation and urban alcoholism treatment programs for American Indians (Mason et al., 1985). Most of these programs have generally evolved out of the Office of Economic Opportunity (OEO) efforts in the late 1960s to provide federal funding to reservation programs. They were than transferred to NIAAA in 1971 and from NIAAA to IHS. In 1976 the number of programs grew when the Office of Alcoholism Programs was established by IHS to oversee and assume financial responsibility for federally funded Indian treatment programs for alcohol problems (see Chapter 4).

As the programs administered and funded by IHS developed, guidelines were established; however, carrying out these standards has been problematic at the very least (May, 1985). In consequence, the results reported for treatment programs targeted at American Indians vary considerably, and published success rates range from 16 percent to 73 percent (Ferguson, 1968; Shore and Von Fumetti, 1972; Wilson and Shore, 1975; Armor, et al., 1978; Westermeyer and Peake, 1983). Despite such variations in program effectiveness, Walker and his colleagues (1985) reported a high rate of alcohol problems treatment use in a sample of urban American Indians, with more than three-quarters of the males and one-half of the females in the sample having a history of treatment for alcoholism.

Even though program developers have made an effort to update guidelines and standards to increase treatment effectiveness, there have been few studies that systematically evaluated alcoholism treatment outcome for American Indians (Shore and Kofoed, 1984). Until recently, treatment outcome studies have been limited to those with the Chippewa (Westermeyer, 1972), the Navajo (Ferguson, 1970) and the Makah (Shore and Von Fumetti, 1970). In these studies, treatment occurred more than ten years ago and the findings indicated successful treatment outcome was elusive. Too, federally funded IHS treatment programs were not included in these studies. In a more recent evaluation of the IHS alcohol treatment programs, Raymond and Raymond (1984) reported that only 8 per cent of these programs performed any outcome evaluation and that the programs in general lacked any guiding philosophy of treatment.

Comparative data for several urban American Indian samples drawn from detoxification, inpatient, halfway house, and outpatient alcoholism treatment settings revealed that successful outcome was infrequent, despite the type of treatment or extended periods in treatment for most persons (Walker et al., 1985). Similar findings were reported from a study of this same sample of American Indians admitted to a detoxification unit: persons continued to experience serious problems with alcohol despite repeated treatment in both medical detoxification and inpatient rehabilitation settings (Kivlahan, et al., 1985).

Many researchers have postulated that a single treatment modality for the American Indian alcoholic will be unsuccessful because of differences in the drinking patterns of the various American Indian groups and the type of psychosocial situations in which they exist (Walker, 1981). To complicate the issue further, researchers generally agree that cultural factors are related to patterns of alcohol abuse; there is little consensus, however, on the precise nature and implications of this relationship (Walker and Kivlahan, 1984). Most treatment programs include combinations of AA principles and traditional activities and religious notions; however, this combination approach, although it may be the most successful programming method, can present difficulties when faced with the rigid constraints of funding requirements (Lewis, 1982). Consequently, there have been calls for a new multimodal approach to treatment, and, to some degree, for a multidisciplinary approach; that is, an approach designed to meet the needs of the individual client (Mail, 1980; Walker, 1981; Young, 1988).

Overall, each of the treatment modalities (AA, religion, medicine, psychology, and traditionalism) contributes in some way to successful treatment outcome for the American Indian with alcohol problems (Mail, 1980). However, in the relative absence of treatment evaluation, it is difficult to assess the strengths and weaknesses of each of these modalities. Without assessing and evaluating specific types of programs, the likelihood of successful treatment outcome is limited. There are, at present, endless questions about the American Indian with alcohol problems that need to be addressed. Such questions include specifying programs that produce successful treatment outcome; identifying individual or blends of treatment modalities that work best for particular subtypes of American Indian patients; and determining the importance of the interplay of sociocultural factors with successful treatment outcome. A wide range of programs has been funded. It is time to step back and very carefully evaluate their functioning to find the answers to these questions.

Asian Americans and Pacific Islanders

Since the studies of Wolff (1972, 1973) and Ewing and coworkers (1974) which suggest that Asians tend to metabolize alcohol faster than other ethnic groups, there has been a commonly held perception that Asian Americans do not abuse alcohol as often as Caucasians. However, some recent studies have shown that there is a great deal of variation among the approximately 20 different nationality groups which are included in the Asian American/Pacific Islander special population category (McGough and Hindman, 1986; USDHHS, 1987; Yamimoto, 1988). Other studies have found that some subgroups have consumption rates approaching those of Caucasians (e.g., Murakami, 1984; Clark, 1985; Ahern; 1985).

Unfortunately, hard data about alcohol use and abuse by Asian Americans and Pacific Islanders are sparse; they consist of a small group studies done in Hawaii and in California noted above and by several others including R. C. Johnson and coworkers at the University of Hawaii (1984). There is a consistent pattern that Caucasians, as a generalization, tend to drink more heavily than persons from other groups. The next heaviest drinkers are the native Hawaiians, followed by (depending on the study) the Asians, either the Japanese or the Filipinos. The number of other Asian groups have not been studied in significant numbers.

The different nationalities represent distinct cultures whose drinking practices are governed by differing traditions, community values, degrees of acculturation, and utilization of community resources for problem solving. McGough and Hindman (1986) identify 9 nationalities from this population that are likely to be seen in U.S. treatment programs and whose cultural response to drinking and to treatment must be taken into account. They are the Chinese, Japanese, Hawaiians, Samoans, Koreans, Cambodians, Thais, Vietnamese, and Filipinos.

There are many interesting questions related to the use and abuse of alcohol by Asians and Pacific Islanders because of genetic differences that have been described by Goedde and others (1980, 1983, and 1985). Aldehyde dehydrogenase (ALDH) isoenzyme negativity in Asians varies from 50 percent in the Han Chinese and 44 percent in the Japanese, to 45 percent among the Zhuang, 30 percent among the Mongols, and 25 percent among the Koreans. The enzyme's absence leads to a buildup of acetaldehyde when alcohol is ingested with very uncomfortable somatic symptoms; therefore, it has been hypothesized that individuals who are ALDH negative will not abuse alcohol. However, some do, and this area is certainly one that should be further studied to determine whether there are additional biological or cultural factors that differentiate these groups and that might be useful for developing prevention and treatment strategies.

In addition to these genetic factors, the influence of traditional cultures in the Orient must be noted. There is a significantly lower prevalence of alcohol use and abuse by females in these groups until they acculturate over several generations. Even then, the prevalence rates may be lower than those found among Caucasian females.

The importance of these factors to the development and treatment of alcohol problems among Asian Americans and Pacific Islanders may also have ramifications for American Indians and Alaska native peoples because of their genetic similarities with Asians. A comprehensive research plan for investigating these questions is very much needed. Thus far, studies on the effectiveness of treatment for alcohol problems for Asian Americans have been minimal. The focus in research has been on the nature and distribution of alcohol problems among the various cultural groups and on broader considerations in the treatment of Asian Americans in psychotherapy (e.g., Sue and Zane, 1987; Sue, 1988). The emphasis in recent years with this special population has been on the establishment of separate, culturally specific and culturally-administered treatment programs that will eliminate barriers and increase utilization (e.g., McGough and Hindman, 1986). As national survey data indicate, there are now a number of such programs (Reed and Sanchez, 1986), but their organization, utilization, and effectiveness have not yet been evaluated.

Blacks

Blacks make up the largest ethnic minority in the United States, about 12 percent of the total population. As with the other special populations that have been discussed, epidemiological surveys and descriptive studies of treatment, along with descriptions of clinical experience, constitute the majority of the research literature available. In contrast to previous editions, the most recent official report to Congress on alcohol and health did not address race/ethnicity as a person characteristic related either to treatment outcome or to access (USDHHS, 1987). Nor was race included as a salient individual characteristic in a recent summary of key issues in treatment outcome evaluation (Longabaugh and Lewis, 1988). The neglect of research on blacks who receive treatment for alcohol problems addressed by King (1981), Saxe and coworkers (1983), and Lex (1985) continues; there have been no studies that have attempted to determine directly through clinical trials which, if any, of the culturally sensitive strategies that are now in use are more effective so that there can be replication and dissemination. In addition, although numerous recommendations have been made regarding separate, culturally specific programs for blacks (e.g., Rogan, 1986), there is disagreement about what a culturally sensitive program should be, given the heterogeneity among blacks in socioeconomic status and residence (urban, rural; North, South) (Harper, 1979). Although blacks who experience alcohol problems are as heterogeneous a group as whites in terms of social class, age, gender, and other such factors, the major focus in prescriptions for culturally relevant treatment has been on the poor, unemployed male.

Researchers continue to report that blacks experience high rates of alcohol-related physical problems, especially black men, who are at higher risk for such disorders as liver cirrhosis and cancer of the esophagus (USDDHS, 1987). National surveys have also found that find blacks of both sexes have higher rates of abstention from alcohol than whites White men were more likely than black men to be heavy drinkers, whereas black women were more likely than white women to be heavy drinkers. Age trends vary: white men appear to drink more heavily at younger ages and then taper off in their drinking; black men report that their drinking rises after the age of 30. In another national survey, a difference was found between white men and black men in terms of the relationship between drinking behavior and income. Among white men, increases in heavy drinking were found to be related to increasing income levels; among black men decreasing income was found to be related to heavier drinking.

There are regional differences in admission rates to treatment that are interpreted as reflecting the increasing urbanization of blacks. Herd (1989) reports on regional variations in admissions to treatment for whites and blacks. The proportions of each in treatment vary by region, with the proportion of blacks in treatment being two to three times higher than their proportion in the state's population in the urban Northeast. In the interior southern states, the proportion in treatment was generally about the same as the state's population. Blacks tended to enter treatment at a younger age than whites even though the age of onset of heavy drinking was later. The implications of these epidemiological findings for treatment design is not immediately evident.

In the past, National Alcohol Profile Information System (NAPIS) data submitted by the NIAAA grantees revealed that more blacks were being treated in predominantly white treatment programs than in those that identified themselves as being black programs (Ferguson and Kirk, 1979). Blacks treated in each of the NIAAA funded special population grant programs were more like the nonblacks seen in that grant program than like blacks seen in other program categories: when compared with blacks being treated in NIAAA funded drinking driver, poverty, or comprehensive treatment programs, blacks being treated in public inebriate programs reported the lowest income and the highest number of years of heavy drinking and average drinking per day just as their nonblack counterparts did; blacks being treated in drinking driver programs had the highest average household income and the lowest average amount of alcohol consumed per day. With the advent of the alcohol, drug abuse, and mental health services block grant, NIAAA funded treatment programs for blacks and other special populations were shifted to state support, and the ability to make such comparisons of person characteristics was lost. Analyses of existing state data bases, similar to those previously performed for the NAPIS data base and similar to those recently completed for Hispanics (Gilbert and Cervantes, 1986, 1988), may be a helpful first step in understanding patterns of utilization and linking these patterns with the epidemiological data to provide suggestions for treatment design.

Hispanics

Diversity is again the main characteristic of this special population group, which is the nation's fastest growing ethnic minority because of new immigrants from Mexico and Central America (Rogler et al., 1987). Of the estimated 18 million Hispanics in the United States in 1986 (U.S. Bureau of the Census, 1987), the majority (60 percent) are Mexican Americans. Puerto Ricans (13 percent) are the next largest group. Each nationality group has a distinct cultural background that results in variations in their attitudes toward drinking and toward treatment for alcohol problems. Indeed, some investigators see no value in even using the general Hispanic category, given these differences (M. J. Gilbert University of California, Los Angeles, personal communication, October 7, 1988). There is also great variation within each nationality group in education, occupation, income, health status, and degree of acculturation. Degree of acculturation is often determined by language (i.e., whether the individual is bilingual or monolingual). Acculturation is seen as a significant factor in treatment response.

Mexican Americans are concentrated in the Southwest, Cubans, in Florida, and Puerto Ricans, on the east coast but mainly in New York (Lex, 1985). These national groups differ in their drinking patterns, with Mexican American men having the highest rates of heavy drinking when compared to the other groups (Caetano, 1988). Differences in drinking patterns are also found between those born in this country and those born in the country of origin. Age variations in self reported problems were more similar to those for black men than for whites: the rates did not drop at 30 years of age but remained high until they were over the age of 40.

Again, research on treatment effectiveness is lacking; there have been no major studies to determine whether culturally sensitive treatment is more effective than treatment in mainstream programs (Gilbert and Cervantes, 1986, 1988). Different approaches have been advocated for the different nationality groups. Given the variations, services researchers see a need for treatment agency data collection systems to distinguish among the nationality groups rather than labeling them all "Hispanic" (Gilbert and Cervantes, 1986).

Gilbert and Cervantes (1986) studied utilization patterns of Mexican Americans, by analyzing national and state data bases, which contain information on publicly funded programs. They found that variations in utilization among states reflected an age differentiation between Mexican Americans (who were younger) and the white population. There were also other determinants involved, For example, more of the Mexican Americans in treatment than the whites in treatment had been referred by the courts; these clients were most likely to be male. It was hypothesized that discriminatory practices in policing rather than differences in prevalence might account for the utilization patterns. Mexican Americans were more likely than other groups to be in outpatient than inpatient or residential treatment when compared to other groups. Gilbert and Cervantes suggested that this difference might be due either to the lack of culturally sensitive programs, the continued involvement of the problem drinker in an extended family network, or the lack of financial resources. They stressed the need to examine closely the effectiveness of various outpatient modalities for Mexican Americans being treated for alcohol problems.

As with the other special population groups, reports of clinical impressions or descriptive studies constitute the majority of the treatment literature for Hispanics. Many of these reports emphasize the importance of the family in all of the Hispanic groups and the need to include the family in treatment (e.g., Panitz, 1983). The form that this involvement should take has been most often based on clinical experience with a subgroup, however; applicability across nationality groups requires empirical testing.

Accessibility to culturally sensitive treatment for Hispanics is the major concern. Researchers and clinicians working in the area recommend that all programs that serve Hispanics of all nationality groups provide bilingual/bicultural staff. An important consideration in the assignment to culturally sensitive treatment is the degree of acculturation—the more acculturated an individual is,the less likely he or she is to need culturally sensitive treatment (Rogler et al. 1987). The committee suggests that large-scale studies of specific treatment approaches and their applicability to the diverse Hispanic population are necessary to go beyond the "findings" of the current impressionist literature.

Summary and Conclusions

There are several common themes that emerge from the literature on the treatment of special populations defined by structural characteristics. These themes are particularly applicable to the ethnic and racial minority groups. First, program designers and clinicians must be wary of defining a given person only in terms of his or her gender, age, or racial or ethnic group membership; members of these special populations vary on other important dimensions that have implications for treatment outcome: socioeconomic status, education level, employment status, income level, presence of physical and psychiatric comorbidities, and degree of acculturation and assimilation to the majority culture.

There are many possible examples of the importance of recognizing the heterogeneity that exists within these special populations. In his critique of the literature on black alcoholism, Harper (1979) noted the focus on drinking practices and treatment of lower income black males in the majority of available studies and criticized the practice of generalizing about treatment needs for all blacks (including black women and upper income blacks) based on data from this subgroup. Many reviewers of the research on particular ethnic groups have noted that Hispanics as well as Asian Americans come from many different countries, each of which has developed different attitudes about drinking practices and about appropriate treatment; they caution about generalizing from one culture to the other in designing treatment programs to overcome barriers because the sources of resistance to treatment may vary. Generational considerations are also important: third generation descendants of refugees typically differ from current immigrants in their responses. Tribal affiliation is a similar variable for American Indians; there are more than 280 different recognized tribes that have developed unique cultures and individualized norms around drinking and help-seeking behavior.

Second, a major factor involved in the perception of underutilization of alcohol problems treatment facilities by racial and ethnic minorities is the lack of means to pay for treatment. For example, Fisher (1978) reported that blacks and Hispanics in a sample of people calling a referral service in New York City were less likely than whites to have insurance coverage for alcohol problems treatment; this lack influenced the nature of the referral made. More recent studies of the extent of insurance coverage for all Americans indicate that members of these racial and ethnic minority groups are more likely to be uninsured and to depend on Medicaid or some other form of public funding (state or local public assistance, local and/or state categorical funding) for their health care (USDHHS, 1985; U.S. Comptroller General, 1987).

Third, persons with alcohol problems who come from minority cultures are perceived as "less likely" to enter majority-run treatment programs. Westermeyer (1982) reviewed a series of studies demonstrating that Hispanics, blacks, and American Indians were less likely to enter white run treatment programs. However, he also found that for those ethnic minority patients who did enter the white-run generic programs, treatment outcomes appeared to be good; in fact, they were equal to those for whites. These findings implied that there was an absence of bias in the treatment process itself and that there need to be further differentiation among the reasons for not entering treatment and for succeeding in treatment. These findings also suggested a rationale for continuing to invest in special population programs:

> While long term careful independent evaluations of these [minority-run] programs have not yet been widely done, early findings indicate that outcomes are comparable to those of majority-run programs. The advantages of ethnically oriented programs appear not so much that something particularly efficacious happens in treatment, but rather that the attraction to treatment is greater when one can join peers in a familiar setting. (Westermeyer, 1982:43)

Fourth, biomedical treatment of alcohol problems is seen as consistent across sex, age, ethnic, and racial groups and does not appear to require specialized culturally sensitive and culturally managed programs (Lex, 1985). Culturally specific psychotherapeutic and sociotherapeutic approaches also appear to be similar across ethnic and racial groups but are believed to help reduce the cultural isolation caused by alcohol problems when applied by therapists from the same cultural group. This belief serves as another reason for continuing to invest in such programs, although these concepts have yet to be empirically tested; it may be that both culturally specific, separately managed and culturally sensitive integrated programs, in which all staff are trained about the cultural backgrounds of the persons entering treatment, are appropriate and equally successful.

Despite the importance attached to structural characteristics in discussions of the need for culturally relevant services and despite the development of treatment strategies based on clinical experience and theories about the etiology of alcohol problems within a special population, there have been few studies testing the validity of these approaches. There is an inexcusable lack of systematic research on the application of specific treatment approaches to each of the special populations defined by structural characteristics. There have been few studies of the advantages and disadvantages of providing separate programs and of the difficulties to be encountered in their administration (Maypole and Anderson, 1987). Despite the recurrent interest in legislation, clinical practice, and program development, there have been no tests of the comparative effectiveness of the various approaches that are advocated. The majority of the literature is descriptive, based either on surveys of clinical or community populations, reports of utilization, or on clinical experience. There are very few data that can be seen as offering guidance to policymakers regarding which treatment approaches are effective with which special populations.

Because the majority of persons needing treatment for alcohol problems will continue to be treated in mainstream programs, age, gender, race, and ethnicity are critical individual characteristics to be considered in developing assessment, matching, and outcome monitoring schemes for mainstream treatment programs. Matching algorithms developed through research and the consensus process described in Chapter 11 should take these characteristics into account as well the degree of acculturation of a minority individual to the majority culture.

REFERENCES

Ahern, F. M. 1985. Alcohol use and abuse among four ethnic groups in Hawaii: Native Hawaiians, Japanese, Filipinos, and Caucasians. Paper presented at the National Institute on Alcohol Abuse and Alcoholism Conference on Epidemiology of Alcohol Use and Abuse among U.S. Minorities, Bethesda, Md., September 11-14.

Amaro, H., L. J. Beckman, and V. E. Mays. 1987. A comparison of black and white women entering alcoholism treatment. Journal of Studies on Alcohol 48:220-228.

American Bar Association. 1986. American Bar Association Policy Recommendation on Youth Alcohol and Drug Problems with Accompanying Report of the Advisory Commission on Youth Alcohol and Drug Problems, ABA Section of Individual Rights and Responsibilities. Washington, D.C.: American Bar Association.

Anderson, G. L. 1979. The Student Assistance Program: An Overview. Madison, Wisc.: Wisconsin Bureau of Alcohol and Other Drug Abuse.

Armor, D. J., J. M. Polich, and H. B. Stambul. 1978. Alcoholism and Treatment. Santa Monica: John Wiley and Sons.

Atkinson, R. M., J. A. Turner, L. L. Kofoed, and R. L. Tolson. 1985. Early versus late onset alcoholism in older persons: preliminary findings. Alcoholism: Clincial and Experimental Research 9:513-515.

Barnes, G., and J. Welte. 1986. Adolescent alcohol abuse: Subgroup differences and relationships to other problem behaviors. Journal of Adolescent Research 1:79-94.

Barr, H. L., and D. Antes. 1981. Seven years after treatment: A follow-up study of drug addicts and alcoholics treated in Eagleville Hospital's inpatient program. Eagleville Hospital, Eagleville, Penn.

Beckman, L. J. 1984. Treatment needs of women alcoholics. Alcoholism Treatment 1:101-114.

Beckman, L. J., and H. Amaro. 1984. Patterns of women's use of alcohol treatment agencies. Alcohol Health and Research World 9:14-25.

Beckman, L. J., and H. Amaro. 1986. Personal and social difficulties faced by women and men entering treatment. Journal of Studies on Alcohol 47:135-145.

Beckman, L. J., and K. M. Kocel. 1982. The treatment delivery system and alcohol abuse in women: Social policy implications. Journal of Social Issues 38:139-151.

Blum, R. W. 1985. The adolescent dialectic: A developmental perspective on social decision-making. Psychiatric Annals 15:614-618.

Blum, R. W. 1987. Adolescent substance abuse: Diagnostic and treatment issues. Pediatric Clinics of North America 34:523-537.

Blum, R. W. 1988. Executive summary: Adolescent alcohol treatment. Prepared for the Committee for the Study of Treatment and Rehabilitation Services for Alcoholism and Alcohol Abuse, June.

Blume, S. B. 1986. Women and alcohol: A review. Journal of the American Medical Association 256:1467-1469.

Blume, S. B. 1987. Executive summary: Treatment and rehabilitation for alcoholism and alcohol abuse. II. Treatment for women. Prepared for the IOM Committee for the Study of Treatment and Rehabilitation Services for Alcoholism and Alcohol Abuse, December.

Braiker, H. B. 1982. The diagnosis and treatment of alcoholism in women. Pp. 111-139 in Special Population Issues, J. de Luca, ed. Washington, D.C.: U.S. Government Printing Office.

Braiker, H. B. 1984. Therapeutic issues in the treatment of alcoholic women. Pp. 394-368 in Alcohol Problems of Women: Antecedents, Consequences, and Interventions, S. Wilsnack and L. J. Beckman, eds. New York: Guilford.

Butynski, W., N. Record, P. Bruhn, and D. Canova. 1987. State Resources and Services for Alcohol and Drug Abuse Problems: Fiscal Year 1986—An Analysis of State Alcohol and Drug Abuse Profile Data. Prepared for the National Institute on Alcohol Abuse and Alcoholism and the National Institute on Drug Abuse. Washington, D.C.: National Association of State Alcohol and Drug Abuse Directors.

Caetano, R. 1988. Alcohol use among Hispanic groups in the United States. American Journal of Drug and Alcohol Abuse 14:293-308.

Caetano, R., and M. E. Medina Mora. 1988. Acculturation and drinking among people of Mexican descent in Mexico and the United States. Journal of Studies on Alcohol 49:462-471.

Clark, W. B. 1985. Drinking patterns among Americans of Japanese ancestry in two study sites. Alcohol Research Group, University of California, Berkeley Calif., September.

Costello, R. M. 1987. Hispanic alcoholic treatment considerations. Hispanic Journal of Behavioral Sciences 9:83-89.

Dawkins, M. P., and F. D. Harper. 1983. Alcoholism among women: A comparison of black and white problem drinkers. International Journal of the Addictions 18:333-349.

Donovan, J. E., and R. Jessor 1978. Adolescent problem drinking: Psychosocial correlates in a national sample study. Journal of Studies on Alcohol 39:1506-1524.

Donovan, J. E., R. Jessor, and L. Jessor. 1983. Problem drinking in adolescence and young adulthood: A follow-up study. Journal of Studies on Alcohol 44:109-137.

Douglas, R. L., E. O. Chuster, and S.C. McLelland. 1988. Drinking patterns and abstinence among the elderly. International Journal of the Addictions 23:399-415.

Durst, M. E. 1988. Statement presented on behalf of the National Council of Juvenile and Family Court Judges at the open meeting of the IOM Committee for the Study of Treatment and Rehabilitation Services for Alcoholism and Alcohol Abuse, Washington, D.C., January 25.

Emrick, C. D. 1975. A review of psychologically oriented treatment of alcoholism: II. The relative effectiveness of treatment versus no treatment. Journal of Studies on Alcohol 36:88-108.

Ewing, J. A., B. A. Rouse, and E. D. Pellizari. 1974. Alcohol sensitivity in ethnic background. American Journal of Psychiatry 131:206-210.

Ferguson, F. N. 1968. Navaho drinking: Some tentative hypotheses. Human Organization 27(2):159-167.

Ferguson, F. N. 1970. A treatment program for Navaho alcoholics: Results after four years. Quarterly Journal of Studies on Alcohol 31:898-919.

Ferguson, L., and J. Kirk. 1979. Statistical report: NIAAA-funded treatment programs, Calendar Year 1978. National Institute on Alcohol Abuse and Alcoholism, Rockville, Md.

Fillmore, K. M., E. Hartka, B. M. Johnstone, R. Speiglman, and M. T. Temple. 1988. Spontaneous remission from alcohol problems: A critical review. Prepared for the IOM Committee for the Study of Treatment and Rehabilitation Services for Alcoholism and Alcohol Abuse, June.

Filstead, W. J., and C. L. Anderson. 1983. Conceptual and clinical issues in the treatment of adolescent alcohol and substance misusers. Child and Youth Services 2:103-116.

Filstead, W. J., and C. L. Anderson. 1985. Characteristics of youth receiving treatment for alcohol and substance abuse problems. Presented at the Annual Meeting of the Research Society on Alcoholism, Isle of Pines, S.C., May 28-June 1.

Finlayson, R. E., R. D. Hurt, L. J. Davis, and R. M. Morse. Alcoholism in elderly persons: A study of the psychiatric and psychosocial features of 216 inpatients. Mayo Clinic Proceedings 63:761-768.

Fisher, J. 1978. An Analysis of People Calling for Help. New York: New York Affiliate, National Council on Alcoholism.

Gilbert, M. J., and R. C. Cervantes. 1986. Alcohol services for Mexican Americans: A review of utilization patterns, treatment considerations and prevention activities. Hispanic Journal of Behavioral Sciences 8:1-60.

Gilbert, M. J., and R. C. Cervantes. 1988. Alcohol treatment for Mexican Americans: A review of utilization patterns and therapeutic approaches. Pp. 199-231 in Alcohol Consumption among Mexicans and Mexican Americans: A Binational Perspective, M. J. Gilbert, ed. Los Angeles: Spanish Speaking Mental Health Research Center, University of California, Los Angeles.

Goedde, H. W., D. P. Agarwal, and S. Harada. 1980. Genetic studies on alcohol-metabolizing enzymes: Detection of isozymes in human hair roots. Enzyme 25:281-286.

Goedde, H. W., D. P. Agarwal, and S. Harada. 1983. The role of alcohol dehydrogenase and aldehyde dehydrogenase isozymes in alcohol metabolism, alcohol sensitivity, and alcoholism. Isozymes: Current Topics in Biological and Medical Research 8:175-193.

Goedde, H. W., D. P. Agarwal, R. Eckey, and S. Harada. 1983. Population genetic and family studies on aldehyde dehydrogenase deficiency and alcohol sensitivity. Alcohol 2:383-390.

Gomberg, E. L. 1981. Women, sex roles, and alcohol problems. Professional Psychology 12:146-155.

Graham, K. 1986. Identifying and measuring alcohol abuse among the elderly: Serious problems with existing instrumentation. Journal of Studies on Alcohol 47:322-326.

Graham, K. 1987. Executive summary: Special consideration regarding assessment and assignment to treatment of elderly persons who have substance problems. Prepared for the IOM Committee for the Study of Treatment and Rehabilitation Services for Alcoholism and Alcohol Abuse, December.

Halikas, J. A., M. Lyttle, C. Morse, et al. 1984. Proposed criteria for diagnosis of alcohol abuse in adolescence. Comprehensive Psychiatry. 25:581-585.

Hall, R. L. 1986. Alcohol treatment in American Indian populations: An indigenous treatment modality compared with traditional approaches. Annals of the New York Academy of Sciences 472:168-178.

Harper, F. D. 1979. Alcoholism Treatment and Black Americans. Rockville, Md.: National Institute on Alcohol Abuse and Alcoholism.

Harrison, P. A., and C. A. Belille. 1986. Women in treatment: Beyond the stereotype. Journal of Studies on Alcohol 48:574-578.

Harrison, P. A., and N. G. Hoffmann. 1987. CATOR 1987 Report: Adolescent Residential Treatment: Intake and Follow-up Findings. Saint Paul, Minn.: Chemical Abuse/Addiction Treatment Outcome Registry, Ramsey Clinic.

Heckler, M. M. 1985. Report of the Secretary's Task Force on Black and Minority Health. Washington, D.C.: U.S. Department of Health and Human Services.

Herd, D. 1989. The epidemiology of drinking patterns and alcohol-related problems among U.S. blacks. Pp. 3-50 in Alcohol Use Among U.S. Ethnic Minorities: Proceedings of a Conference on the Epidemiology of Alcohol Use and Abuse Among Ethnic Groups, September 1985, D. L. Spiegler, D. A. Tate, S. S. Aitken, and C. M. Christian, eds. Rockville, Md.: U.S. Department of Health and Human Services.

Hoffmann, N. G., J. A. Halikas, and D. Mee-Lee, 1987. The Cleveland Admission, Discharge, and Transfer Criteria: Model for Chemical Dependency Treatment Programs. Cleveland, Ohio: The Greater Cleveland Hospital Association.

Hurt, R. D., R. E. Finlayson, R. M. Morse, and L. J. Davis. Alcoholism in elderly persons: Medical aspects and prognosis of 216 inpatients. Mayo Clinic Proceedings 63:753-760.

Indian Health Service (IHS). 1980. Alcohol-related Discharges from Indian Health Service and Contract General Hospitals: Fiscal year 1977. Rockville, Md.: Indian Health Service.

Janik, S. W., and R. G. Dunham. 1983. A nationwide examination of the need for specific alcoholism treatment programs for the elderly. Journal of Studies on Alcohol 44:307-317.

Jessor, R., J. A. Chase, and J. E. Donovan. 1980. Psychosocial correlates of marijuana use and problem drinking in a national sample of adolescents. American Journal of Public Health 70:604-613.

Johnson, S. 1979. Cirrhosis mortality among American Indian women: Rates and ratios, 1975 and 1976. Pp. 455-463 in Currents in Alcoholism, vol. 7, M. Galanter, ed. New York: Grune and Stratton.

Johnson, R. C., C. T. Nagoshi, S. Y. Schwitters, K. S. Bowman, F. M. Ahern, and J. R. Wilson. 1984. Further investigation of racial/ethnic differences and familial resemblances in flushing in response to alcohol. Behavior Genetics 14:171-178.

Johnston, L. D., P. M. O'Malley, and J. G. Bachman. 1987. National Trends in Drug Use and Related Factors among American High School Students and Young Adults: 1975-1986. Rockville, Md.: National Institute on Drug Abuse.

Kandel, D., and J. Logan. 1984. Patterns of drug use from adolescence to young adulthood. I. Period of risk for initiation, continued use, and discontinuation. American Journal of Public Health 74:660-667.

King, L. M. 1979. Alcoholism: Studies regarding black Americans 1977-1980. Pp. 385-407 in Special Population Issues, J. de Luca, ed. Washington, D.C.: U.S. Government Printing Office.

Kitano, H. H. L., and I. Chi. 1986/1987. Asian Americans and alcohol use: Alcohol Health and Research World 11(2):42-47.

Kitano, H. H. L., and I. Chi. 1989. Asian Americans and alcohol: The Chinese, Japanese, Koreans and Filipinos in Los Angeles. Pp. 373-382 in Alcohol Use Among U.S. Ethnic Minorities: Proceedings of a Conference on the Epidemiology of Alcohol Use and Abuse Among Ethnic Groups, September 1985, D. L. Spiegler, D. A. Tate, S. S. Aitken, and C. M. Christian, eds. Rockville, Md.: U.S. Department of Health and Human Services.

Kivlahan, D. R., R.D. Walker, D. M. Donovan, and H. D. Mischke. 1985. Detoxification recidivism among urban American Indian alcoholics. American Journal of Psychiatry 142:1467-1470.

Kofoed, L. L., R. L. Tolson, R. M. Atkinson, R. L. Toth, and J. A. Turner. 1987. Treatment compliance of older alcoholics: An elder specific approach is superior to "mainstreaming." Journal of Studies on Alcohol 48:47-51.

Lemert, E. M. 1982. Drinking among American Indians. Pp. 80-95 in Alcohol, Science, and Society Revisited, E. L. Gomberg, H. R. White, and J. A. Carpenter, eds. Ann Arbor, Mich.: University of Michigan Press.

Levy, J. E., and S. J. Kunitz. 1981. Economic and political factors in the use of basic research findings in Indian alcoholism programs. Journal of Studies on Alcohol Suppl. 9:60-72.

Lewis, R. G. 1982. Alcoholism and the Native American—A review of the literature. Pp. 315-328 in Special Population Issues, J. de Luca, ed. Washington, D.C.: U.S. Government Printing Office.

Lex, B. W. 1985. Alcohol problems in special populations. Pp. 89-187 in The Diagnosis and Treatment of Alcoholism, J. H. Mendelson and N. K. Mello, eds. New York: McGraw-Hill.

Longabaugh, R., and D. C. Lewis. 1988. Key issues in treatment outcome studies. Alcohol Health and Research World 12:168-175.

Mail, P. D. 1980. American Indian drinking behavior: Some possible causes and solutions. Alcohol and Drug Problems Association of North America 26(1):28-39.

Mail, P. D., and D. R. McDonald, eds. 1980. Tulapi to Tokay: A Bibliography of Alcohol Use and Abuse Among Native Americans of North America. New Haven, Conn.: HRAF Press.

Maloney, S. K. 1976. Guide to Alcohol Programs for Youth. Rockville, Md.: National Institute on Alcohol Abuse and Alcoholism.

Marden, P. G., and K. Kolodner. 1977. Alcohol Use and Abuse among Adolescents. Rockville, Md.: National Institute on Alcohol Abuse and Alcoholism.

Mason, R. D., P. D. Mail, I. Palmer, and R. L. Zephier. 1985. Briefing Book for the Alcoholism Program Review. Alberquerque, New Mexico: Indian Health Service, Alcoholism Program Branch.

May, P. A. 1982. Substance abuse and American Indians: Prevalence and susceptibility. International Journal of the Addictions 1982 17:1185-1209.

May, P. A. 1985. Alcohol and drug abuse prevention programs for American Indians: Needs and opportunities. Presented at the National Institute on Alcohol Abuse and Alcoholism and National Institute on Drug Abuse Conference on Prevention, Rockville, Md., June 22-24, 1983, and the Indian Health Service Alcoholism Program Review, Denver, Col., May 1.

Mayer, J. E., and W. J. Filstead. 1979. Adolescence and Alcohol. Cambridge, Mass.: Ballinger.

Maypole, D. E., and R. A. Anderson. 1986/1987. Alcohol programs serving minorities: Administrative issues. Alcohol Health and Research World 11(2):62-65.

McGough, D. P., and M. Hindman. 1986. A Guide to Planning Alcoholism Treatment Programs. Rockville, Md.: National Institute on Alcohol Abuse and Alcoholism.

Millman, R. B., and E. T. Khuri. 1982. Alcohol and adolescent psychopathology. Pp. 163-178 in Alcoholism and Clinical Psychiatry, J. Solomon, ed. New York: Plenum Press.

Mishara, B. L. 1985. What we know, don't know, and need to know about older alcoholics and how to help them: models of prevention and treatment. Pp. 243-261 in The Combined Problems of Alcoholism, Drug Addiction, and Aging, E. Gottheil, K. A. Druley, T. E. Skoloda, and H. M Waxman, eds. Springfield, Ill.: Charles C. Thomas.

Moos, F. D., E. Edwards, M. E. Edwards, F. V. Janzen, and G. Howell. 1985. Sobriety and American Indian problem drinkers. Alcoholism Treatment Quarterly 2:81-96.

Murakami, S. R., J. S. Raymond, L. Sine, and F. Ahern. 1984. Point prevalence rates from the Hawaii Epidemiological Survey: Psychiatric symptomatology, drug and alcohol use. Presented at the Hawaii Public Health Association Annual Meeting, Honolulu, Hawaii, May 18.

National Council on Alcoholism (NCA). 1987. A Federal Response to a Hidden Epidemic: Alcohol and Other Drug Problems Among Women. New York: National Council on Alcoholism.

National Council of Family Court Judges. 1987. Juvenile and family substance abuse: A judicial perspective. National Council of Family Court Judges, Reno, Nevada.

Owen, P., and L. Nyberg. 1983. Assessing alcohol and drug problems among adolescents: Current practices. Journal of Drug Education 13:249-254.

Panitz, D. R., R. D. McConchie, S. R. Sauber, and J. A. Fonseca. 1983. The role of machismo and the Hispanic family in the etiology and treatment of alcoholism in Hispanic American males. The American Journal of Family Therapy 11:31-42.

Raymond, M., and E. V. Raymond. 1984. Identification and Assessment of Model Indian Health Service Alcoholism Projects. Minneapolis, Minn.: First Phoenix American Corporation.

Reed, P. G., and D. S. Sanchez. 1986. Characteristics of Alcoholism Services in the United States-1984: Data from the September 1984 National Alcoholism and Drug Abuse Program Inventory. Rockville, Md.: National Institute on Alcohol Abuse and Alcoholism.

Rhoades, E. R., R. Mason, P. Eddy, E. M. Smith, and T. R. Burns. The Indian Health Service approach to alcoholism among American Indians and Alaskan Natives. Public Health Reports. 103:621-627.

Rogan, A. 1986. Recovery from alcoholism: Issues for black and Native American Alcoholics. Alcohol Health and Research World 11(1):42-44.

Rogler, L. H., R. G. Malgady, G. Costantino, and R. Blumenthal. What do culturally sensitive mental health services mean: The case of Hispanics. American Psychologist 42:565-570.

Roman, P. 1988. Women and Alcohol Use: A Review of the Research Literature. Rockville, Md.: National Institute on Alcohol Abuse and Alcoholism.

Saxe, L., D. Dougherty, K. Esty, and M. Fine. 1983. The Effectiveness and Costs of Alcoholism Treatment. Washington: U.S. Congress, Office of Technology Assessment.

Schuckit, M. A., and E. R. Morrisey. 1976. Alcoholism in women: Some clinical and social perspectives with an emphasis on possible subtypes. Pp. 5-35 in Alcoholism Problems in Women and Children, M. Greenblatt and M. A. Schuckit eds. New York: Grune and Stratton.

Schuckit, M. A., E. R. Morrisey, N. J. Lewis, and W. T. Buck. 1976. Adolescent problem drinkers. Pp. 325-355 in Currents in Alcoholism, vol. 2, F. Sexias ed. New York: Grune and Stratton.

Schuckit, M. A., and E. R. Morrisey. 1978. Minor in possession of alcohol: What does it mean? Pp. 339-356 in Currents in Alcoholism, vol. 4, F. A. Seixas, ed. New York: Grune and Stratton.

Shore, J. H., and L. Kofoed. 1984. Community intervention in the treatment of alcoholism. Alcoholism 8:151-159.

Shore, J. H., and R. N. von Fumetti. 1972. Three alcohol programs for American Indians. American Journal of Psychiatry 128:1450-1454.

Skinner, H. A. 1981. Assessment of alcohol problems: Basic principles, critical issues, and future trends. Pp. 319-369 in Research Advances in Alcohol and Drug Problems, vol. 6, Y. Israel, F. Glaser, H. Kalant, R. Popham, R. G. Smart, and W. Schmidt, eds. New York: Plenum Press.

Smart, R. G. 1979. Young alcoholics in treatment: Their characteristics and recovery rates at follow-up. Alcoholism: Clinical and Experimental Research 3:19-23.

Sue, S. 1988. Psychotherapeutic services for ethnic minorities: Two decades of research findings. American Psychologist 43:301-308.

Sue, S., and N. Zane 1987. The role of culture and cultural techniques in psychotherapy: A critique and reformulation. American Psychologist 42:37-45.

Towle, L. H. 1975. Alcoholism treatment outcomes in different populations Pp. 112-133 in Proceedings of the Fourth Annual Conference of the National Institute on Alcohol Abuse and Alcoholism, M. Chafetz, ed. Rockville, Md.: National Institute on Alcohol Abuse and Alcoholism.

U.S. Department of Health and Human Services (USDHHS). 1981. Fourth Special Report to the U.S. Congress on Alcohol and Health. Rockville, Md.: National Institute on Alcohol Abuse and Alcoholism.

U.S. Department of Health and Human Services (USDHHS). 1985. Fifth Special Report to the U.S. Congress on Alcohol and Health. Rockville, Md.: National Institute on Alcohol Abuse and Alcoholism.

U.S. Department of Health and Human Services (USDHHS). 1987. Sixth Special Report to the U.S. Congress on Alcohol and Health. Rockville, Md.: National Institute on Alcohol Abuse and Alcoholism.

U.S. Department of Health, Education, and Welfare (USDHHS). 1971. First Special Report to the U.S. Congress on Alcohol and Health. Rockville, Md.: National Institute on Alcohol Abuse and Alcoholism.

Vannicelli, M. 1984. Treatment outcome of alcoholic women: The state of the art in relation to sex bias and expectancy effects. Pp. 369-412 in Alcohol Problems in Women: Antecedents, Consequences, and Interventions, S. C. Wilsnack and L. J. Beckman, eds. New York: Guilford.

Vannicelli, M. 1988. Executive summary: Key Issues related to the treatment of alcoholic women. Prepared for the IOM Committee for the Study of Treatment and Rehabilitation Services for Alcoholism and Alcohol Abuse, March.

Walker, R. D. 1981. Treatment strategies in an urban Indian alcoholism program. Journal of Studies on Alcohol Suppl. 9:171-184.

Walker, R. D., D. M. Donovan, D. R. Kivlahan, and M. R. O'Leary. 1983. Length of stay, neuropsychological performance, and aftercare: Influences on alcohol treatment outcome. Journal of Consulting and Clinical Psychology 51:900-911.

Walker, R. D., and D. R. Kivlahan. 1984. Definitions, models, and methods in research on sociocultural factors in American Indian use. Substance and Alcohol Actions/Misuse 5:9-19.

Walker, R. D., A. H. Benjamin, D. Kivlahan, and P. S. Walker. 1989. American Indian alcohol misuse and treatment outcome. Pp. 301-311 in Alcohol Use Among U.S. Ethnic Minorities: Proceedings of a Conference on the Epidemiology of Alcohol Use and Abuse Among Ethnic Groups, September, 1985, D. L. Spiegler, D. A. Tate, S. S. Aitken, and C. M. Christian, eds. Rockville, Md.: U.S. Department of Health and Human Services.

Weibel, J. C. 1982. American Indians, urbanization, and alcohol: A developing urban Indian drinking ethos. Pp. 331-358 in Special Population Issues, J. de Luca, ed. Washington, D.C.: U.S. Government Printing Office.

Weibel-Orlando, J. 1984. Substance abuse among American Indian youth. Journal of Drug Issues 14(2):313-335.

Welte, J., and G. Barnes. 1987. Alcohol use among adolescent minority groups. Journal of Studies on Alcohol 48:329-336.

Westermeyer, J. 1972. Chippewa and minority alcoholism in the Twin Cities: A comparison. Journal of Nervous and Mental Diseases 155:322-327.

Westermeyer, J. 1974. The drunken Indian: Myths and realities. Psychiatric Annals 4:29-35.

Westermeyer, J. 1982. Ethnic factors in treatment. Pp. 709-717 in Encyclopedic Handbook of Alcoholism, E. M. Pattison and E. Kaufman, eds. New York: Gardner Press.

Westermeyer, J. 1986. A Clinical Guide to Alcohol and Drug Problems. Philadelphia: Praeger, 1986.

Westermeyer, J. 1988. Executive summary: Culture, special populations, and alcoholism treatment. Prepared for the IOM Committee for the Study of Treatment and Rehabilitation Services for Alcoholism and Alcohol Abuse, April.

Westermeyer, J., and J. Baker. 1986. Alcoholism and the American Indian. Pp. 273-282 in Alcoholism Development, Interventions, and Consequences, N. J. Estes and M. E. Heineman, eds. St Louis: Mosby.

Westermeyer J., and J. Neider. 1988. Social networks and psychopathology among substance abusers. American Journal of Psychiatry 145:1265-1269.

Westermeyer, J., and E. Peake. 1983. A ten year follow-up of alcoholic Native Americans in Minnesota. American Journal of Psychiatry 140:189-194.

Westermeyer, J., and R. D. Walker. 1982. Approaches to treatment of alcoholism across cultural boundaries. Psychiatric Annals 12:434-439.

Westermeyer, J., R. D. Walker, and E. Benton. 1981. A review of some methods for investigating substance abuse epidemiology among American Indians and Alaskan Natives. White Cloud Journal 2:13-21.

Williams, E. P. 1985. Older alcoholics in treatment. Prepared for the New Jersey Division of Alcoholism and the Connecticut Alcohol and Drug Commission, Rutgers University Center of Alcohol Studies, Piscataway, N.J.

Wilson, L. G., and J. M. Shore. 1975. Evaluation of a regional Indian alcohol program. American Journal of Psychiatry 132:255-258.

Winters, K. C., and G. A. Henly. 1988. Executive summary: Assessment of adolescent substance involvement. Prepared for the IOM Committee for the Study of Treatment and Rehabilitation Services for Alcoholism and Alcohol Abuse.

Wolff, P. 1972. Ethnic differences in alcohol sensitivity. Science 175:449-450.

Wolff, P. 1973. Vasometer sensitivity to alcohol in diverse mongoloid populations. American Journal of Human Genetics 25:193-199.

Woltzen, M. C., W. J. Filstead, C. L. Anderson, S. Twadell, C. Sisson, and P. Zoch. Clinical issues central to the residential treatment of alcohol and substance misusers. Advances in Adolescent Mental Health 2:271-282.

Yamimoto, J. 1988. Executive summary: Alcohol use and alcohol-related problems in Asian Americans. Prepared for the IOM Committee for the Study of Treatment and Rehabilitation Services for Alcoholism and Alcohol Abuse, May.

Yamoguchi, K., and D. Kandel. 1984. Patterns of drug use from adolescence to young adulthood. II. Sequence of progression. American Journal of Public Health 74:668-672.

Young, T. J. 1988. Substance use and abuse among Native Americans. Clinical Psychology Review 8:125-138.

Zimberg, S. 1974. Evaluation of alcoholism treatment in Harlem. Quarterly Journal of Studies on Alcohol 35:550-557.

Zimberg, S. 1983. Comprehensive model of alcoholism treatment in a general hospital. Bulletin of the New York Academy of Medicine 59(2):222-229.

Zimberg, S. 1985. Principles of alcoholism psychotherapy. Pp. 3-22 in Practical Approaches to Alcoholism Psychotherapy, S. Zimberg, J. Wallace, and S. B. Blume, eds. New York: Plenum Press.

16 Populations Defined by Functional Characteristics

The special populations discussed in this chapter are those who share a common social, clinical, or legal status. There has been general agreement in the field that these groups have been seen to require "culturally sensitive" specialized treatment services that also take into account the unique characteristics that distinguish the members of a particular group, even though these individuals may not identify themselves with the group. The groups used as examples in this chapter are people referred to treatment as a result of a drinking-and-driving arrest; the homeless and chronic public inebriate; the person with a coexisting psychiatric condition; college students; and children of alcoholic parents. Other groups that have been identified as special populations on the basis of a functional characteristic include the physically impaired, the deaf, and inmates of correctional facilities. Occupational groups (e.g., military personnel, physicians, migrant workers) have also been seen as socially defined special populations, and there are specialized programs which have been designed to meet their unique needs. For some of these functionally defined special populations (e.g., drinking drivers and skid row public inebriates), specialized agencies have developed and form a discrete subsystem within the specialist alcohol treatment sector described in Chapter 4.

Drinking Drivers

Drinking drivers, a special population defined solely in terms of their common legal status, are those persons who have been arrested for an alcohol-related driving offense. Most often, the offense is a violation of a driving-under-the-influence statute, although at times a vehicular homicide charge is also involved. A nationwide network of drinking-driver assessment and case management programs has been created to identify, classify, and refer drinking drivers to intervention and treatment; generally these programs use the methodology developed under the Alcohol Safety Action Program (ASAP), a joint effort of NIAAA and the National Highway Traffic Safety Administration (NHSTA) (Kisko, 1976; Fridlund, 1977; U.S. Department of Transportation, 1979a; Reis, 1984). A network of specialty alcohol education and treatment agencies for drinking drivers has also been developed. Concerns have been expressed that the influx of drinking drivers into community-based treatment settings have shifted their orientation away from working with persons who have severe and substantial alcohol problems and converted community-based agencies into extensions of the criminal justice system (Weisner and Room, 1984; Weisner, 1986). Whether these concerns are justified is open to question because there has been no recent review of the structural and operating characteristics of these individual state "DWI program" networks across the nation or any recent comprehensive evaluation of their effectiveness.

There is no doubt that drinking drivers are a heterogeneous lot, and there have been numerous efforts to define subtypes as a way to improve treatment matching (e.g., Selzer et al., 1977; Steer et al., 1979; Zung, 1979; Donovan and Marlatt, 1982; Donovan et al., 1985; Snowden and Campbell, 1986; Wells-Parker et al., 1986; Mann, 1988). Arrestees typically have been divided into two groups—problem drinkers and social drinkers—on the basis of their drinking behavior and problem status. Problem drinkers were those offenders who had lost control of their drinking and suffered severe social, physical and psychological consequences. Social drinkers were those offenders who drank occasionally but suffered no undue consequences as a result of their consumption prior to their arrest for driving after drinking (U.S. Department of Transportation, 1979a).

Following these characterizations, drinking-driver rehabilitation programs were differentiated into a short-term, didactic, lecture-oriented component for social drinkers and a treatment component for problem drinkers. The educational components were usually based on the original ASAP model and consisted of a limited number of sessions (usually 4 to 8) in which information on alcohol effects, traffic safety, and alcohol problems was provided in small group or lecture formats (Malfetti and Winter, 1976). The treatment components were most often short term, fixed-length group counseling (12 to 16 sessions). Progress was monitored by the courts, generally by a specially trained probation officer.

Initial evaluation data on the ASAP suggested that for social drinkers minimal intervention consisting of educational presentations of factual information, discussions, and the threat of future punishment if rearrested was effective in preventing repeat arrests; for problem drinkers a more intensive treatment experience was required involving affective education, individual and group counseling, and other therapies and supportive services if change was to be effected in their drinking-and-driving behaviors (Scoles and Fine, 1977; U.S. Department of Transportation, 1979a,b). Today, the program's treatment component continues to include didactic information presentations, but these presentations occur in smaller, interactive discussion groups rather than in large lecture sessions. Additional differentiation has taken place, such as the development of long-term individually oriented counseling programs and more intensive residential treatment programs targeted at multiple offenders (Mann et al., 1983; Wells-Parker et al., 1986; McCarty and Argeriou, 1988).

From 1971 until 1982 NIAAA sponsored a categorical grant program to serve drinking drivers; the program ended with the advent of the block grant. Although the federal policy emphases have changed, states have continued to support these programs; however, the focus has shifted from the state or local government directly funding education or treatment (or both) to its licensing programs that are supported by court-mandated fees and fines and its provision of financial assistance for indigent offenders (Weisner and Room, 1984). The system in most states is very similar to that described for Minnesota in Chapter 4: DWI programs provide intervention and treatment according to protocols that are often codified in legislation and licensure standards. The precise nature of this network of DWI programs varies from state to state and has not been studied recently. There is evidence that suggests that this rapid increase in treatment programs dependent on the courts for "coerced" referrals has markedly changed the nature of treatment for alcohol problems as many agencies become more involved in the criminal justice system than they are in the health care system (Weisner, 1986; see Appendix D).

In a typical DWI referral network, drinking drivers are classified into three subgroups: (1) social drinkers; (2) incipient problem drinkers; and (3) problem drinkers. (This categorization uses the methodology originally developed for the ASAP projects.) Screening is done either by court personnel or by the licensed program using a combination of interview data, driving history data and screening instruments, most often the Mortimer-Filkins Interview (Filkins et al., 1973; Wendling and Kolody, 1982) or the Michigan Alcoholism Screening Test (Selzer et al., 1977), or both (Mann, 1988). Some jurisdictions have modified the methodology extensively (e.g., Pisani, 1986), while others have maintained or added to it (e.g., Booth, 1986). In some jurisdictions, drinking drivers are beginning to be classified at the initial screening as either first offenders or repeat offenders; repeat offenders are more likely than first offenders to be referred to intensive treatment (Reis, 1984; Hagen, 1985; McCarty and Argeriou, 1988; Mishke and Venneri, 1987; Beerman et al., 1988; Mann, 1988).

Jurisdictions also vary in who carries out the screening and referrals; sometimes an employee of the court functions in a modified probation officer role, and sometimes this task is handled by a contract agency. Jurisdictions vary in the amount of discretion given to the court to use in referrals to assessment and treatment as a sentencing option. There has been a move toward increasing the severity of DWI penalties, particularly for multiple offenders, led by such advocacy groups as Mothers Against Drunk Driving (MADD) (Ungergleider and Bloch, 1987) and the Presidential Commission on Drunk Driving (1983).

Despite the increased focus on the deterrence of drinking and driving which led to the initiation of the ASAP and similar programs, this behavior persists as a major social and public health problem. Primary and secondary prevention efforts with young drivers, the subgroup with the highest risk of a DWI offense, have been relatively ineffective (Donovan, 1988). Driver training programs that attempt to provide young drivers with better driving skills appear to have little or no impact in reducing the number of accidents per licensed driver. In fact, such training programs, by encouraging youth to become licensed at an earlier age, may increase their exposure to driving risks and inadvertently lead to an increase in accidents.

Educational counseling programs that focus on drinking and driving among youth have had mixed results, and it is not yet possible, no matter how promising they seem intuitively, to state with any certainty how effective they are. The most effective method of reducing alcohol-related accidents appears to be to increase the legal age at which alcohol can be purchased. Well-designed studies indicate that increases in this age are associated with notable decreases in accidents in the affected age groups; furthermore these reductions have been found to persist over periods of up to six years. The upper limits of this intervention may now have been reached because all of the states have increased the legal drinking age to 21. One strong incentive for such action was provided by the federal government: states that failed to raise the legal drinking age risked a loss of 10 percent of federal highway funds (Donovan, 1988).

Secondary prevention attempts using general deterrence strategies also have been of limited success. The general deterrence model is based on the assumption that the penalties contingent on the arrest for a drunk driving offense will be swift, certain, and severe. The clearest finding related to this approach is that if the perceived risk of arrest and punishment for drunk driving is sufficiently increased, there appears to be some deterrence of drinking-driving and a reduction of accidents that appear to be related alcohol (H. L. Ross, 1984; Waller, 1985; Donovan, 1988). These reductions appear to be relatively short-lived, however, and rates return to or sometimes exceed preintervention baselines over time.

The least costly and most effective specific deterrents appear to be license suspension and revocation (Hagen, 1985). Although a large number of individuals who have lost their licenses continue to drive, they drive less frequently, for fewer miles, and more cautiously. Studies comparing license actions with rehabilitation programs have suggested that the licensing actions are more effective in reducing subsequent DWI recidivism and accidents. Such findings question the rationale for and effectiveness of "diversion" programs (e.g., deferred prosecution) that allow DWI offenders to seek treatment as a substitute for court-ordered punitive sanctions (e.g., jail, license suspension). Indeed diversion programs may be similar to a double-edged sword. On the one hand, they encourage offenders to enter treatment. On the other hand, by allowing the offender to avoid or circumvent what appear to be particularly effective deterrent licensing sanctions, the programs may actually be counterproductive. It has been argued that alcohol education and rehabilitation should be used in conjunction with and not as a substitute for licensing sanctions, that is, as a complementary rather than a competing approach (Hagen, 1985).

Hagen's conclusions from his review of the research on the effectiveness of education and rehabilitation as a "sanctions" for reducing recidivism (i.e., reducing repeated offenses of driving while impaired) are consistent with those of other reviewers (i.e., Vingilis, 1983; Mann, 1988). These investigators argue that too much emphasis had been placed on this sanction (i.e., education and treatment) alone and that it should be conceptualized in conjunction with other sanctions, particularly license suspension.

Referral to education for social drinkers or to treatment for problem drinkers remains an important and widely used countermeasure to reduce drinking and driving, even though it cannot be said to be a particularly effective means to achieve this purpose. Indeed without more research, no approach can be viewed as preeminent; more systematic studies are needed on the effects of the different penalty and referral systems now in place and on the different strategies for matching DWI referrals to appropriate settings, modalities, and intensities of treatment. Hagen (1985) vividly described the multiplicity of prevailing approaches for solving this particular alcohol problem:

> Sanctions for the drunken driving offender vary throughout the world, ranging from the typical monetary fines, jail sentences and licensure controls to a variety of options collectively called education and rehabilitation. The latter may range from a 2-hr didactic education course to a full blown alcoholism treatment involving psychotherapy. The orchestrator for the administration of this elaborate permutation of sanctions lies with the judiciary, with the application being the responsibility of the service providers—be it a correctional facility, licensing agency or the treatment-educational facility. (p. 79)

In contrast to these more negative findings regarding the effectiveness of education and treatment for DWI offenders, evaluation reports from state programs continue to emphasize the successes that have been achieved (e.g., Booth, 1986; Hoffmann et al., 1987; McDonnell and Fortinsky, 1987).

The evaluation of the effects of educational and rehabilitation programs on treatment outcome has been plagued by an array of methodological problems that make unequivocal interpretation of the results difficult (Mann, 1988; Donovan, 1988). Even more recent treatment outcome studies that have provided more appropriate experimental control, such as those conducted by Reis (1984) in California and by Landrum et al. (1983) in Mississippi, have led to equivocal results. One important aspect that must be taken into account in such evaluations is that the DWI population is not homogeneous in nature. Rather, this population appears to consist of a number of groups whose distinguishing characteristics may have meaning for determining the most effective way to prevent DWI offenses. Subtypes have been identified through analysis of arrest histories, personality assessments, and other data. Subtypes have been based on a number of dimensions, including sociodemographic variables, personality structure, anger and hostility, driving- related attitudes, psychopathology, drinking-behavior-related variables, and both general and driving-related arrest records. Current research efforts focus on determining whether treatment (education or rehabilitation) outcomes among DWI offenders may be enhanced by more effective matching of differential interventions to such legally defined or empirically derived subtypes. For example, McCarty and Argeriou (1988) have recently reported initial positive results for an intensive short-term residential primary treatment jail alternative for multiple offenders.

The most elaborate drinking driver classification system yet proposed for differential treatment planning includes seven groups or subtypes (Steer et al., 1979). Using four indexes of alcohol impairment, records for a pool of 1,500 male DWI arrestees that had been seen in NIAAA-funded treatment programs were cluster analyzed. Clinical experience and knowledge of the literature led the investigators to describe suggested interventions and treatment regimens for each of the seven groups. The groups varied in severity of impairment; the intensity of the interventions varied concomitantly, from license restrictions plus instruction in safe driving skills to license revocation plus court-mandated hospitalization for forced withdrawal followed by probationary supervision and psychotropic medication.

Although there has been no definitive experimental evaluation of the effectiveness of drinking driver programs, most of the studies that have been conducted support their general effectiveness in decreasing abusive drinking and improving psychosocial functioning; they cannot, however, shed light on whether such programs reduce drinking-related traffic violations. Additional studies are needed where different types of drinking drivers are assigned to different tailored treatment modalities on the basis of pretreatment assessment (U.S. Department of Transportation, 1979a,b; Swenson et al., 1981; Wells-Parker et al., 1986; Donovan, 1988; Mann, 1988). Evaluation of efforts to date suggests that treatment of the drinking driver is clearly not a substitute for civil sanctions and criminal penalties, but that treatment is a valuable supplement, although perhaps only for clearly specified subgroups. Further progress depends on developing better subgroup classification systems, better referral and matching procedures, better follow-up procedures, and more specific treatment methods.

Dual-Diagnosis Psychiatric Patients

A special population that has been receiving a great deal of attention recently is the so-called "dual-diagnosis" patient (Harrison et al., 1985; Blume, 1987; Galanter et al., 1987; Rounsaville, 1988). Advocates of the "disease model" of alcoholism totally rejected psychiatric concepts and methods of treatment during the initial effort to distinguish alcoholism as a primary disorder in and of itself (see Chapter 3). They rejected the conceptualization that alcohol problems were merely a symptom of an underlying psychiatric condition requiring psychoanalytically oriented dynamic psychotherapy or psychopharmacological treatment. Initially, many of the recovering alcoholics who were involved in developing what was then the "new" Minnesota model intensive residential and hospital-based treatment programs and specialist halfway houses avoided any relationships with psychiatrists and the specialty mental health system. This avoidance came in part as a reaction to a history of ineffective psychotherapy and the use of drugs that were themselves addictive (Rounsaville, 1988). "Alcoholism is not a Valium deficiency" was a common critique heard of the psychiatric approach to treatment of long-term alcohol problems.

The recent attention to the "dual-diagnosis" patient has resulted from the recognition of both alcohol and mental health specialist groups that there was a subgroup with whom neither sector worked well and a concern that the number of individuals in this group was growing (Galanter et al., 1987; Penick et al., 1988). These individuals often require treatment for the use of other drugs as well as alcohol, and mention increasingly is made of the "mentally ill chemical abuser" who is disruptive to the milieu of a standard treatment program (e.g., New York Division of Alcoholism and Alcohol Abuse, 1988). Persons with mental illness in addition to alcohol problems have seldom found a ready welcome in the specialty alcohol treatment sector. Minnesota model programs have tended to exclude those with overt psychopathology, whereas those working in the traditional mental health sector either referred persons with alcohol problems to a specialty agency or continued to treat them. When mental health practitioners did treat persons with alcohol problems, they used either the older, symptomatic approach or one of the newer treatment methods that blend psychodynamic approaches with approaches that focus specifically on drinking behavior (e.g., Khantzian, 1981, 1985). There has been continuing interest in the relationships between specific psychiatric syndromes and alcohol problems, primarily depression and antisocial personality disorder. As one means of differentiating which individuals should be seen in which sector, Schuckit (1985) has made a distinction between those persons with an alcohol problem who were found to have a preexisting psychiatric condition and those whose psychiatric problem emerged subsequent to the onset of heavy drinking.

As with other special populations, many of the available studies on dual-diagnosis patients have focused on epidemiological and diagnostic considerations—that is, on determining how many of the persons seen in various community and treatment settings have concomitant DSM-III diagnoses of alcohol dependence and "another" psychiatric disorder, including dependence on other drugs (Hesselbrook et al., 1985; H. E. Ross et al., 1988a,b). The development of more precise diagnostic criteria and assessment instruments have helped to identify those persons entering treatment who are experiencing both an alcohol problem and a psychiatric condition. Estimates of the size of the population being seen in each treatment sector vary, ranging from over 5 percent of those entering standard alcohol treatment programs to over 70 percent of those entering psychiatric programs. The conditions that have received the most attention are depression (affective disorders), antisocial personality disorders, and schizophrenia. The prevalence of antisocial personality disorders has been reported as ranging from 20 to 79 percent in persons treated for alcohol problems (Hesselbrock et al., 1985; Rounsaville, 1988). The prevalence of antisocial personality disorder and alcohol problems in the general population has been estimated to be about 7 percent. Anxiety disorders in combination with alcohol problems have also been found in high numbers, especially panic and phobic disorders; however, the prognostic significance of this combination for either condition is not clear (Rounsaville, 1988).

Major depression also has been reported as having a wide range in samples of persons being treated for alcohol problems, with lifetime rates ranging from 18 to 52 percent and current rates of 9 to 38 percent; these findings contrast with community rates which are around 6 percent to 7 percent for lifetime and 2 to 3 percent for current status. Studies are now being carried out to determine whether there are any systematic differences in outcome using different treatment protocols (e.g., treatment of the depression with an antidepressant drug and targeted psychotherapy) to determine whether methods that have been shown to be effective in treating depression alone can be used with dual-diagnosis patients.

Efforts have been made to develop specialized treatments for each of the dual-diagnosis subgroups (e.g., depression plus alcohol problems) as well as separate treatment units (Harrison et al., 1985), because the standard psychiatric approaches have had a high success rate (Galanter et al., 1987). Several states (e.g., Illinois, New York, New Jersey, Colorado) have developed special funding categories, but there are still numerous unanswered questions about diagnosis and treatment (Rounsaville, 1988). Several studies have shown that adding psychotherapy, when it is carried out by an experienced psychotherapist, as a component in a more standard alcohol/drug counseling program can improve the chances for successful outcome in those persons who have been assessed as having severe psychological problems (McLellan et al., 1983; Rounsaville et al., 1987). It has been suggested that psychiatric diagnosis can be an important matching variable even if no specific treatment for that combination is found. For example, an individual with alcohol problems and antisocial personality disorder might respond better to an alcohol problems treatment program that uses very structured limits-setting than to a more open, less rigorously structured treatment environment even though there is currently no demonstrated effective treatment for antisocial personality disorder.

Homeless Persons: The New Public Inebriates

Concern for the homeless person with alcohol problems has replaced concern for the chronic public inebriate, although they may truly be the same individual (Finn, 1985; Shandler and Shipley, 1987). The current status of treatment availability has been partially reviewed in a recent IOM report (1988), which distinguished among the temporarily homeless, the episodically homeless, and the chronically homeless. The third group were most likely to comprise either chronically mentally ill persons or "chronic substance abusers"—in the committee's terms, a person with chronic disabling alcohol problems. There are no well-defined surveys of the homeless population, but it is estimated that 30 to 40 percent are persons with chronic alcohol problems (IOM, 1988). The likelihood of a comorbid psychiatric disorder is also very high, placing a large number of the homeless within the dual-diagnosis special population. The recent literature on alcohol problems among the older inhabitants of skid rows and the "new homeless" was reviewed by Fisher (1987).

With the disappearance of skid rows in the 1970s, the termination of the NIAAA categorical grant program, and the deinstitutionalization of chronically mentally ill and alcoholic persons, concern with the chronic public inebriate at the national level of public policy began to dissipate. The public inebriate problem had not been resolved (Scrimegour and Palmer, 1976a,b; Diesenhaus, 1982; Finn, 1985), but it apparently was not seen as needing continued national focus. This view is supported by the lack of designated set-aside funds in the block grant. Efforts to deliver services within the fragmented services network continued in major cities with state and local support but without the resources considered necessary by those working with this special population (e.g., Finn, 1985; Sadd and Young, 1986; Shandler and Shipley, 1987).

The hub of these efforts was the network of nonhospital, nonmedical detoxification centers that replaced "drunk tanks" for public inebriates in the early 1970s. These centers were established following a state's passage of the Uniform Act or its enactment of a change in policy to come into conformity with court decisions decriminalizing public intoxication. The increase in the "recovery rate" that many thought would result from moving the "processing" of the public inebriate out of the criminal justice system and into the health care system did not occur. The expectation that such recovery could take place was challenged on theoretical and practical grounds by some (e.g., Room, 1976; Pisani, 1977; Pittman, 1977); and it was verified empirically by others (e.g., Annis and Smart, 1978). The detoxification center had merely replaced the drunk tank as a "revolving door." The explanation given for the failure to see dramatic change in public inebriety was the inadequacy of the resources committed to meeting the extensive needs for health care, supportive living arrangements, gradual but consistent engagement in treatment by meeting survival needs as well as treating the drinking behavior (Blumberg et al., 1973; Finn, 1985). Gradually, agencies serving public inebriates began to develop the added social support, health care, and vocational counseling services required to supplement the specific treatment modalities they offered to reduce problem drinking (e.g., Moos et al., 1978).

Thus, the current emphasis in this area of alcohol problems treatment appears to be on developing a comprehensive treatment system that deals with all of the health care and social support needs of homeless persons, including alcohol problems (Breakey, 1987). A design for the integrated continuum of care thought to be needed to provide such services has been summarized by Shandler and Shipley (1987); it comprises emergency medical care for the intoxicated, hospital or nonmedical detoxification, psychosocial evaluation, inpatient or residential formal treatment that focuses on developing job skills and on seeking housing, outpatient treatment, partial hospitalization, and aftercare. Detoxification lasts five to seven days, inpatient/residential treatment lasts about four months and outpatient or partial hospital treatment lasts six months.   The model anticipates the need to repeat the full cycle of treatment several times before success is achieved, and clients are urged to return if they lose control of their drinking. This model is based on over 20 years of experience gained by the Philadelphia Diagnostic Center, one of the nation's pioneering public inebriate programs.

Such programs are designed to break through the disaffiliation, or lack of personal linkages to social and family groups, that is a crucial characteristic of the chronically homeless. Distrust of authority, another key characteristic of homeless people, is also seen as complicating the development of a sustained treatment relationship. Homeless persons and chronic public inebriates move in and out of treatment for alcohol problems; services must be designed with due recognition of this characteristic (Morgan et al., 1985; Fagan and Mauss, 1986; Fisher, 1987).

There is some debate as to whether homelessness is a cause or consequence of being on the street (Dennis, 1987). It is likely that it is both. Therefore, another important aspect of treatment for the homeless is the provision of long-term supportive living arrangements in an alcohol free living environment (Fisher, 1987; Korenbaum and Burney, 1987).

At present, there is a major NIAAA initiative under way to evaluate effective treatment for the homeless person with chronic alcohol problems (Lubran, 1987; NIAAA, 1987). Although a number of descriptive studies have been performed, there have been no clinical trials to establish which treatment methods have the most success in moving an individual out of both the homeless and the problem drinking conditions. The specific configuration of services needed, the possibility that different configurations are necessary for different subgroups, and the effectiveness of involuntary commitment have not been empirically tested despite the almost 20 years of identification of the public inebriate and skid row alcoholic as a special population.

College Students

Recently, college students as a subgroup of adolescents have become identified as a new special population. The common characteristics are age, life situation, and legal status. There are several reasons for this development. First, the focus on drinking and driving with attention being drawn to the high incidence of alcohol-caused accidents among adolescents and young adults has led to federal and state legislation raising the legal drinking age to 21. This change has created even more dissonance and concern on college campuses, which already had trouble enforcing the laws on underage drinking within their mixed-age populations. Second, an increase in the number of highly publicized tragedies associated with on-campus parties and fraternity hazing has led universities to review their policies and practices. Third, although there have been some encouraging results from the studies on primary prevention strategies, primarily those using education and awareness campaigns (Goodstadt and Caleekal-John, 1984; USDHHS, 1987), there have been questions raised about the effectiveness of these efforts, both from a methodological and practical perspective (e.g., Moskowitz, 1986). Finally, the college campus is in many respects a closed community with many unique aspects; one of those aspects is that the student is a transient member who becomes the responsibility of the permanent administration and faculty functioning *in loco parenti* for many aspects of daily living.

For example, on February 18, 1988, the *New York Times* published an editorial entitled "Drinking Themselves to Death." The editorial described the recent death of a freshman at Rutgers University who suffered an overdose of alcohol at an initiation party. This death followed by less than a week a near fatality at Princeton University, in which a student drank himself into a coma during an initiation party at an eating club. The editorial quoted Rutgers' president, Edward Bloustein, who observed that there appears now to be "a growing trend of abusive use of alcohol" on campuses, in part, according to some experts, because alcohol is seen by students as a safe and generally legal alternative to illicit drugs. The editorial concluded that most universities have adopted a "hands-off" attitude toward student drinking, particularly when it occurs in off-campus facilities such as fraternity houses. "Except where they are hosts or landlords, institutions cannot do much except advise and educate their students on the responsible use of alcohol. Whether to follow the advice is for the students to decide," the editorial concluded. Growing concern over college student drinking has been expressed in colleges and universities all over the country. Newspaper articles document the increasing number of alcohol-related accidents and overdose fatalities. To take still another example, at the University of Washington in Seattle, several students have died of alcohol-related accidents (e.g., falls from fraternity house windows) in the past several years (Marlatt, 1988).

Research efforts in this area to date have primarily focused on surveys of drinking practices and the distribution of problems (e.g., Engs and Hanson, 1985; Anderson and Gadeleto, 1985; Saltz and Elandt, 1986) and the evaluation of primary prevention strategies. A recent assessment of student drinking patterns in one University of Washington fraternity found (after evaluating two weeks of daily self-monitoring of alcohol intake by fraternity members) that the average house member consumed 16 drinks per week with an average maximum blood-alcohol level (BAL) of .16 percent, well above the legal intoxication level of .10 percent. In addition, the average member reported being intoxicated (BAL > .10 percent) for 8.4 hours per week. Another sample of heavy-drinking college students reported driving an automobile while under the influence of alcohol an average of 7.5 times in the past year (Marlatt, 1988).

These findings are representative of other college drinking studies. In a review of 38 studies published between 1976 and 1985, Saltz and Elandt (1986) reported that 47 percent of the students surveyed reported being at risk of a DWI or driving under the influence (DUI) citation; 24 percent reported injuries or alcohol-related injuries. Data reported in the same review showed that the prevalence of college student drinking appeared to be growing in recent years. Compared with data reported by Straus and Bacon in their classic 1953 study (showing that 80 percent of college men and 61 percent of women were drinkers), Saltz and Elandt (1986) indicate that the range of reports on the incidence of male college drinking was 81 to 98 percent, whereas that of female college drinking was 78 to 98 percent.

As described by Marlatt (1988), the college-age drinker is unique in several respects. First, most college students who drink are engaged in an illegal activity to the extent that they are under the legal drinking age of 21. Their drinking behavior is often excessive and uncontrolled because many students are "naive" and inexperienced drinkers. However, their legal status presents a problem for programs that attempt to teach responsible drinking behaviors for this age group. Opposition to "responsible drinking" as a goal for underage drinkers has been stated by several national groups, including the National Council on Alcoholism and the National Institute on Alcohol Abuse and Alcoholism. Second, college students have flexible class and work schedules and are under minimal supervision while on campus. Most of their drinking occurs in social or "party" situations, frequently associated with bouts of heavy drinking over relatively short periods (e.g., weekend evenings). As a result, their drinking is influenced primarily by peer behavior and attitudes toward drinking. Prevention programs geared toward influencing peer drinking norms would seem to be most appropriate in this regard. Third, although many college students drink very heavily, most do not qualify as "alcoholics" in the traditional sense; they do not usually show sign of physical dependence on alcohol (e.g., withdrawal symptoms). As a result, most students reject the idea that their drinking behavior can be described as a "disease" and that abstinence is the preferred solution to this problem. Therefore, they do not seek help from traditional intervention and treatment programs.

These characteristics suggest that college-age problem drinkers may respond more positively to brief interventions that are geared toward a goal of moderate or safe drinking. Studies that have followed students longitudinally from college on to post-college life show that the vast majority "mature out" of their heavy drinking patterns as they become more involved in family and employment roles (e.g., Fillmore et al., 1979). Programs designed to inculcate moderate or safe drinking practices for the college age drinker can be considered attempts to "speed up" this natural process of maturity and increased personal responsibility. The college campus which is concerned with drinking among its students becomes a natural community setting for testing the system of generalist and specialist treatment outlined in Chapter 13.

Because few students see themselves as having a problem with alcohol, the main problem facing the administrators of alcohol prevention, intervention, and treatment programs targeted at the college-age population is one of motivating students to participate. Marlatt (1988) has described what may be the necessary characteristics of a college intervention program, identifying possible ways to enhance motivation and to carry out the brief intervention component of a comprehensive program by tying the intervention to ongoing campus primary prevention efforts:

- Programs should be based on an educational approach rather than on a medical or disease model of alcoholism because students are more likely to attend a class or course on alcohol issues than they are to attend a "clinic for alcoholics."

- Programs should reach out to students who are children of alcoholic parents, have a special interest in the topic of alcohol education, and are at particular risk for developing problems.

- Educational and prevention programs should employ student-peer leaders and invite the participation of interested student groups and campus leadership.

- College alcohol education programs should recognize that alcohol affects males and females in different ways and work with gender differences. Materials distributed by these programs should focus on the role of alcohol in social and sexual behavior, including risk behavior associated with sexual aggression and sexually transmitted diseases (especially AIDS).

- Rather than adopting a moralistic approach, prevention and intervention programs for college drinkers should provide students with personalized feedback concerning their drinking behavior and associated health risks that contains non-judgmental normative information indicating the student's drinking level and the risks that go along with a particular level.

- The "tone" of educational programs should be one of optimism and the opportunity to acquire self-mastery and self-management skills. Approaches that are primarily negative and attempt to increase fear of negative consequences (e.g., becoming an alcoholic in the future) are unlikely to motivate student participation.

College students can be considered a unique high-risk special population for alcohol problems. They are, however, heterogeneous on the other key variables that have served to identify special populations (gender, race and ethnicity, social class, living situation, personality type), and this heterogeneity must be considered in program planning

(White and Mee-Lee, 1988). The majority of college students would probably be assessed as having only mild or moderate alcohol problems and would benefit the most from brief intervention efforts which use an educational model and a moderation approach. Indeed this population presents a unique opportunity for utilizing—and evaluating—the brief intervention strategies described in Chapter 9 and the comprehensive system described in Chapter 13. A program based on these principles is now being tested at the University of Washington (Marlatt, 1988). Other colleges and universities have already established primary prevention programs, and a few have established their own special population treatment programs (e.g., Rutgers). Such programs may take several forms, ranging from courses offered for academic credit to self-help materials and specialist led group therapy. There is an opportunity to introduce secondary prevention programs as well as treatment programs for students who show signs of substantial or severe alcohol problems. However, as a newly recognized special population, there have been few studies evaluating the effectiveness of either singular or comprehensive strategies. To avoid the problems that have occurred in defining treatment models for other special populations, recent concerns over college drinking should lead to rigorously evaluated demonstrations of alternative models before recommendations are made that all colleges invest in such efforts.

Children of Alcoholics

The special population group most recently singled out for attention is children of alcoholics (USDHHS, 1983, 1987; Children of Alcoholics Foundation, Inc., 1984; Waite and Ludwig, 1985). Children of persons with alcohol problems are considered to be at increased risk of developing alcohol problems both because of possible genetic linkages and environmental influences. The major assumption underlying the identification of this group as a special population is that parental alcohol problems and family dysfunction create an environment that can lead to psychosocial problems for children and to abusive drinking at an early age, even in the absence of a genetically transmitted susceptibility (USDHHS, 1987).

Interest in providing prevention and intervention services to children of alcoholics has grown rapidly among people working in the field, and there are increasing numbers of articles on this subject in the popular literature. In addition, a strong and vital national advocacy movement has been created to lobby for increased services and research (Woodside, 1988; Blane, 1988). The Children of Alcoholics Foundation and the National Association for Children of Alcoholics are prominent advocacy and educational organizations in the field. Differentiations are made among the needs of child, adolescent, and adult children of alcoholics (Blane, 1988). The Children of Alcoholics Foundation estimates that there are 28.6 million children of alcoholics in the United States and that 22 million of them are adults (Woodside, 1988). Self-help and group therapy approaches predominate at the adult level; for children and adolescents, two general approaches are the most used: school-based primary prevention and secondary prevention efforts and treatment-based interventions. School-based efforts are focused on identifying children of alcoholics and the interventions are targeted at them. Treatment-based interventions tend to be targeted at the family, with the youth participating in family therapy. Other treatment activities such as peer support groups are also used in both environments.

The advocacy movement noted earlier has a strong self-help ethic and borrows many of its principles from Alcoholics Anonymous, Al-Anon, and Alateen. It includes a national network of author-lecturers who have written popular books aimed at children of alcoholics and who present their strategies for prevention or treatment at professional and popular workshops (Blane, 1988). There has been an increasing demand for specialized treatment for adult children of alcoholics, with the emphasis on group therapy. A variety of intervention and specialized treatment strategies and programs have been developed using clinical experience rather than research (Russell et al., 1985; Waite and Ludwig, 1985; Cermak, 1986; Brown, 1988). The Children of Alcoholics Foundation recently identified 235 programs in 34 states that had been specifically designed to serve either young or adult children of alcoholics. The programs were small and relatively new—approximately three-fourths had been in operation less than four years (Woodside, 1988).

The concern for children of alcoholics is one aspect of the more general concern for the families of persons with alcohol problems. This concern arose from the conceptualization that "alcoholism is a family disease" and that the same principles of recovery apply to all members of the family. In the early years of development of treatment for alcohol problems, there was a movement toward requiring participation in formal treatment or self-help efforts, or both, by all family members as essential for recovery. This emphasis has led to an increase in the of treatment services offered to other family members, even when the person with the identified problem is not engaged in treatment. The justification for treatment for these groups is based predominantly on their risk of developing problems with alcohol themselves and the potential detrimental effects that may be incurred from their involvement with a person experiencing problems with alcohol.

This new—and growing—treatment focus has been labeled codependency, the term now in frequent use for the psychological and adjustment problems of other members of the family of the person with alcohol problems. The concept of codependency seems to be fairly well established. Representatives of many of the states who attended the Joint Federal and State Agency Meeting on Alcohol and Drug Data Collection, conducted by the National Association of State Alcohol and Drug Abuse Directors in March 1989, indicated that agencies in their states were identifying codependent persons as primary clients and including them in their reports to federal and state agencies, including the SADAP and the NDATUS (see Chapter 7). The recommendations from those meetings were to include codependency status as part of the national uniform minimal data set. In the private sector, the area is sufficiently established that there are specific codependency treatment programs and codependency units in alcohol programs (Cermak, 1984, 1986).

Yet, the treatment of children of alcoholics and other codependents is an area where definitions are unclear and research pertaining to etiology or outcome is lacking. Martin (1988) found a wide variety of conceptualizations in her review of the popular literature on codependency. Some writers in the field advocate an independent official diagnosis of codependency personality disorder be recognized (Cermak, 1986) as well as a biological model of the condition (Laign, 1989a).

The main body of research on treatment outcome to this point comes predominantly from clinical practice and frequently consists of case study reports that focus on model building, personality profiles, or treatment strategies (Brown, 1988; Cermak, 1986; Wegscheider-Cruse, 1985). There are only the very beginnings of a research-based literature. For example, Parker and Harford (1988) have analyzed national survey data on adult children of alcohol abusers, Cutter and Cutter (1987) have studied adult children of alcoholics in Al-Anon groups, and Ackerman (cited in Laign, 1989b) has recently conducted a survey of adult daughters of alcoholics.

What many of these studies show is that the same methods used to treat the person with alcohol problems are being used to treat codependents. Yet the appropriateness of these methods has not been justified, nor has the differential (marginal) effectiveness of these specialty approaches been evaluated in a series of clinical trials. There have also been no studies that compare specialized programs for adult children of alcoholics with standard programs that incorporate specialized techniques as suggested by

Russell and coworkers (1985). A number of the problems involved in developing a body of research (e.g., the lack of retrievable data sources) have been identified by Woodside (1988) and Roman (1988).

Because an investigation of codependency—whether spouses or children of alcoholics—was not specifically part of the committee's mandate, it has chosen not to make a specific recommendation about this issue. However, the committee is concerned about the lack of clarity that such reporting practices create (in terms of who is being treated) and the effects on the access to treatment for persons with alcohol problems of the increasing numbers of codependents who are being seen as primary clients. Clarification and improved definitions are needed before policy recommendations can be made.

Summary and Conclusions

The conclusions that emerge from a review of the literature on the treatment of special populations defined by functional characteristics are not substantially different from those reached by looking at groups defined by structural characteristics. Again, however, the committee cautions policymakers, program designers, and clinicians to be wary of defining a given person only in terms of his or her special population group membership. Members of each of these functionally defined special populations also vary on other important dimensions that have implications for treatment outcome—including those structural characteristics discussed in the previous chapter. Despite the importance that has been attached to the defining characteristics of a special population in developing treatment strategies based on clinical experience and theories about the etiology and maintenance of alcohol problems within each population, there have been few studies that test the differential effectiveness of these approaches.

The conclusion that there is an inexcusable lack of systematic research on the application of specific treatment approaches holds for those special populations defined by functional characteristics as well as for those defined by structural characteristics. Again, the recurrent interest in legislation, clinical practice, and program development for these populations is not followed by tests of the comparative effectiveness of the various approaches that have been advocated. Without such test policymakers are at a loss for the empirically based guidance necessary in making needed refinement and improvements.

REFERENCES

Anderson, D. S., and A. F. Gadaleto. 1986. College alcohol survey: 1985, 1982, and 1979. Alcohol Health and Research World 9:46-47,71.

Annis, H. M., and R. G. Smart. 1978. Arrests, readmissions, and treatment following release from detoxication centers. Journal of Studies on Alcohol 39: 1276-1283.

Argeriou, M. 1979. Reaching problem drinking blacks: The unheralded potential of drinking driving programs. International Journal of Addictions 13:443-459.

Beerman, K. A., M. M. Smith, and R. L. Hall. 1988. Predictors of recidivism in DUIIs. Journal of Studies on Alcohol 49:443-449.

Berkowitz, A. D., and H. W. Perkins. 1986. Problem drinking among college students: A review of recent research. Journal of American College Health 35:21-28.

Blane, H. T. 1988. Prevention issues with children of alcoholics. British Journal of Addiction 83:793-798.

Blumberg, L., T. Shipley, and I. W. Shandler. 1973. Skid Row and Its Alternatives. Philadelphia: Temple University Press.

Blume, S. B. 1987. Executive summary: Treatment and rehabilitation for alcoholism and alcohol abuse. Prepared for the IOM Committee for the Study of Treatment and Rehabilitation Services for Alcoholism and Alcohol Abuse, December.

Booth, R. 1986. Education/Treatment Intervention among Drinking Drivers and Recidivism. Prepared for the Colorado Alcohol and Drug Abuse Division. Denver, Col.: Colorado Department of Health.

Breakey, W. R. 1987. Treating the homeless. Alcohol Health and Research World 11(3):42-46,90.

Brown, S. 1988. Treating Adult Children of Alcoholics: A Developmental Perspective. New York: John Wiley and Sons, 1988.

Cermak, T. L. 1984. Children of alcoholics and the case for a new diagnostic category of codependency. Alcohol Health and Research World 8(4):38-42.

Cermak, T. L. 1986. Diagnosing and Treating Codependence. Minneapolis, Minn.: Johnson Institute.

Children of Alcoholics Foundation, Inc. 1984. Report of the Conference on Research Needs and Opportunities for Children of Alcoholics, April. New York: Children of Alcoholics Foundation.

Cutter C. G., and H. S. G. Cutter. 1987. Experience and change in Al-Anon family groups: Adult Children of Alcoholics. Journal of Studies on Alcohol 48:29-32.

Dennis, D. L., ed. 1987. Research Methodologies Concerning Homeless Persons with Serious Mental Illness and/or Substance Abuse Disorders. Proceedings of a two-day conference sponsored by the Alcohol, Drug Abuse, and Mental Health Administration, July 13-14. Rockville, Md.: Alcohol, Drug Abuse, and Mental Health Administration.

Diesenhaus, H. I. 1982. Current trends in treatment programming for problem drinkers and alcoholics. Pp. 219-290 in Prevention, Intervention, and Treatment: Concerns and Models, J. de Luca, ed. Washington, D.C.: U.S. Government Printing Office.

Donovan, D. M. 1988. Executive summary: Drinking drivers as a special population. Prepared for the IOM Committee for the Study of Treatment and Rehabilitation Services for Alcoholism and Alcohol Abuse, April.

Donovan, D. M., and G. A. Marlatt. 1982. Personality subtypes among Driving-While-Intoxicated offenders: Relationship to drinking behavior and driving risk. Journal of Consulting and Clinical Psychology 50:241-249.

Donovan, D. M., H. R. Quiesser, P. M. Salzberg, and R. L. Umlauf. 1985. Intoxicated and bad drivers: Subgroups within the same population of high risk men drivers. Journal of Studies on Alcohol 46:375-382.

Engs, R. C., and D. J. Hanson. 1985. The drinking patterns and problems of college students:1983. Journal of Alcohol and Drug Education 31:65-83.

Fagan, R. W., and A. L. Mauss. 1986. Social margin and social reentry: An evaluation of a rehabilitation program for skid row alcoholics. Journal of Studies on Alcohol 47:413-425.

Filkins, L. D., Mortimer, R. G., D. V. Post, and M. M. Chapman. 1973. Field Evaluation of Court Procedures for Identifying Problem Drinkers. Final Report. Prepared for the U.S. National Highway Traffic Safety Administration. Ann Arbor, Mich.: University of Michigan, Highway Safety Institute.

Fillmore, K. M., S. D. Bacon, and M. Hyman. 1979. Final Report: The 27 Year Longitudinal Panel Study of Drinking by Students in College, 1949-1976. Rockville, Md.: National Institute on Alcohol Abuse and Alcoholism.

Finn, P. 1985. Decriminalization of public drunkenness: Response of the health care system. Journal of Studies on Alcohol 46:7-22.

Fisher, P. J. 1987. Alcohol problems among contemporary American homeless populations: An analytic review of the literature. Prepared for the IOM Committee on Health Care for Homeless People, May.

Fridlund, G. 1977. Summary, Conclusions, and Recommendations of the Final Report on Problem Drinking Driver Programs Funded by NIAAA. Prepared for the National Institute on Alcohol Abuse and Alcoholism. Stanford Research Institute, Menlo Park, Calif.

Galanter, M., R. Castenada, and J. Ferman. 1987. Substance abuse among general psychiatric patients: Place of presentation, diagnosis, and treatment. American Journal of Drug and Alcohol Abuse 14:211-235.

Gilbert, M. J., and R. C. Cervantes. 1986. Alcohol services for Mexican Americans: A review of utilization patterns, treatment considerations and prevention activities. Hispanic Journal of Behavioral Sciences 8:1-60.

Gilbert, M. J., and R. C. Cervantes. 1988. Alcohol treatment for Mexican Americans: A review of utilization patterns and therapeutic approaches. Pp. 199-231 in Alcohol Consumption among Mexicans and Mexican Americans: A Binational Perspective, M. J. Gilbert, ed. Los Angeles: Spanish Speaking Mental Health Research Center, University of California, Los Angeles.

Goodstadt, M. S., and A. Caleekeel-John. 1984. Alcohol education programs for university students: A review of their effectiveness. International Journal of the Addictions 19:721-741.

Hagen, R. E. 1985. Evaluation of the effectiveness of educational and rehabilitation efforts: opportunities for research. Journal of Studies on Alcohol Suppl. 10:179-183.

Harper, F. D. 1979. Alcoholism Treatment and Black Americans. Rockville, Md.: National Institute on Alcohol Abuse and Alcoholism.

Harrison, P. A., J. A. Martin, V. B. Tuason, and N. G. Hoffmann. 1985. Conjoint treatment of dual disorders. Pp. 367-390 in Substance Abuse and Psychopathology, A. I. Alterman, ed. New York: Plenum Press.

Hesselbrock, M. N., R. E. Meyer, and J. J. Keener. 1985. Psychopathology in hospitalized alcoholics. Archives of General Psychiatry 42:1050-1055.

Hoffmann, N. G., F. Ninonuevo, J. Mozey, and M. G. Luxenberg. Comparison of court-referred DWI arrestees with other outpatients in substance abuse treatment. Journal of Studies on Alcohol 48:591-594.

Institute of Medicine. 1988. Homelessness, Health, and Human Needs. Washington, D.C.: National Academy Press.

Khantzian, E. J. 1981. Some treatment implications of the ego and self-disturbances in alcoholism. Pp. 163-188 in Dynamic Approaches to the Understanding and Treatment of Alcoholism, M. H. Bean and N. E. Zinberg, eds. New York: Free Press.

Khantzian, E. J. 1985. Psychotherapeutic interventions with substance abusers—the clinical context. Journal of Substance Abuse Treatment 2:83-88.

Kisko, J. A. 1976. Comparison of NIAAA's drinking driver programs with other types of alcoholism programs. Pp. 41-43 in DWI Rehabilitative Programs. Proceedings of the National DWI Conference, Lake Buena Vista, Fla., May 9-12. Falls Church, Va.: AAA Foundation for Traffic Safety.

Korenbaum, S., and G. Burney. 1987. Program planning for alcohol-free living centers. Alcohol Health and Research World 11(3):68-74.

Laign, J. 1989a. Codependency "disease: Tied to neurotransmitters. The U.S. Journal of Drug and Alcohol Dependence 13(4):19.

Laign, J. 1989b. Daughters of alcoholics are different—Ackerman study. The U.S. Journal of Drug and Alcohol Dependence 13(4):19.

Landrum, J. R., S. Miles, R. Neff, T. Pritchard, J. Roebuck, E. Wells-Parker, and G. Windham. 1983. Mississippi DUI Probation Follow-up Project. Prepared for the National Highway Traffic Safety Administration. Publication DOT HS 806-274. Springfield, Va.: National Technical Information Service.

Larson, E. W., and D. E. McAlpine. 1988. Treating the hearing-impaired in a standard chemical dependence unit. Journal of Studies on Alcohol 49:381-383.

Lubran, B. G. 1987. Alcohol-related problems among the homeless: NIAAA's response. Alcohol Health and Research World 11(3):4-6,73.

Malfetti, J. L., and D. J. Winter. 1976. Counseling Manual for DWI Counterattack Programs. Falls Church, Va.: AAA Foundation for Traffic Safety.

Mann, R. E. 1988. Executive summary: Assessing and treating the convicted drinking driver. Prepared for the IOM Committee for the Study of Treatment and Rehabilitation Services for Alcoholism and Alcohol Abuse.

Mann, R. E., G. Leigh, E. R. Vingilis, and K. DeGenova. 1983. A critical review of the effectiveness of drinking-driving rehabilitation programs. Accident Analysis and Prevention 15:441-461.

Marlatt, G. A. 1988. Executive summary: College students as a high risk group. Prepared for the IOM Committee for the Study of Treatment and Rehabilitation Services for Alcoholism and Alcohol Abuse, April.

Martin, D. 1988. A review of the popular literature on codependency. Contemporary Drug Problems 15:383-399.

McCarty, D., and M. Argerieu. 1988. Rearrest following treatment for repeat offender drunken drivers. Journal of Studies on Alcohol 49:1-6.

McDonnell, P., and R. Fortinsky. 1987. A Study of OUI in Maine: Participation in DEEP, Rearrest and Perceptions of OUI Laws, Enforcement and Services. Prepared for the Division of Driver Education Evaluation Programs, Maine Department of Human Services Bureau of Rehabilitation. Portland, Me.: University of Southern Maine Center for Research and Advanced Study Human Services Development Institute.

McLellan, A. T., G. E. Woody, L. Luborsky, C. P. O'Brien, and K.A. Druley. 1983. Increased effectiveness of substance abuse treatment: A prospective study of patient-treatment "matching." Journal of Mental Diseases 171:597-605.

Mischke, H. D., and R. L. Venneri. 1987. Reliability and validity of the MAST, Mortimer-Filkins, and CAGE in DWI assessment. Journal of Studies on Alcohol 48:492-501.

National Institute on Alcohol Abuse and Alcoholism (NIAAA). 1987. Request for Applications: Community Demonstration Grant Projects for Alcohol and Drug Abuse Treatment of Homeless Individuals, RFA AA-87-04. Rockville, Md.: NIAAA.

Morgan, R., E. I. Geffner, E. Kiernan, and S. Cowles. 1985. Alcoholism and the homeless. Pp. 131-150 in Health Care of Homeless People, P. W. Brickner, L. K. Scharer, B. Conan, A. Elvy, and M. Savarese, eds. New York: Springer.

Moos, R. H., B. Mehren, and B. S. Moos. 1978. Evaluation of a Salvation Army alcoholism treatment program. Journal of Studies on Alcohol 39:473-490.

Moskowitz, J. M. 1989. The primary prevention of alcohol problems: A critical review of the research literature. Journal of Studies on Alcohol 50:54-88.

New York Division of Alcoholism and Alcohol Abuse (NYDAAA) 1989. Five Year Comprehensive Plan for Alcoholism Services in New York State: 1989-1994. Albany, N.Y.: NYDAAA.

Parker, D. A., and T. C. Harford. 1988. Alcohol-related problems, marital disruption and depressive symptoms among adult children of alcohol abusers in the United States. Journal of Studies on Alcohol, 49:306-314.

Pisani, V. D. 1977. The detoxication of alcoholics—aspects of myth, magic or malpractice. Journal of Studies on Alcohol 38:972-985.

Pisani, V. D. 1986. DUI recidivism: Implications for public policy and intervention. [no page nos.] in Zeroing-in on Repeat Offenders: A Summary of Conference Proceedings: Papers Presented at the Conference on Recidivism, September 16. Washington, D.C.: National Commission Against Drunk Driving.

Pittman, D. 1977. Barriers to the effective implementation of the Uniform Intoxication Treatment Act. Paper presented at the Fourth Annual Summer Conference of the Alcoholism and Drug Abuse Institute, Seattle, Wash.

Penick, E. C., B. J. Powell, B. J. Liskow, J.. Jackson, and E. J. Nickel. 1988. The stability of coexisting psychiatric syndromes in alcoholic men after one year. Journal of Studies on Alcohol 49:395-405.

Presidential Commission on Drunk Driving. 1983. Final Report. Washington, D.C.: U.S. Government Printing Office.

Reis, R. E. 1984. The effects of DUI education and counseling programs on recidivism. Presented at the NIAAA and NHTSA Workshop on Alcohol and the Drinking Driver, Bethesda, Md.: May 2-4.

Room, R. 1976. Comment on "The Uniform Alcoholism and Intoxication Treatment Act." Journal of Studies on Alcohol 37:133-144.

Ross, H. L. 1984. Deterring the Drinking Driver: Legal Policy and Social Control. Lexington, Maine: Lexington Books.

Ross, H. E., F. B. Glaser, and T. Germanson. 1988. The prevalence of psychiatric disorders in patients with alcohol and other drug problems. Archives of General Psychiatry 45:1023-1-31.

Ross, H. E., F. B. Glaser, and S. Stiasny. 1988. Sex differences in the prevalence of psychiatric disorders in patients with alcohol and other drug problems. British Journal of Addictions 83:1179-1192.

Rounsaville, B. J., Z. S. Dolinsky, T. S. Babor, and R. E. Meyer. Psychopathology as a predictor of treatment outcome in alcoholics. Archives of General Psychiatry 44:505-513.

Rounsaville, B. 1988. Executive summary: Psychiatric comorbidity in alcoholics. Prepared for the IOM Committee for the Study of Treatment and Rehabilitation Services for Alcoholism and Alcohol Abuse, June.

Russell, M., C. Henderson, and S. B. Blume. 1985. Children of Alcoholics: A Review of the Literature. New York: Children of Alcoholics Foundation.

Sadd, S., and D. W. Young. 1986. A Controlled Study of Detoxification Alternatives for Homeless Alcoholics. New York: Vera Institute of Justice.

Saltz, R., and D. Elandt. 1986. College student drinking studies, 1976-1985. Contemporary Drug Problems 13:117-159.

Shandler, I. W., and T. E. Shipley. 1987. New focus for an old problem: Philadelphia's response to homelessness. Alcohol Health and Research World 11:54-56.

Schuckit, M. A. 1985. The clinical implications of primary diagnostic groups among alcoholics. Archives of General Psychiatry 42:1043-1049.

Schutt, M. 1985. Wives of Alcoholics: From Codependency to Recovery. Pompano Beach, Florida: Health Communications.

Scoles, P. E., and E. W. Fine. 1977. Short term effects of an education program for drinking drivers. Journal of Studies on Alcohol 38:633-637.

Scoles, P. E., E. W. Fine, and R. A. Steer. 1984. Personality characteristics of high risk drivers never apprehended for driving while intoxicated. Journal of Studies on Alcohol 45:411-416.

Scrimegour, G. J. 1976. Report on the Impact Study of the Uniform Alcoholism and Intoxification Treatment Act. Washington, D. C.: Council of State and Territorial Alcoholism Authorities.

Scrimegour, G. J., and J. Palmer. 1976. Executive Summary: Guidance Manual for Implementation of the Uniform Alcoholism and Intoxication Treatment Act. Bloomington, Ind.: University of Indiana Institute for Research in Public Safety.

Selzer, M. L., A. Vinokur, and T. D. Wilson. 1977. A psychosocial comparison of drunken drivers and alcoholics. Journal of Studies on Alcohol 38:1292-1312.

Snowden, L. R., and D. Campbell. 1986. Validity of an MMPI classification of problem drinker-drivers. Journal of Studies on Alcohol 47:344-347.

Steer, R. A., E. W. Fine, and P. E. Scoles. 1979. Classification and treatment implications. Journal of Studies on Alcohol 40:159-182.

Straus, R., and S. D. Bacon. 1953. Drinking in College. New Haven, Conn.: Yale University Press.

Swenson, P. R., D. L. Struckman-Johnson, V. S. Ellinstad, T. R. Clay, and J. L. Nichols. 1981. Results of a longitudinal evaluation of court-mandated DWI treatment programs. Journal on Studies of Alcohol 42:642-653.

Ungergleider, S., and S. A. Bloch. 1987. Perceived effectiveness of drinking-driving countermeasures: An evaluation of MADD. Journal on Studies of Alcohol 49:191-195.

U.S. Department of Health and Human Services (USDHHS). 1983. Fifth Special Report to the U.S. Congress on Alcohol and Health. Rockville, Md.: National Institute on Alcohol Abuse and Alcoholism.

U.S. Department of Health and Human Services (USDHHS). 1987. Sixth Special Report to the U.S. Congress on Alcohol and Health. Rockville, Md.: National Institute on Alcohol Abuse and Alcoholism.

U.S. Department of Transportation. 1979a. Summary of National Alcohol Safety Action Projects, vol. 1. Washington, D.C.: U.S. Government Printing Office.

U.S. Department of Transportation. 1979b. Results of National Alcohol Safety Action Projects, vol. 2. Washington, D.C.: U.S. Government Printing Office.

Vingilis, E. 1983. Drinking drivers and alcoholics: Are they from the same population? Pp. 299-342 in Research Advances in Alcohol and Drug Problems, vol. 7, R. G. Smart, F. B. Glaser, Y. Israel, H. Kalant, R. E. Popham, and W. Schmidt, eds. New York: Plenum Press.

Waite, B. J., and M. J. Ludwig. 1985. A Growing Concern: How to Provide Services for Children from Alcoholic Families. Rockville, Md.: U.S. Department of Health and Human Services.

Wegscheider-Cruse, S. 1985. Choicemaking: For Codependents, Adult Children and Spirituality Seekers. Pompano Beach, Florida: Health Communications.

Weisner, C. 1986. The social ecology of alcohol treatment in the United States. Pp. 203-243 in Recent Developments in Alcoholism, vol. 5, M. Galanter, ed. New York: Plenum Press.

Weisner, C. and R. Room. 1984. Financing and ideology in alcohol treatment. Social Problems 32:167-184.

Wells-Parker, E., P. J. Cosby, and J. W. Landrum. 1986. A typology for drinking driving offenders: methods for classification and policy implications. Accident Analysis and Prevention 18:443-453.

Wendling, A., and B. Kolody. 1982. An evaluation of the Mortimer-Filkins test as a predictor of alcohol-impaired driving recidivism. Journal of Studies on Alcohol 43:751-766.

White, W. T., and D. Mee-Lee. 1988. Substance use disorders and college students: Inpatient treatment Issues--A model of practice. Journal of College Student Psychotherapy 2(3/4):177-204.

Woodside, M. 1988. Research on children of alcoholics: Past and future. British Journal of Addiction 83:785-793.

Zung, B. J. 1979. Sociodemographic correlates of problem drinking among DWI offenders. Journal of Studies on Alcohol 40:1064-1072.

17 The Treatment of Special Populations: Conclusions and Recommendations

What is most apparent from the committee's examination of the research and clinical literature on special populations is that, in some ways, every individual is "special" in this sense; that is, if the demarcations of special population groups are based on demographic, social, legal, economic, and biological factors, there is really no person who would be excluded from one or more groupings. These groupings appear logical, yet it is not known whether the concept of special populations always has heuristic value for providing treatment for alcohol problems that speaks to a group's particular needs. The concept has undoubtedly helped some individuals by providing more attractive, culturally specific, and relevant treatment organizations. Given the absence of adequate studies, however, it is not possible to determine whether programs targeted toward a special population are any more effective than an integrated mainstream program in reducing alcohol problems. The committee has tried to determine whether there are data available to resolve such questions about the need for special programs and for special emphases. Like Saxe and colleagues (1983), however, it found that there has been little evaluation of efforts to develop treatment programs tailored to the diverse needs of special populations. There have been no additional studies since the Saxe review to change the conclusion that *the evidence is not available to resolve the ongoing disagreement between those who believe that it is important to provide culturally specialized treatment programs using staff who share the cultural background (and language, when appropriate) of the individuals being treated and those who believe treatment should focus on the alcohol problem itself.* The situation today is perhaps even more complex with the emergence of additional special population groups, defined in terms of functional as well as structural characteristics.

A useful notion that has recently evolved is that problem drinking in special population groups is multidimensional. As is emphasized in other sections of this report, professionals are beginning to understand that alcohol problems do not constitute a unitary disease process but are more analogous to cancer or diabetes, with the occurrence and manifestation of symptoms that are unique to each individual. The emergence of this perspective has led to the identification of key subgroups within special populations using variables to categorize the subgroups that are the same as those used to define other special populations (e.g., Gilbert and Cervantes' [1988] discussions of the differential treatment needs of Mexican American males and females and of Mexican American male drinking drivers and Caucasian male drinking drivers; Argeriou's [1979] discussion of the differential treatment needs of black drinking drivers and black public inebriates; Bander and colleagues' [1983] study of the difference in response to treatment for women varying in socioeconomic status).

Despite the current emphasis on subtype variability, the treatment blend of individual characteristics, attitudes, traits, and special population membership nuances has yet to be empirically determined. There is general agreement that members of the identified special populations vary considerably on characteristics that are relevant to treatment outcome; the assumption is made that group members would benefit from some homogeneous treatment based on practices, values, or beliefs that reflect their special population membership. Yet, interdependent factors germane to the individual are also known to influence the way persons use or abuse alcohol. Many, perhaps even most persons in treatment have certain general or common identities as well as one or more special identities. Some examples that were encountered at one treatment facility over a brief period included the following:

- a 32-year-old college-educated, employed male with special identities: he is single, Native American, and homosexual;

- a 28-year-old married female with special identities: she is pregnant and has a bipolar disorder;

- an 18-year-old single female college student with special identities: she has a social phobia and is depressed;

- a 25-year-old married employed male with special identities: he had an alcoholic mother, is legally blind, and is of borderline intelligence (i.e., as a result of fetal alcohol effect).

The personal and situational heterogeneity encountered among persons with alcohol problems suggests that identifying the key structural or functional characteristic to use in determining referral to a special population program is difficult in many cases. It is clear that an individual can be a member of numerous special population groups, depending on the definitions and focuses used.

Following this logic, if alcohol problems are heterogeneous and it is recommended that treatment for the general population should be heterogeneous, then treatment for special population groups should also be heterogeneous. The committee recognizes, however, that there is a limit on the number of separate programs that can be funded. Therefore, it has considered whether efforts should be focused on improving the match between individuals and well-specified treatment regimens, regardless of a person's special population membership, rather than on developing additional separate special population programs.

Cautiously, the committee has concluded that the concept of special populations is a dynamic one and that it is necessary to consider all of the factors in an individual's life that may or may not contribute to a positive treatment outcome. In other words, numerous considerations must be addressed in the planning of effective treatment for alcohol problems for any member of a special population, or, in fact, for any person with alcohol problems. One cannot say: "Here is a woman, and because she is a woman, she will benefit from Treatment X." A clinician may be confronted with a woman who is a white, unmarried, deaf mother of two children, or one who is a married, Asian American housewife with no children. Where should the treatment emphasis lie? Which characteristic of special populations requires the most emphasis? How does the clinician adequately assess an individual's characteristics and life circumstances to provide the best treatment?

Providing culturally specific programming is not simply the identification of an individual's special population status or cultural orientation and other personal characteristics and the subsequent provision of a clearly indicated treatment. Treatment in this case involves a complex interplay of forces including administrative and funding issues (Maypole and Anderson, 1986/1987). Such factors as racial and ethnic group identification of the target population and of the program staff, service locations, the structure and programs of the service delivery system, the source and means of financing, and the racial and academic backgrounds of administrators of minority service programs are important variables to be considered in providing culturally specific programming. The committee recognizes that total reliance on isolated treatment programs, each serving a particular subpopulation that has been defined as "special," is neither cost-effective nor realistic at best, and, may be anti-therapeutic at worst. The committee, therefore, has sought to take account of individual uniqueness and special population membership but not to advocate only for increasing the number of separately run programs. It sees a need to continue the emphasis on special populations to improve access to treatment but at the same time decries the lack of adequate research on the extent to which these programs have actually improved either access or effectiveness.

Matching persons seeking treatment to particular types of therapists and particular treatment modalities can have a far reaching effect in improving retention in treatment and outcome of treatment for special populations. Thus far, matching efforts have had little clinical impact in working with special populations because matching schemes are complex and not readily implemented in the current funding environment. However, adoption of the committee's recommendations regarding outcome monitoring, independent assessment, and funding for all clinically effective interventions will make such matching more appropriate in treatment for special populations.

The committee originally began its review of the current status of programming, research findings, clinical observations, and legislative actions involving special populations in order to provide recommendations for future services development. Yet the lack of adequate data has led instead to our emphasis on the need for more adequate study of existing practice. *The committee recommends that funding should be provided for discrete evaluations of special population intervention and treatment programs.* The federal government, through NIAAA, should fund national, multicenter studies of treatment process and outcome that are designed to investigate the factors that determine positive treatment outcome for each of the major special populations. These studies could be patterned after the current research demonstrations being carried out to evaluate treatment for the homeless with alcohol problems (Lubran, 1987; NIAAA, 1987) and to study matching (NIAAA, 1989).

Because there continue to be unanswered questions regarding the effectiveness of customized, culturally relevant treatment, it is recommended that study groups be specifically created to pursue these issues for each of the major special populations and to design a specific services research agenda for each. These groups should begin by undertaking reviews and analyses of the existing literature and data. The current research on special populations leaves much to be desired. Little is known regarding the impact on outcome of culturally specific treatments whether implemented in culturally specific programs or generic mainstream programs. There is also limited information on the comparative effectiveness of mainstream treatment for different special population groups and on whether the increased availability of special treatment programs encourages those within the targeted population who are in need of treatment to seek it.

Considering the literature on special populations and the many outstanding questions that have emerged, it seems more than likely that there is a need for novel research strategies to examine the complexities treatment issues for these groups. Much of the current research being funded by the federal government has no direct relevance to treatment decisions, planning, or intervention with these groups. Instead the emphasis in these efforts has been either on "theory rich" research that might uncover new theories of etiology or on specific treatments. After two decades, this strategy has added much to our understanding of the mechanisms of alcohol abuse and dependence but relatively little to treatment efforts. What is needed now is a new research direction that is characterized by being "theory poor," in the sense that it is aimed not at new theories or interventions but at demonstrating the applied utility of current theory and practice. On the other hand, this new research direction should be "method rich"—or at least "method complex"—in requiring careful sampling, precise descriptions of treatment, random assignment to controlled interventions, long-term interventions persisting over several months to a few years, and the longitudinal study of outcome beyond the treatment period. The research program that is shaped by these new emphases must provide representative coverage of each of the major special population groups and not limit work only to one group.

The extent to which culturally specific treatment programs enhance the probability of successful outcome for their target populations is the critical question to be answered regarding treatment for special populations. A major effort should be undertaken to encourage existing special population programs and mainstream programs that serve large numbers of special population members to participate in multisite comparative trials. It will then be possible to compare treatment process and treatment outcome for the special population in culturally specific and mainstream programs. The design of such studies should also include identification of the unique and specific elements of treatment in culturally relevant treatment programs. The use of multisite naturalistic and quasi-experimental studies and clinical observation to identify characteristics of special population members who respond differently to mainstream or culturally sensitive treatment approaches will allow the formulation of more practical recommendations for treatment design and funding. These initial quasi-experimental trials can then be followed by more precise multisite clinical trials. These trials can test the program models that are potential candidates for replication and identify the characteristics of those special population members for whom a specific treatment approach is appropriate.

Consideration should be given to developing clinical trials to test the effectiveness and appropriateness of culturally relevant treatment. Such trials should evaluate the following: (a) comparative outcomes of members of the special population and other Americans involved in the same treatment programs; (b) comparative outcomes of members of the special population and other Americans receiving the same treatments but in culturally segregated groups; (c) comparative outcomes of members of the special population assigned to culturally oriented treatment programs and those assigned to non-culturally specific treatment programs; and (d) treatment outcomes for special populations stratified by structural and functional characteristics (e.g., gender, age, class, and acculturation).

Any attempt at effective matching of members of a special population group to a specific treatment, whether culturally specific or not, is premature at this time. Each of the special populations itself is heterogeneous. There may well be various culturally specific treatments that are appropriate for different population subgroups, but the assessment of what constitutes an alcohol problem and the grading of problem severity need further refinement to determine the appropriate measurement techniques and cut-off points for each special population. It is obvious that different concepts apply to different population extremes (e.g., adolescents and the elderly). The assessment tools that are currently available have been developed for and with adults, primarily white males, and their applicability to other special population groups requires empirical verification. It is extremely important that any effort to match adolescents and young adults to appropriate types and levels of treatment be preceded by an effort to develop distinct assessment and referral tools. It is also important that assessment and referral tools be validated for each of the special population groups in which they will be employed; the need for such validation is particularly acute for the referral and matching of persons from each of the racial and ethnic minorities.

Exclusive special population programs may be feasible and desirable in some facets of treatment but impractical or suboptimal in others. In the early stages of treatment (detoxification, crisis intervention, and the process of self-assessment), persons with alcohol problems, regardless of their special demographic, legal, social, or clinical characteristics, have similar needs. Thus, sensitivity to cultural issues is not pivotal in the first stages of recovery (Moos et al., 1985; Westermeyer, 1988). During this period, the individual is coming to terms with his or her problems, and drinking-related factors assume a greater importance than personal or social factors. It is during this period in the treatment sequence that matching a person either to a generic or to a special population rehabilitation and maintenance program appears critical.

Clinical observations indicate that members of special populations tend to use generic treatment programs when their need is great and special population resources are not available. Yet once the crisis is past, many special population members are apt to reject further recovery in mainstream programs in which they are uncomfortable because of their special identity or that do not meet their special needs. The predictable result is a high rate of dropout from treatment and a high rate of readmission to crisis-oriented treatment—the so-called "revolving door" problem (Westermeyer and Peake, 1983; Kivlahan et al., 1985; Babor and Mendelson, 1986).

It is in the assessment and referral, rehabilitation, and maintenance phases of treatment for alcohol problems that the individual's status as a member of one or more special populations appears to gain in importance. For example, members of the person's social network, who often belong to special demographic populations themselves, are key to adequate social assessment and may prove valuable in aiding the person's rehabilitation. The person in treatment who is undergoing rehabilitation (and later, maintenance) is acquiring and solidifying a new identity as a person who no longer drinks hazardously. He or she is faced with two difficult social tasks: (1) dropping social network members (mostly heavy drinkers) whose company is an occasion for excessive alcohol use and (2) replacing them with new members. If recovery requires that the person develop alternative coping mechanisms and an identity that is not based on alcohol use, it is important that, while in rehabilitation, the person have access to other recovering individuals with whom they can identify. This identification is made easier when those persons are members of the same special population (Favazza and Thompson, 1984; Westermeyer and Neider, 1988).

It is also important for treatment staff to be able to establish a rapport with the person's network members and involve them in recovery (including the amelioration of codependence problems, if appropriate). In addition, as treatment and rehabilitation progress, staff must know the resources available in the community to meet individuals' special needs. In the case of special populations, the establishment of rapport with social network members and intimate knowledge of community resources may depend on staff themselves being part of the special population with which the person in treatment is identified.

This objective can be achieved either by increasing special population representation among treatment staffs or by increasing the heterogeneity of staff and broadening their training accordingly. The committee prefers to see both avenues pursued. Yet it is doubtful that full representativeness can ever be achieved. Staff who are conducting assessments, making referrals, and carrying out specific treatments must understand the problems presented by special population members in order to deal with them constructively. A married, middle-class suburban male staff member may have difficulty in empathizing with—or confronting, when appropriate—a single parent, inner-city mother of five children. This level of understanding can be facilitated by staff who share some of the same characteristics as the persons in treatment, but obviously, treatment staff cannot totally share the identities of all persons whom they treat. There appears to be some critical level of identity that enables an individual seeking treatment to view a particular program's staff as acceptable; however, its parameters are not known. To what extent should the staff demographically resemble those whom they treat? Does each program require a solo parent, a paraplegic, a fundamentalist Christian, and an HIV-seropositive homosexual on staff? Even if this were desirable—and it is not clear that this arrangement is therapeutically advantageous (e.g., Padilla et al., 1975; Sue, 1988)—the diversity of special populations makes it impossible to achieve staff representativeness in large, mainstream programs that serve multiethnic, diverse special populations.

Given the current resources available, the committee recognizes that many members of special population groups will continue to be treated in majority-run, mainstream programs. Thus, expanded training, incorporating the most recent developments in clinical practice and research findings, is required. *The committee recommends that there be a major effort to train staff working in these mainstream programs in the skills and sensitivity needed to identify and work with the special populations that can be expected to seek treatment in their programs. This recommendation is based on a twofold need: to improve existing services and to provide opportunities to study whether such training can improve treatment outcome for special population members who receive treatment in these programs.* Questions of staff and program representativeness can and should be addressed by future research efforts about the contribution of therapist characteristics to treatment effectiveness (see Chapters 4 and 11).

To avoid misinterpretation, the committee believes it prudent to emphasize that the conclusion it noted at the beginning of this chapter regarding the lack of more refined knowledge on the effectiveness of culturally specific treatments should not be taken as a rationale for discontinuing the funding of such programs. Even though there is no definitive evidence at this time that these programs provide more effective treatment, the committee has concluded that there is evidence that access to treatment has been improved for members of special populations, in many cases simply because of the development of these additional culturally sensitive programs. *Thus, the committee recommends that there be continuation of funding for special population treatment programs in order to to facilitate access to treatment and to provide the basis for examining effectiveness.* These examinations can be carried out both through special studies and through the routine outcome monitoring the committee wishes to see conducted by every treatment program as a condition of funding. The committee also urges that there be predictable funding on a long-term basis for these studies, so that clinicians and researchers alike are given appropriate opportunity to investigate the relevant questions, provide comparisons, and address issues related to special population groups.

REFERENCES

Argeriou, M. 1979. Reaching problem drinking blacks: The unheralded potential of drinking driving programs. International Journal of Addictions 13:443-459.

Babor, T. F., and J. H. Mendelson. 1986. Ethnic/religious differences in the manifestations and treatment of alcoholism. Annals of the New York Academy of Sciences 472:46-59.

Bander, K. W., N. A. Stilwell, E. Fein, and G. Bishop. 1983. Relationship of patient characteristics to program attendance by women. Journal of Studies on Alcohol 44:318-327.

Favazza, A. R., and J. J. Thompson. 1984. Social networks of alcoholics: Some early findings. Alcoholism: Clinical and Experimental Research 8:9-15.

Gilbert, M. J., and R. C. Cervantes. 1988. Alcohol treatment for Mexican Americans: A review of utilization patterns and therapeutic approaches. Pp. 199-231 in Alcohol Consumption among Mexicans and Mexican Americans: A Binational Perspective, M. J. Gilbert, ed. Los Angeles: Spanish Speaking Mental Health Research Center, Univerity of California, Los Angeles.

Kivlahan, D. R., R. D. Walker, D. M. Donovan, and H. D. Mischke. 1985. Detoxification recidivism among urban American Indian alcoholics. American Journal of Psychiatry 142:1467-1470.

Lubran, B. G. 1987. Alcohol-related problems among the homeless: NIAAA's response. Alcohol Health and Research World 11(3):4-6,73.

Maypole, D. E., and R. B. Anderson. 1986/1987. Alcoholism programs serving minorities: Administrative issues. Alcohol Health and Research World 11(2):62-65.

Moos, F., D. E. Edwards, M. E. Edwards, F. V. Janzen, and G. Howell. 1985. Sobriety and American Indian problem drinkers. Alcoholism Treatment Quarterly 2:81-96.

National Institute on Alcohol Abuse and Alcoholism (NIAAA). 1987. Request for Applications: Community Demonstration Grant Projects for Alcohol and Drug Abuse Treatment of Homeless Individuals, RFA AA-87-04. Rockville, Md.: NIAAA.

National Institute on Alcohol Abuse and Alcoholism (NIAAA). 1989. Request for Cooperative Agreement Applications: Matching Patients to Alcoholism Treatments, RFA AA-89-02a, Coordinating Center. Rockville, Md.: NIAAA.

Padilla, A., R. Ruiz, and R. Alverez. 1975. Community mental health services for the Spanish-speaking/surnamed populations. American Psychologist 30:892-9050.

Saxe, L., D. Dougherty, K. Esty, and M. Fine. 1983. The Effectiveness and Costs of Alcoholism Treatment. Washington, D.C.: U.S. Congress, Office of Technology Assessment.

Sue, S. 1988. Psychotherapeutic services for ethnic minorities: Two decades of research findings. American Psychologist 43:301-308.

Westermeyer, J. 1988. Executive summary: Culture, special populations and alcoholism treatment. Prepared for the IOM Committee for the Study of Treatment and Rehabilitation Services for Alcoholism and Alcohol Abuse, April.

Westermeyer, J., and E. Peake. 1983. A ten year follow-up of alcoholic Native Americans in Minnesota. American Journal of Psychiatry 140:189-194.

Westermeyer J., and J. Neider. 1988. Social networks and psychopathology among substance abusers. American Journal of Psychiatry 145: 1265-1269.

18 The Evolution of Financing Policy

As treatment has advanced and become more specialized, there have been significant changes in the financing and organization of treatment services. Financing the treatment—or perhaps more accurately the custodial care—of persons with alcohol problems was previously seen as primarily the responsibility of the states as part of their mental health program. Until the early 1970s, the majority of individuals admitted for inpatient treatment of alcohol problems went to state mental hospitals, fewer than 10 percent of which had special wards or programs for such treatment. Indeed, in the 1960s, up to 40 percent of all the admissions to state hospitals were "chronic problem drinkers" (Glasscote et al., 1967; Plaut, 1967). There were few general hospitals that had special wards or programs; those that did have such units provided primarily emergency care and detoxification. Most private psychiatric hospitals also lacked separate programs; persons with alcohol problems (who constituted approximately 6 percent of admissions) were treated in their general psychiatric units (Glasscote et al., 1967). By 1986, the situation had changed dramatically: in a survey conducted by the American Hospital Association, there were 1,097 hospitals reported offering treatment for alcohol problems in a specialized program (1,039 general, psychiatric, and other specialty hospitals had designated units and 58 specialty hospitals offered "alcoholism/chemical dependency treatment") (AHA, 1987).

The number of outpatient and nonhospital residential facilities and programs has seen similar growth. There were only 130 outpatient clinics and 100 halfway houses and recovery homes which specialized in providing care for alcohol problems when the original survey was conducted in 1967 (Glasscote et al., 1967). Many of the halfway houses surveyed were privately funded clinics that provided safe withdrawal and supportive care for the well-to-do; others had been started by AA members as Twelfth Step houses to provide similar services on a voluntary basis. In contrast, in 1987, there were over 5,700 distinct specialty programs that reported providing treatment for alcohol problems within an identifiable unit (NIDA/NIAAA, 1989). More than 2,000 were outpatient facilities, and more than 1,300 were residential facilities (e.g., halfway houses, recovery homes).

Since the early 1970s and the first efforts to develop separate funding and organizational structures for specialty, high-quality treatment for alcohol problems, the mechanisms for funding such treatment have undergone a number of shifts. The first shift was from state and local undifferentiated funding to state, local, and federal government categorical grants and contracts. (Categorical grants and contracts are funds targeted to meet a specific need of a specific population through an application process with tightly defined program and administrative requirements.) Indeed, categorical government appropriations became the major sources of funding for treatment of persons with alcohol problems (Booz-Allen and Hamilton, Inc., 1978; USDHHS, 1981; Akins and Williams, 1982; Cahalan, 1987; Butynski and Canova, 1988). With this change came a different notion of what treatment should be. Financing treatment for alcohol problems was formerly seen as the responsibility of state and local governments; they were most likely to fund emergency care for public inebriates in jails and in public hospital emergency rooms and custodial care for chronic alcoholics in state mental hospitals. Together with the shift toward government categorical funding of treatment came the concept of a shared federal-state responsibility to develop a continuum of specialist treatment services in each community. The federal government thus provided categorical grants for community-based services and encouraged the states to increase their categorical funding of these programs (President's Commission on Law Enforcement, 1967a,b; Boche, 1975; Weisman, 1988).

The second important shift in funding that has occurred since the 1970s has been the move toward increased coverage of specialized treatment for alcohol problems as a separate, discrete benefit by public and private third-party payers. As a result, financing treatment for alcohol problems is now accepted, albeit not without reservations, as also the responsibility of the federal government (acting on behalf of the categorically needy, the elderly, and the chronically disabled) and of private insurers (acting on behalf of employers and individuals who purchase health insurance) (e.g., Leland et al., 1983; Sievert, 1983).

As discussed in Chapter 8, initiating these shifts in funding sources and developing a stable financing base have been major priorities of the voluntary associations and governmental agencies involved in specialty treatment for alcohol problems. All of these groups placed major emphasis on moving the financing of treatment for alcohol problems into the mainstream of health care financing; their efforts have led to a substantial increase in the total contribution of private health insurance, state and local categorical funds, and self-payment. There is continuing involvement of the federal government as a source of financing as well, but its relative contribution through both categorical funds and public health insurance has diminished. One consequence of the lessening of the federal role has been a substantial variability in sources and level of funding among the states and within the public and private specialist sectors (Jacob, 1985; Institute for Health and Aging, 1986; USDHHS, 1987).

Major questions are now being raised about whether current financing and reimbursement policies provide for access to the most cost-effective treatments (Freeborn, 1988). These policies have evolved over the last 20 years through a combination of government initiatives, research findings, and advocacy efforts. Recently, they have come into conflict with policies relating to cost containment and have been faced with questions regarding the effectiveness of current strategies (Gordis, 1987; Holden, 1987; Wallace, 1987; Gibson, 1988; Lewis, 1988). It may be helpful to look briefly at some of the noteworthy points along this evolutionary path for a historical perspective on the current state of funding policy.

Development of a National Policy

The recommendations of the Joint Commission on Mental Illness and Health (1961) are a good starting point for observing the development of a national policy on funding of treatment for alcohol problems. These recommendations were the driving force behind the shifts from state-dominated operation and financing of institutional services toward an increasing role for, first, the federal government (through categorical grants for community-based services) and, then, for public and private health insurance in financing a continuum of community-based treatment services for all mental disorders, including alcohol problems. Similar efforts of the Cooperative Commission on the Study of Alcoholism were aimed at removing the financial barriers to treatment of problem drinkers in community-based traditional hospital and nontraditional social model residential settings. One of the commission's most far-reaching recommendations was that a national organization be supported which would provide leadership in developing a coordinated approach to research, prevention, manpower development, and treatment throughout the United States (Plaut, 1967; Chafetz, 1976; Lewis, 1982; Burney, 1987).

The major impetus for change in both the financing and organization of treatment for all mental illness came in 1963, with the passage of the Mental Retardation Facilities and Community Mental Health Centers Construction Act of 1963 (P.L. 88-164). The major impetus for similar change in treating alcohol problems came in 1970 with the passage of the "Hughes Act," the Comprehensive Alcohol Abuse and Alcoholism Prevention, Treatment, and Rehabilitation Act of 1970 (P.L. 91-616). With this legislation came establishment of the National Institute of Alcohol Abuse and Alcoholism as the focal point for the coordination of federal activities and for the development of national policies and priorities (USDHEW, 1971; USGAO, 1977; NIAAA, 1984; Cahalan, 1987; Lewis, 1988a).

Important contributions to a national policy were made by the Task Force on Drunkenness of the President's Commission on Law Enforcement (1967b) and by a series of court decisions that supported the disease concept of alcoholism (Hart, 1977; Lewis, 1982). These efforts focused on the ineffective and inhumane handling of public inebriates within the criminal justice system, recommending that such individuals be treated within a public health model. The President's Commission on Law Enforcement (1967a) recommended that a network of detoxification centers be established to replace local jail facilities for public inebriates.

One important factor in bringing about the recommended changes was the efforts of Senator Harold Hughes (as chair of the Special Subcommittee on Alcoholism and Narcotics), Senator Harrison Williams, Congressman Paul Rogers, and a coalition of constituent groups led by the National Council on Alcoholism and the North American Association of Alcohol Problems. As a result of their efforts, the National Center for the Prevention and Control of Alcoholism was established in 1969 within the NIMH Division of Special Mental Health Programs. In 1970 the center was upgraded and renamed the Division on Alcohol Abuse and Alcoholism to give added visibility to the federal effort.

The Establishment of the National Institute on Alcohol Abuse and Alcoholism

The advocates of the new "problem drinking approach" embodied in the reports of the commissions noted above were not content with the establishment of the Division on Alcohol Abuse and Alcoholism. They were pushing for an even more visible and independent federal alcohol control agency which would not be dominated by the larger mental health establishment (Lewis, 1982, 1988; Neiberding, 1983; Cahalan, 1987; Weisman, 1988). Their goal was to redefine alcoholism as a primary illness rather than a symptom of mental illness (its position at that time). Their strategy was to create a network of specialist treatment facilities linked within a continuum of care (D. J. Anderson, 1981). With the early support of President Johnson and his assistant, Joseph Califano, who was later to become secretary of health, education and welfare, Senator Hughes and the constituent groups sought and ultimately received congressional authorization for a program of direct federal funding of alcohol treatment and prevention programs. This authorization was embodied in the Comprehensive Alcohol Abuse and Alcoholism Prevention, Treatment, and Rehabilitation Act of 1970.

This legislation, known as the Hughes Act (P.L. 91-616), established the National Institute of Alcohol Abuse and Alcoholism (NIAAA) as an independent institute within the National Institute of Mental Health (NIMH). NIAAA's mission was to administer the new programs which were authorized by the Hughes Act as well as those already established through amendments to the Community Mental Health Centers Act (P.L. 90-574 and P.L. 91-211). The secretary of health, education, and welfare, acting through NIAAA, was required to develop and conduct comprehensive health education, training, research, and planning programs for the prevention and treatment of alcohol abuse and alcoholism.

Using Federal Grants to Increase Treatment Resources

The Hughes Act also established two major new programs with significance for the development of alcohol treatment services. The first was a program of formula grants (i.e., allotments to states according to a formula involving population, per capita income, and need). States were to use these grants for planning, establishing, and maintaining prevention and treatment programs. The second program was a two pronged approach comprising project grants to public agencies and nonprofit organizations and contracts with public or private organizations or individuals.

The formula grant program required preparation of state plans outlining needs and resources for alcoholism programs and containing a description of the activities for which the federal funds were to be used. The initial plan submitted by a state was to identify a single agency, the state alcoholism authority (SAA) to administer the plan. The plan was required to contain assurances that federal funds would supplement, not replace, state and other nonfederal funds that were already being spent to support alcoholism programs.

In 1971, only a few of the states had oversight agencies in place that were similar to the proposed SAA (i.e., that could develop and monitor specialty programs for treatment of alcohol problems). (More than 40 states had separate alcohol programs, but the programs were primarily engaged in public education; only a few states operated a specialty inpatient program or provided funds for community-based outpatient clinics.) Most alcohol treatment services were provided by the state mental health authorities, either directly in state hospitals or through grants and contracts to newly developing community-based programs. The formula grant program provided the means for all of the states and territories to develop a new specialty oversight agency, the SAA, or to strengthen an existing agency; whichever proved to be the case, the resulting agency would then directly provide categorical funds for specialized treatment services and coordinate and monitor funds expended by other state agencies. NIAAA also provided financial support for the development of a national organization, the Council of State and Territorial Alcoholism Authorities, to promote the exchange of programming and financing strategies; this organization later merged with a similar group founded by directors of state drug abuse agencies to become the National Association of State Alcohol and Drug Abuse Program Directors (NASADAD). NASADAD has become the major vehicle by which the states interact with the federal government on policies for federal financing of treatment for alcohol problems (Akins and Williams, 1982; Butynski et al., 1987; Butynski and Canova, 1988).

The initial appropriation for the NIAAA formula grants program was made during the federal government's fiscal year 1972 and represented 35 percent of the institute's appropriation for all activities that year. By the end of the fiscal year, all of the states had submitted their required plans and received formula grant awards. The formula grant program ended in 1981. Approximately 80 percent of the formula grant expenditures over the years were for intervention, treatment, and rehabilitation services.

The second new program authorized by the Hughes Act consisted of project grants and contracts (awarded and administered by the secretary acting through NIAAA) to conduct demonstration, service, and evaluation projects. The initial focus of the program was on the use of project grants to demonstrate the feasibility of providing community-based intervention and treatment that was oriented toward the integration of services and the provision of comprehensive services. Through these projects, combined with the education and training of personnel, and cooperation with other agencies, NIAAA was to assume the leadership role in developing treatment capacity across the nation. Indeed the new institute's highest priority was the expansion of available treatment for persons with alcohol problems within their home communities (USDHEW, 1971). The major barriers to accomplishing this goal were the stigma attached to alcoholism, which was still viewed as a moral failing rather than as a disease; general ignorance about the condition; general hospital admission practices that excluded persons with alcohol problems; and the exclusion of alcohol-related disorders from health insurance coverage.

The strategy DHEW and NIAAA adopted was to expand treatment resources as rapidly as possible through categorical grants to states, local governments, and local community groups for treatment and rehabilitation services. The primary target population for these initial categorical grant programs were uninsured persons with alcohol problems (i.e., public inebriates, poverty area residents, and ethnic minorities). The initial appropriation for the categorical grants program was made in federal fiscal year 1972. In addition to the new grants for treatment services, staffing grants for comprehensive community alcoholism programs had previously been awarded under amendments to the Community Mental Health Centers Act. These grants were now also to be administered by NIAAA. Originally, these staffing grants utilized the initial community mental health centers model, which called for five essential services organized within a continuum of care to a delineated catchment or service area; the five services are: (1) inpatient care; (2) outpatient care; (3) intermediate care such as halfway houses and day or night hospitals; (4) emergency care; and (5) consultation and education services (see Chapter 3). These staffing grants were later redefined and became NIAAA's cross-population demonstration program, keeping the concept of the continuum of care but eliminating the catchment area concept and the concept of five essential services (Booz-Allen and Hamilton, Inc., 1978).

In keeping with its mission as the central federal agency for alcohol-related activities, other programs also moved under NIAAA's control. When the Office of Economic Opportunity was abolished in 1972, NIAAA assumed the administration of almost 200 grants serving residents of low income areas, American Indians, and Alaskan natives. These projects were originally funded under the Economic Opportunity Amendments of 1968 and 1969 and were the first federal grants for services to persons with alcohol problems; they provided primarily outreach and linking services or outpatient care, or both. The largest group of grantee agencies funded under this program comprised community action agencies, whose activities focused on social advocacy and linking poor persons with alcohol problems to treatment providers. The poverty grant program became the largest of NIAAA's special population categorical program areas, constituting approximately 54 percent of all such grants. Problems were encountered when the transfer occurred because the program's social advocacy and social services approach was not consistent with the field's effort to integrate treatment of person's with alcohol problems into more traditional health care financing mechanisms. These poverty grantees were seen as the group least likely to continue to receive funding if categorical grants were discontinued because their approach was not consistent with the treatment approach favored by state or third-party funders (Booz-Allen and Hamilton, Inc., 1978).

During the lifetime of this categorical project grant mechanism, grants for treatment and rehabilitation services to special, or underserved, populations received priority as a way to complement the "generic" treatment provided through the community mental health services approach (comprehensive services to a designated catchment area) (USDHEW 1971; see section IV). In addition to the cross-population, poverty, and Indian grants, additional programs were created to fund demonstrations of effective services for Hispanics, blacks, women, youth, the elderly, drinking drivers, criminal justice clients, gays and lesbians, migrant farmworkers, physically handicapped persons, and public inebriates. NIAAA prepared guidelines for grant applications to identify those elements that were thought to be essential components of treatment services for each of the special populations (e.g., child care services to enable women to enter inpatient residential treatment; vocational counseling and job training for low-income ethnic minorities; outpatient counseling for youth).

A third treatment oriented grant program was established in 1974. The incentive or uniform act grant program was designed to provide additional financial support for treatment services to those states that decriminalized public intoxication and provided treatment rather than jails for intoxicated persons (Grad et al., 1971; USDHEW, 1971; Finn, 1985; Burney, 1987). As an additional encouragement to this trend of treatment rather than jail, NIAAA supported the development of the Uniform Alcoholism and Intoxication Treatment Act by the National Conference of Commissioners on Uniform State

Laws (see Chapter 3 and Appendix D). When the NIAAA program ended in 1981, 34 states had passed an acceptable version of the Uniform Act and received incentive grants (Finn, 1985).

Despite NIAAA's effort to strengthen the SAAs through the formula and incentive grant programs, the early years of the NIAAA categorical grant program were marked by a lack of communication and coordination about funding priorities with the SAAs (USGAO, 1977; Booz-Allen and Hamilton, Inc., 1978). To improve cooperation, the states and NIAAA collaborated in the development of a demonstration program, in which the SAA would become the grantee for all project grants, assume responsibility for monitoring the adequacy of treatment, and provide data on accomplishments (Akins and Williams, 1982). While this project grant mechanism was still in the demonstration phase, however, the alcohol, drug abuse, and mental health services block grant was established by statute. The block grant consolidated the project and formula grant and contract programs administered by NIAAA and transferred responsibility for administration of these services funds to the Alcohol, Drug Abuse, and Mental Health Administration (ADAMHA). The leadership role in treatment capacity and services development was transferred to each of the states in keeping with the intent of the legislation to allow states the flexibility to set and carry out their own priorities (ADAMHA, 1984). There was also a cutback in the level of federal funds (Sharfstein, 1982; Robertson, 1988). The determination of the level and form of treatment services and their financing is fairly well left to each state. The block grant mechanism is still in place today, and states now allocate block grant funds according to the same policies by which they allocate state appropriations (USGAO, 1984; ADAMHA, 1988).

Efforts to Increase Public and Private Health Insurance

A second major emphasis in early NIAAA activities was on demonstrating that treatment of the employed individual who was experiencing alcohol problems was beneficial to both the individual and the employer; the primary mechanisms for these efforts were grants for the establishment of occupational alcoholism programs (now known as employee assistance programs) and the creation of an alcoholism counseling service for federal employees (Trice, 1986; Roman, 1988). In addition, NIAAA offered grants to each SAA to develop its own statewide program of consultation and technical assistance to local businesses and government agencies that were considering the establishment of occupational alcoholism programs. In particular, the state consultation programs highlighted the cost savings to be achieved through the adoption of company policies for identifying, referring, and treating the employee with alcohol problems in concert with the adoption of a specific health insurance benefit that encouraged early intervention for employees whose job performance was impaired by alcohol problems. A significant part of NIAAA's effort in this area was support for research on the development and testing of model health insurance benefit packages (e.g., Berman and Klein, 1977a, Hallan and Holder, 1983; Holder and Blose, 1986).

Working with the major voluntary association, the National Council on Alcoholism (NCA), and representatives from the insurance industry, NIAAA sponsored the development and dissemination of a model benefit package in 1973 (USDHEW, 1974; Williams, 1981). The suggested benefit structure was developed through a review of the existing coverage of treatment services for alcoholism and alcohol-related conditions offered by both private insurers and public insurers (Medicare and Medicaid) and by analyzing the costs and practice patterns of current NIAAA grantees (USDHEW, 1974). NIAAA offered the model benefit plan to insurers and companies purchasing health insurance as a basis for projecting a reasonable range of possible costs to use in their negotiations. The model was also seen as a guide for future studies of the impact of providing coverage on the cost of insurance coverage.

The cost estimates in the model were derived from analyses of 27 treatment programs offering treatment in more than 60 settings. The model was designed to reflect the continuum of care with a projected length of stay for each setting required for treatment: inpatient emergency care—6 days; inpatient care—14 days; intermediate care, short term—30 days; intermediate care, long term—60-90 days; and outpatient care—30 visits. When it distributed the package, NIAAA noted that costs varied significantly among the variety of settings in which equivalent care or treatment was provided (e.g., general hospital inpatient emergency care was found to cost from 2 to 10 times as much as other emergency care settings), a factor that continues to require consideration today (Holder and Hallan, 1983; Holder et al., 1988) (see Chapter 8).

This original benefit design attempted to incorporate then current expert opinion on effective treatment regimens and to promote alternatives to inpatient hospital treatment, including treatment in residential or partial care settings. NIAAA continued to encourage the development and adoption of model benefit packages working with the voluntary sector, professional associations, and state agencies; its role shifted in the late 1970s from advocating a specific model benefit to sponsoring research and providing information on which employers, third party payers, and other policymakers can base decisions on the extent and nature of coverage (Luckey, 1987; USDDHS, 1987). In recent years, however, the leadership role in encouraging the adoption of a model benefit has been shifted to the SAAs, which are working with the voluntary and professional interest groups in the field to obtain voluntary expansions of benefits or to have such coverage mandated by law (Alcohol and Drug Problems Association Task Force on Treatment Financing, 1983; Butynski, 1986; Oregon State Health Planning and Development Agency, 1986; Massachusetts Special Commission, 1988; New Jersey Department of Insurance, 1988).

During the 1970s, the federal role in financing treatment for alcohol problems—as with other physical and mental illnesses—was developmental: using the categorical grant mechanism, federal efforts were directed toward capacity building and resource development, embodied in such activities as basic and clinical research, professional training, and services demonstration. In general, this support was seen as a temporary measure, to be used only until the "more conventional" third-party financing mechanisms (particularly the expected national health insurance) could be brought into play. This view was expressed in a report by a study committee organized by the American Hospital Association (Advisory Panel on Financing Mental Health Care, 1973:59):

> Personal services for alcohol abuse should be financed through the same mechanisms as treatment for all other illnesses, even though some categorical support for direct services may be necessary in initial states of program development. The establishment of categorical administrative structures and funding structures at the Federal level, while providing a justifiable and necessary focus for the development of resources and the coordination of existing ones, should represent a temporary mode of approach. Fragmentation of authority and financing mechanisms within the mental health field, unquestionably has contributed to increased costs and reduced effectiveness. In the long run, federal programmatic support for the control of alcohol abuse should not be separated from Federal funding for all mental health programs.

Thus it was assumed that conventional third-party reimbursers (public insurance for the indigent and private insurance for the employed and their families) would begin to support these federally initiated alcohol treatment projects. Grantees were encouraged to seek out funding from a variety of third-party payers, ranging from private health insurance, to Medicaid, to Title XX Social Services funds (Morrison, 1978). The Health Services Funding Regulations and Guidelines [42 CFR, Sec. 50.101-107] adopted in 1974 specified the steps to be taken to capture these funds. In addition, technical assistance was offered to grantees through workshops, consultants, and manuals (Boche, 1975; Morrison, 1978). The goal was for projects to become financially self-sufficient, replacing federal categorical grant funds with other third-party sources by the end of the demonstration period. However, concerns began to surface about whether such a goal was realistic, and several studies suggested that many NIAAA-funded categorical projects could not expect to capture third party funds and to survive in the existing funding environment without significant changes to meet the medical model requirements of third-party payers (Boche, 1975; Booz-Allen and Hamilton, Inc., 1978; President's Commission on Mental Health Task Panel on Alcohol-Related Problems, 1978; Creative Socio-Medics Corporation, 1981).

Contemporary NIAAA reports sound the same theme as the American Hospital Association committee report while continuing to seek separate alcohol-specific third-party financing mechanisms. One of the agency's major objectives was to promote changes in the practices of health insurers who were seen to discriminate against persons with alcohol problems. This theme is consistently presented in each of NIAAA's early reports to Congress, which also detail the agency's efforts to demonstrate that effective treatment of alcohol problems is possible, that direct treatment of alcohol problems reduces other health care and productivity costs, and that treatment for alcohol problems can be brought into the "mainstream"—that is, included in existing health and social care systems (USDHEW, 1971; USDHEW, 1974; Chafetz, 1976; USDHHS, 1986). Despite NIAAA's advocacy, however, there were questions raised as to whether such mainstreaming was possible given the nature of the services needed (supportive social as well as medical services) and the continuing doubts of insurers and policymakers regarding the effectiveness of treatment (Boche, 1975; Booz-Allen and Hamilton, Inc., 1978; Leyland et al., 1983; Saxe et al., 1983; Sievert, 1983; Hurst, 1987).

To aid the survival of its grantees and to further demonstrate the validity of its approach, NIAAA funded a variety of projects aimed at addressing the concerns of Congress, the states, and the insurance industry regarding quality of treatment delivered, the effectiveness of treatment, and the costs of adding treatment of alcohol problems as a covered benefit. For example, NIAAA awarded a contract to the Blue Cross/Blue Shield Association to study the feasibility of offering a comprehensive benefit that would include the new nontraditional settings for treatment as eligible providers, allow counselors as well as physicians, psychologists, and social workers to be included in coverage, and provide coverage for the newer psychosocial modalities (e.g., family treatment) (Berman and Klein, 1977a). Another contract supported the development of accreditation standards for alcoholism treatment facilities by the Joint Commission on the Accreditation of Hospitals (now the Joint Commission on the Accreditation of Health Care Organizations). Such standards could be used to demonstrate that providers of treatment for alcohol problems could meet the traditional quality control measures used by the insurance industry in defining provider eligibility (Joint Commission on the Accreditation of Hospitals, 1979, 1983). In addition, a combined management information and treatment evaluation system was developed and its use made a requirement for NIAAA funding; these data were considered by peer review committees in determining whether to continue NIAAA funding of individual projects. Another NIAAA project was aimed at credentialing personnel; here, the agency chose to develop model standards to be used by the states and voluntary organizations in licensing or accrediting counselors (Birch and Davis Associates, Inc., 1984).

While NIAAA was pursuing these avenues, state alcoholism authorities were encouraging the nontraditional agencies they funded to attempt to bring in a mix of patients and funding sources by conducting outreach to employers and by obtaining accreditation from the Joint Commission on Accreditation of Hospitals. A number of states also strengthened their own licensing requirements. Their efforts brought some progress. Insurers began to recognize state licensure of certain nonhospital programs as a substitute for accreditation (Leyland et al., 1983). However, efforts to obtain similar recognition by Medicare and Medicaid were unsuccessful (Noble et al., 1978; Saxe et al., 1983; Lawrence Johnson and Associates, Inc., 1983, 1986).

The Current Situation

The Shifting Leadership Role

In 1982 the alcohol, drug abuse, and mental health services block grant established by the 1981 Omnibus Budget Reconciliation Act (P.L. 97-35) replaced the NIAAA formula, incentive, and project services grant programs. The action was taken as a result of general congressional and administration concerns about the proliferation of categorical programs that served many of the same client populations and the often duplicative and burdensome federal reporting requirements (Agranoff and Robins, 1982; USGAO, 1982; Grupenhof, 1983). Still in place today, the block grant is administered by the Alcohol, Drug Abuse, and Mental Health Administration (ADAMHA), the umbrella agency established in 1974 to oversee NIMH, NIAAA, and NIDA; the grant provides funds to the states for redistribution to local governments or agencies to carry out the general aims of the legislation but with minimal federally directed requirements. The initial award was based on the amount of funds which a state was receiving under the NIAAA categorical grant programs, less 25 percent. Since the initial award, however, there have been several adjustments in the level of the funding and in the formula because of concerns about inequities in the distribution of funds among the states (W. J. Anderson, 1984; USGAO, 1985, 1987b; Institute for Health and Aging, 1987).

The block grant was designed to be more flexible than NIAAA's categorical and formula grants program in its application, administration, and reporting requirements. There are relatively few restrictions placed on any of the block grants, although in some cases monies have been "set aside" for specific purposes (ADAMHA, 1984, 1988; USGAO, 1987a). The alcohol, drug abuse and mental health services block grant provides set asides for primary prevention and increased treatment availability for women (NCA, 1987). There is also a restriction on the amount of the block grant that can be used to support state administrative costs and a prohibition against using block grant funds to pay for hospital treatment of alcohol and drug problems.

With the shift to block grant funding for treatment services, the leadership previously exercised by NIAAA in the development of the network of specialist programs and enhanced financing for treatment devolved upon the states (Lewis, 1982, 1988; Cahalan, 1987). NIAAA's role has become primarily to fund and conduct research; to disseminate research findings to improve the prevention and treatment of alcohol-related problems; and to provide technical assistance in the development of effective alcohol abuse prevention and treatment programs and activities (USDHHS, 1986; Butynski and Canova, 1988; NASADAD, 1988). The momentum for continued resource development and capacity building has been shifted to the states and local communities, to advocacy groups, and to professional associations.

State and Local Government Activities

Today, each state has an identifiable unit charged with overseeing the development, funding, and regulating of specialist treatment for alcohol problems and of monitoring the quality of such treatment (USDHHS, 1986; NASADAD, 1988). As noted earlier in this chapter, the concept of a state alcoholism authority with specific functions was introduced as part of the requirements to obtain federal formula grants under the Hughes Act; these requirements were reduced with the passage of the block grant. Yet the SAAs have remained in place, carrying out most of the same functions and continuing to provide funding for treatment of low-income persons and other special populations.

The organizational placement, statutory structure, and functioning of the SAAs vary from state to state (NASADAD, 1988). In some states the SAA is part of an independent agency that also serves as the single state authority for drug abuse (e.g., Connecticut); in others it may be a component of a state mental health agency (e.g., Virginia, Alabama, Illinois), of a health department (e.g., Ohio, Pennsylvania), or of a human resources superagency (e.g., California, Minnesota). In fiscal year 1986, there were 14 states in which the state health agency served as the SAA to receive the alcohol portion of the federal block grant; all but one of these agencies were also the designated recipients of the drug abuse portion of the block grant. In only 6 states were the state alcoholism, state drug abuse, and state mental health authorities placed within the public health department (Public Health Foundation, 1988).

Funding practices and program administration vary considerably among the states and territories (Butler and Littlefield, 1985). Although each state and territory has an agency designated as responsible for funding and monitoring alcohol problem treatment activities, this agency may not be the only state entity to expend such funds. In three states (the District of Columbia, Indiana, and Montana), other state agencies are reported to provide more funding to publicly supported specialty programs than does the SAA (Butynski et al., 1987). As discussed in Chapter 8, funding varies among the states in terms of per capita levels and the relative proportion of funds available from state and local government appropriations as well as from public and private health insurance. The determinants of this variation are not clear. Additional empirical studies of the complex funding environments that exist are required to understand the sources of variation.

The SAA usually provides categorical funds to specialty providers but generally does not directly manage other funds for treatment in hospitals, correctional facilities, and social services agencies. Some states contract directly with provider agencies (e.g., Colorado, Connecticut, Missouri); other states provide funds to counties or regional coordinating agencies to use for provider contracting (e.g., Michigan, New York, California, Pennsylvania, Virginia). In addition, some states that contract with counties also have programs for contracting directly with providers on demonstration and other special projects (e.g., New York, California).

Most state governments are the largest single purchaser in their state of treatment services for alcohol problems through the categorical programs administered by the SAA. The NDATUS and SADAP survey data reported in Chapter 8 suggest that states provide more than 50 percent of the funds available to nonprofit specialty programs, which primarily serve the indigent and uninsured. The continuum of care supported by the benefit package in each state program differs from that of other states; within states, benefit plans of the Medicaid agency, the state employee health insurance program, and the SAA programs also differ. For example, Medicaid continues primarily to support a medical model of hospital-based detoxification and rehabilitation, whereas the SAA more often supports a mixed medical and social model that also includes social services, relapse prevention, and extended care in nontraditional, nonhospital settings (Lawrence Johnson and Associates, Inc., 1986; Butynski and Canova, 1988). Both public- and private-sector programs reflect the dominance of the Minnesota model discussed in Chapter 3 (inpatient primary rehabilitation followed by extended care or aftercare of decreasing intensity and frequency and using a blend of AA and professional services).

The trends toward decentralization in funding decisions that were noted in the last comprehensive study of the sources of and barriers to financing of treatment for persons with alcohol problems have continued (Booz-Allen and Hamilton, Inc., 1978); consequently, the current environment is extremely complex, with large interstate and intrastate variation in both funding levels and funding policies (Weisner and Room, 1984; Weisner, 1986). The role of substate units (e.g., counties, regional coordinating agencies) has continued to grow in importance as more states require local matching funds as a condition of receiving state-appropriated funds or federal "pass-through" monies (i.e., block grant or Medicaid funds). This shift is reflected in the SADAP annual reports of state alcohol and drug abuse agencies: there are six states in which the county or other local government share is 20 percent or more of the total expenditures for treatment of alcohol problems (Butynski et al., 1987).

Another factor in the development of coverage and reimbursement policies is the trend toward combined alcohol and drug treatment programs and state and county authorities. Reflecting both a desire for administrative simplicity and the perception that more and more of the persons being seen in treatment have problems related to both alcohol and other drugs, all but four of the states now have combined alcohol and drug abuse state agencies (NASADAD, 1988). Some states with combined agencies still have separate funding mechanisms and policies for alcohol problems treatment (e.g., California, Colorado, New York); others have the same mechanisms (an addictions, chemical dependency, or substance abuse orientation as in Connecticut, Minnesota, and Michigan). Still others administer their funds for treatment of alcohol problem as part of a combined alcohol, drug, and mental health funding mechanism (e.g., Virginia's Community Services Boards; Alabama's integrated community services).

The diversity in funding policies and organization that exists among the states can be best communicated by describing several of the current state programs. California represents the administrative combination of distinct drug and alcohol programs into a single department within a large human resources agency. The California SAA has adopted a social model in its funding of specialist treatment for alcohol problems. Minnesota and Oregon represent combined alcohol and drug programs which have adopted mixed medical and social model concepts and administrative requirements. The three SAAs are attempting to deal with the issues of improving provider accountability and increasing the availability of appropriate treatment using different mechanisms.

California   The California SAA, the Alcohol Program Division within the Department of Alcohol and Drug Programs, represents an increasingly common administrative pattern (California Department of Alcohol and Drug Programs, 1988). The California SAA has an annual budget of approximately $64 million for treatment. Funds are primarily distributed through county agencies that serve as county alcohol authorities and purchase specific services from local providers. The state's Alcohol Program Division assists counties in the planning, development, implementation, coordination, and funding of local prevention, treatment, and rehabilitation programs. The state agency identifies statewide objectives and priorities that serve as guidelines to the counties in the preparation of their county alcohol plans. The county plans are then used as the basis for receiving state funding.

The continuum of services for treatment of persons with alcohol problems administered by the California State Department of Alcohol and Drug Programs includes three categories of residential programs (detoxification, short term and extended-term residential treatment, and short term and extended-term recovery homes) and three categories of nonresidential services (treatment/recovery, vocational rehabilitation, and drinking driver). The SAA has no formal relationship with hospital-based programs that provide treatment for alcohol problems nor with any private program that does not receive governmental funds or drinking driver referrals. The SAA estimates that 60 percent of the specialist programs in the state receive its funding (Butynski and Canova, 1988).

Although the services supported by the California SAA vary, their orientation is primarily nonmedical, reflecting the California model of social recovery. The model stresses an alcohol-free environment and participant responsibility for recovery as described in Chapter 3 (S. Blacksher, California Alcohol Program Division, personal communication, December 30, 1987). Most staff in programs funded by the state and county authorities are nondegreed counselors, and many are recovering individuals. Costs are lower as a result. The state requires all social model providers of direct alcohol services to have medical backup, which is not paid for by the state and federal block grant categorical funding. In addition, all funded programs must be capable of identifying those persons who need medical attention for physical complications or other comorbid conditions (e.g., mental illness, problems with other drugs, or mental retardation) and of referring them to the appropriate resource.

Participants in SAA-funded services tend to be persons with chronic severe alcohol problems who have limited financial, health, vocational or social resources and little in the way of spiritual reserves. Therefore, many of the programs incorporate other goals such as getting off welfare, becoming employed, and sustaining independent living in addition to the goal of eliminating alcohol use (Costello, 1982; Borkman, 1983, 1988; Weisner, 1986; Reynolds and Ryan, 1988) (see Chapter 3).

Minnesota The continuum of care supported by the Minnesota SAA as described in Chapter 4 comprises detoxification, assessment, primary treatment, extended care, halfway houses, and aftercare. Community services block grant funds are used to cover certain services and, in contrast to California, hospital programs can also be reimbursed for providing appropriate services (Minnesota Chemical Dependency Program Division, 1987, 1989a). Minnesota is currently unique in its implementation of a consolidated chemical dependency treatment fund, administered by the Chemical Dependency Program Division organizationally housed within the Department of Human Services (Minnesota Chemical Dependency Program Division, 1987, 1989b). Initiated in 1988, amid concern that hospital and residential primary rehabilitation was being overutilized, the fund covers outpatient and inpatient primary treatment, extended care, and halfway houses; it combined $27 million in state appropriations for treatment of alcohol and drug abuse from six sources or funding areas: (1) general assistance, (2) general assistance medical care, (3) medical assistance (Medicaid), (4) regional treatment centers, (5) the alcohol, drug abuse, and mental health block grant, and (6) state categorical appropriations. The funds are allocated to counties based on population, income, and welfare caseload; they are distributed to Indian reservations based on population. A 15 percent county match is required (i.e., the county must provide 15 percent of the total in matching funds). One of the major advantages of the consolidated fund mechanism is that it removes eligibility restrictions on the types of treatment service providers that are eligible for reimbursement (e.g., freestanding residential facilities and halfway houses for Medicaid recipients). In this way, persons who are eligible to receive state public assistance in paying for treatment for alcohol (or other drug) problems can be treated in the most appropriate and economical manner. The county agency administering the mix of state, federal, and local funds assigns individuals to treatment using legislatively defined, uniform placement criteria and an assessment and referral methodology approved by the SAA.

Oregon States vary not only in the continuum of care they fund but in the mechanisms and criteria they use to monitor contractor performance. Some states have imposed fairly stringent performance contracting requirements on providers (e.g., Oregon,

Indiana, Colorado), even when funding is channeled through counties or regional coordinating agencies; others impose minimal contract obligations.

The policies developed by the Oregon SAA for a performance contracting reimbursement mechanism are an example of the attempts by the SAAs to develop both process and outcome objectives which can be used to monitor treatment providers' performance (Oregon State Health Planning and Development Agency, 1986; Oregon Office of Health Policy, 1988; J. Kushner, Oregon Office of Alcohol Programs, personal communication, August 1, 1988). The Oregon SAA has established specific performance criteria for each service element in the continuum of care under its funding authority. The elements are detoxification, CIRT (community intensive residential treatment), residential care, and outpatient treatment, all of which take place in nonhospital settings. Like the California SAA, the Oregon SAA does not fund or monitor hospital-based detoxification or rehabilitation programs. Oregon's three rehabilitation programs warrant some description because they are representative of the nontraditional, Minnesota model-based mixed social and medical model programs now favored by many of the SAAs after almost 20 years of experience.

CIRTs provide rehabilitation services to persons who are severely impaired by their alcohol problems and who have typically been unsuccessful in maintaining sobriety after completing less intensive treatment programs. CIRTs resemble the freestanding primary care facilities in Minnesota, Illinois, Colorado, New York, and other states and are based on the original Minnesota model programs described in Chapter 3. Oregon requires the CIRT to meet certain program standards. The CIRT program is designed to last an average of 28 days. The services the providers must offer to qualify for reimbursement include a minimum of 30 hours of structured therapy per week (a minimum of 6 hours a day for 5 days, 14 hours of structured recreational activities over the full 7-day week, and 2.5 hours of alcohol-and-drug specific education per week (Hubbard and Anderson, 1988).

Oregon's alcohol residential treatment (ART) programs are designed to provide 24-hour care within a structured environment that emphasizes group therapy and minimal individual therapy. Other activities to be made available as part of an individualized treatment plan are educational or vocational counseling or training, referral for job placement, consumer living skills training, creative recreational activities, and family counseling. Unlike the CIRT, the state does not specify the hours required for each activity. Although the CIRT and the ART both are rehabilitation programs in terms of the stage model introduced in Chapter 3, the CIRT can be seen as offering only primary care, while the ART is a combination primary care and extended care facility. The ART program represents the professionalized halfway house, in which staff provide both supportive care and treatment for persons who cannot live independently in the community without relapsing (Rubington, 1974).

Oregon's alcohol outpatient treatment programs (AOPs) provide assessment and treatment services for persons who are not in need of 24-hour supervision. The target populations for AOPs are described as persons who are less severely impaired by their alcohol problems. The treatment activities offered by these programs are individual, group, and family therapy or counseling and chemotherapy (e.g., Antabuse); the ancillary, or supportive, services offered are educational and vocational training, consumer living skills training, and recreational therapy. The state does not specify a set number of hours for any of the activities.

There are four contractor performance criteria applicable to all four service elements: (1) program participants must take part in a self-help group during treatment; (2) participants must be referred to a self-help group at discharge; (3) participants must be referred to another element in the continuum of care upon discharge; and (4) participants must show benefits from treatment as measured by completion of at least two-thirds of a mutually agreed upon treatment plan. Detoxification programs must meet an additional criterion: the individual in treatment cannot be readmitted to the same treatment center within one year.

There are five additional program performance criteria applicable to the three rehabilitation elements (CIRT, residential treatment, and outpatient treatment): (1) participants who are not employable at their admission to the program must be employable at discharge; (2) if employed, their employment status must be maintained or improved while they are participating in treatment; (3) their educational status must be maintained or improved while participating in treatment; (4) they must not be arrested during treatment; and (5) they must be abstinent/drug free during the 30 days prior to discharge.

The criteria used by the Oregon SAA to judge the performance of funded programs are representative of those used by other states to monitor outcome and determine funding priorities. The criteria incorporate the broad definition of treatment for alcohol problems combining direct and supportive services (see Chapter 3). There have been no studies, however, of the impact of these performance contracting strategies on the accessibility of treatment services or on outcome. Little is known about the reasons for the differential utilization of resources among the states and whether differences in organization and financing, including the use of performance contracting, play a role in creating this differential. Many SAAs do have in place a treatment outcome monitoring system for program evaluation, although the use made in program planning and funding varies considerably (Lewin/ICF, 1988a,b; Kusserow, 1989).

Federal Government Activities

The federal government continues to finance treatment for alcohol problems through a variety of mechanisms. It supports agencies that operate their own networks of treatment programs for alcohol problems (e.g., the Veterans Administration, the military services within the Department of Defense, and the Indian Health Service) (see Chapters 4 and 8). It also supports treatment through agencies that serve as third-party payers: the Health Care Financing Administration (HCFA), the Department of Defense, and the Office of Personnel Management. Agencies that provide block grant funding used to support treatment and ancillary supportive services for persons with for alcohol problems are the Alcohol, Drug Abuse,and Mental Health Administration and the Office of Human Services (i.e., the social services block grant). Operating within statutorily defined parameters, each agency sets its own policy on the type and level of services to be provided (Macro Systems, Inc., 1980; NIAAA, 1984). Each agency responds to different congressional oversight committees. Since the repeal of the statutory requirement for the existence of the Interagency Committee on Alcohol Abuse and Alcoholism in 1982, there has been no systematic review of the different approaches; nor does there appear to be an ongoing effort within either the congressional or executive branches to coordinate the methods used by the various programs in deciding which treatments are to be supported financially (Grupenhoff, 1983; Cahalan, 1987).

In addition to the block grant funding, which can now be considered a state-determined activity, the three major sources of federal funding for treatment of alcohol problems are Medicare, Medicaid, and the Federal Employees Health Benefits Program.

Medicare As discussed in Chapter 8, Medicare is the federally administered health insurance program that covers most elderly Americans, aged 65 and older, and certain disabled individuals under the age of 65, who meet specific criteria or have chronic kidney disease. Under Medicare, treatment for alcohol problems continues to be included in the general category of psychiatric health services rather than being treated as a discrete benefit (as desired by the field). Medicare coverage for inpatient care within a psychiatric hospital is limited to 190 lifetime days; there no limit on inpatient psychiatric care within a general hospital. (This limit was originally included in the Medicare benefit design to ensure that only active treatment under a physician's supervision and evaluation, and not "custodial care," would be covered. This restriction reflected a concern that federal funds would be used to supplant state funds for long term care in state mental hospitals.) Coverage is not available for treatment in the newer freestanding residential facilities supported by the majority of SAAs (Noble et al., 1978; Lawrence Johnson and Associates, Inc., 1983, 1986; Saxe et al., 1983). Coverage for outpatient treatment is similarly limited.

The major policy issues confronted by Medicare are cost containment and ensuring the effectiveness of the treatment that is delivered. In 1983 Medicare introduced its new prospective payment system (PPS) as a cost containment measure (Sloan et al., 1988). (Prior to late 1983, Medicare paid hospitals on a cost-based retrospective basis; that is, charges were incurred by patients and then submitted to Medicare for reimbursement.) A similar cost-containment system was introduced in 1986 for hospital costs in the Veterans Administration and in 1988 for the military's CHAMPUS health care plan. Several states and private insurers have also adopted this method of payment in the general effort to reduce costs.

Under the Medicare PPS, more than 20,000 medical conditions are classified into one of 468 diagnosis related groups (DRGs). Hospitals are then reimbursed a specific predetermined amount for all admissions within that group; the amount reimbursed is based on a complex formula including adjustments for "case mix," length of stay, complications, section of the country, status as a teaching hospital, etc. If hospitals routinely use more resources than the standard recognized by the PPS reimbursement, they are penalized (i.e., the amount reimbursed is less than the cost to the hospital); if they use less resources, they are rewarded (i.e., the amount reimbursed is more than the cost to the hospital). Only psychiatric, rehabilitation, and long term care facilities were originally exempted by the legislation authorizing PPS.

The original DRGs for psychiatric illnesses included four for alcohol problems: (1) 433—substance use and substance-induced organic mental syndrome, left against medical advice; (2) 436—alcohol dependence; (3) 437—alcohol use except dependence; (4) 438—alcohol- and substance-induced organic mental syndrome. These initial DRGs would have allowed an average of $2,165 per admission to cover both detoxification and rehabilitation. As one would expect, they met with much resistance from treatment providers and advocacy groups (e.g., NAATP, Inc., 1987) In fact, all of the psychiatric DRGs were roundly criticized as being less predictive of resource utilization (length of stay, costs) than were the DRGs for physical illnesses or surgical cases (Taube et al., 1985; McGuire et al., 1987; Taube et al., 1988). A major criticism of the alcohol-related DRGs was that the length of stay used to develop the reimbursement available for cases classified in DRG 436 was based on limited data; it reflected detoxification-only services offered by the hospitals that provided the data base of Medicare patients used in constructing the original DRGs. As a result of these concerns, the secretary of health and human services in 1984 granted exemptions to certain alcohol and drug problem treatment units while a study was being conducted of the fairness of the relevant DRGs and a review of clinical practice undertaken to develop a more appropriate DRG configuration for these conditions. Alcohol specialty units in general hospitals and specialty hospitals were exempted from the PPS policy; admissions to a regular medical/surgical bed of a general hospital (so-called "scatter" beds) were not exempted. Similar exemptions were granted to specialty units treating drug abuse and all psychiatric disorders (Taube et al., 1985; McGuire et al., 1987).

Applying the original DRGs to a much broader sample of hospitals, Taube and colleagues (1985) obtained evidence to support the argument that the original data base had been too limited. They found a wide range of differences among unit and nonunit hospitals (i.e., hospitals with specialty treatment units and hospitals without such units) for DRGs, lengths of stay, patient characteristics, and other variables. Consistent with other studies, there was a higher percentage of discharges in all four DRGs from hospitals without a specialty unit than from those with a specialty unit (40.1 percent of total discharges versus 18.2 percent, respectively). "Organic mental problems" was the predominant discharge diagnosis. Taube and coworkers suggested that the short length of stay found for the majority of the admissions was due to detoxification being the treatment of choice in both unit and nonunit hospitals included in both data bases. Qualifying this conclusion, they noted that the length of stay for DRG 436, alcohol dependence, was three times the usual two- to five-day detoxification period. This finding suggested that some rehabilitation was taking place for persons in this category in both unit and nonunit hospital settings.

In 1985 the alcohol-related DRGs were modified to include the distinction between detoxification and rehabilitation as recommended by NIAAA. The exemption for treatment of alcohol and drug problems in hospital settings was ended in 1987 after a joint ADAMHA-HCFA review that generated a second revised set of DRGs more acceptable to both practitioners and payers. Yet concerns are still being voiced (as is the case with DRGs for other physical and psychiatric disorders) that inadequate attention has been paid to variables that contribute significantly to the process of treatment and resource utilization—for example, age, physical comorbidities, psychiatric comorbidities, severity of dependence, dependence on multiple substances, and level of social stability or deterioration.

The DRGs adopted in 1987 continue to differentiate between detoxification and rehabilitation, although alcohol and drug problems are combined: (1) 433—alcohol/drug abuse or dependence, left against medical advice; (2) 434—alcohol/drug abuse or dependence, detoxification or other symptomatic treatment with complications or comorbidity; (3) 435—alcohol/drug abuse or dependence, detoxification or other symptomatic treatment without complications or comorbidity; (4) 436—alcohol/drug dependence with rehabilitation; and (5) 437—alcohol/drug dependence with detoxification and rehabilitation.

Supporters of prospective payment have predicted that the use of such a system would decrease the average length of stay and the number of admissions to covered settings. There have been no studies published as yet, however, that describe the impact of the shift to prospective payment in regard to the treatment of alcohol problems in covered hospital settings either for detoxification or rehabilitation.

Medicaid As previously discussed (see Chapter 8), Medicaid is a jointly financed federal-state entitlement program, the major public insurance mechanism for providing medical assistance to low-income persons in federally supported welfare programs. States can also choose to make Medicaid available to other persons who are not eligible for the federal welfare programs and are unable otherwise to access health care. The states administer Medicaid within broad federal guidelines that establish required and optional services as if it were an insurance program. Each state designs its own unique Medicaid program, and the coverage of treatment for alcohol problems can, and does, vary from state to state (Macro Systems, Inc., 1980; Sharfstein, 1982; Toff, 1984; Howell et al., 1988).

Like Medicare, Medicaid does not have a specific benefit for the treatment of alcohol problems and does not necessarily provide coverage for the educational, vocational, and psychosocial services that are considered by most treatment providers as an essential part of rehabilitation and relapse prevention, particularly for low-income persons. Medicaid, like Medicare and other health insurance plans, still categorizes the treatment of alcohol problems under the mental disorders rubric. It provides federally mandated coverage for inpatient hospital treatment of alcohol-related diagnoses except in institutions for mental disorders or tuberculosis. (Medicaid does provide coverage for children, adolescents, and young adults under the age of 22 treated as inpatients in psychiatric hospitals.) A state can include physician-supervised nonhospital residential services and outpatient care in its package of optional services, and some have done so (Cooper, 1979; Toff, 1984); however, Medicaid coverage of outpatient treatment for alcohol problems does not appear to be a significant funding resource in most states, although there are exceptions (e.g., New York, in which the state has elected the clinic option to cover eligible individuals being treated in state-aided and state-operated outpatient programs).

There have been no recent detailed studies of the benefits currently available among the states for treatment of alcohol problems independent of generic mental health coverage. (The routine reporting of services available state by state does not include this level of description.) In many states, reporting on psychiatric expenditures includes reporting about the treatment of alcohol problems among a limited set of eligible providers. Recent surveys of state practices in funding mental health services, as well as earlier studies specific to the treatment of alcohol problems, suggest that Medicaid reimbursement for the nontraditional forms of treatment supported by SAAs is lacking (Toff, 1984). Indeed, because Medicaid was originally designed as a decentralized program, there has been little detailed information available at the national level to monitor performance and expenditures (Howell et al., 1988).

The Federal Employees Health Benefits Program   The Federal Employees Health Benefits Program (FEHBP), which was established in 1959, offers health insurance to federal government and postal service employees, retirees, and their dependents. FEHBP is the largest employer-sponsored health insurance program in the nation. The Office of Personnel Management (OPM) administers the program and contracts annually with various health plans to provide coverage for different employee groups. Each of these health plan varies in its provisions, covered benefits, and premiums. In 1985, there were about 300 plans participating in the FEHP; the plans collected premiums of approximately $6 billion to cover 10 million enrollees. The cost of the premiums is shared by the federal government and its employees. The government's share of the premiums is anticipated to be approximately $2 billion in fiscal year 1989. (The Office of Personnel Management is also responsible for overseeing the development and operation of appropriate counseling and assistance services for federal civilian employees; however, this employee assistance program is distinct from the FEHP [OPM, 1988].) In recent years, several of the major plans have cut back on the level of benefits available for treatment for alcohol, drug, and mental problems (Hustead et al., 1985).

The U.S. General Accounting Office (GAO) (1986) compared the coverages offered in 1985 by the FEHBP with that offered by private-sector employers and found that 53 percent of federal employees were covered for alcohol and drug abuse care, whereas 68 percent of private-sector enrollees were covered for alcohol problems treatment and 61 percent were covered for drug abuse treatment. GAO studied the benefits provided in the 18 plans that had a total enrollment more than 20,000 for each of the six years under review and noted that all of the plans covered medical and hospital services for acute care or detoxification; 14 of the 18 had some coverage for rehabilitation. (In 1987, the remaining four plans added the benefit.) GAO did not study the specific coverages offered. In some plans the alcohol problems benefit is distinct; in others it is included in a substance abuse benefit or a mental health benefit. Outpatient care and coverage for treatment by nontraditional social model providers appear to be limited. In general, the level of coverage has declined for all mental health benefits since 1980 and also for coverage of the treatment of alcohol problems.

In 1983, at the request of Congress, the Office of Technology Assessment undertook a review of the effectiveness of treatment for alcohol problems specifically to make recommendations about whether to continue support for the system that had evolved (Saxe et al., 1983). The study found that the research evidence was not conclusive in regard to the effectiveness of specific modalities and could provide little guidance for reimbursement policies. It noted that HCFA and NIAAA were supporting a four year demonstration to test the effectiveness of less costly social model treatment settings (e.g., freestanding inpatient and outpatient facilities, halfway houses) and to assess whether nonmedical personnel could carry out detoxification and rehabilitation effectively (Lawrence Johnson and Associates, Inc., 1983, 1986). The evaluation of this demonstration was not completed in time for committee review, although preliminary findings do suggest that these facilities and staff can provide equivalent services to those generally offered under the traditional medical model (e.g., Becker and Sanders, 1984; Reutzel et al., 1988). In fact, the states involved (Michigan, Connecticut, Illinois, Oklahoma, New York, and New Jersey) have attempted to implement the preliminary findings of the demonstration in their treatment policies for alcoholism problems. There are a number of methodological problems with the evaluation, however, and these problems again make it difficult to suggest that Medicare and Medicaid reimbursement policies should be based on its findings. If there are concerns remaining regarding the appropriateness of the mixed medical and social model that has adopted by the states, HCFA and NIAAA should conduct a more adequately designed clinical trial using random assignment. The committee's review of the literature, however, suggests that there is sufficient information regarding the effectiveness of these strategies to propose some general principles for the revision of all benefit structures of federal agencies that fund treatment for alcohol problems (see Chapter 20).

Private Health Insurance Activities

It is generally assumed that health insurance coverage makes treatment more accessible to those who need it by lowering the effective price (i.e., the out-of-pocket cost) at the time care is sought (Morissey and Jensen, 1987; American Hospital Association, 1988; Freeborn, 1988). Private health insurance was originally seen as the major target of efforts to expand coverage for the treatment of alcohol problems to ensure equal access to all who desired such treatment and not just care for the physical consequences of alcohol use (Hallan, 1972; USDHEW, 1978; Regan, 1981; USDHHS, 1981). Yet early studies of the availability of coverage for the treatment of alcohol problems found that both insurers and providers actively discriminated against persons with alcohol problems through exclusions and limitations (Rosenberg, 1968; Holder and Hallan, 1983).

Initial efforts in the field to overcome resistance to developing a specific nondiscriminatory public and private insurance health benefit for the treatment of alcohol problems focused on obtaining coverage for inpatient hospital treatment of alcohol withdrawal and dependence. These efforts have been fairly successful. Basic coverage now no longer excludes the treatment of alcohol-related physical illnesses and trauma or detoxification in general hospital settings. Rehabilitation, which is defined as the treatment of alcohol abuse and dependence, is most often still an add-on benefit that is included in major medical coverage or as an additional rider with an extra premium cost. Advocates of a specific benefit for treatment for alcohol problems have used two major strategies to obtain increased private insurance coverage: (1) demonstrations of cost savings through analysis and simulation of claims experience and (2) legislative mandates. NIAAA sponsored the development of model benefit packages and studies on the cost of adding insurance coverage as well as on the health care cost offsets (i.e., savings in other health care expenditures) to be obtained by providing coverage for treatment of alcohol problems (Holder and Hallan, 1983; Holder et al., 1985; Holder, 1987). The research emphasis has been on demonstrating that the addition of a discrete benefit, even when very liberal, would not lead to a dramatic rise in costs that would lead to a premium increase. (Any premium increases were expected to be offset by the decrease in costs associated with the use of other health services [Holder et al., 1985; Holder, 1987]). An NIAAA-sponsored study examined the cost implications of six model insurance benefit plans through simulations of utilization and costs (Holder and Hallan, 1983). The coverage provided by the six plans ranged from a limit of 14 days of hospitalization only to a combination of up to 30 days of hospital care with up to 30 days of intermediate (transitional) care and up to 45 outpatient sessions. The different models were associated with substantial differences in benefits paid over a five-year period and with sufficient cost offsets to decrease the amount of the monthly premium increase that would be required to add the benefit. The outcomes of these studies and simulations have not been widely accepted, however, because of their design and because of questions about the value of long term offsets to the insurer and employer (Luckey, 1987; IOM, 1989) (see Chapter 19).

A number of studies have found that the largest proportion of direct expenditures for the treatment of alcohol problems is spent on services provided in short-term community general hospitals (Harwood et al., 1985a; Davis, 1987). Some of the services in community hospitals are provided in specialized units, but the bulk of such services utilize "scatter" beds in hospitals that do not have a designated unit. Treatment activity in general hospitals includes detoxification and rehabilitation, but it still emphasizes treating related health problems and the direct consequences of excessive alcohol use for such illnesses as cancers, and ulcers as well as cirrhosis, pancreatitis, and cardiopathies, and trauma resulting from accidents. Other studies suggest that the primary treatment for alcohol problems that is currently available in community hospitals is still oriented toward detoxification rather than rehabilitation (Harwood et al., 1985a; Blue Cross of Greater Philadelphia, 1987).

Proponents of expanding a discrete benefit for the treatment of alcohol problems interpret the above data on the numbers of persons admitted to hospitals only for detoxification and treatment of alcohol-related physical illnesses as reflecting a continuing failure to recognize the value of such treatment in reducing future health care and social costs (Fein, 1984; Davis, 1987). This practice is seen as related to the current structure of benefit designs, which continue to emphasize acute treatment in inpatient hospital settings (McAullife et al., 1987; Freeborn, 1988; New Jersey Department of Insurance, 1988).

Despite efforts to demonstrate the value of having a specific benefit for the treatment of alcohol problems, there has not been full acceptance by health insurers of the insurability of treatment of alcohol problems. It has been estimated that only a limited number of the persons at risk have private health insurance that also includes coverage of such treatment (Fein, 1984; USDHHS, 1986). Surveys of private health insurance benefit packages reveal that coverage for treatment of alcohol problems varies greatly and is still frequently limited to inpatient medical procedures. Most private insurance and public insurance plans continue to place stringent restrictions and limits on the range of services covered, the providers eligible, and the level of coverage offered for the direct treatment of alcohol problems (the primary rehabilitation and maintenance stages) (Davis, 1987). Private insurance expenditures continue to appear to be primarily for treatment of related disorders and consequences and for acute intervention and detoxification, although the number of plans which offer a separate benefit for rehabilitation has been greatly expanded (Morissey and Jensen, 1988).

Insurers as a group have not all been opposed to providing insurance benefits for the treatment of alcohol problems. The Kemper Insurance Companies have pioneered providing coverage of treatment for alcohol problems, establishing an employee alcoholism program in 1962 for their own employees (Graham, 1981). Kemper added coverage to their employee accident and health plan offerings in 1964; the first Blue Cross plans providing coverage appeared in 1969.

Yet, as noted by Jensen and Gabel (1988), treatment for alcohol problems is still considered by many private health insurers to be a "fringe service." Although some coverage is provided and is not likely to be dropped totally because of employers' interest, broader coverage is constrained because of concerns over treatment costs and effectiveness. This reluctance of insurers to cover the treatment of alcohol problems at the same level as that for physical illnesses has remained consistent even though the percentage of employers providing some form of coverage has grown from 36 percent in 1981 to 68 percent in 1985 in the medium and large firms covered by the biannual Bureau of Labor (BLS) Statistics Employee Benefits Survey (Morissey and Jensen, 1988). Preliminary data from the 1988 survey show a continuing increase in plans that offer a specific benefit for alcohol treatment: 86 percent of the plans surveyed provided some form of coverage (Bureau of Labor Statistics, 1989). A larger proportion of HMO plans (96 percent) versus non-HMO plans (78 percent) included some coverage. The pattern of benefits also differed between HMO and indemnity plans. In addition, HMO plans are more likely to offer coverage for inpatient detoxification and outpatient treatment (more than 90 percent offered such coverage); non-HMO plans, on the other hand, tend to offer these benefits in addition to inpatient rehabilitation, although not in the same proportion—approximately 60 percent (Bureau of Labor Statistics, 1989). Size is a factor in determining whether a firm will provide a benefit for treating alcohol problems; larger firms tend to offer such a benefit (more than 75 percent of Fortune 500 firms do so) (Davis, 1987).

A major problem with the BLS survey, however, is that it only establishes whether the coverage was in place and not the breadth and depth of that coverage. Studies are needed of the actual coverage that is offered by specific plans and how this coverage varies throughout the country (Morissey and Jensen, 1988). Given the pattern of interstate variation of such reimbursement to specialist programs as seen in the most recent NDATUS data (see Chapter 8), studies are also needed to determine utilization and costs over a wide range of plans, industries, and geographically dispersed service areas.

There have been a number of analyses of the sources of the resistance of third-party payers, whether representing public or private interests, to provide the same level and type of coverage for the treatment of alcohol problems as is provided for physical illnesses (e.g., Boche, 1975; Butynski, 1982, 1986; Sieverts, 1983; Fein, 1984; Sharfstein, et al., 1984; Morissey and Jensen, 1988; New Jersey Department of Insurance, 1988). Proponents of expanded coverage argue that insurers have questioned—and continue to question—whether alcohol problems are truly diseases, or rather represent self-inflicted injury and therefore not eligible for coverage. Proponents also contend that insurers remain uncomfortable with the many nontraditional settings and organizational arrangements in which and by which treatment services for alcohol problems are now delivered.

The development of freestanding residential facilities and clinics, which have adopted the social model of treatment mixing medical and social support services, have, indeed, created questions and concerns among insurers regarding the appropriateness of health insurance for these services (Booz-Allen and Hamilton, Inc., 1978; Noble et al., 1978; Lawrence Johnson and Associates, Inc., 1983, 1986; Leyland et al., 1983; Sieverts, 1983). The majority of treatment services outside the traditional hospital facilities and clinic or private practice settings are delivered increasingly by nonphysician case managers and counselors, both with and without physician supervision. As a result, insurers have questioned the professional status of the treatment providers in these settings. Many insurers now provide coverage for rehabilitation and detoxification in such facilities only if they conform to the traditional medical model practices embodied in licensure and accreditation standards.

Another source of the resistance of insurers arises from their perception of providers as treatment entrepreneurs. They believe providers create a market for their services by being overinclusive in their definition of who needs treatment and by overtreating those they do identify. The expansion of inpatient services described earlier in the chapter has not necessarily been welcomed, however, and questions are now being raised by researchers as well as public and private payer regarding the necessity for inpatient detoxification and rehabilitation and the cost of such services (e.g., Miller and Hester, 1986; Harrison and Hoffmann, 1986; Annis, 1987; Saxe and Goodman, 1988; Yahr, 1988; Klerman, 1989).

Insurers see the model benefit package advocated by treatment providers, with its emphasis on fixed-length inpatient primary rehabilitation programs as the preferred treatment strategy, as creating demand for unnecessary services. Insurers and employers continue to have concerns about the lack of hard cost data about the cost-effectiveness of contemporary practices. Where once insurers preferred to view "alcoholism" as an acute disorder and pay for "short-term" treatment with definite time limits (i.e., 28-day inpatient programs and no-cost aftercare), the cost-effectiveness of this pattern is now being questioned and alternatives are being sought (Walsh and Egdahl, 1984; Hurst, 1987; Lebenluft and Lebenluft, 1988; Shadle and Christiansen, 1988).

In response to insurers' concerns about the lack of quality control and credentialing procedures for treatment facilities, programs, and personnel, efforts were undertaken to develop standards that would be acceptable to them (Gualtieri, 1977; Gunnersen and Feldman, 1978; Birch and Davis, Inc., 1984). States were encouraged to develop licensing procedures, to be administered either by the SAA or the health facilities regulatory agency. In addition, NIAAA contracted with the Joint Commission on the Accreditation of Hospitals (JCAH) to develop standards acceptable to insurers (JCAH, 1974). Now known as the Joint Commission on the Accreditation of Health Care Organizations (JCAHO), it accredits approximately 800 specialty residential and outpatient facilities and specialty units in general and psychiatric hospitals (M. McAnnich, JCAHO, personal communication, 1988). The Commission on Accreditation of Rehabilitation Facilities (CARF) has recently developed accreditation standards that are seen as more compatible with the mixed social and medical model of treatment now offered by the majority of nonhospital programs in both the public and private sectors (CARF, 1988). The program began in 1986, and CARF now accredits 42 programs. CARF accreditation is recognized by a number of Blue Cross/Blue Shield plans and is accepted by six states as part of their licensure process (J. Schacht, CARF, personal communication, 1988).

Mandated Private Health Insurance

The concerns about decreasing the discrimination in the health insurance industry against persons with alcohol problems have led to calls from the field for federal and state legislative mandates requiring insurance carriers to provide coverage for alcohol problems similar to the coverage provided for other diseases (Hallan, 1972; Butynski, 1982, 1986; Holder and Hallan, 1983; Toff, 1984; McAuliffe et al., 1988). Originally, a joint NIAAA-NCA task force rejected the notion of pushing for mandates, choosing instead to work voluntarily with the insurance industry and employers to implement the model benefit package that they had developed (see the discussion earlier in this chapter) (National Council on Alcoholism Task Force on Health Insurance, 1974). However, for many in the field, the perception of a lack of progress toward the goal of achieving broader private insurance coverage for alcohol problems led to pressing for mandated coverage at both the state and federal levels with the National Council on Alcoholism assuming a leadership role in 1977 (Seesel, 1988).

Mandates are generally opposed by insurers and employers as adding costs and restricting flexibility in designing a set of benefits tailored to the specific population at risk. Indeed, this ongoing push for mandated coverage from the alcohol treatment community has created a continuing adversarial relationship between the insurers and providers (e.g., Alkire, 1987; Hurst, 1987; New Jersey Department of Insurance, 1988). As a result, success from the perspective of the field has been achieved only at the state level. Thirty-seven states and the District of Columbia (comprising 85 percent of the nation's population) have now legislatively mandated that private health insurance plans offer some form of coverage for the treatment of alcohol problems. (The number of states is up from the 33 states reported in 1982 [Butynski, 1982] and up from the 19 states having any mandate in 1977 [Booz-Allen and Hamilton, Inc., 1978]). Twenty-five of the 37 states and the District of Columbia have laws in place that mandate the provision of benefits for treatment of alcohol problems; the remaining 12 states have laws that require health insurance companies to offer these treatment benefits for purchase. Mandates vary from state to state: some are very specific and set out a minimum number of days or sessions to be covered or a dollar value to be provided; others simply require that a benefit be offered for sale. The benefit structure elements spelled out in mandates may or may not be related to actual practice (Frank and Lave, 1985); they may include both requirements and restrictions (e.g., reimbursable days per admission, per year, or per lifetime; modalities covered or excluded; providers, facilities, and personnel eligible to receive reimbursement).

In 1981 the National Association of Insurance Commissioners (NAIC) adopted a recommended model act for the coverage of alcohol and drug dependence by group health insurance contracts and policies. The act requires insurers to offer benefits for sale that are not less favorable than those offered for physical illness: dollar limits, treatment duration limits, deductibles, and coinsurance factors are to be the same (NAIC, 1981). The act also requires insurers to pay for treatment in nonhospital treatment centers if the centers are affiliated with a hospital, licensed by the appropriate governmental agency, or accredited by the JCAHO and there is a treatment plan approved and monitored by a physician. Not included in the act but endorsed nevertheless by the NAIC is a model benefit structure for treatment of alcohol problems that provides for 30 days of inpatient care and 30 outpatient visits.

Although the state mandates now in place are seen as an indication of some progress in expanding private insurance coverage, advocates contend that much remains to be done. For one thing, the mandates do not include all third party payers. Medicare and Medicaid are exempted from state mandates, as are employers who are self-insurers under the federal employee retirement act (ERISA) (Sharfstein et al., 1984; AHA, 1988; Jensen et al., 1988). There is concern that, absent mandates, self-insured companies are less likely to provide coverage for treatment of alcohol problems (e.g., New Jersey Department of Insurance, 1988). Although there is some evidence to support this contention, the presence or absence of a state mandate appears to be less important as a predictor of coverage than are other company characteristics such as the industry, the size of the company, and the makeup of the work force (Morrissey and Jensen, 1988). In fact, Morrissey and Jensen found that 65 percent of the self-insured companies that participated in the 1985 Bureau of Labor Statistics Survey of Employee Benefits did have some coverage for the treatment of alcohol problems and that coverage grew faster among self-insured employers from 1981 to 1985 than among firms that purchased coverage from insurance carriers.

Another difficulty with the state mandates is that they vary widely in their provisions (Butynski, 1986). Some states cover both group and individual contracts; in other states, only group contracts may be covered. HMOs may or may not be included in the scope of the legislation. The type of treatment setting (hospital, residential and/or outpatient) covered by the mandates varies, as does the type of individual provider (physician, social worker, psychologist, or other professionals). Vermont's mandate now includes certified substance abuse counselors as an eligible individual providers. Statutes also vary in their requirements regarding physician-provided or physician-supervised services. In addition, the mandates may specify benefit minimums or limits, or both, expressed as dollars or units of service. It is commonly accepted that the nature of the coverage available shapes the treatment available and used (Cahallan, 1987; Freeborn, 1988; see Chapters 7 and 8).

Although the structure of the mandates vary, most are derived from the model benefit packages developed in the early 1970s. These models did not reflect the continuum of care outlined in the Uniform Act or in the original NCA-NIAAA benefit package but rather the modal treatment approach being implemented at that time: 30 days of inpatient hospital or nonhospital residential detoxification and primary rehabilitation, followed by (minimal) outpatient aftercare. This pattern reflected the spread of the Minnesota model hospital-based programs described in Chapter 3.

Typically mandates are structured to promote the treatment form currently seen as necessary for the treatment of all persons with alcohol problems. Thus, earlier mandates emphasized a 30-day stay in a hospital setting; later legislation has added freestanding residential facilities as a lower cost alternative when the facilities are licensed by the state or accredited by the Joint Commission on Accreditation of Hospitals. (CARF is now seeking similar recognition.) This shift to encourage the use of less expensive inpatient detoxification and rehabilitation in nonhospital or freestanding residential facilities is the result of efforts by the SAAs to obtain third-party coverage for persons admitted to the modified medical and social model programs that had been developed (through both federal and state efforts) to implement the continuum of care defined in their state plans (DenHartog, 1982; Diesenhaus, 1982; Saxe et al., 1983; Butynski, 1986). Private health insurers have also begun to reimburse these facilities (Leyland et al., 1983; McGuire et al., 1986; ICF, Inc., 1987). Despite these efforts, however, the most recent NDATUS data suggest that the majority of health insurance funds are still expended for inpatient hospital treatment (see Chapter 8).

Initially, in the field of treatment for alcohol problems, insurers were more comfortable with the fixed-length primary care program structure that stressed active treatment of a finite duration in hospital settings with familiar operations and quality assurance mechanisms under medical supervision. The fixed length of stay program was seen as an important means of developing a reasonable, acceptable model benefit. Insurers preferred to view alcohol dependence as an acute disorder and pay for short-term treatment with definite time limits (i.e., 28-day inpatient programs) rather than accepting the providers' view of dependence: a condition having a high potential for relapse and requiring long-term support and repeated episodes of treatment in some cases. Now, however, concerns about the overutilization of the hospital and increasing distrust of physician practice patterns in all areas of medicine, coupled with controversial evidence on the marginal effectiveness of fixed-length inpatient programs have led to increased questioning of the need for mandates and for the emphasis on hospital rehabilitation (Walsh and Egdahl, 1984; Alkire, 1987; New Jersey Department of Insurance, 1988).

The primary arguments for and against legislation to require mandatory insurance for the coverage of treatment for alcohol problems have been well reviewed in a 1982 study sponsored by NIAAA (Butynski, 1982). Mandates are supported by those who believe that health insurers discriminate against the treatment of persons with alcohol problems because of the stigma associated with alcoholism as a self-inflicted condition. Mandates are also supported as a means to provide a broader and more stable financial base for the treatment of alcohol problems (Fein, 1984). They are seen as increasing the accessibility and availability of treatment, especially for employed individuals and their dependents , as promoting resource development by bringing in private-sector providers that offer those services that will be reimbursed (McAuliffe et al., 1988). Mandates are also supported as a way to cut health care costs over the long run, by decreasing the excessive use of all health care services by persons with chronic, severe alcohol problems.

Employers and insurers oppose mandates on the grounds that they need flexibility to purchase a tailored benefit package. They maintain that decisions regarding what is to be covered should be left to the purchasers after evaluating the needs of the persons to be covered and the data on treatment appropriateness. In this way, purchasers are not forced to pay for coverage that they do not want or need or that is not of proven efficacy. Mandates are also opposed on the grounds that they will increase costs and premiums to the extent that benefits for other conditions may be endangered and because of questions about the effectiveness of treatment for alcohol problems and concerns about the mix of services to be provided. Furthermore, current mandated insurance coverage has several structural limitations that may interfere with its ultimate purpose of increasing the availability and accessibility of services. Recent reviews suggest that outpatient benefits tend to be low, and very few states include an intermediate care option. The mandates also tend to be rigid in structure and do not permit trading off between different kinds of benefits as a way to take advantage of alternative treatments and settings. Finally, the typical mandate does not provide for outpatient assessment and diagnostic testing services that are required if placing the individual in the appropriate level of care or setting and matching to the appropriate modalities are to be possible.

Recently, McAuliffe and colleagues (1988) conducted a review of the impact of mandated benefits for alcoholism and drug abuse treatment on the availability and utilization of treatment. They concluded that statutory mandates do increase the availability of and access to services for employed persons without adversely affecting the insurance industry. They also concluded that such mandates do not similarly increase access and availability for indigent persons or for persons who have exhausted their private benefits and must therefore be covered by either public insurance (i.e., Medicaid and Medicare) or by state and federal categorical funds.

Comparisons of per capita expenditures between those states with mandates and those without suggest that the mandates have played a role in increasing private health insurance expenditures (Butynski, 1986). Median per capita expenditures for private insurance were found to be higher in those states that mandated benefits than in those states that only required that they be offered or in those that did not have mandate legislation (Butynski, 1986). This same pattern is found in the 1987 NDATUS; however, the large interstate variation in all three groups of states makes such an analysis by itself meaningless. There is no way to determine whether the increase in the amount of reimbursement by private health insurance is due to the passage of mandated benefits legislation, to changes in attitudes about the ability to treat alcohol problems successfully, or to the specific industries and companies located in a state (Morrissey and Jensen, 1988). In addition, Butynski's median analysis does not successfully capture the wide range of variation in per capita expenditures among the states that is found in the most current NDATUS data and described in Chapter 8. More sophisticated studies are required to determine which factors are at work (Morrisey and Jensen, 1987).

Many features of the mandates currently in place in this country are reflected in the recommended model benefit design recently proposed by the National Council on Alcoholism and the Legal Action Center. This design, which is for coverage of both alcohol and drug problems, is based on a survey of the mandated benefit laws in place in states that require coverage be included or offered in all group health plans. The survey revealed that the majority of states (28) mandate coverage in terms of days of treatment per year rather than in terms of dollar limits. The majority of states have also added coverage for treatment in nonhospital freestanding residential facilities (when they are appropriately licensed) to reflect the movement away from hospital services that is favored by the majority of state agencies. The proposed model is based on the median coverage in the states that mandate such coverage in days of active treatment per year. It comprises three elements: (1) inpatient detoxification for up to 7 days per year in a hospital or detoxification facility; (2) inpatient rehabilitation for up to 30 days per year in a hospital or residential facility; and (3) outpatient rehabilitation for up to 60 days per year. The benefits are renewable each year. The model has been proposed for inclusion in any federal legislation that sets up minimum standards for health insurance coverage (Flavin, 1988). It is designed for the socially stable person with alcohol problems and reflects provider preferences rather than the continuum of care considered necessary for treating heterogeneous subgroups of both socially advantaged and socially disadvantaged persons (see Chapter 3).

McAuliffe and colleagues (1988) studied the effect of mandates on the utilization and cost of treatment for alcohol and drug abuse problems. Following their review, they recommended to the Rhode Island State Alcohol/Drug Authority that it follow the lead of Oregon and play an aggressive role in restructuring its mandated benefit legislation to provide realistic incentives for outpatient and residential treatment and in implementing the legislation through regulation. They recommended using tighter licensing requirements and monitoring of all treatment programs, public and private alike. They also recommended that the state authority actively participate with insurance carriers in efforts to develop utilization review criteria, as was done in Oregon. Oregon has recently adopted mandate legislation that favors outpatient services and that includes provisions for an aggressive utilization review system, including preadmission certification and continuing stay review (Oregon State Health Planning and Development Agency, 1986; Oregon Office of Health Policy, 1988; J. Kushner, Oregon Office of Alcohol Programs, personal communication, August 1, 1988). The Oregon SAA, the insurance carriers, and the providers are working together to develop and refine the criteria and procedures.

Similarly, an ad hoc advisory committee has been exploring the need to revise the 1977 New Jersey law mandating treatment for alcohol problems and recently recommended that any facility that offered only detoxification without an affiliated rehabilitation program or that offered only inpatient rehabilitation without an outpatient equivalent not be eligible to receive reimbursement under the proposed mandate (New Jersey Department of Insurance, 1988). The committee's report stressed the need to provide the full continuum of care, with three stages identified as detoxification, rehabilitation, and aftercare/relapse prevention. The advisory committee concluded that the structure of the current mandate had unnecessarily increased costs by emphasizing inpatient hospital treatment for all rather than only for those whose clinical status required this level of care. The committee therefore recommended that a revised mandate statute require that rehabilitation be available in all four of the settings discussed in its proposed model benefit (outpatient, day care, residential inpatient, and hospital inpatient). The committee also recommended not licensing facilities that offer only one level of care for rehabilitation; these facilities therefore would not be eligible for reimbursement by third party payers. The ad hoc committee recommended that any inpatient facility, whether hospital or residential, be required to provide day-care and outpatient rehabilitation (primary care) to qualify for licensure and reimbursement by private and public third party payers.

Finally, the ad hoc committee also recommended that the revised mandate include provisions for managing treatment in the most appropriate and cost-effective setting. In that regard, it emphasized the need for preadmission and continuing stay authorizations by qualified practitioners experienced in treating alcohol and drug problems. The report indicates that insurance industry and employer representatives on the committee agreed with the need for these provisions but did not agree that the continuation of a mandate was the desired pathway to achieve the objectives of broad and stable coverage in the most cost-effective setting. This report reflected the changes taking place throughout the nation as funders and providers reevaluate current programs in light of continued cost increases (Arnett and Trapnell, 1984).

Changes in Health Care Financing Policy:
The Recent Emphasis on Cost Containment

In its 1977 study of the feasibility of a comprehensive benefit for the treatment of alcohol problems, the Blue Cross Association stressed the need for concern about the overall environment of rising health care costs:

> With health care costs in the United States rising about 14 percent a year, third party payors cannot tamper with the structure of their benefits and risk drawing costs still higher unless they know the change will enhance community health within tolerable new costs and/or will generate more efficient use of health resources. (Berman and Klein, 1977b:A2-4)

Recent developments in the financing of all health care—an emphasis on cost containment by restricting benefits or changing practice patterns by utilization review, or both; prospective pricing; sharing risk; the encouragement of competition among insurers and providers; and the development of new forms of practice—have led to modifications that affect coverage for the treatment for alcohol problems. The growth of HMOs and of managed care arrangements represent modifications in private insurance that illustrate the changing climate in which financing policy is now being determined.

Since the early 1980s employers have reacted to increases in insurance premiums with efforts to cut costs: participating in business coalitions that share data in order to bargain for improved rates, shifting to full or partial self-insurance, contracting with managed care administrators who cut down on (inappropriate) utilization through a variety of mechanisms (e.g., concurrent review, case management), increasing employee cost sharing (e.g., increased deductibles, copayments, maximum limits on claims recovery), and excluding payments for procedures whose effectiveness is questionable. Insurers and employers as major purchasers of care are looking for solid answers to questions about which of the treatments available for a particular condition will produce the best results for the least cost (Jensen et al., 1988). Yet there are few data, especially in the case of treatment for alcohol problems, on which to base such answers.

Cost containment has become the dominant theme in the delivery of all health care services. Today, the emphasis is on monitoring the costs of treating patients and on the modification of provider practice patterns to decrease costs by providing fiscal incentives for valued procedures and disincentives for questioned procedures (e.g., Tsai et al., 1988). In such a climate, the treatment of alcohol problems has become a popular target, with complaints regarding the rise in treatment costs being the most prominent. For example, a large manufacturer was reported to have experienced an 81 percent increase in one year of its benefit costs for mental health and chemical dependence treatment; other firms report similar increases of 10 percent to 40 percent (Walsh and Egdahl, 1984; Rodriguez and Maher, 1986; Hurst, 1987; Muszynski, 1987).

There is continuing uneasiness with the certification of rehabilitation as "medically necessary" because the psychosocial and behavioral treatments involved in many current programs do not fit the traditional health insurance definitions of "procedures" (Sieverts, 1983; Wenzel, 1988). Insurers continue to question whether contemporary treatments can bring about long-term behavioral changes in drinking behavior, and therefore they tend to anticipate unpredictable and uncontrollable costs for repeated rehabilitation episodes (Holder, 1987). As noted by Goldman (1986) in a discussion of financing long-term psychiatric care, "Financing mechanisms, such as Medicare and most private insurance, favor high skill, medically oriented treatment benefits excluding from coverage maintenance and custodial care services as well as lower intensity treatment alternatives, such as psychosocial rehabilitation." (p. 6) Health insurers typically focus on services offered by traditional providers (i.e., hospitals, physicians) and have not become comfortable with the new specialty providers that also treat alcohol withdrawal and excessive alcohol use (e.g., detoxification and rehabilitation in freestanding residential facilities that are not always under physician direction). Those in the field see private and public health insurers as trying to apply acute care treatment models and financing mechanisms to problems which require chronic care or episodic care models and financing strategies.

The current troubled relationship between providers of treatment for alcohol problems and representatives of employers and insurers—for example, benefit administrators—stems to a large degree from the benefit administrators' perception that the dramatic increase in the demand for inpatient treatment, whether in a hospital or freestanding residential setting, reflects the providers' marketing efforts rather than the true need for these services. This perception is reenforced by the fact that providers of treatment for alcohol problems have been among the pioneers and leaders in advertising medical services on television and in newspapers; for example, the Television Bureau of Advertising reported that CompCare Corporation, one of the larger firms operating and managing specialty programs, spent $6.3 million on TV advertising in 1985, whereas the Kaiser Health Plans spent just over $1 million and Humana, the fourth largest hospital chain, was reported to have spent $1.5 million (Modern Healthcare, 1987). In addition, administrators view with a great deal of skepticism any claims by providers regarding the effectiveness of the procedures being marketed (Hurst, 1987; Saxe and Goodman, 1988).

Reflexively, providers (many of whom are themselves recovering persons) believe that the benefit administrators' concerns reflect the stigma borne by persons with alcohol problems who are perceived as untreatable and as undeserving of treatment. Providers see the increase in treatment episodes as merely the expression of a latent need previously ignored by payers who excluded treatment of alcohol problems from their benefit packages; insurers see the increase in treatment episodes as an expression of moral hazard, the tendency to seek treatment because insurance is available to pay for it (T. Doherty, Recovery Centers of America, personal communication, January 21, 1988; Ford, 1988; Shulman, 1988). The history of efforts to develop a discrete benefit for the treatment of alcohol problems in HMOs can illustrate the effects of such concerns regarding expanded options for treatment and for cost containment.

Health Maintenance Organizations

HMOs are becoming a significant factor in all health care and an increasingly significant source of funding for treatment of alcohol problems (Shadle and Christianson, 1988). HMOs are prepaid health insurance plans that use a per capita or "capitation" approach to provide comprehensive health services to a voluntarily enrolled and defined population (Burton, 1984). They attempt to combine the delivery and financing of health care services into a single organization. The HMO assumes all or some portion of the financial risk or gain in the delivery of comprehensive care. In contrast to the indemnity or services plan that purchases care from independent providers, HMOs provide health care directly to their subscribers through their own facilities and staff. They may employ their own medical staff (the staff model of organization) or they may contract with a group of practitioners to provide care in the HMO's facilities or in the practitioners' own offices (the individual practice association, or IPA, model). Except under certain conditions (e.g., emergencies, traveling outside the service area, the need for a service the HMO does not offer), treatment provided to enrollees by nonparticipating facilities or practitioners is not covered by the HMO or is covered at a reduced level.

HMOs are an alternative to private indemnity health insurance plans which offer a schedule of benefits for the treatment of various illnesses on both an inpatient and outpatient basis. In HMOs, the basic inpatient and outpatient coverages available in private plans are typically included as basic benefits that are generally covered in full; supplemental services are subject to additional controls such as special copayments or limits on volume or frequency. In many instances in which an HMO has not developed a capacity for treating a specific condition (e.g., alcohol problems), it will contract with one or more facilities in the community to provide specified services on direct referral from the person's primary care physician or another HMO employee "gatekeeper" (e.g., a psychologist, social worker, counselor). The payment mechanism is also likely to be a capitation fee—that is, a fixed amount for each enrollee—and the specialty provider is at risk along with the HMO if utilization is greater than anticipated when the fee is negotiated (Korchok, 1988). Fees are based on estimates of the number of enrollees who will require inpatient care, outpatient treatment, family counseling, and so forth; the fee is calculated by estimating the units of service that will be required for each projected admission (Hunter and Rowe, 1982).

Although prepaid group practices have been in operation for years, interest in HMOs has recently been heightened because of the continuing escalation of health care costs and employer fringe benefit costs (Plotnick et al., 1982; Fein, 1984; Bitker, 1985). The HMO option was developed as a more cost-efficient means of providing medical care, primarily through control of hospitalization rates. Traditionally, HMOs have emphasized outpatient services, utilization review, and conservative practice patterns and have been promoted by both the federal government and by health policy analysts as providing less costly alternatives to conventional indemnity insurance arrangements. It is assumed that there are extra (possibly unnecessary) services performed under the conventional indemnity arrangement in which the fee for each unit of service is paid by a third party (an insurance company; an employer; a federal, state, or local government agency) rather than the patient; the reasons given for the provision of these extra services range from practice patterns based on untested clinical experience, income maximizing on the part of unscrupulous providers, overly cautious practice patterns owing to a fear of malpractice suits, providers' desires to meet patient and family expectations "to do something", and so on. Because HMOs are not paid more for providing these extra services, it is assumed that there is an economic incentive to provide as few services as possible; this position is counterbalanced by an incentive to provide the appropriate number of services which arises from the influence of professional and ethical norms, the threat of malpractice suits, and the threat of loss of patients to competing systems. In past years, HMOs have shown reduced medical care costs, largely because of reduced inpatient use (Manning and Wells, 1986; Luft, 1988).

The federal government has actively promoted and subsidized the formation of new HMOs since 1973, when legislation was enacted to provide federal grants, loans, and loan guarantees. The legislation also gave HMOs access to the full market for health insurance by requiring certain employers to offer a federally qualified HMO along with any other health insurance. The most well known of the models existing prior to the passage of the federal legislation were the Kaiser Foundation Health Plans, the Group Health Association of Washington, D.C., and the Puget Sound Health Cooperative. HMO membership is distributed unevenly throughout the country with concentrations in such states as Minnesota and California. Most major health insurers, including Blue Cross and Blue Shield, have now introduced their own HMOs as a way to remain competitive and to offer both indemnity and HMO options to employers, associations, and individuals seeking to purchase the best plan for their needs. Although HMOs primarily are seen as serving the private sector, increasing numbers of public sector agencies (e.g., government agencies that purchase HMO coverage for their employees, as well as Medicare and Medicaid) have been testing the feasibility of using private HMOs as the vehicle for treating their beneficiaries (e.g., Temkin-Geser and Clark, 1988).

The earlier growth in enrollment, however, has now begun to slow as competition has increased among HMOs and as other forms of health insurance have adopted many of the HMO cost-cutting strategies through such mechanisms as utilization management and preferred provider organizations (in which providers agree to participate at fixed rates and to accept more stringent constraints on hospital admissions, expensive procedures, and lengths of stay). To remain competitive, HMOs have had to raise premiums, to cut back on the services they offered, and to institute new controls (Luft, 1988). IPAs, in which the physician is an independent solo or group practitioner and not an employee, have had the most difficulties in keeping costs down.

The federal government's continuing uncertainty over the best means to promote the availability of treatment for alcohol problems can be seen in the debate over whether to include coverage in HMO's as a mandate or as an option; the compromise was to include minimum coverage. From 1973 to 1986, federal legislation, as interpreted by regulation, required only those HMOs that were seeking federal funds or approval for loans to include within their basic benefits provisions for detoxification (either inpatient or outpatient) and for the treatment of alcohol-related medical problems and referral services for alcohol dependence; other benefits for treatment of alcohol dependence (both nonmedical ancillary services such as vocational rehabilitation and counseling as well as rehabilitation in a specialized inpatient or hospital facility) could be offered on an optional or supplemental basis (Hunter and Rowe, 1982). Only about 60 percent of the new HMOs that were being established sought federal approval and thus came under these requirements; those that did were often encouraged by health insurance analysts to provide only the minimum benefit for alcohol problems, drug abuse and mental disorders that was necessary to remain competitive and in compliance (Sutton, 1981).

Thus the benefits available through HMOs for treating alcohol problems, along with those for treating mental disorders and drug abuse, have tended to be more restricted than the benefits for treating general medical conditions (Burton, 1984), although this situation is now changing. In a 1982 national survey of 205 HMOs in operation for more than one year, treatment for alcohol problems was provided as a limited supplemental benefit by 96 percent of the plans; only detoxification and emergency treatment were covered by almost half the plans offering coverage (Levin et al., 1984). In a 1985 national survey of 286 HMOs, more than 95 percent of the plans offered at least one benefit package that covered treatment for alcohol problems. All these plans offered a broad range of services and outpatient treatment was stressed. Treatment for alcohol problems constituted 1.2 percent of the reporting HMOs' total costs. The average benefit was 34 days of inpatient treatment and 28 outpatient visits. Approximately 17 percent of those treated received inpatient services (Shadle and Christiansen, 1988).

To encourage HMOs to provide coverage for treatment of alcohol problems, the federal government, through NIAAA, had sponsored a series of studies that many believe are a successful demonstration that HMOs can profit from providing a comprehensive treatment program for alcohol problems as part of their basic benefits (Hunter and Rowe, 1982; Plotnick et al., 1982). Working with the Group Health Association of America, Inc. (the national HMO organization), NIAAA sponsored studies and developed a handbook for HMOs that wanted to implement a "realistic" benefit package or treatment component (Hunter and Rowe, 1982). The package was based on the results from the demonstration of the feasibility of the benefit in five plans that used in-house staff and services; the program is outpatient oriented for both detoxification and rehabilitation, deemphasizing the utilization of hospital or residential inpatient care in favor of outpatient counseling and follow-up using both alcohol counselors and medical/nursing personnel.

Another area that has been stressed in HMO practice is preventative services, routine health checkups, and early case finding. The NIAAA sponsored studies have also demonstrated that routine screening for alcohol problems and early referral to specialty treatment can decrease the utilization of other health services (e.g, Putnam, 1982).

As a relatively new and rapidly growing major segment of the health care system, there is still a relative paucity of data on performance, although a recent case study comparing treatment for alcohol problems in HMOs and through conventional indemnity plan fee-for-service programs suggests that HMOs have cut hospital utilization significantly (Shadle and Christianson, 1988). The study examined data from Minnesota, one of the states in which HMOs have captured a significant market share and found a differential utilization of hospital days by residents of the Saint Paul-Minneapolis area. Residents enrolled in HMOs used 14 alcohol and other drug abuse inpatient days per 1,000 persons, whereas residents not enrolled in HMOs used 68 inpatient days per 1,000 persons.

Preferred Provider and Managed Care Arrangements

Another cost-cutting strategy that has developed in recent years is the preferred provider arrangement, a network of service providers that may be organized in a variety of ways. These networks may be assembled by an insurer to offer services to potential industrial clients at a discounted rate, or they may be assembled directly by a large corporate purchaser. Preferred provider arrangements originally differed from HMOs in that they retained a fee-for-service orientation, offering discounted services and adherence to standards of care, rather than shared risk through capitation. Insurers offered financial incentives to the employees and their families for using members of the preferred provider network; copayments and deductibles were usually lowered when treatment was delivered by a preferred provider. These arrangements have been evolving: groups of providers create their own networks and negotiate with the third party payers for their services and other preferred provider reimbursement methods (e.g., capitation, per case payments) have been introduced.

A relatively recent innovation has been the managed care firm, which offers a variety of services that range from serving as an external utilization review agent for an insurer or corporation, to providing case management, to organizing and administering a preferred provider arrangement (Rodriguez and Maher, 1986; Goldstein et al., 1988). The managed care contractor assumes the responsibility for establishing provider eligibility criteria (that must be met by facilities and practitioners in order to receive referrals of eligible beneficiaries), recruiting participant practitioners and organized programs, and negotiating contracts. Contracts typically include a discounted rate for services, referral policies, and agreement to abide by the firm's standards of performance and its hospital admission and length-of-stay review procedures. Each of the firms has developed its own criteria for admission, length of stay, and treatment procedures (Hoffmann et al., 1987; Weedman, 1987; Goldstein et al., 1988; Korchok, 1988; Tsai et al., 1988).

Managed care plans achieve their cost-cutting objectives by limiting the choices available to patients and providers in charting the course of treatment for a given illness episode. Heretofore, the major limitation imposed by this type of plan has been curtailment of the use of the most expensive component of treatment: the inpatient hospital stay. Some of the mechanisms used for this purpose have been preadmission screening, continued stay reviews, retrospective claims reviews, discharge planners, and prospective payment systems. Now managed care firms are directing similar attention to an examination and questioning of the appropriateness and cost-effectiveness of specific procedures used in physical medicine (e.g., Rodriguez, 1983, 1984; Lohr et al., 1988; Wennberg, 1988).

Managed care firms in the private sector offer the same types of external control and monitoring services to third party payers (insurance companies, employers) that were initially developed by professional standards review organizations for the Medicare program (Rodriguez and Maher, 1986). The managed care firm usually offers a menu of services, ranging from utilization review, preadmission certification, second opinion programs, and concurrent review to case management and a capitation plan to provide and monitor all inpatient and outpatient treatment. Most managed care firms still include treatment of alcohol problems under their psychiatric program. Recently, a number of companies have been formed which provide only psychiatric managed care; others that had been primarily serving as contract employee assistance program providers now offer specialized substance abuse services. There is considerable debate among employee assistance practitioners about whether they are to become financial case managers or to continue their advocacy of clinically appropriate services for employees in need of treatment (Googins, 1986; Mahoney, 1987). Such advocacy has often brought employee assistance personnel in conflict with benefit administrators, who view them as in appropriately unconcerned with the overall effect of the cost of the treatment on the costs of health insurance benefits (Walsh and Egdahl, 1984; Tison, 1989).

Managed care firms have gone beyond the quality assurance, peer review and second opinion techniques used by other such entities to introduce "case management" in a form which involves the external reviewer more actively with the primary counselor or physician in the evaluation of the individual's clinical and psychosocial status and treatment needs. More and more, reviewers are active in the formulation of the short- and long-term treatment plans, in the development of a discharge and aftercare plan, and in referrals for additional services. Clinicians and programs have tended to question the experience and training of the case managers as well as the adequacy of the various firms' uniquely developed and applied decision rules about treatment options and lengths of stay (Lewis, 1988b; Shulman, 1988). Treatment providers see these efforts, which are a prominent feature in the marketing strategies used by managed care firms, as indicative of their emphasis on cost reduction, a less appropriate focus (in the providers' view) than the delivery of adequate, high-quality treatment (Rodriguez and Maher, 1986; Muszynski, 1987; Korchok, 1988; Wenzel, 1988; Altman, 1989).

In the application of managed care to psychiatric services as well as to physical medicine, firms have tended to emphasize outpatient services rather than hospital services; the firms stress that their focus is on obtaining the least intensive level of care that is medically necessary. This principle has led these firms to turn more readily to the lower cost freestanding, medically supervised residential facilities offering detoxification and rehabilitation for persons with alcohol problems and to devise mechanisms for admitting persons to the appropriate "level of care" (i.e., setting). The impact of these recent innovations for the treatment of alcohol problems has not been systematically studied (Shadle and Christianson, 1988). Much of the information on the impact of these private cost-containment efforts is anecdotal and nonsystematic, although studies are beginning to appear that suggest that costs are being reduced (Feldstein et al., 1988; Goldstein et al., 1988; Tsai et al., 1988).

The concern of providers regarding the actions of case managers in the treatment arena has led them to develop their own mechanisms for treatment management. An example of such a mechanism is a placement system currently being tested, the Cleveland Admission, Discharge, and Transfer Criteria (Hoffmann et al., 1987). (The appendix to Chapter 11 is a sample of these criteria.) The system was developed under the auspices of an areawide association of treatment providers who sought to provide clear and consistent guidelines for assigning adolescents and adults in need of substance abuse treatment to the appropriate "level of care." The providers were concerned with the lack of a standardized nomenclature and classification for treatment approaches and with the proliferation of idiosyncratic setting and modality definitions (as well as nonempirically supported treatment assignment criteria) being introduced by third party payers: "Some third party payers have specific criteria for determining appropriate utilization of services, but because no single uniform set of criteria have been adopted by the insurance industry, treatment providers are confronted by an array of confusing and conflicting treatment placement guidelines" (Hoffmann et al., 1987:1).

The criteria the providers developed reflect their review of available programs nationally and of clinically developed assignment criteria currently in use. The criteria make use of empirical work in process to develop an assessment tool, the Recovery Attitude and Treatment Evaluator, that can be used for making placements to the appropriate level and intensity of care at each stage of treatment (Mee-Lee, 1988; White and Mee-Lee, 1988). From their review, the providers developed six levels of care ranging from mutual self-help to intensive inpatient programs. Placement decisions were to be made using seven common dimensions for evaluating an individuals clinical status: (1) acute alcohol and/or drug intoxication and/or potential withdrawal; (2) physical condition or complications; (3) psychiatric condition or complications; (4) life area impairments (behavioral, social, academic, legal); (5) treatment acceptance or rejection; (6) loss of control and extent of relapse crisis; and (7) nature of the recovery environment (supportive, remedial vs. pathogenic, destructive). The status of an individual on these dimensions is determined either through a 3 to 6 hour assessment (for applicants who are socially and behaviorally stable and compliant) or an inpatient assessment lasting approximately one week (for noncompliant, socially unstable applicants). The six levels of care to which an individual may be assigned are: (1) mutual/self help; (2) low intensity outpatient treatment; (3) intensive outpatient treatment; (4) structured all-day treatment; (5) medically supervised intensive inpatient treatment; and (6) medically managed, intensive inpatient evaluation unit.

As is evident in these six levels of care, a major concern for the providers is the organization and setting in which the treatment takes place. The outpatient, intermediate (day care), and inpatient settings are included as potential levels of care for each stage of treatment (see Chapter 3). The Cleveland criteria are designed to address recent concerns about overreliance on the inpatient setting as a result of the dramatic increase in the number of hospital units and freestanding residential facilities for treating alcohol problems (Saxe et al., 1983; Annis, 1986, 1987; Miller and Hester, 1987; Allo et al., 1988; Mintzes, 1988; Saxe and Goodman, 1988; Yahr, 1988). Clinicians, however, continue to press for the use of 24-hour care programs with various lengths of stay to remove individuals from pathogenic, nonsupportive environments. What is needed is an empirically tested set of criteria which payers, managed care firms, providers, and clinicians can agree upon.

State Agencies

Private insurers and managed care firms are not the only bodies seeking to control access to inpatient primary care. The Minnesota, Oregon, and New Jersey SAAs have also prepared initiatives as described in the discussion of mandated benefits earlier in this chapter. Confronted with the same evidence—and lack of evidence—regarding the effectiveness of various treatment modalities, the Michigan SAA has recommended that a common set of guiding principles should be adopted by all "prudent" purchasers of cost-effective treatment for alcohol problems (Nischan et al., 1986; Allo et al., 1988; Mintzes, 1988). Its proposal is an outline of a clinical management system similar to the comprehensive treatment system recommended by the committee in Chapter 13 of this report:

I.   Every client, where possible, should receive a thorough assessment (using standardized assessment techniques).

II.   Program services provided to sustain substance abuse clients should be carefully defined with specific goals against which they should be measured.

III.   Service planning for each client should be based on that client's goals, resources, diagnosis and prognosis at that time as derived from the thorough assessment of that client.

IV.   Clients should be impartially assigned to services in response to individual goals, resources, diagnoses and prognoses and the specific capabilities of each particular service.

V.   Whenever possible and appropriate, the substance abuse network of care should help clients draw upon resources in other human service organizations.

VI.   Aftercare, planned and matched with the same care and deliberation as the initial service should be a standard part of treatment planning and assignment.

VII.   Purchasers of service should give careful attention to outcomes so that programs can be improved based on what is learned from those outcomes (Mintzes et al., 1987/1988:112).

The Michigan SAA implements these principles by purchasing a continuum of care that includes assessment and screening services as well as residential detoxification, residential primary rehabilitation, and outpatient counseling services (Nischan et al., 1986; Mintzes, 1988). The continuum of care described by the SAA is a multidimensional concept that actually comprises a number of continua: (1) the sequential continuum, which begins with assessment and matching and continues through aftercare and follow up; (2) the continuum of range across the kinds of services provided in each step of the sequential continuum; and (3) a continuum of intensity for each kind of service.

To construct the necessary outcome monitoring mechanism, the Michigan SAA has contracted with a group of investigators at Michigan State University to develop an integrated client outcome evaluation system. This study, which is currently in process, is the seen as the first step in the development of a statewide client-treatment matching study (Stoffelmayer, 1988). Both person characteristics and agency characteristics (including treatment ideology) have been incorporated into the evaluation design because of the research findings regarding their importance in predicting outcome. Results from this and several other studies currently in progress (Walsh et al., 1986; T. A. McClellan, Philadelphia VA Medical Center, personal communication, May 25, 1989) will be useful in developing a common framework that could be used by payers and providers for level of care and treatment modality assignment strategies.

Conclusions and Recommendations

The past twenty years has seen the development of a national network of over 5,000 specialty programs for the treatment of alcohol problems. These programs have been established in the form of freestanding units and as components of general health, mental health, and social services agencies. This growth from the 300 or so specialty programs identified by the Cooperative Commission in 1967 (Plaut, 1967) has been made possible primarily through the formula and categorical grant programs introduced by the federal government which have been complemented by matching funds from state and local governments. These efforts have been supplemented with those of the state alcoholism authorities which provide categorical funding to serve mainly indigent persons who lack other resources (e.g., public or private health insurance). Some of the progress made in establishing this network of specialty programs is a result of the success that has been achieved in removing the barriers formerly found in coverage for treatment of alcohol problems in private and public health insurance.

Yet the field's hopes for a nondiscriminatory policy of financing treatment for alcohol problems have not yet been fully realized. Concerns continue to be expressed that the level of services which is still considered to be inadequate to meet the identified need and that the benefit cutbacks of public and private third-party payers for such treatment. It is difficult to respond to these concerns because there has been no ongoing program to monitor the development of the service delivery system—neither from the standpoint of capacity and utilization nor of financing. As outlined in several earlier chapters, there are insufficient data on the current level of services, on the characteristics of the treatment organizations, and on how these characteristics influence the delivery and outcome of treatment; thus, the committee is constrained from agreeing or disagreeing with these concerns. Similarly, there has been insufficient study of the public and private insurance mechanisms by which these services are funded and of the impact of alternative financing and reimbursement strategies on the availability and effectiveness of services. What data exist suggest uneven development of financing for treatment, together with continued uncertainty on the part of all funders about which treatments to support.

The recent report to Congress from the Advisory Board to the Alcohol, Drug Abuse, and Mental Health Administration (1987) also identified the lack of adequate information on the cost of treatment services as a serious problem. Without such data, it is not even possible to identify the sources of funds available to groups of potential treatment seekers and providers; it is also impossible to develop estimates of the cost-effectiveness of alternative treatment models, settings, and modalities.

The Current Funding Environment

In the past, the overall pattern of funding for specialty programs that provide treatment for alcohol problems has varied from that found for all health care settings: for alcohol treatment, state and local governments were the most prominent source of funds, and private and public health insurance did not contribute an equivalent share (Harwood et al., 1984, 1985b; Davis, 1987). Today, the most recent NDATUS findings suggest that, nationally, the proportion of funds contributed by private insurance varies only slightly from that found for overall health care expenditures (see Chapter 8). Nevertheless, there is wide interstate variation in the availability of third party funds. In many states, the dominant source of support for the treatment of alcohol problems is state and local categorical funding, which incorporates federal block grants. Nationally, there is still a lower proportion of direct patient payments and federal public insurance funds available for alcohol problems treatment when compared to expenditures for all health services. There has been a steady increase of additional private insurance coverage in selected states but little success overall in obtaining increased public insurance coverage. These differences are not explained by the presence or absence of mandated benefit legislation, and additional research on the effect of mandating benefits is needed.

Although the model benefit packages that have been tested have included both inpatient and outpatient services, state mandates have tended to be more oriented toward support for fixed-length inpatient rehabilitation programs. Recent efforts aim to develop revised mandates emphasizing outpatient treatment and the matching of persons to the appropriate level of care. These efforts parallel the implementation of cost-containment strategies by all third party payers, whether public or private, and exemplified most strongly by HMOs and managed care firms.

As discussed in Chapters 4 and 7, there has been a dramatic increase in the number of specialty, nontraditional community-based treatment facilities for alcohol problems as well as an increase in the availability of treatment in more traditional hospital alcohol detoxification and rehabilitation units. The 1987 NDATUS data (reviewed in Chapter 8), suggest that these hospital-based units are receiving the majority of the available private and public health insurance funding; state and local categorical funds (including the federal alcohol, drug abuse and mental health block grant) are going primarily to residential and outpatient treatment facilities. These differences reflect the variations in the policies adopted by these third party payers: a classical medical model for the public and private insurers and a mixed medical-social model for the state and local funding agencies. Legislation to mandate private health insurance coverage for treatment, which encouraged development of inpatient facilities, also played a role in the development of this pattern of funding.

The increase in the availability of specialized treatment for alcohol problems has been marked by the proliferation of uncoordinated, inconsistent, and increasingly complex sets of public and private financing strategies, reimbursement mechanisms, and cost-containment schemes. The committee received materials and heard presentations about the impact of these variations. There appears to be no general agreement about which mechanisms are effective, little consistency among payment sources across states, ownership categories, and settings. There is also a clear lack of well-designed studies to guide policymaking (regarding the structure of benefits) and individual decision making (regarding placement in an appropriate level of care or matching to a cost-effective treatment regimen). The end result is that a coherent financing policy has not emerged, even though this has been one of the major aims of the federal and state agencies charged with the development of the treatment resources.

The one note of consistency among all payers has been in the effort to introduce cost-containment mechanisms; the strategies used, however, vary widely and are not yet based on sound empirical tests of the effectiveness of alternative treatments. There is no consensually developed framework for matching persons in need of treatment to a given setting, orientation, stage, or modality. The current situation in paying for the treatment of alcohol problems parallels that of persons whose health care needs are covered by Medicaid: similar people in similar circumstances but in different states have access to different types of care because of the sources of payment and treatment network options available to them. A major issue is whether coverage will be provided in alternative settings which do not adhere to the classical medical model. The limited data available reflect the shift of SAAs away from paying for hospital-based and medically directed services for alcohol problems treatment to the use of social model services that provide for medical involvement and backup. A number of state alcoholism authorities (SAAs) have moved to purchase only nonhospital detoxification and rehabilitation (e.g., Oregon, California) or to require preadmission screening (e.g., Minnesota), whereas the private insurance and public insurance payers, including Medicare and Medicaid, continue to emphasize treatment in hospital settings. Several states (e.g., Minnesota, Oregon, Nevada, Michigan, New Jersey) are actively involved in efforts to persuade all payers to follow their lead in developing cost-containment strategies that would decrease the use of hospital-based units for detoxification and rehabilitation.

Taken together, the NDATUS and SADAP findings (see Chapter 8) suggest that state and local categorical funding administered by SAAs appears to have replaced the more traditional sources of public insurance (Medicaid and Medicare) in the majority of states as the primary source of public funds for low-income persons with alcohol problems. At the same time a segment of the private sector, involving both for-profit and not-for-profit hospitals, appear to have been developing more traditional hospital-based programs to serve insured persons and those with sufficient financial resources to pay fees. The data also suggest the continuing lack of adequate reimbursement, by all funding sources, for ambulatory or nonhospital residential detoxification and rehabilitation, a trend that has resulted in a markedly uneven distribution in availability of treatment options across the nation.

These interpretations, based on preliminary data from the NDATUS, the few available health services research studies, and a review of the evolution of financing policies, must be considered tentative until the necessary follow-up studies are carried out. There are currently no adequate studies available, for example, on which to base a recommendation that a financing and reimbursement mechanism follow either the medical model of rehabilitation favored by insurance carriers or the social model of recovery favored by some of the state and county alcoholism authorities, or the mixed medical and social model favored by most SAAs. Any such recommendation must await the conduct of well-designed studies that will provide a clearer view of the cost-effectiveness of these models in treating persons with alcohol problems.

The Need for Better Data on Funding and the Costs of Treatment

As noted in Chapter 8, there is no adequate data base and few reported studies that can be used to establish the total level of expenditures for the treatment of alcohol problems and to describe who is paying for which treatment services. The two major national surveys, the NDATUS and SADAP, do not provide sufficiently detailed information to establish the specific sources of payment available for each stage of treatment and in each of the multiple settings available, either on a national or state-by-state basis. *Additional surveys and studies are needed to provide information not only on who is paying for the treatment of alcohol problems but also which types of treatment are being covered in which settings.* NIAAA's recent request for applications for grants which has been issued to stimulate investigator interest in such surveys is a minimal initial step in the direction of obtaining such data (NIAAA, 1988).

It is difficult to answer questions about who pays for treatment and about the financing and reimbursement policies followed by different payers when there has been no regular monitoring program to follow the development of the service delivery system. As outlined in several earlier chapters, there are few data in hand on the level of treatment services available, funding levels and patterns, and the characteristics of provider organizations and how these characteristics influence the delivery and outcome of treatment. Without adequate data on these and other topics, formulating financing policy is an exercise in fantasy. What is required to bring policymaking back to the "real" world is the reestablishment of comprehensive national data collection efforts of relevance to the treatment of alcohol problems. One element of such efforts should be a comprehensive, ongoing description of the treatment delivery system that captures all of its variability and complexity, the characteristics of the individuals being seen, the alcohol problems they bring to treatment, and the costs being expended on their treatment in each component of the system.

Rather than constructing a separate data collection system *de novo,* existing survey mechanisms could be used, provided they could be adapted to obtain alcohol treatment-specific data in the relevant domains. The reintroduction of financial and other policy-oriented questions in the 1987 NDATUS is a limited beginning toward achieving the data collection objectives noted above; however, a client-based data collection system like National Medical Care Expenditures Survey may be more valuable. Other possible vehicles include the National Hospital Discharge Survey, and the National Nursing Home Survey, all of which are conducted by the National Center for Health Statistics.

The Anti-Drug Abuse Act of 1988 (P.L. 100-690, Sec. 2052) named the Department of Health and Human Services as responsible for the annual collection of data to monitor the incidence and prevalence of alcohol problems and provide information on the service delivery system for the treatment of alcohol problems. The funding mechanism it chose for this purpose was a variable percentage of the block grant. However, some SAAs have criticized this use of block grant funding as counter to the block grant's purpose of supporting service delivery. Some have even suggested that the use of such a mechanism places the data collection activity in competition with service delivery in the public sector.

Given this history, the committee recommends that critical data on the provision and financing of services for persons with alcohol problems be obtained through the modification of existing service surveillance mechanisms or, if existing mechanisms prove inadequate, through the creation of a new mechanism. The ongoing services and financing surveillance programs now being carried out should be expanded. The NDATUS should be supplemented with sample surveys which monitor service delivery in more detail within the specialty alcohol treatment sector and which monitor services in related health care, social services, criminal justice, and educational sectors. These surveys should include both facility censuses (e.g., NDATUS) and discharge and episode surveys modeled after the National Hospital Discharge Survey and the National Nursing Home Survey. There should be ongoing monitoring of the activities in each setting and sector, and intervention as well as treatment activities should be covered. Samples should be drawn from specialty treatment units reporting on the NDATUS as well as from those facilities in nonspecialist sectors in which a significant number of persons with alcohol problems are treated (e.g., general hospitals without designated specialty units, employee assistance programs that offer diagnostic and treatment services, correctional facilities). The samples should be stratified by size, geographic location, and other relevant variables (e.g., treatment stage, ideology, setting, ownership). For a detailed review of financing sources, data should be collected from a sample of facilities (using a client-based system complementary to that for service provision) rather than conducting a census of all facilities.

The effort to develop and implement such a comprehensive surveillance system should begin, first, by convening services researchers, evaluation and management information system administrators, and epidemiologists to define the system's parameters and its data elements. Representatives of the public and private insurance carriers should also be included, as well as the state and federal government agencies involved in categorical funding.

Second, the federal government, through ADAMHA, and working with the SAAs through NASADAD, should establish a format for standardized reporting for data on treatment services supported through the alcohol, drug abuse, and mental health block grant funds and appearing on the SADAP. Introducing a requirement for reporting on services within a standard format will provide accountability for the expenditure of block grant funds that does not now exist. The NDATUS, the block grant application and report of activities, and the SADAP currently do not use the same data elements, which leads to inconsistent findings that are difficult to interpret. In addition, the format should be consistent with that used in the surveys that are part of the national surveillance program. All surveys in the national surveillance programs should use common definitions and response categories. Furthermore, data on sources of funding should be collected in sufficient detail that the relevant sources can be independently tracked.

Another potential source of data is data collection systems of the various states. The data gathered by these systems are not now being aggregated through the existing reporting requirements. There has been some discussion about developing a methodology to accept the data from the state's own system and translate the records into a common metric; further exploration of this proposal is needed. Utility would be limited in the same manner that the SADAP is limited (i.e., cover only programs funded by the SAA), so this method would not negate the need for other surveys. The SAAs in conjunction with ADAMHA can gather this data as part of the annual block grant application process and provide some of the data needed for ongoing policy review.

As important as discovering the current level of services and the funding that supports them is the need to determine the level of resources that are actually needed--that is, the prevalence of alcohol problems. The states presently employ a variety of methods, as do federal agencies and other third-party payers, to develop need estimates for treatment planning and budgeting. Each payer system has its own methodology for projecting how many beds are needed for detoxification or rehabilitation, how many outpatient slots are needed, and how many personnel are required. State and county alcoholism authorities are also concerned with how many maintenance stage beds must be provided for supportive living for use by persons with chronic, severe alcohol problems (e.g., halfway houses, recovery homes, custodial-domiciliary facilities) (Costello and Hodde, 1981; Brown University Center for Alcohol Studies, 1984; Manov and Beshai, 1986; Reynolds and Ryan, 1988; Wittman and Madden, 1988; New York Division of Alcoholism and Alcohol Abuse, 1989).

These estimates have cost implications that must be considered in developing financing policies—the greater the number of persons needing inpatient detoxification or rehabilitation, or both, the higher the costs; the more persons who are appropriately matched to brief interventions, the lower the costs. Such estimates are critical in developing capitation rates and insurance premiums. What is needed is a common framework to describe prevalence and the number of persons who will need and want treatment during a year. There has been some communication among the states on this issue and backup support available from NIAAA's Alcohol Epidemiology Data System (AEDS). *A new effort is needed, however, and thus the committee recommends that a consensus activity be carried out to gain adoption of a common set of prevalence indicators and consequent treatment needs and costs.* Currently available state or individual insurer estimates, although useful, cannot now be aggregated to provide a comprehensive national picture because of the incompatibility of definitions and data sets. Bringing the states and other payers together to review the various methods now used for prevalence, resource allocation, utilization, and cost estimation as a first step in developing a common methodology is a much needed endeavor. A consensually developed prevalence, utilization, and cost estimating method would be useful for national evaluations of the adequacy of the level of treatment availability for persons with alcohol problems.

Another area in which consensus and commonality is needed is in the development of criteria for assigning individuals in treatment to the appropriate level of care (see Chapter 20). These efforts have has proceeded on a fragmented basis without guidance from a comprehensive model for describing the treatment delivery system that captures all of the existing variations in orientations and settings in each of the states. Each managed care firm, third-party payer, and provider has developed its own system for justifying or denying admission to a given level of care based on "medical necessity." Each has developed unique criteria by interpreting the literature on treatment effectiveness and cost as best it can. Several of the existing approaches were described earlier in this chapter (e.g., the Cleveland Criteria, the Minnesota consolidated fund, the Oregon SAA approach). Although each approach addresses the same issues, definitions of the various treatment settings differ as do the matching variables. As discussed in Chapters 10 and 11, there are now procedures and variables that can be used to create matches between persons seeking treatment and the appropriate treatment regimens. *The committee thus recommends that a consensus activity be conducted to develop a common set of criteria for determining the appropriate level of care (setting) and the appropriate treatment orientation, and modality for an individual at each stage of treatment.* Bringing together researchers, practitioners, funders, and regulators in an expert committee for a systematic review of the various methods currently in use and of the experiences of both payers and providers in applying those methods could lead to the adoption of a common framework and a reduction in the confusing array of criteria systems that now confronts purchasers and providers of services alike. Although additional research is required on the effectiveness of specific treatment matches, the committee believes that there is now sufficient data and experience for the development of a common framework. What has been lacking is a neutral and ongoing forum for such an endeavor. The consensus activity the committee recommends could provide such a forum and could continue on a regular basis (perhaps in the form of an expert committee, as described in Chapter 11) offering an opportunity for researchers, payers, and providers to review and consider matching approaches based on the results of outcome monitoring activities and experimental studies. Such an endeavor could also clarify the conditions under which the medical model and the social model are most appropriate for use.

In addition to a surveillance program, there should be expanded support of health services research programs that are currently investigating financing policy issues. There are a number of such programs that are funded at a minimal level; with appropriate modifications these research programs could provide the necessary data for planners and policymakers to use in making decisions regarding the allocation of resources and choices among competing modalities and settings. The following research is needed: studies on the impact of the structure of insurance benefits and of alternate cost-containment strategies on the availability and outcome of treatment for alcohol problems; in-depth studies of the differences among payers in policies and experiences in funding treatment of alcohol problems; in-depth investigations of the variation among the states in the sources of funding available to different types of providers; research on the impact of the availability of insurance benefits on the level of treatment utilization in distinct populations; and effectiveness studies that routinely include the mode of payment and cost data in their data collection and analyses.

Currently, the research funded by the federal government on the financing of treatment for alcohol problems is minimal. NIAAA's (1988) recently issued program announcement soliciting investigator-initiated research on economic and socioeconomic issues in prevention, treatment, and epidemiology is a step in the right direction, but as currently structured the program is too small to stimulate sufficient attention and produce the volume of data that is needed. The committee strongly endorses the establishment of visibility and priority for research on financing policy in the appropriate federal agencies. The committee also recommends that NIAAA take the lead in these efforts, just as it has led in the establishment and evolution of financing policy in previous years. Now, however, the agency is positioned to play a key role in the refinement of that policy by sponsoring more rigorous research and a broader program of studies to capture the data required for sound decision making.

REFERENCES

Advisory Panel on Financing Mental Health Care. 1973. Financing Mental Health Care in the United States. Rockville, Md.: National Institute on Mental Health

Agranoff, R., and L. Robins. 1982. How to make block grants work: An intergovernmental perspective. New England Journal of Human Services 2:36-46.

Akins, C., and D. Williams. State and local programs on alcoholism. Pp. 325-352 in Prevention, Intervention, and Treatment: Concerns and Models, J. de Luca, ed. Washington, D.C.: U.S. Government Printing Office.

Alcohol and Drug Problems Association Task Force on Treatment Financing. 1983. A Position Paper on Public and Private Insurance Financing of Treatment Services for those Addicted to Alcohol and/or Drugs. Washington, D.C.: Alcohol and Drug Problems Association.

Alcohol, Drug Abuse, and Mental Health Advisory Board (ADAMHA). 1987. First Report to Congress. April, 1987. Rockville, Md.: Alcohol, Drug Abuse, and Mental Health Administration.

Alcohol, Drug Abuse, and Mental Health Administration (ADAMHA). 1984. Alcohol and Drug Abuse and Mental Health Services Data: Report to Congress, January, 1984. Rockville, Md.: Alcohol, Drug Abuse, and Mental Health Administration.

Alcohol, Drug Abuse, and Mental Health Administration (ADAMHA). 1988. Alcohol and Drug Abuse Treatment and Rehabilitation Block Grant: Report to Congress, May, 1988. Rockville, Md.: Alcohol, Drug Abuse, and Mental Health Administration.

Alkire, A. 1987. A research based approach to curbing mandates. Business and Health 3(4):7-9.

Allo, C. D., B. Mintzes, J. A. Nischan, and R. A. Brook. 1988. Purchasing Substance Abuse Treatment: Toward a System for Enhancing Positive Outcomes. Lansing, Mich.: Michigan Office of Substance Abuse Services.

Altman, L. S. 1989. Preferred provider organization: A historical perspective, legal considerations, and special issues. The ALMACAN 19(3):22-27.

American Hospital Association (AHA). 1988. Promoting Health Insurance in the Workplace: State and Local Initiatives to Increase Private Coverage. Chicago: AHA.

American Hospital Association (AHA). 1987. Hospital Statistics. Chicago: AHA.

Anderson, W. J. 1984. Improvements in the alcohol, drug abuse, and mental health services block grant distribution formula can be made now and in the future (letter report). U. S. General Accounting Office, Washington, D.C., June.

Anderson, D. J. 1981. Perspectives on Treatment: The Minnesota Experience. Center City, Minn.: Hazelden Foundation.

Annis, H. M. 1987. Effective treatment for drug and alcohol problems: What do we know? Presented at the Annual Meeting of the Institute of Medicine, Washington, D.C., October 21.

Annis, H. M. 1986. Is inpatient rehabilitation of the alcoholic cost effective? Con position. Advances in Alcohol and Substance Abuse 5:175-190.

Arnett, R. H., and G. R. Trapnell. 1984. Private health insurance: New measures of a complex changing industry. Health Care Financing Review 6(2):31-42.

Becker, F. W., and B. K. Sanders. 1984. The Illinois Medicare/Medicaid Alcoholism Services Demonstration: Medicaid Cost Trends and Utilization Patterns. Prepared for the Illinois Department of Alcohol and Substance Abuse. Springfield Ill.: Center for Policy Studies and Program Evaluation, Sangamon State University.

Berman, H., and D. Klein. 1977a. Project to Develop a Comprehensive Alcoholism Benefit through Blue Cross: Final Report of Phase I. Prepared for the National Institute on Alcohol Abuse and Alcoholism. Chicago: Blue Cross Association.

Berman, H., and D. Klein. 1977b. Project to Develop a Comprehensive Alcoholism Benefit through Blue Cross: Final Report of Phase I. Appendices. Prepared for the National Institute on Alcohol Abuse and Alcoholism. Chicago: Blue Cross Association.

Birch and Davis Associates, Inc. 1984. Development of Model Professional Standards for Counselor Credentialing. Rockville, Md.: National Institute on Alcohol Abuse and Alcoholism. (Reprinted 1986, Dubuque, Iowa: Kendall/Hunt Publishing.)

Bitker, T. E. 1985. Health maintenance organizations and prepaid psychiatry. Pp. 119-129 in The New Economics and Psychiatric Care, S. S. Sharfstein and A. Beigel, eds. Washington, D.C.: American Psychiatric Press.

Blue Cross of Greater Philadelphia. 1987. Community Data Report: Extending the Influence Beyond the Source. Philadelphia: Blue Cross of Greater Philadelphia.

Boche, H. L., ed. 1975. Funding of Alcohol and Drug Programs: A Report of the Funding Task Force. Washington, D.C.: Alcohol and Drug Problems Association of North America.

Booz-Allen and Hamilton, Inc. 1978. The Alcoholism Funding Study: Evaluations of the Sources of Funds and Barriers to Funding Alcoholism Treatment Programs. Prepared for the U.S. Department of Health Education and Welfare. Washington, D. C.: Booz-Allen and Hamilton, Inc.

Borkman, T. 1983. A Social-Experiential Model in Programs for Alcoholism Recovery: A Research Report on A New Treatment Design. Rockville, Md.: National Institute on Alcohol Abuse and Alcoholism.

Borkman, T. 1988. Executive summary: Social model recovery programs. Prepared for the Committee for the Study of Treatment and Rehabilitation Services for Alcoholism and Alcohol Abuse, May.

Brown University Center for Alcohol Studies. 1984. Care for the Chronic Inebriate: Analysis and Recommendations. Prepared for the Rhode Island Department of Mental Health, Retardation, and Hospitals, Division of Substance Abuse. Providence, R.I.: Brown University Center for Alcohol Studies.

Bureau of Labor Statistics (BLS). 1989. Prepublished data from the Employee Benefits Survey for the National Institute on Alcohol Abuse and Alcoholism: Health insurance plan counts. Bureau of Labor Statistics, Washington, D.C., January.

Burney, G. L. 1987. NIAAA Remembers: Milestones in the History of the Alcoholism Field. Rockville, Md.: National Institute on Alcohol Abuse and Alcoholism.

Burton, J. L. 1984. Coverage Policies for Alcohol, Drug Abuse, and Mental Health Care under Major Health Care Financing Programs. Prepared for the ADAMHA Reimbursement Task Force. Rockville, Md.: Alcohol, Drug Abuse, and Mental Health Administration.

Butler, P., and C. Littlefield. 1985. Health Care Cost Containment in the Alcohol and Drug Abuse Division. Prepared for the Alcohol and Drug Abuse Division, Colorado Department of Health, Denver, Col., December.

Butynski, W. 1982. Status of State Legislation and Research on Health Insurance Coverage for Alcoholism Treatment. Prepared for the National Institute on Alcohol Abuse and Alcoholism. Washington, D.C.: Scientific Management Corporation.

Butynski, W. 1986. Private health insurance coverage for alcoholism and drug dependency treatment services: State legislation that mandates benefits or requires insurers to offer such benefits for purchase. NASADAD Alcohol and Drug Abuse Report Special Report: January/February:1-28.

Butynski, W., N. Record, P. Bruhn, and D. Canova. 1987. State Resources and Services for Alcohol and Drug Abuse Problems: Fiscal Year 1986—An Analysis of State Alcohol and Drug Abuse Profile Data. Prepared for the National Institute on Alcohol Abuse and Alcoholism and the National Institute on Drug Abuse. Washington, D.C.: National Association of State Alcohol and Drug Abuse Directors.

Butynski, W., and D. Canova. 1988. Alcohol problem resources and services in state supported programs, FY 1987. Public Health Reports 103:611-620.

Cahalan, D. 1987. Understanding America's Drinking Problem: How to Combat the Hazards of Alcohol. San Francisco: Jossey-Bass.

California Department of Alcohol and Drug Programs (CAPD). 1988. California Alcohol Program State Plan: Fiscal Year 1987-1988. Sacramento: California Department of Alcohol and Drug Programs.

Chafetz, M. E. 1976. Alcoholism. Psychiatric Annals 6:107-141.

Commission on Accreditation of Rehabilitation Facilities (CARF) 1988. Program Evaluation in Alcoholism and Drug Abuse Treatment Programs. Tucson, Arizona: CARF.

Cooper, M. L. 1979. Private Health Insurance Benefits for Alcoholism, Drug Abuse, and Mental Illness. Washington, D.C.: Intergovernmental Health Policy Project, George Washington University.

Costello, R. M. 1982. Evaluation of alcoholism treatment programs. Pp. 1197-1210 in Encyclopedic Handbook of Alcoholism, E. M. Pattison and E. Kaufman, eds. New York: Gardner Press.

Costello, R. M., and J. E. Hodde. 1981. Costs of comprehensive alcoholism care for 100 patients over 4 years. Journal of Studies on Alcohol 42:87-93.

Creative Socio-Medics Corporation. 1981. An Analysis of Third Party Funding in the Alcoholism Treatment Delivery System in the United States. Prepared for the National Institute on Alcohol Abuse and Alcoholism. Vienna, Va.: Creative Socio-Medics Corp.

Davis, K. 1987. The organization and financing of alcohol and drug abuse services. Presented at the annual meeting of the Institute of Medicine, Washington, D.C., October 21.

DenHartog, G. L. 1982. "A Decade of Detox:" Development of Non-hospital Approaches to Alcohol Detoxification—A Review of the Literature. Substance Abuse Monograph Series. Jefferson City, Mo: Division of Alcohol and Drug Abuse.

Diesenhaus, H. I. 1982. Current trends in treatment programming for problem drinkers and alcoholics. Pp. 219-90 in Prevention, Intervention, and Treatment: Concerns and Models, J. de Luca, ed. Washington, D.C.: Government Printing Office.

Fein, R. 1984. Alcohol in America: The Price We Pay. Newport Beach, Cal.: CareInstitute.

Feldstein, P. J., T. M. Wickizer, and R. C. Wheeler. 1988. Private cost containment: the effects of utilization review programs on health care use and expenditures. New England Journal of Medicine 318:1310-1314.

Finn, P. 1985. Decriminalization of public drunkenness: Response of the health care system. Journal of Studies on Alcohol 46:7-22.

Flavin, D. 1988. Health insurance coverage for alcoholism and other drug dependencies. Testimony presented before the U.S. House of Representatives Committee on Energy and Commerce, Subcommittee on Commerce, Consumer Protection, and Competitiveness hearing regarding insurance coverage of drug and alcohol abuse treatment, National Council on Alcoholism, Washington, D.C., September 8.

Ford, M. 1988. Statement presented to the open meeting of the IOM Committee for the Study of Treatment and Rehabilitation Services for Alcoholism and Alcohol Abuse, Washington, D.C., January 25.

Frank, R. G. and J, R. Lave. 1985. The impact of Medicaid design on length of hospital stay and patient transfers. Hospital and Community Psychiatry 36:749-753.

Freeborn, D. K. Executive summary: Insurance coverage and the treatment of alcoholism. Prepared for the IOM Committee for the Study of Treatment and Rehabilitation Services for Alcoholism and Alcohol Abuse.

Gibson, R. W. 1988. The influence of external forces on the quality assurance process. Pp. 247-264 in Handbook of Quality Assurance in Mental Health, G. Stricker and A. Rodriguez, eds. New York: Plenum.

Glasscote, R. M., T. F. A. Plaut, D. W. Hammersley, F. J. O'Neil, M. E. Chafetz, and E. Cumming. 1967. The Treatment of Alcohol Problems: A Study of Programs and Problems. Washington, D.C.: Joint Information Service of the American Psychiatric Association and the National Association of Mental Health.

Goldman, H. H. 1986. Financing long term psychiatric care. Business and Health 3(3):5-7.

Goldstein, J. M., E. L. Bassuk, S. K. Holland, and D. Zimmer. 1988. Identifying catastrophic psychiatric cases: Targeting managed care strategies. Medical Care 26:790-799.

Googins, B. 1986. EAPs and cost containment. The ALMACAN 16(11):18-19.

Gordis, E. 1987. Accessible and affordable health care for alcoholism and related problems: Strategy for cost containment. Journal of Studies on Alcohol 48:579-585.

Grad, F. P., A. L. Goldberg and B. A. Shapiro. 1971. Alcoholism and the Law. Dobbs Ferry, N. Y.: Oceana Publications.

Graham, G. 1981. Occupational programs and their relation to health insurance coverage for alcoholism. Alcohol Health and Research World 5(4):31-34.

Grupenhoff, J. T. 1983. Congressional support for alcohol and substance abuse programs. Advances in Alcohol and Substance Abuse 2:5-13.

Gualatieri, P. K. 1977. State Issues in Drug and Alcohol Abuse: A Sourcebook. Washington, D.C.: Georgetown University Health Policy Center.

Gunnersen, U., and M. L. Feldman. 1978. Alcohol and Alcoholism Programs: A Technical Assistance Manual for Health Systems Agencies. San Leandro, Calif.: Human Services, Inc..

Hallan, J. B. 1972. Health Insurance Coverage for Alcoholism. Prepared for the National Institute on Alcohol abuse and Alcoholism. Rockville, Md: National Institute on Alcohol abuse and Alcoholism.

Harrison, P. A., and N. G. Hoffmann. 1986. Chemical Dependency Inpatients and Outpatients: Intake Characteristics and Treatment Outcome. Prepared for the Chemical Dependency Program Division, Minnesota Department of Human Services. St. Paul, Minn.: St Paul-Ramsey Foundation.

Hart, L. 1977. A review of treatment and rehabilitation legislation regarding alcohol abusers and alcoholics in the United States: 1920-1971. International Journal of the Addictions 12:677-678.

Harwood, H. J., J. V. Rachal, and E. Cavanaugh. 1985a. Length of stay in treatment for short term hospitals. Prepared for the National Institute on Alcohol Abuse and Alcoholism. Research Triangle Institute, Research Triangle Park, N.C.

Harwood, H. J., P. Kristiansen, and J. V. Rachal. 1985b. Social and Economic Costs of Alcohol Abuse and Alcoholism. Prepared for the National Institute on Alcohol Abuse and Alcoholism. Research Triangle Park, N.C.: Research Triangle Institute.

Harwood, H. J., D. M. Napolitano, P. L. Kristiansen, and J. J. Collins. 1984. Economic Costs to Society of Alcohol and Drug Abuse and Mental Illness: 1980. Prepared for the Alcohol, Drug Abuse, and Mental Health Administration. Research Triangle Park, N.C.: Research Triangle Institute.

Hoffmann, N. G., J. A. Halikas, and D. Mee-Lee, 1987. The Cleveland Admission, Discharge, and Transfer Criteria: Model for Chemical Dependency Treatment Programs. Cleveland, Ohio: The Greater Cleveland Hospital Association.

Holden, C. 1987. Alcoholism and the medical cost crunch. Science 235:1132-1133.

Holder, H. D., and J. B. Hallan. 1983. Development of Cost Simulation Study of Alcoholism Insurance Benefit Packages. Prepared for the National Institute on Alcohol Abuse and Alcoholism. Rockville, Md.: National Institute on Alcohol Abuse and Alcoholism.

Holder, H. D., R. Longabaugh, and W. R. Miller. 1988. Cost and effectiveness of alcoholism treatment using best available information. Prepared for the IOM Committee for the Study of Treatment and Rehabilitation Services for Alcoholism and Alcohol Abuse.

Holder, H. H. 1987. Alcoholism treatment and potential health care cost saving. Medical Care 25:52-71.

Holder, H. D., J. O. Blose, and M. J. Gasiorowski. 1985. Alcoholism Treatment Impact on Total Health Care Utilization and Costs: A Four Year Longitudinal Analysis of the Federal Employees Health Benefit Program with Aetna Life Insurance Program. Prepared for the National Institute on Alcohol Abuse and Alcoholism. Chapel Hill, N.C.: H-2, Inc.

Howell, E. M., M. Rymer, D. K. Baugh, M. Ruther, and W. Buczko. 1988. Medicaid tape-to-tape findings: California, New York, and Michigan, 1981. Health Care Financing Review 9(4):1-29.

Hubbard, R. L., and J. Anderson. 1988. Final Report: A Followup Study of Individuals Receiving Alcoholism Treatment. Prepared for the Oregon Office of Alcohol and Drug Programs. Research Triangle Park, N.C.: Research Triangle Institute.

Hunter, H. R., and J. C. Rowe. 1982. Alcoholism Services Handbook for Prepaid Group Plans. Washington, D.C.: Group Health Association of America, Inc.

Hurst, R. A. 1987. Alternative delivery systems perspective. Presented at the National Association of Addiction Treatment Programs Workshop on Trends and Issues in the Reimbursement of Chemical Dependency Treatment Programs, Houston, Texas, September 15.

Hustead, E., S. Sharfstein, S. Muszynski, J. Brady, and J. Cahill. 1985. Reductions in coverage for mental and nervous illness in the federal employees health benefits program, 1980-1984. American Journal of Psychiatry 142:181-186.

ICF, Inc. 1987. Analysis of Treatment for Alcoholism and Chemical Dependency. Irvine, Ca.: National Association of Addiction Treatment Providers.

Institute of Medicine. 1989. Research Opportunities in the Prevention and Treatment of Alcohol-Related Problems. Washington, D. C.: National Academy Press.

Institute for Health and Aging (IHA). 1986. Review and Evaluation of Alcohol, Drug Abuse and Mental Health Services Block Grant Allotment Formulas: Final Report. Prepared for the Alcohol, Drug Abuse, and Mental Health Administration. San Francisco, Calif.

Jacob, O. 1985. Public and Private Sector Issues on Alcohol and Other Drug Abuse: A Special Report with Recommendations. Prepared for the National Institute on Alcohol Abuse and Alcoholism. Rockville, Md.: Alcohol, Drug Abuse, and Mental Health Administration.

Jensen, G. A., and J. R. Gable. 1988. The erosion of purchased health insurance. Inquiry 25:328-343.

Jensen, G. A., M. A. Morrisey, and J. W. Marcus. 1988. Cost-sharing and the changing pattern of employee-sponsored benefits. The Milbank Quarterly 65(4) 521-550.

Joint Commission on the Accreditation of Hospitals (JCAH). 1974. Accreditation Manual for Alcoholism Programs. Chicago: JCAH.

Joint Commission on the Accreditation of Hospitals (JCAH). 1983. Consolidated Standards Manual for Child, Adolescent and Adult Psychiatric, Alcoholism, and Drug Abuse Facilities. Chicago: JCAH.

Joint Commission on Mental Illness and Health. 1961. Action for Mental Health. New York: Basic Books.

Klerman, G. L. 1989. Treatment of alcoholism. New England Journal of Medicine 320:394-395.

Korchok, M. 1988. Managed Care and Chemical Dependency: A Troubled Relationship. Providence, R.I.: Manisses Communications Group, Inc.

Kusserow, R. P. 1989. An Assessment of Data Collection for Alcohol, Drug Abuse, and Mental Health Services. Office of the Inspector General, U.S. Department of Health and Human Services, Washington, D.C.

Lawrence Johnson and Associates, Inc. 1983. Evaluation of the HCFA Alcoholism Services Demonstration: Final Evaluation Design. Prepared for the Office of Research and Demonstrations, Health Care Financing Administration. Washington, D.C.

Lawrence Johnson and Associates, Inc. 1986. Evaluation of the HCFA Alcoholism Services Demonstration: Final Second Analytic Report. Prepared for the Health Care Financing Administration. Washington, D.C.

Lebenluft, E., and R. F. Lebenluft. 1988. Reimbursement for partial hospitalization: A survey and policy implications. American Journal of Psychiatry 145:1514-1520.

Levin, B. L., J. H. Glaser, and R. E. Roberts. 1984. Changing patterns in mental health service coverage within health maintenance organizations. American Journal of Public Health 74:453-458.

Lewin/ICF. 1989a. Analysis of State Alcohol and Drug Data Collection Instruments, Volumes I through VI. Prepared for the Office of Finance and Coverage Policy, National Institute in Drug Abuse. Washington D.C.

Lewin/ICF. 1989b. Feasibility and Design of a Study of the Delivery and Financing of Drug and Alcohol Services. Prepared for the National Institute on Drug Abuse, Alcohol, Drug Abuse, and Mental Health Administration. Washington, D. C.

Lewis, J. S. 1982. The federal role in alcoholism research, treatment and prevention. Pp. 385-401 in Alcohol, Science and Society Revisited, E. Gomberg, H. White, and J. Carpenter, eds. Ann Arbor, Mich. and New Brunswick, N.J.: University of Michigan Press and Center of Alcohol Studies, Rutgers University.

Lewis, J. S. 1988a. Congressional rites of passage for the rights of alcoholics. Alcohol Health and Research World 12:241-251.

Lewis, J. S. 1988b. Growth in managed care forcing providers to adjust. Alcoholism Report 16(24):1.

Leyland, A. Jr., V. Paukstys, and T. Raichel. Substance Abuse Treatment Benefits: A Guide for Plans. Chicago: Blue Cross and Blue Shield Association, 1983.

Lohr, K. N., K. D. Yordy, and S. O. Thier. 1988. Current issues in the quality of care. Health Affairs 7(1):5-18.

Luckey, J. W. 1987. Justifying alcohol treatment on the basis of cost savings: The offset literature. Alcohol Health and Research World 12:8-15.

Luft, H. S. 1988. HMOs and the quality of care. Inquiry 25:147-156.

Macro Systems, Inc. 1980. Final Report: Federal Activities on Alcohol Abuse and Alcoholism: FY 1978. Prepared for the National Institute on Alcohol Abuse and Alcoholism. Silver Spring, Md.: Macro Systems, Inc.

Mahoney, J. J. 1987. EAPs and Medical Cost Containment. The ALMACAN 17(5):16-20.

Manning, W. G., and K. B. Wells. 1986. Preliminary results of a controlled trial of the effect of a prepaid group practice on the outpatient use of mental health services. Journal of Human Resources 21:293-320

Manov, W. F., and N. N. Beshai. 1986. Alcohol-free living centers: Long term, low cost, alcohol recovery housing. Presented at the 114th Annual Meeting of the American Public Health Association, September 28-October 2.

Massachusetts Special Commission Relative to the Admission and Denial of Drug and Alcohol Patients in Hospitals and Other Facilities. 1986. First Interim Report of the Special Commission Relative to the Procedures of Admitting Certain Drug-Alcohol Patients for Detoxification and Rehabilitation by Insurance Companies. Submitted to the Legislature, Commonwealth of Massachusetts under Chapter 2 of the Resolves of 1985. Boston: The Commission.

McAuliffe, W. E., P. Breer, N. White, C. Spino., L. Goldsmith, S. Robel, and L. Byam. 1988. A Drug Abuse Treatment and Intervention Plan for Rhode Island. Cranston, R.I.: Rhode Island Department of Mental Health, Retardation, and Hospitals.

McGuire, T. G., B. Dickey, G. E. Shively, and I. Strumwasser. 1987. Differences in resource use and cost among facilities treating alcohol, drug abuse, and mental disorders: Implications for design of a prospective payment system. American Journal of Psychiatry 144:616-620.

Mee-Lee, D. 1988. An instrument for treatment progress and matching: The Recovery Attitude and Treatment Evaluator (RAATE). Journal of Substance Abuse Treatment 5:183-186.

Miller, W. R., and R. K. Hester. 1986. Inpatient alcoholism treatment: Who benefits? American Psychologist 41:794-805.

Minnesota Chemical Dependency Program Division. 1987. Biennial Report to the Governor and the Minnesota Legislature. St. Paul: Minnesota Department of Human Services.

Minnesota Chemical Dependency Program Division. 1989a. Directory of Chemical Dependency Programs in Minnesota. St. Paul: Minnesota Department of Human Services.

Minnesota Chemical Dependency Program Division. 1989b. Report to the State Legislature on the Status of the Consolidated Chemical Dependency Treatment Fund. St. Paul: Minnesota Department of Human Services.

Mintzes, B. 1988. Statement on behalf of the Michigan Office of Substance Abuse Services and the National Association of State Alcohol and Drug Abuse Directors. Presented to the open meeting of the IOM Committee for the Study of Treatment and Rehabilitation Services for Alcoholism and Alcohol Abuse, Washington, D.C., January 25.

Mintzes, B., C. Allo, and R. C. Brook. 1987/1988. Cost containment in the purchasing of substance abuse services. Drugs and Society. 2(2):110-123.

Modern Healthcare. 1987. Healthcare marketing. Modern Healthcare 17(7):27.

Morrisey, M. A., and G. A. Jensen. 1988. Employer-sponsored insurance coverage for alcoholism and drug-abuse treatments. Journal of Studies on Alcohol. 49: 456-461.

Morrison, L. 1978. Title XX Handbook for Alcohol, Drug Abuse, and Mental Health Treatment Programs. Prepared for the Alcohol, Drug Abuse, and Mental Health Administration. Washington, D.C.: U.S. Government Printing Office.

Muszynski, I. L. 1987. Trends in health care financing and reimbursement of chemical dependency programs. Presented at the National Association of Addiction Treatment Programs Workshop on Trends and Issues in the Reimbursement of Chemical Dependency Treatment Programs, Houston, Texas, September 15.

National Association of Addiction Treatment Providers, Inc. 1987. NAATP will oppose DRGs for the fourth time. NAATP News 8(4):1, 6.

National Association of Insurance Commissioners (NAIC). 1981. Report of the National Association of Insurance Commissioners' Task Force on Alcoholism, Drug Addiction, and Insurance. Washington, D.C.: NAIC.

National Association State Alcohol and Drug Abuse Program Directors (NASADAD). 1988. Summary of Alcohol and Drug Agency Locations Within the State Systems. Washington, D.C.: NASADAD.

National Council on Alcoholism Task Force on Health Insurance. 1974. Recommendations for Health Insurance Coverage for Alcoholism (memorandum). National Council on Alcoholism, Washington, D.C., January.

National Council on Alcoholism (NCA). 1987. A Federal Response to a Hidden Epidemic: Alcohol and Other Drug Problems Among Women. New York: National Council on Alcoholism.

National Institute on Alcohol Abuse and Alcoholism (NIAAA). 1984. Report to the U.S. Congress on Federal Activities on Alcohol Abuse and Alcoholism: FY 1981 and FY 1982. Rockville, Md.: NIAAA.

National Institute on Alcohol Abuse and Alcoholism (NIAAA). 1988. Program Announcement: Research on Economic and Socioeconomic Issues in the Prevention, Treatment, and Epidemiology of Alcohol Abuse and Alcoholism. Rockville, Md.: NIAAA.

National Institute on Drug Abuse/National Institute on Alcohol Abuse and Alcoholism (NIDA/NIAAA). 1989. Highlights from the 1987 National Drug and Alcoholism Treatment Unit Survey (NDATUS). Rockville, Md.: NIDA/NIAAA.

Neiberding, S. 1983. The evolution of the National Institute on Alcohol Abuse and Alcoholism. Advances in Alcohol and Substance Abuse 2:15-21.

New Jersey Department of Insurance. 1988. Report of Governor's Cabinet Working Group's Ad Hoc Advisory Committee on Funding Sources for Treatment for Alcoholism and Drug Abuse. Trenton, N.J.: New Jersey Department of Insurance.

New York State Interagency Task Force on Insurance. 1988. Mandating Health Insurance Coverage of Inpatient Treatment of Alcoholism and Substance Abuse: A Report to the Legislature as Required by Chapter 444 of the Laws of 1987. Albany, N.Y.: New York State Interagency Task Force on Insurance.

New York Division of Alcoholism and Alcohol Abuse (NYDAAA) 1989. Five Year Comprehensive Plan for Alcoholism Services in New York State: 1989-1994. Albany, N.Y.: NYDAAA.

Nischan, J. A., C. D. Allo, and R. C. Brook. 1986. Continued evolution in the substance abuse services network of care. Michigan Office of Substance Abuse Services, Lansing, Mich., February.

Noble, J. A., P. Widem, H. Malin, and J. R. Coakley. 1978. Medicare Coverage for the Treatment of Alcoholism: Excerpts from DHEW's 1978 Report to Congress on the Advantages and Disadvantages of Extending Medicare Coverage to Mental Health, Alcohol, and Drug Abuse Centers. Rockville, Md.: National Institute on Alcohol Abuse and Alcoholism.

Office of Personnel Management (OPM). 1988. Report on Title V of Public Law 99-570: The Federal Employee Substance Abuse Education and Treatment Act of 1986. Washington, D.C.: Office of Personnel Management.

Oregon State Health Planning and Development Agency. 1986. Second Report on Oregon's Experience with Remodeling Insurance Benefits for Mental Health and Chemical Dependency. Report to the 64th Oregon Legislative Assembly on Implementation of Chapter 601, Oregon Laws, 1983. Salem, Oregon: Oregon State Health Planning and Development Agency.

Oregon Office of Health Policy. 1988. Model admission and continued stay criteria for chemical dependency treatment of adults (memorandum). Department of Human Resources, Salem, Oregon, June.

Plaut, T. F. A., ed. 1967. Alcohol Problems: A Report to the Nation. New York: Oxford University Press.

Plotnick, D. E., K. M. Adams, H. R. Hunter, and J. C. Rowe. 1982. Alcoholism Treatment Programs within Prepaid Group Practices: A Final Report. Rockville, Md.: National Institute on Alcohol Abuse and Alcoholism.

President's Commission on Law Enforcement and Administration of Justice. 1967a. The Challenge of Crime in a Free Society. Washington, D.C.: U.S. Government Printing Office.

President's Commission on Law Enforcement and Administration of Justice. 1967b. The Challenge of Crime in a Free Society, Task Force Report: Drunkenness. Washington, D.C.: U.S. Government Printing Office.

President's Commission on Mental Health Task Panel on Alcohol Related Problems. 1978. Report of the Liaison Panel on Alcohol Related Problems. Pp. 2078-2092 in Appendix: Task Panel Reports. Vol. 4 of the Report to the President from the President's Commission On Mental Health, Washington, D. C.: U.S. Government Printing Office.

Public Health Foundation. 1988. Public Health Agencies 1988: An Inventory of Programs and Block Grant Expenditures. Washington D. C.: Public Health Foundation.

Putnam, S. 1982. Short-term effects of treating alcoholics for alcoholism: Utilization of medical care services in a health maintenance organization. Group Health Journal 3(1):19-30.

Regan, R. 1981. The role of federal, state, local, and voluntary sectors in expanding health insurance coverage for alcoholism. Alcohol Health and Research World 5(4):22-26.

Reutzel, T. J., F. W. Becker, and B. K. Sanders. 1988. Expenditure effects of changes in Medicaid benefit coverage: An alcohol and substance abuse example. American Journal of Public Health 77:503-504.

Reynolds, R. I., and B. E. Ryan. 1988. Executive summary: Policy implications of social model alcohol recovery services. Prepared for the IOM Committee for the Study of Treatment and Rehabilitation Services for Alcoholism and Alcohol Abuse, July.

Robertson, A. D. 1988. Federal and state support for alcohol and drug abuse services. Testimony on behalf of the National Association of State Alcohol and Drug Abuse Directors. Presented to the U.S. Senate Committee on Governmental Affairs hearing regarding overview of federal activities on alcohol abuse and alcoholism, National Association of State Alcohol and Drug Abuse Directors, Washington, D.C., May 25.

Rodriguez, A. R. 1983. Psychological and psychiatric peer review at CHAMPUS. American Psychologist 38:941-947.

Rodriguez, A. R., and J. J. Maher. 1986. Psychiatric case management offers cost, quality control. Business and Health 3(5):14-17.

Rodriguez, A. R. 1984. Peer review program sets trends in claims processing. Business and Health 1(10):21-25.
Roman, P. 1988. Growth and transformation in workplace alcoholism programming. Pp.131-158 in Recent Developments in Alcoholism, vol. 6, M. Galanter, ed. New York: Plenum Press.

Rosenberg, N. 1968. Survey of Health Insurance for Alcoholism. Prepared for the National Center for Prevention and Control of Alcoholism. Bethesda, Md.: National Institute of Mental Health.

Rubington, E.. 1974. The role of the halfway house in the rehabilitation of alcoholics. Pp. 351-383 in Treatment and Rehabilitation of the Chronic Alcoholic. Vol. 5 of The Biology of Alcoholism, B. Kissin and H. Begleiter, eds. New York: Plenum Press.

Saxe, L., D. Dougherty, K. Esty, and M. Fine. 1983. The Effectiveness and Costs of Alcoholism Treatment. Washington, D.C.: U.S. Congress, Office of Technology Assessment.

Saxe, L., and L. Goodman. 1988. The effectiveness of outpatient vs. inpatient treatment: Updating the OTA report. Center for Applied Social Science, Boston University, Boston, Mass., June.

Seesel, T. 1988. Statement presented on behalf of the National Council on Alcoholism to the open meeting of the IOM Committee for the Study of Treatment and Rehabilitation Services for Alcoholism and Alcohol Abuse, Washington, D.C., January 25.

Shadle, M., and J. B. Christianson. 1988. The Organization and Delivery of Mental Health, Alcohol, and Other Drug Abuse Services within Health Maintenance Organizations. Final Report. Prepared for the Alcohol, Drug Abuse, and Mental Health Administration. Minneapolis: Interstudy.

Sharfstein, S. S. 1982. Medicaid cutbacks and block grants: Crisis or opportunity for community mental health? American Journal of Psychiatry 139:466-470.

Sharfstein, S. S., S. Muszynski, and G. M. Arnett. 1984. Dispelling myths about mental health benefits. Business and Health 1(10):7-11.

Shulman, J. 1988. Statement presented on behalf of the National Association of Addiction Treatment Providers to the open meeting of the IOM Committee for the Study of Treatment and Rehabilitation of Alcoholism and Alcohol Abuse, Washington, D. C., January 25.

Sieverts, S. 1983. Third party reimbursement for alcoholism services. Bulletin of the New York Academy of Sciences 59(2)211-215.

Sloan, F. A., M. A. Morrisey, and J. Valona. 1988. Effects of the Medicare prospective payment system on hospital cost containment: An early appraisal. The Milbank Quarterly 66(2):191-220.

Stoffelmayer, B. 1988. The treatment environment—lessons from the field. Statement presented to the open meeting of the IOM Committee for the Study of Treatment and Rehabilitation Services for Alcoholism and Alcohol Abuse, Washington, D.C., January 25.

Sutton, H. L. 1981. Estimating the costs of alcoholism treatment services in HMO programs. Presented to the Conference on Financing of Alcoholism Services in HMOs, Washington, D.C., June.

Taube, C. A., H. H. Goldman, and E. S. Lee. 1988. Use of specialty psychiatric settings in constructing DRGs. Archives of General Psychiatry 45:1037-1040

Taube, C. A., J. W. Thompson, B. J. Burns, P. Widem, and C. Prevost. 1985. Prospective payment and psychiatric discharges from general hospitals with and without psychiatric units. Hospital and Community Psychiatry 36:754-760.

Temkin-Geser, H., and K. T. Clark. 1988. Ethnicity, gender, and utilization of mental health services in a medicaid population. Social Sciences in Medicine 26:989-996.

Tison, T. 1989. Defining the relationship between EAPs and benefit departments. The ALMACAN 19(4):19-25.

Toff, G. E. 1984. Mental Health Benefits under Medicaid: A Survey of the States. Washington, D.C.: Intergovernmental Health Project, George Washington University.

Toff, G. E. 1984. States concerned about cost, impact of mandated mental health benefits. Business and Health 1(10):50-51.

Tsai, S. P., S. M. Reedy, E. J. Bernacki, and E. S. Lee. 1988. Effect of curtailed insurance benefits on the use of mental health care: The Tenneco Plan. Medical Care 26:430-440.

U.S. Department of Health and Human Services (USDHHS). 1981. Fourth Special Report to the U.S. Congress on Alcohol and Health. Rockville, Md.: National Institute on Alcohol Abuse and Alcoholism.

U.S. Department of Health and Human Services (USDHHS). 1987. Sixth Special Report to the U.S. Congress on Alcohol and Health. Rockville, D.C.: National Institute on Alcohol Abuse and Alcoholism.

U.S. Department of Health and Human Services (USDHHS). 1986. Toward a National Plan to Combat Alcohol Abuse and Alcoholism. Report submitted to the United States Congress. Rockville, Md.: National Institute on Alcohol Abuse and Alcoholism.

U.S. Department of Health, Education, and Welfare (USDHEW). 1971. First Special Report to the U.S. Congress on Alcohol and Health. Rockville, Md.: National Institute on Alcohol Abuse and Alcoholism.

U.S. Department of Health, Education, and Welfare (USDHEW). 1974. Second Special Report to the U.S. Congress on Alcohol and Health. Rockville, Md.: National Institute on Alcohol Abuse and Alcoholism.

U.S. Department of Health, Education, and Welfare (USDHEW). 1978. Third Special Report to the U.S. Congress on Alcohol and Health. Rockville, Md.: National Institute on Alcohol Abuse and Alcoholism.

U.S. General Accounting Office (USGAO). 1977. Progress in Treating Alcohol Abusers. Washington, D.C.: USGAO.

U.S. General Accounting Office (USGAO). 1982. A Summary and Comparison of the Legislative Provisions of the Block Grants Created by the 1981 Omnibus Reconciliation Budget Reconciliation Act. Washington, D.C.: USGAO.

U.S. General Accounting Office (USGAO). 1984. States Have Made Few Changes in Implementing the Alcohol, Drug Abuse, and Mental Health Services Block Grant. Washington, D.C.: USGAO.

U.S. General Accounting Office (USGAO). 1985. Block Grants: Overview of Experiences to Date and Emerging Issues. Washington, D.C.: USGAO.

U.S. General Accounting Office (USGAO). 1986. Health Insurance: Comparison of Coverage for Federal and Private Sector Employees. Washington, D.C.: USGAO.

U.S. General Accounting Office (USGAO). 1987a. Block Grants: Federal Set-Asides for Substance Abuse and Mental Health Services. Rockville, Md.: USGAO.

U.S. General Accounting Office (USGAO). 1987b. Block Grants: Proposed Formulas for Substance Abuse, Mental Health Provide More Equity. Washington, D.C.: USGAO.

Wallace, C. 1987. Employers turning to managed care to control their psychiatric care costs. Modern Healthcare 9(7):82.

Walsh, D. C., and R. H. Egdahl. 1984. Treatment for chemical dependency and mental illness: Can this utilization be managed? Health Affairs 3(3):130-135.

Walsh, D. C., R. W. Hingson, and D. M. Merrigan. 1986. A randomized trial comparing inpatient and outpatient alcoholism treatments in industry—A first report. Presented at the Annual Meeting of the Alcohol Epidemiology Section of the International Council on Alcohol and Addictions, Dubrovnik, Yugoslavia, June 9-13.

Weedman, R. D. 1987. Admission, Continued Stay, and Discharge Criteria for Alcoholism and Drug Dependence Treatment Services. Irvine, Calif.: National Association of Addiction Treatment Providers.

Weisman, M. N. 1988. Musings on the art of treatment. Alcohol Health and Research World 12:282-87.

Weisner, C., and R. Room. 1984. Financing and ideology in alcohol treatment. Social Problems 32:167-184.

Weisner, C. 1986. The social ecology of alcohol treatment in the United States. Pp. 203-243 in Recent Developments in Alcoholism, vol. 5, M. Galanter, ed. New York: Plenum Press.

Wennberg, J. E. 1988. The medical care outcome problem. Health Affairs 7(10):5-18.

Wenzel, L. 1988. Mental health options under HMOs. Business and Health 5(4):30-33.

White, W. T., and D. Mee-Lee. 1988. Substance use disorder and college students: Inpatient treatment issues—a model of practice. Journal of College Student Psychotherapy 2(3/4):177-203.

Williams, W. G. 1981. Nature and scope of benefit packages in health insurance coverage for alcoholism. Alcohol Health and Research World 5(4):5-11.

Wittman, F. D., and P. A. Madden. 1988. Alcohol Recovery Programs for Homeless People: A Survey of Current Programs in the U.S. Prepared for the National Institute on Alcohol Abuse and Alcoholism. Rockville, Md.: National Institute on Alcohol Abuse and Alcoholism.

Yahr, H. T. 1988. A national comparison of public- and private-sector alcoholism treatment delivery system characteristics. Journal of Studies on Alcohol 49:233-239.

19 Cost-Effectiveness

Information that compares the net medical cost of treatment for a person with alcohol problems with the treatment effect or effects is necessary for judging the desirability of support for such treatment and of insurance coverage for it. This analysis of costs and effects furnishes "cost-effectiveness" data that can be used in decision making.

Cost-effectiveness analysis as a decision aid is, at base, a comparative tool. No strategy is literally cost-effective in isolation; the most that can be said is that one strategy is more cost-effective than another. If, for instance, strategy A is more costly and no more effective than strategy B, one can say that B is cost-effective compared with A. However, the information on costs and effectiveness of the two strategies cannot tell us that strategy B is cost effective in isolation or in comparison, let us say, to a strategy of no intervention. The comparative aspect of cost-effectiveness is an important point, especially when different treatment strategies are analyzed. Strictly speaking, cost-effectiveness analysis as such can only provide information about *relative* desirability and not about whether anything at all should be done. There is, however, one common and natural use of the term *cost-effectiveness* as an absolute concept that is relevant to the treatment of alcohol problems. If a costly medical treatment lowers medical costs elsewhere in the system (either simultaneously or in the future), if it does so to such an extent that the value of the cost savings more than offsets the cost of the treatment, and if the treatment at least does no harm, then it might legitimately be said that the treatment is "cost effective" and obviously desirable in the sense that it leads to negative net medical costs compared with a "no treatment" alternative.

The cost-effectiveness analysis of treatment for alcohol problems has, to a considerable extent, pursued this question of cost offset (IOM, 1989). In addition to the question of whether treatment itself actually saves money, compared with no treatment, there is the additional particular question of which treatment to select. The net cost of treatments varies; some treatment strategies may have higher net costs than others but may also have greater effectiveness. This situation then poses the classic cost-effectiveness question: how does the additional cost compare with the additional effectiveness?

The discussion that follows, examines both of these cost-effectiveness questions: the possibility of cost offsets (and a negative net cost) of some treatment compared with no treatment and the cost-effectiveness of one treatment compared with another.

Studies of Costs and Cost Offsets

Because alcohol problems and alcohol dependence are associated with positive medical costs—for example, from alcohol-related illness and from accidents and injuries—it might be expected that successful treatment would lower those costs and an offset would occur. Jones and Vischi (1979) carried out an early review that displayed the pattern shown in subsequent research. They reviewed 25 studies that examined whether treatment for mental illness, alcohol abuse, or drug abuse reduced subsequent utilization of health services. Twelve of the 25 studies involved alcohol abuse; Jones and Vischi concluded that these studies showed that reductions did take place in either medical care utilization measures (e.g., hospital days, outpatient visits) or surrogate measures (e.g., sick days, sickness and accident benefits paid). They also observed reductions in the subsequent use of health services that ranged from 26 percent to 69 percent, with a median reduction of 40 percent. Methodological problems were noted in all 12 studies (e.g., limited time spans, small samples, lack of appropriate comparison groups); in addition, none of the studies was a randomized clinical trial that could have served to suggest causality. A further methodological problem was that a majority of the reviewed studies were conducted in HMOs or employer-based programs. This factor led the reviewers to raise questions about the generalizability of the findings as well as about the specific cause of the observed subsequent reductions in utilization (i.e., the cause may have been a characteristic of the treatment setting rather than of the treatment itself).

Jones and Vischi discussed the implications of the findings for three areas of policy concern: (1) the setting in which treatment takes place, (2) the linkage of treatment for alcohol and drug abuse and mental disorders with general health services, and (3) health insurance coverage. They made no specific recommendations because of the limitations of the studies they reviewed. Their review, however, set the stage for continued studies of cost offsets in subsequent health services utilization and in insurance costs as a major strategy for obtaining improved coverage for treatment of persons with alcohol or drug problems or mental disorders. Some of these more recent studies are reviewed by Saxe and coworkers (1983), Holder (1987), and Holder and colleagues (1988). These analysts attempted to determine whether treatment for alcohol problems provides any cost offsets and, if it does, whether the offsets are large enough to produce a negative net cost for treatment.

The types of cost offset studies that have been conducted and the nature of the results differ by the form of insurance coverage for treatment, the characteristics of the population at risk, and the process by which people are induced to seek treatment. Because there is reason to believe that the cost offset may vary depending on the process that stimulates treatment, it will be useful to treat each group of studies separately.

Early studies of cost offsets looked at the experience of employee assistance programs (EAPs). These programs identified workers who were problem drinkers and assisted and encouraged them in seeking treatment. A number of studies of (EAPs) have compared medical costs, disability costs, and sick days before and after an employee was successfully referred for treatment (e.g., Alander and Campbell, 1975). There was consistent and unequivocal evidence of a change in outcome after treatment, either compared with the employee's previous behavior or compared with trends among a control group of persons with alcohol problems who did not seek treatment. Among the treated employees, sick days and injury days fell, and inpatient costs dropped. Sometimes the savings in the medical costs over the one- to two-year follow up period exceeded (in present value terms) the cost of the program; sometimes the offset was not complete. However, these studies typically followed small groups over a limited time period and did not measure all medical costs.

A later set of studies used data from insurance and HMO plans and permitted longer follow-up periods and larger samples of employees and dependents. Holder and colleagues (Holder and Hallan, 1976, 1986; Holder and Blose, 1986) examined several large samples (in one case, more than 1,500 observations) of persons with alcohol problems. Using sophisticated statistical models, they compared the total medical cost levels of the participants before and after treatment initiation. The Holder team found a universal pattern of decreases in hospital admission rates and average total medical costs, compared with past trends and with trends in a control group. Over a two- to three-year period, the full cost of the treatment was more than offset. Other studies (Brock and Boyajy, 1978; Sherman et al., 1979) showed similar results.

The third group of studies involved were people who were receiving treatment from publicly funded programs (both the Veterans Administration and Medicaid) (Magruder-Habib et al., 1985; Calkins et al., 1986). These studies failed to find a cost offset and may in fact have found a cost increase. This finding is in contrast to those from earlier studies of public clients (JWK International Corporation, 1976; Gregory et al., 1982; Becker and Sanders, 1984); however, those studies projected substantial cost offsets but were not based on actual total expense data. Luckey (1987) conjectures that the differences among the populations in these studies of publicly funded programs, compared with the EAP and insurance company studies, may explain the difference in results; that is, lower income people may have more chronic health problems before they initiate treatment and may have fewer incentives (or less opportunity) to maintain recovery.

Thus, the overall picture regarding cost offsets is one of cost declines after treatment for people who are not poor, declines which are frequently large enough to offset the cost of treatment (Luckey, 1987). Do these studies conclusively demonstrate that there is a negative net cost? Does the remarkable consistency of documented reductions in health care costs among insured groups strongly suggest the decreases are real?

Unfortunately, despite the consistency of the results and the large sample sizes, there is still a methodological Achilles heel to the findings. In all of the studies, treatment recipients selected treatment for themselves (self-selection) and were not randomly assigned. That is, the studies do not tell us how those individuals would have fared had they not obtained treatment, information that could have been provided through the use of random assignment to experimental and control groups. The comparisons that were actually used in the studies were based either on the prior experience of those who sought treatment or on the experience of other control groups. As a result, the studies cannot report with confidence that treatment caused a difference in outcome (i.e., enabled later cost offsets) because the studies use two different groups of people for comparison: those who sought treatment and those who did not.

Yet a question remains: If the treatment did not necessarily cause the decline, what did? One possible answer is that the people who sought treatment were ready to stop drinking anyway, with or without help. The other possibility is the statistical phenomenon called "regression to the mean," in which periods of unusually high levels of anything (whether it be rainfall, temperature, or the Dow-Jones index) are most likely to be followed by a return to the average: because an episode of treatment for alcohol problems is accompanied by high costs for all medical care, it is to be expected that low costs would follow.

Some reviewers nevertheless conclude that there is some evidence to support the hypothesis that treatment for alcohol problems is cost-beneficial (Saxe et al., 1983; Holder, 1987; Luckey, 1987). The benefits of treatment for alcohol problems are cautiously seen to be in excess of the cost of providing such treatment even if they fall short of what may be claimed. The caution stems from the subjective judgments that the reviewers must conjecture about the degree of spurious causation in the studies they reviewed because neither the studies nor the reviews provide any objective basis for determining the seriousness of the problem of spurious causation.

One way out of this impasse would be to use the kind of reasoning suggested earlier. There are no controlled trials of cost offsets in real world settings, but there are the many before-and-after studies reviewed (Holder, 1987; IOM, 1989). There are the many controlled trials of the effectiveness of treatment in clinical settings reviewed for this report. Can one link the two sets of results to come to a reasonable conclusion? There are two reasons why the answer may still be negative. One answer is brief and theoretical; the other is longer and is based on empirical fact.

The theoretical problem is that the effectiveness demonstrated in controlled trials of treatment alternatives (there have been no controlled trials of cost-effectiveness) may not carry with it the kind of cost offset (at least in terms of size) suggested by the uncontrolled studies. This objection might be dismissed by appeal to the ethical and practical difficulties of randomizing large numbers of persons with alcohol problems to a long-term no-treatment trial. However, the strength of such an appeal is lessened by the fact that there have been some additional large sample studies that do use a type of real-world random assignment and that failed to find any cost offset (e.g., Hayami and Freeborn, 1981; Manning et al., 1986).

It is usually not easy to assign people who seek treatment to a no-treatment control group, nor is it possible to assign people who do not seek treatment to treatment. Considering the difficulties involved in randomized controlled trials, it will necessarily be impossible to get a reliable estimate of the cost offset for treatment of an "average" person with alcohol problems. In any case, because there is no way to compel that person to seek treatment, such an estimate does not really answer the relevant policy question: whether there is a cost offset for the type of person who can be induced to enter treatment by feasible policy interventions (e.g., better insurance coverage, the use of an EAP, court orders, an especially powerful way of marketing treatment). This question can be explored using a different methodology from that of randomized trials. Although one cannot assign individuals to treatment and no treatment study conditions, one can assign populations containing persons with alcohol problems to policy interventions that are thought to provide a stronger stimulus to such treatment than is provided in other environments. An example of such a study is provided by the Hayami and Freeborn (1981) analysis of different levels of out-of-pocket payment. This study raises serious questions about the existence of a relevant cost offset.

In the Hayami and Freeborn study, more than 20,000 members of the Kaiser-Portland health plan were randomly assigned to different levels of out-of-pocket payment for subsequent treatment for alcohol problems. Half of the population was "assigned" to receive coverage for such care free of charge (i.e., full insurance coverage); the others received the standard benefit of 50 percent coverage.

Regardless of the level of insurance coverage, only a small percentage of the plan's members who were eligible for treatment of alcohol problems actually sought such treatment. The free care group used significantly more treatment services than the copayment group and also showed a modest improvement in condition. However, there was no difference between the two groups in the use of medical services in the posttreatment period. That is, there was no evidence of a cost offset associated with more generous insurance coverage and the higher level of use associated with it.

A study that examined a wider range of insurance coverage but for mental health services in general and not just for alcohol problems treatment, is the RAND Corporation health insurance study carried out by Manning and coworkers (1986). This study employed a randomized design that assigned 5,800 people to levels of insurance coverage ranging from free care to very high copayments. Compared with those who had free care, those who had copayments were less than half as likely to use mental health services. The follow-up period in this study (up to five years) was longer than in the Hayami-Freeborn study, but again no posttreatment cost offset was found.

Yet these studies also have certain limitations that may affect the meaning one ascribes to their results. The follow-up period in the Hayamai-Freeborn study was short (although the follow-up period in the Manning study was not); the Manning team's study was not limited to treatment for alcohol problems. These limitations mean that one can only say that these studies failed to find any cost offset, not that a cost offset does not exist. Nevertheless, these results raise serious questions about the inevitability of cost offsets from more extensive insurance coverage, and they surely do not prove that better coverage saves enough money to offset its cost.

It would be possible to reproduce these studies, even in private insurance settings, by phasing in more generous benefits for treatment of alcohol problems on a random or nonsystematic basis. Alternatively, it would be possible to examine the experience of people with other, exogenous influences on their use of services (e.g., the distance to or availability of treatment facilities, mandated referrals by the criminal justice system) to carry out population-based real world analysis of cost offsets. In the current state of knowledge, however, there is still some doubt that the net cost of treatment for alcohol problems would surely be negative for some population. "Probably" is a reasonable adverb to attach to cost offsets, but reasonable people can differ. One should hasten to add that suspecting that treatment might have a net positive medical cost hardly suggests that treatment is undesirable. It only means that attention must be focused on the other benefits to be gained from reducing alcohol problems. Those benefits, in terms of increased productivity, reduced danger to others, and the value placed by the person with an alcohol problem and his or her family on the reduction or elimination of that problem, are all surely positive. It is on the value of these benefits that one should rest the case for the advantage of treatment for alcohol problems (Harwood et al., 1984; Harwood, 1988).

Cost-Benefit and Cost-Effectiveness Analysis

The discussion above indicated that there is some, although not conclusive, evidence that spending money on treatment today lowers future medical costs. Whether there is, in any case, sufficient cost savings in the future to more than offset current costs is not known. Compared with no treatment, the use of some treatment (i.e., brief intervention) has a chance of lowering cost.   But what about treatment beyond the level of brief interventions? More intensive treatment, even if it should be discovered to have some cost offset, almost surely will have a positive net cost. Yet a more costly treatment may still be appropriate if it is more effective, if it provides more overall person and social benefit. Conversely, a treatment that provides some additional benefit may still not be desirable if it costs too much. For effective judgements, what we need to know is the cost effectiveness of alternative forms of treatment, a comparison of additional costs and additional benefits (Luckey, 1987).

There has been almost no formal examination of the cost-effectiveness of alternative treatments (Pauly, 1988). As discussed in Chapter 5, there is substantial uncertainty about whether interventions beyond the brief intervention level have any additional benefit when indiscriminately applied; there has been virtually no analysis of their additional cost. It is probably plausible to assume that brief interventions are cost-effective compared with no treatment. (The cost of a brief intervention is so low that a negative net cost is achieved through only a small cost offset. Moreover, even if it should have a positive net cost, that cost is likely to be low enough that the benefit provided by such interventions would usually be judged to be worth the cost.) Beyond brief interventions, however, there is simply no basis for determining the additional costs compared with the additional benefits because there is much uncertainty about benefits and virtually complete ignorance about costs. Thus, it is not known whether there are any additional cost offsets attached to treatment offered at levels beyond that of brief intervention. Also at issue is whether positive costs, if present, are exceeded by benefits.

Holder and colleagues (1988) have indicated the sort of study needed to answer this question: one with standard measures of outcomes, standard means of treatment, and random assignment.   Absent this type of analysis, one is forced to make informal comparisons by relying on the effectiveness literature and guessing what the comparative costs would be.

The best (and most conclusive) example of such an analysis is based on the "more intensive—less intensive" split. As noted earlier (see Chapter 5 and Appendix B), when forms of care that are more intensive than brief interventions are applied to undifferentiated populations of people with alcohol problems, there is usually no significantly greater effect than there would have been using less intense treatments. Under the reasonable assumption that more intensive care is more costly than brief interventions or outpatient care, one could conclude that more intensive care is less cost-effective than those less costly alternatives. This is not a tautology; if the improvement in effect with more intensive, more costly care had been positive and large, one might well have concluded that more costly care was more cost-effective. With zero effects and high costs, however, it is a foregone conclusion that it more costly care is not more cost-effective. More generally, given any set of treatment approaches that yield comparable outcomes—and this uniformity is the rule rather than the exception in effectiveness studies for alcohol treatment—the least costly intervention in the set is always the one to be preferred on cost-effectiveness grounds.

Holder and colleagues (1988) suggest some possible exceptions to this conclusion. They note that "it may be that certain types of programs/facility combinations better retain persons with chronic, severe alcohol problems in treatment or some form of institutional care (24-hour care) is necessary for patients with more severe physical disability resulting from chronic drinking" (p. 7). They conclude, however, that at present "this is more speculation than science."

Are there circumstances requiring qualifications to the conclusion that residential/inpatient care is less cost-effective than outpatient alternatives? Most of the argument, as usual, turns out to be about effectiveness, and not about cost. Many of the studies that show no differences are old and do not represent the type of treatment program currently being used in many residential programs. Others reveal that certain kinds of persons may do better in a residential setting, especially persons with less social stability (Kissin et al., 1971) or with a dysfunctional family or work relationships (McLellan et al., 1982). There was one random assignment study where residential care proved more effective for socially disadvantaged persons (Wanberg, Horn, and Fairchild, 1974). Against these exceptions, however, is mounted a group of studies that show that outpatient or day treatment settings offer effective treatment that is at least as good as—if not better than—that offered in inpatient/residential settings.

The finding that an inpatient program is sometimes more effective does not, of course, mean that it is also cost-effective. Put more bluntly, if residential programs for people with dysfunctional family relationships are a little better but a lot more costly than outpatient programs, they may still be undesirable because the benefits are not worth the cost, that is, are not large enough to "justify" the cost. To know for sure, it is necessary to assign values to benefits, something health care analysts try to avoid if at all possible. Yet ducking the value judgment may not always be an option. The value judgement may need to incorporate considerations other than cost effectiveness. For example, for persons with severe and chronic alcohol problems, Holder and colleagues (1988), concluded that there is no treatment intervention with a full cost offset.

Although residential or inpatient settings may be more costly and no more effective than outpatient approaches for people who have already decided to initiate treatment, they may attract more people into treatment than the "live in the community/face your friends" alternative. If treatment does have a cost offset, spending more per person to attract more people to treatment may actually result in a lower net cost for a given population of people with alcohol problems. However, this "marketing" or "attractiveness" dimension—which reflects the benefits individuals perceive will be forthcoming from a particular treatment—has not been investigated at all. More evidence may show that this ability to attract persons to treatment could be the strongest argument, if there is to be any strong argument to be made, for treatment in the residential setting.

The intensity of treatment (as distinct from the treatment setting) again displays the "no difference" results. There have been few direct comparisons of brief interventions (e.g., brief counseling) compared with intensive residential treatment. A recent study by Chick and coworkers (1988) showed better outcomes for extended treatment by the second follow-up year but did not provide estimates of the difference in the cost of the two approaches. Finally, even informal comparisons of treatment methods are simply not possible on cost-effectiveness grounds (Holder et al., 1988).

In summary, for a heterogeneous group of persons with alcohol problems, no one treatment has been shown to be more effective than any other, whether the treatment variable used for study is the setting, intensity, modality, technique, or process. Thus, it cannot be ruled out that, even in some of the cases in which more intensive treatment is effective, the cost per unit of "effect" is disproportionately large. Better information is sorely needed.

Matching and Cost-Effectiveness

Matching individuals with alcohol problems to particular treatments seems to increase average treatment effectiveness. Matching is the strategy preferred by this committee. However, there is no literature that bears on the question of cost-effectiveness in matching programs because there is relatively little evidence on the question of the effectiveness of matching itself (Holder et al., 1988). Posing the cost-effectiveness question requires first that one specify both the total level of resources to be applied to a population of persons with alcohol problems who have different needs and how those resources are distributed among different individuals. One might imagine that in theory there is some distribution, given a resource constraint, that "maximizes effectiveness"—but what is it? Without such knowledge, the allocation of resources based on clinical judgment about appropriate matching could lead to lower aggregate "effectiveness" than if there were no matching.

A related issue concerns the cost-effectiveness of various matching procedures. The "best" treatment for a particular individual, given his or her condition, may not be the most cost-effective one. As the dismal comment of the previous paragraph suggests, it may even be best to do nothing, or to do very little, rather than match treatment to someone for whom the most effective treatment has nevertheless low effectiveness and high cost.

Still a third cost-effectiveness question concerns the cost of matching itself. Careful assessments use up real resources, and the benefits from better matching may not be worth the cost of determining who needs which treatment. One suspects this may be particularly the case with less severe problems, where it may be less costly to give everyone a standard brief intervention and perform assessments much later and only for those people who seem to be responding poorly. Conclusions here all depend on information that has not even been a subject of speculation, much less an object of fact: the cost of assessment; the consequences (in both cost and outcome) of mismatches, whether false positives or false negatives; and the cost in real-world settings of managing clinically ideal matching programs.

If overlaid on the problem is the notion that, from a policy perspective, all one can do is encourage matching or try to structure insurance and financing policy to permit matching, the situation becomes even more complex. How effective, and how cost effective, would it be to replace blanket 28-day program insurance coverage with coverage for managed care? Would case managers really be able to avoid enough long inpatient stays to pay for easier access to outpatient care? Or would one see the more common real-world setting in which outpatient treatment expands when coverage is extended but the long inpatient stays fail to contract?

Conclusions and Recommendations

Although there are some critical findings from cost-effectiveness research that have helped the committee to formulate its recommendations on financing treatment for alcohol problems, it is painfully obvious that much of what we need to know is not known. Defensible measures of the cost-effectiveness of treatment beyond brief interventions for particular populations are simply not available; consequently, the data on cost-effectiveness are still insufficient for unambiguous policy guidance. Accordingly, the committee sees it as appropriate to recommend an intensive program of research to determine the costs of alternative treatments for persons with alcohol problems relative to the benefits of such treatments. *The committee recommends that the federal government sponsor an expanded program of research and analysis directed at discovering the costs, effectiveness, and responsiveness to insurance coverage of the various treatment strategies now in use and the matching strategy, which the committee favors, that is now being introduced.* The program should include studies of the impact of all types of third party funding on the utilization of different forms of treatment for alcohol problems. Agencies which should be involved in developing this program of research would appropriately include the National Center for Health Services Research, the Health Care Financing Administration, and the National Institute on Alcohol Abuse and Alcoholism.

None of these agencies currently has such an effort under way. The recent NIAAA (1988) program announcement outlining areas of interest and requesting applications for research on financing issues and the costs of various treatment services and settings represents an initial step toward developing such a program. Much more, however, needs to be done (Wallen, 1988: IOM, 1989). In particular, studies should be undertaken to determine the question of whether it is necessary to provide discrete coverage for brief interventions in order to bring more persons into treatment and to compare alternative detoxification and primary rehabilitation strategies.

As recommended in Chapter 18, there should also be an expansion of the federal government's services research effort to establish the cost-effectiveness of alternative strategies and models for treating alcohol problems. Studies of treatment effectiveness should not be undertaken without a consideration of the comparative cost-effectiveness questions (Holder et al, 1988). Thus, treatment outcome studies should routinely include mode of payment and cost data in order to begin to define the relative cost-effectiveness of various approaches to treatment of alcohol problems.

REFERENCES

Alander, R., and T. Campbell. 1975. An evaluative study of an alcohol and drug recovery program, a case study of the Oldsmobile experience. Human Resources Management 14:14-19.

Becker, F. W., and B. K. Sanders. 1984. The Illinois Medicare/Medicaid Alcoholism Services Demonstration: Medicaid Cost Trends and Utilization Patterns—Managerial Report. Prepared for the Illinois Department of Alcohol and Substance Abuse. Center for Policy Studies and Program Evaluation, Sangamon State University. Springfield, Ill.

Brock, C.P., and T. G. Boyajy. 1978. Alcoholism within Prepaid Group Practice HMO's. Prepared for the National Institute on Alcohol Abuse and Alcoholism. Washington, D.C.: Group Health Association of America.

Calkins, R., E. Kemp, J. Lock, J. Ramsey, and M. Cohen. 1986. Enhanced Evaluation of the Michigan Medicare/Medicaid Alcoholism Services Demonstration Project—Medicaid Costs and Utilization. Prepared for the Michigan Department of Substance Abuse Services. Lansing, Mich.: Michigan Department of Substance Abuse Services.

Chick, J., B. Ritson, J. Connaughton, A. Stewart, and J. Chick. 1988. Advice versus treatment for alcoholism: A controlled trial. British Journal of Addictions 83:159-170.

Gregory, D., R. Jones, and R. Rundell. 1982. Feasibility of an alcoholism health insurance benefit. Pp. 195-202 in Currents in Alcoholism: Recent Advances in Research and Treatment. vol. 7, M. Galanter, ed. New York: Grune and Stratton.

Harwood, H. J., D. M. Napolitano, P. L. Kristiansen, and J. J. Collins. 1984. Economic Costs to Society of Alcohol and Drug Abuse and Mental Illness: 1980. Prepared for the Alcohol, Drug Abuse, and Mental Health Administration. Research Triangle Park, N. C.: Research Triangle Institute.

Harwood, H. J. 1988. The burden of alcoholism on business: A simulation of alternative policies. Prepared for the IOM Committee to Study Treatment and Rehabilitation Services for Alcoholics and Alcohol Abusers.

Hayami, D. E., and D. K. Freeborn. 1981. Effect of coverage on use of an HMO alcoholism treatment program, outcome, and medical care utilization. American Journal of Public Health 71:1133-1143.

Holder, H. D., 1987. Alcoholism treatment and potential health care cost saving. Medical Care 25:52-71.

Holder, H. D., and J. B. Hallan. 1976. A Study of Health Insurance Coverage for Alcoholism for California State Employees: Two Year Experience Summary Report. Prepared for the National Institute on Alcohol Abuse and Alcoholism. Raleigh, N.C.: H-2, Inc.

Holder, H. D., and J. B. Hallan. 1986. Impact of alcoholism on total health care costs: A six year study. Advances in Alcohol and Substance Abuse 6(1):1-15.

Holder, H. D., and J. O. Blose. 1986. Alcoholism treatment and total health care utilization and costs: A four year longitudinal analysis of federal employees. Journal of the American Medical Association 256:1456-1460.

Holder, H.D., R. Longabaugh, and W.R. Miller. 1988. Cost and effectiveness of alcoholism treatment using best available information. Prepared for the IOM Committee to Study Treatment and Rehabilitation Services for Alcoholics and Alcohol Abusers.

Institute of Medicine. 1989. Prevention and Treatment of Alcohol Problems: Research Opportunities. Washington, D.C.: National Academy Press.

JWK International Corporation. 1976. Benefit-Cost Analysis of Alcoholism Treatment Centers. Prepared for the National Institute on Alcohol Abuse and Alcoholism (NIAAA). Rockville, Md.: NIAAA.

Jones, K., and T. Vischi. 1979. Impact of alcohol, drug abuse and mental health care utilization. Medical Care 17 (12, Suppl.):1-82.

Kissin, B., A. Plautz, and W. H. Su. 1971. Social and psychological factors in the treatment of chronic alcoholism. Journal of Psychiatric Research 8:13-17.

Luckey, J. W. 1987. Justifying alcohol treatment on the basis of cost savings: The offset literature. Alcohol Health and Research World 12:8-15.

Magruder-Habib, K., J. Luckey, V. Mikow, P. Barrow, and H. Feits. 1985. Effects of Alcoholism Treatment on Health Services Utilization Patterns. Technical Report IIIR-82-026. Washington, D.C.: Veterans Administration.

McLellan, A. T., L. Luborsky, L. O'Brien, C. Woody, and K. S. Druley. 1982. Is treatment for substance abuse effective? Journal of the American Medical Association 247:1423-1428.

Manning, W. G., K. B. Wells, N. Duan, J. Newhouse, and J. Ware. 1986. How cost sharing affects the use of ambulatory mental health services. Journal of the American Medical Association 256:1930-1986.

National Institute on Alcohol Abuse and Alcoholism (NIAAA). 1988. Program Announcement: Research on Economic and Socioeconomic Issues in the Prevention, Treatment, and Epidemiology of Alcohol Abuse and Alcoholism. Rockville, Md.: NIAAA.

Pauly, M. V. 1988. Delivery and financing of alcoholism treatment. Presented at the National Institute on Alcohol Abuse and Alcoholism/National Center for Health Services Research "Workshop on Health Economics of Prevention and Treatment of Alcohol Problems," Rockville, Md., September.

Saxe, L, D. Dougherty, K. Esty, and M. Fine. 1983. The Effectiveness and Costs of Alcoholism Treatment. Washington, D.C.: U.S. Congress, Office of Technology Assessment.

Sherman, R. M., S. Reiff, and A. B. Forsythe. 1979. Utilization of medical services by alcoholics participating in an outpatient treatment program. Alcoholism: Clinical and Experimental Research 3:115-120.

Wanberg, K. W., J. L. Horn, and D. Fairchild. 1974. Hospital versus community treatment of alcoholism problems. International Journal of Mental Health 3:160-176.

20 Paying for the Treatment System

This chapter considers possible changes in the methods that are currently used to pay for the treatment of alcohol problems. As outlined in earlier chapters, the major sources of funding for treatment of alcohol problems are private health insurance and governmental agencies (i.e., tax-financed public insurance or public production of treatment); out-of-pocket reimbursement is a much less dominant source. Under private insurance, a person obtains coverage through the payment of a premium himself or by an employer and enters a risk pool along with others who have purchased the same coverage. Under tax-financed public insurance or public production of treatment, a person obtains coverage through an entitlement—attaining a particular status through illness, age, or a given legal or social condition.

Both methods offer a "benefit plan" to those persons for whom there is coverage of medical care expenses by a third-party payer even if that coverage is not described as a benefit plan. A benefit plan is the specific description of the services that will be paid for, the providers who are eligible to be reimbursed for providing those services, the amounts that will be paid, and the mechanisms by which such services will be authorized and paid for on behalf of the plan's beneficiaries.

From the committee's perspective, for example, the alcohol, drug abuse, and mental health block grant funds given by the federal government to each state for use in purchasing services is a benefit plan with minimum restrictions (e.g., that these funds cannot be used to purchase inpatient hospital treatment). The state determines who will be eligible to receive services purchased with these funds and distributes them to venders; the venders provide the state's list of approved services to eligible clients. In some states, the state passes the funds through to the county to distribute with minimum restrictions; an example is the California Division of Alcohol Programs, which provides a formula allocation of state, county, and federal funds to purchase nonhospital detoxification, residential recovery services, and nonresidential recovery services using a social model to define eligible providers and services. In other states, the block grant is passed through to counties with a very strict legislatively defined method for level of care placement; an example is the Minnesota Chemical Dependency Program Division, which provides a formula allocation to counties to purchase both hospital and nonhospital services for eligible beneficiaries meeting stringent income guidelines. (These funding mechanisms are described in greater detail in Chapters 4 and 18).

An example of a more traditional benefit plan would be that offered by a commercial insurance company that provides employers with coverage for detoxification as part of the company's basic medical plan at no extra premium cost. Such a plan might have the following elements. Detoxification is covered under the same deductible and copayment schedule as other physical illnesses. Coverage for rehabilitation is offered at an additional premium of $1.20 per month per enrollee. Rehabilitation in a hospital or residential setting is covered for up to 30 days with an additional deductible of $200 and a 20 percent copayment requirement; rehabilitation in an outpatient or day care setting or rehabilitation provided in a private practice setting by a physician or licensed clinical psychologist is covered to a maximum of $1,000 per year, and requires a 50 percent copayment.

A benefit plan is, simply, a list of eligible services and venders that the plan will reimburse on behalf of its beneficiaries. To a large extent the criteria to be used for determining whether a benefit plan should provide coverage for a given condition, procedure, or provider are the same regardless of whether insurance or taxation is the source of payment. The coverage criteria are the same for Medicaid, for the categorical funds administered by the state alcoholism authority, for the block grant, or for health insurance offered by a commercial firm, an HMO, or Blue Cross/Blue Shield.

To set the stage for a discussion of past, present, and future financing levels, it would be useful to know what is being spent today, relative to the costs to society of all the damage caused by alcohol problems does (e.g., Harwood et al., 1984). Unfortunately, existing data do not provide a complete picture of total spending. There are reasonably accurate estimates of spending in specialized treatment facilities (see Chapter 8), and it is possible to construct estimates of inpatient costs for persons hospitalized with a primary diagnosis of alcohol abuse and alcohol dependence. What is quite speculative, however, is the cost of treatment of people with alcohol abuse or alcohol dependence who contact the medical care system for some other complaint as well but who receive treatment for their alcohol problems without a recorded diagnosis. The cost of treatment for hospital admissions with an alcohol-related secondary diagnosis can be estimated, but what is not known is what portion of the cost of those hospital episodes represents direct treatment of the alcohol consumption problem, as opposed to the other conditions.

Using 1983 data adjusted for inflation (Harwood et al., 1985; Davis, 1987), the committee estimates that the level of 1988 spending on specific formal treatment of alcohol problems in all health care settings was more than $6 billion. It was not possible to account for the cost of the informal treatment associated with secondary diagnoses that occurred in hospitals, primary care settings, and nursing homes, but it is unlikely that much of these expenditures were for treatment of the alcohol problem; probably most of the expenditure was for treatment of the primary physical problem. Though not included in previous estimates, the cost of informal treatment outside the medical sector (e.g., Alcoholics Anonymous) is estimated as a real cost (even though no money changes hands) of perhaps $1.5 billion. In total, treatment costs for alcohol problems, even using liberal estimates that will yield a high number, will probably not exceed $10 billion. In comparison with these current levels of expenditure, the estimated cost to society of alcohol problems is more than 10 times as high, generally estimated at $117 billion (Davis, 1987; U.S. Department of Health and Human Services, 1987; Gordis, 1987). These estimates are based on a study conducted by the Research Triangle Institute (Harwood et al., 1984; U.S. Department of Health and Human Services, 1986); an update is currently in progress, but the findings will not be available until next year. Nevertheless, it seems possible to come to the firm conclusion that the current cost of treating alcohol problems is quite small relative to the costs to society that could be avoided if alcohol problems were successfully treated.

In the discussion that follows, the committee has considered the changes that will be required in terms of two options: first, the changes that are necessary to improve the current system of specialist treatment with its multiple sources of financing and variety of methods to access the system and, second, the changes that are required to pay for treatment in the proposed ideal comprehensive treatment system outlined in Chapter 13. In that system (as discussed in Chapter 13) access to the appropriate orientation, setting, and modality at each stage would be controlled through assessment, matching, outcome monitoring, and continuity assurance activities.

Financing the Current Treatment System

Developing and implementing the committee's ideal treatment system will take some time, but it is not unrealistic to consider implementation within a five-year period. In the meantime, the current system of treatment should be financed in a way that is more appropriate than at present and which is conducive to the emergence of the ideal system.

There is obviously a connection between the cost-effectiveness of care (and the absence of evidence for cost-effectiveness) and the certainty that coverage is desirable.

Criteria for Evaluating Coverage Appropriateness

Insurance appropriately covers the cost of uncertain medical care expenses. In an ideal world, the best insurance coverage would be coverage that paid only for appropriate care and nothing else. Insurance itself is costly because of the administrative cost associated with collecting premiums and paying benefits. If the cost of appropriate care is sufficiently large and sufficiently uncertain, then risk-averse people will gain from buying insurance coverage against the cost of this care. Out-of-pocket payment is appropriate when the expense is small, when the expense is more nearly certain, or when full insurance coverage would stimulate inappropriate use.

These principles immediately imply that if there were any type of care which was known to be ineffective for a particular type of problem or person, that type of care should not be covered at all for that type of problem or person. When care is known to be effective (in the sense of yielding positive net benefit), coverage is appropriate if the value placed on that benefit is great enough and the expense is sufficiently large and uncertain. If there are two alternative ways of achieving the same benefit, then the benefit plan should cover only the least costly way.

Finally, when a type of care is of uncertain effectiveness and there is no care that is less costly and of certain effectiveness, policy directions become murkier. In instances in which reasonable people differ about the expected benefit to be received from some type of care, coverage will obviously be appropriate for those who think the benefit is great enough. Where the objective evidence is incomplete but is nevertheless regarded as sufficiently compelling to suggest that the type of care is a reasonable gamble, one could say that coverage is, indeed, appropriate. Yet it would not be appropriate to compel someone who reads the evidence in a different way to buy coverage. In instances in which the evidence is more ambiguous, in which one's conclusion about what is a "good bet" depends on how one reads the literature and what subjective probabilities one attaches to some very uncertain relationships, then perhaps the best strategy is to label coverage for that type of care as neither appropriate nor inappropriate but "neutral." Those who are sufficiently convinced of a positive effect should buy the coverage, but policy advice should be neutral on recommending that a benefit plan include coverage for that type of care.

In real insurance settings, the insurance contract cannot specify or monitor the precise set of circumstances in which benefits are to be provided. Variations in the severity of illness, in the type of person, and in individual preferences can all lead to different choices regarding the appropriate level of care. If, however, insurance pays simply on the basis that care has been rendered and costs incurred, there is a chance that more costly care, even if it is not much more effective than some other type of care, will nevertheless be rendered if both types of care are fully covered by insurance.

If it is not possible to write an insurance contract (i.e., benefit plan) that specifies what is covered unequivocally, without any danger of misinterpretation, what other options are available? As discussed in Chapter 18, there are three broad strategies that have been used: (1) develop insurance that provides complete coverage for care that is usually appropriate (i.e., "effective," "the least cost, given its effectiveness," and "effective enough, given the cost"), less complete coverage (coverage with cost sharing through deductibles and copayments) for care that is less frequently appropriate or of uncertain appropriateness, and no coverage for care that is rarely appropriate; (2) develop coverage that nominally pays for a very wide continuum of services but requires prior approval from an insurer-employed case manager; and (3) develop very broad coverage, but set the maximum price that suppliers will receive at a sufficiently low rate that they will tend to supply the more effective forms of care (i.e., use a reimbursement/payment strategy).

These three strategies are not mutually exclusive; they will, however, be treated separately in the discussion below in order to examine the strengths and weaknesses of each. The separation also benefits the committee's development of a comprehensive coverage strategy, as well as recommendations to implement its proposed plan.

Before proceeding, however, it is important to note that none of these three methods are perfect. Imposing cost sharing provisions or failing to cover some services at all necessarily means that insurance will sometimes fail to pay for care that is appropriate. The only way to avoid the "denial of needed care" (actually the "denial of payment for needed care") is to generate more situations in which payment is made for care that is low in value or high in cost. Moreover, in practice, the use of case managers is another imperfect method. Case managers cost money; they may also lack the information needed to judge appropriateness perfectly. Sometimes it is difficult to motivate them to use properly the information they can obtain. Finally, paying providers just enough to do things right means that people who use inefficient providers or who use providers that call the insurer's "bluff" will not get the care they should.

These principles help us judge alternative ways of financing treatment for alcohol problems. Clearly, if a treatment were to prove ineffective under all circumstances, or even to be equally effective but more costly than available alternatives, insurance coverage would not be appropriate. Judgments about the appropriate financing of services of known or possible effectiveness are more difficult because of uncertainties about effectiveness and the extent and need for care, the value of the effect, and the possibility of insurance-induced inappropriate use all of which need to be taken into account. These issues are considered in the following discussion of the three broad coverage strategies noted earlier in this chapter.

Optimal Conventional Coverage

We begin by using these principles to define what might be desirable coverage of the conventional sort, coverage without extensive case management that pays market prices for medical services. This type of insurance uses out-of-pocket payments to affect beneficiary and provider choices. If a type of care is thought to be wholly inappropriate, there is no coverage, and the person who nevertheless still wants the service must pay for it. Thus, out-of-pocket payment serves as a deterrent to inappropriate use. Coverage will be regarded as appropriate either when it covers treatment that is costly but of great benefit to the individual or if it significantly stimulates use that prevents further utilization (and cost) of other types of already insured medical care.

The committee began its review by attempting to separate the types of care into those that are known to be effective, those that are of probable effectiveness, those that are of uncertain effectiveness, and those that are not known to be effective—all compared with lower cost alternatives. The guiding principle in formulating a recommended strategy is that coverage of care of uncertain (or rare) effectiveness will not be desirable—even though the lack of coverage discourages use of care that is occasionally beneficial. This review obviously required a reconsideration of the evidence on effectiveness described in Chapter 5 and Appendix B. Evaluation of the appropriateness of coverage can be no better, and no more certain, than the evidence on the effectiveness of care. *Given the lack of adequate cost-effectiveness studies comparing alternative treatments, it is not possible at this time to say definitively which treatments should and should not be covered.* It is possible to make recommendations on which strategies should be followed in providing coverage.

On effectiveness grounds, brief interventions, as described in Chapter 9, might be highly appropriate candidates for full insurance coverage. However, the cost of brief interventions is so low that such coverage would be efficient only if it stimulated use. The reason is straightforward: most people could afford the small cost of a brief intervention, and the financial risk attached to this low cost is not great. Insurance coverage would only lead to wasteful paperwork. Things are quite different if the use of brief interventions should prove to be responsive to coverage and if there is a substantial cost offset in the form of lower future medical costs. If insurance coverage of brief interventions causes many more people to seek this form of treatment, given the existence of the cost offset, it would be desirable to expand the use of this type of treatment. However, the critical empirical fact—how the demand for brief intervention responds to its user price—is unknown. In addition, the evidence on the cost offset is more in the "probably a good bet" than in the "sure thing" class.

More important than financing per se (i.e., having insurance pay for brief interventions) would be strategies to ensure that such treatment is available for purchase by larger populations and that information about the treatment's usefulness is provided to the public at large so that they can appropriately seek to purchase brief intervention rather than the more expensive intensive interventions. Making brief interventions widely available in the larger community and within the specialized treatment system will require a reorientation of our existing treatment system, training of treatment providers to use these techniques, and extensive campaigns to inform the public of their availability.

Marginal efficacy has been established for selected more intensive treatments but there has been no documentation of the marginal cost of these interventions or, more importantly, of whether the additional benefit is worth the cost. (That is, for some methods and for some cases, it is known that treatment that is more costly than brief interventions is beneficial, but it is not known whether the additional cost is justifiable.) For more intensive treatment of possible but uncertain effectiveness and for more costly treatment locations (e.g., hospitals or other residential settings), the question arises as to whether the additional benefits that may be realized justify the additional expenditures required to achieve them. Answering this question is a task for future research. As an interim measure, the committee suggests that insurance coverage for intensive and costly services should continue to be furnished but that these services should be utilized cautiously and according to explicit guidelines developed through the consensus process recommended in Chapter 18.

These observations suggested to the committee that its recommendations should be designed to encourage financing for a broad range of alternative settings and modalities at each stage in the treatment process and to permit limitation of the more costly settings to persons with conditions for which that setting is generally appropriate. *Thus, with regard to the currently available system of identification and treatment, the committee recommends that public and private insurance should provide coverage for the following: (a) assessment, reassessment, and continuity assurance to facilitate matching to the appropriate level and intensity of treatment at each stage; (b) brief interventions for alcohol problems, if coverage is needed to facilitate the use of the service; (c) detoxification and other forms of acute intervention in the lowest cost setting of appropriate quality; (d) rehabilitation in the lowest cost setting of appropriate quality; (e) maintenance in the lowest cost setting of appropriate quality; and (f) treatment for as long as is clinically necessary with no prespecified number of inpatient days and/or outpatient sessions as part of desired coverage.*

The intent of this recommendation is to encourage financing for a broad range of alternative sites for therapy at each stage in the treatment process, a strategy which would permit limitation of the more costly sites to persons with conditions for which that site is generally appropriate. As transition occurs and financing moves toward a more ideal system in which assessment and matching become a primary guide to appropriateness, then particular restrictions should become unnecessary. For example, given the lack of support for differential effectiveness of the length of stay in an inpatient rehabilitation program for heterogeneous groups, there seems to be no reason to include a prespecified number of inpatient days or outpatient visits as part of the desired coverage. Rather, the goal would be to provide treatment for as long as clinically necessary.

The committee further recommends that coverage for detoxification and other forms of acute intervention, rehabilitation, and maintenance be provided in both social model and medical model programs. If nonmedical professionals are providing appropriate care of high quality, medical supervision should not necessarily be required for provision of the benefit. Medical consultation, however, should be available and covered by the benefit.

Given the findings of studies that found no greater positive outcomes of treatment in medical model programs compared with mixed medical-social model and social model programs, a medical presence should not necessarily be required for coverage of the service. There has been enough clinical experience and research to persuade the committee that appropriate care of high quality has been and can be provided in these "nonmedical" programs under certain conditions: when there is state licensure or professional accreditation, when there are procedures for referring persons with physical and psychiatric comorbidities to the appropriate treatment setting, and when there is matching of persons seeking treatment to the appropriate orientation, setting, and modality.

From a cost-effectiveness perspective, it is desirable to implement a significant redistribution of resource use from more intensive to less intensive medical model and social model treatments. *Therefore, the committee recommends that in each community, the full range of alternative treatments be established and covered by both public and private financing mechanisms.* That such a distribution of alternative treatment is currently not available can be inferred from the uneven distribution of the "types of care" reported in the 1987 NDATUS and described in Chapter 7. The committee anticipates that the availability of such alternatives as brief intervention in community settings, day care programs, residential programs, and intensive primary rehabilitation outpatient programs will result in a significant redistribution of resource utilization.

The committee believes that such a redistribution is consistent with its understanding of appropriate care within current practices. There are several issues regarding the redistribution: the rate at which it would occur, the magnitude, and the way in which the distribution is to be accomplished. It is clear to the committee that, from what we now know of cost-effectiveness, some restraints should be placed on insurance coverage of the more intense hospital- and residential-based treatments. On the other hand, for a meaningful redistribution to occur, it will be necessary to provide incentives for the development of coverage for less intensive options. Changes in coverage—that is, restrictions on coverage for inpatient and residential treatment—should not be put in place prior to the development of coverage for alternatives and the establishment of quality alternative programs. Implementation of these recommendations will require availability of the full range of appropriate resources.

One sort of restriction is to provide coverage but to specify the types of conditions or situations in which resources are to be utilized. Numerous criteria for determining the appropriateness of an individual's admission to a treatment program and for his or her continuing stay are now operative in insurance and government contracts with private and public sector treatment providers. As discussed in Chapter 18, there has been a proliferation of managed care programs, each with its own criteria for determining the appropriate level of care for a person being treated. As yet there is no common framework; the definitions of levels of care and the criteria used by such programs vary.

Committee members held different opinions regarding appropriate criteria for the utilization of the inpatient level of care. Some members suggested that expert clinical determinations of appropriateness should be the primary guide to resource utilization.

Others maintained that sufficient data were at hand to sharply and categorically restrict inpatient coverage options for care. The committee has reviewed a number of the sets of criteria now in use and found none that it could recommend unequivocally.

Two sets of criteria the committee reviewed are examples of the efforts now under way to restrict the use of more expensive hospital and residential settings. One is the criteria developed for the implementation of a consolidated chemical dependency treatment fund, a statewide program recently instituted by the state of Minnesota (see Chapters 10 and 18). In each county, assessors use uniform guidelines established by the state's Chemical Dependency Program Division to determine the level of care placement for persons who meet the financial eligibility requirements for coverage (Minnesota Chemical Dependency Program Division, 1987, 1989; Minnesota Department of Human Services, 1987). Criteria have been developed for placement in either outpatient care, primary residential care in a freestanding facility or in a hospital setting, or extended care in a residential facility or a halfway house. (These components of the Minnesota continuum of care were described in Chapter 4.)

The basic principles of the Minnesota criteria are that persons should be offered rehabilitation in the least restrictive setting consistent with sound clinical judgment and the availability of an appropriate program. Exceptions can be made, for example, if an outpatient program is not available within a 50-mile radius of the home of the person seeking treatment and the assessor and the individual can agree on an alternative placement. Exceptions can also be made when a culturally specific program at the appropriate level of care is not available and the assessor and individual agree on placement in a culturally specific program at a different level.

The placement criteria employ an assessment of a number of factors to determine the appropriate level of care: level of chemical involvement, social and vocational functioning within the past year, physical health status, emotional health status, history of prior treatment for alcohol and other drug problems, history of specific behaviors when under the influence, and family and friends' support for treatment and achieving program goals. Assessors classify applicants for rehabilitation services into four levels of chemical involvement: (1) no apparent problem, (2) at risk of developing future problems, (3) chemical abuse, or (4) chemical dependence. To be referred for treatment, persons must be assessed as a chemical abuser or as chemically dependent. The specific criteria used are contained in Figure 20-1, which is a copy of the placement summary that documents the appropriateness of the level of care placement.

To be placed in a licensed outpatient treatment program, a person must be assessed as capable of functioning in the usual community environment in spite of the existing chemical use. He or she is either assessed as chemically dependent or as a chemical abuser who has experienced either an arrest or other legal intervention related to chemical use in the past year, loss or impairment of employment or education as a result of chemical use, or the deterioration of family relationships due to chemical use. In contrast, to be placed in primary treatment in either a freestanding residential or hospital setting, the person must be assessed as chemically dependent and unable to abstain from chemical use outside a residential facility that controls access to chemicals. He or she must also be experiencing one or more of the following conditions: loss or impairment of employment or education owing to chemical use; lack of family support; an arrest or legal intervention related to chemical use in the past year; or participation in a chemical dependency treatment program within the past year. To be placed in primary treatment in a hospital setting, the person must also be assessed as either having a physical complication that requires more than detoxification or brief or episodic nursing care or having a mental disorder that requires more than brief or episodic nursing care but that does not otherwise prevent the person from participating in and benefiting from treatment.

Preliminary data from the state's first year of experience with these uniform placement criteria suggest that there has been an increased use of outpatient and halfway house programs and a decreased use of inpatient residential and hospital programs (Minnesota Chemical Dependency Program Division, 1989). Unfortunately, there could be no direct comparison of placements under the old system and the new system because the consolidated fund mechanism has brought together for the first time in one billing system diverse funding sources that previously did not report to the state alcoholism authority. Yet the preliminary analysis is that more persons are receiving treatment at a lower per episode cost in a greater variety of licensed programs. The criteria have not yet been rig-

DHS-2794 (7-87)
PZ-02794-02

PLACEMENT SUMMARY
CHEMICAL USE ASSESSMENT

GENERAL GUIDELINE:
Clients should be offered the least restrictive referral consistent with sound clinical judgment. All items checked must be clearly documented in the client file. This form should remain in the client file.

DEFINITIONS:
CHEMICAL ABUSE: A pattern of inappropriate and harmful use which exceeds social or legal standards of acceptability, the outcome of which includes **at least three** of the following: **Circle** those which are documented.

A. Weekly use to intoxication;
B. Inability to function in a social setting without becoming intoxicated;
C. Driving after consuming sufficient chemicals to be considered legally impaired under Minnesota Statutes, section 169.121, whether or not an arrest takes place;
D. Excessive spending on chemicals that results in an inability to meet financial obligations;
E. Loss of friends due to behavior while intoxicated; or
F. Chemical use that prohibits one from meeting work, school schedule, or social obligations.

CHEMICAL DEPENDENCY: Must meet both PART 1 and PART 2.

PART 1: either ☐ markedly increased tolerance **or** ☐ withdrawal syndrome.

PART 2: a pattern of pathological use. This means compulsive use including **at least three** of the following. **Circle** those which are documented.

A. Daily use required for adequate functioning;
B. An inability to abstain from use;
C. Repreated efforts to control or reduce excessive use;
D. Binge use, such as remaining intoxicated throughout the day for at least two days at a time;
E. Amnesic periods for events occurring while intoxicated; and
F. Continuing use despite a serious physical disorder that the individual knows is exacerbated by continued use.

LICENSED OUTPATIENT	LICENSED PRIMARY RESIDENTIAL	LICENSED EXTENDED	LICENSED HALFWAY

☐ Chemically Dependent
 	
OR
 	
☐ Chemical Abuser **PLUS**
    Chemical Use Caused
☐ Legal in Past Year
    OR
☐ Loss/Impair Voc/Educ
    OR
☐ Family Rel. Deterioration
	☐ Chemically Dependent
	PLUS
	☐ Unable to Abstain
	PLUS
	ONE OR MORE
	☐ Loss/Impair Voc/Educ Due to
	    C.D.
	☐ Lacks Family Support
	☐ Legal in Past Year
	☐ C.D. Treatment in Past Year
	    OR
	☐ Hospitalization due to physi-
	    cal or mental disorder
		☐ Chemically Dependent
		PLUS
		FOUR OR MORE
		☐ Prim. Resid. Past 2 Yrs
		☐ Legal in Past Year
		☐ M.D. Documents Physical
		    Deterior Due to C.D.
		☐ Lacks Family Support
		☐ Lost Voc/Educ Due to CD
		☐ Documented Mental Disorder
		    Under Control
		☐ Lacks Recognition of Need to
		    Change
			☐ Chemically Dependent
			PLUS
			☐ Now in Outpt or was in Detox,
			    Primary, Extended
			PLUS
			THREE OR MORE
			☐ Unable to Abstain
			☐ Lacks Family Support
			☐ Lost Voc/Educ Due to CD
			☐ Lacks Helpful Social Network
			☐ Documented Mental Disorder
			    Under Control

☐ *Exception	☐ *Exception	☐ *Exception	☐ *Exception

*SEE BACK AND CHECK WHICH CATEGORY: ☐ 1. ☐ 2. ☐ 3. ☐ 4. ☐ 5. ☐ 6. ☐ 7. ☐ 8. ☐ OTHER (Explain)

FIGURE 20-1 Minnesota Chemical Dependency Program Division Level of Care Placement Form.

orously evaluated; although comprehensive evaluation is currently being undertaken. It should be noted that these criteria are tied to the existing state continuum of care and a county based funding and assessment mechanism as defined in Minnesota and may not be easily transportable to other states.

The so-called Cleveland criteria (which are discussed in Chapters 11, 15, and 18) represent another, more easily transferable example of the kind of level of care placement guidelines that could be used to determine reimbursement availability as well as to provide clinical guidance in the matching of patients to appropriate levels of care (Hoffmann et al., 1987). In this system, there are six levels of care, that differ in intensity, involvement of professional staff, degree of environmental control, and degree of medical and nursing care available. At each level the type of treatment is specified along with a description of the expected programmatic features of the treatment. Levels of care are ordered from the least to the most intensive and the treatment episode is conceptualized in stages in which it is possible to transfer the person from a higher to a lower level of care as treatment progresses, as well as from a lower to a higher level of care if there is deterioration or a lack of progress. Using such a stepped approach, coverage guidelines could be developed requiring less intensive approaches be tried before the more costly and intensive approaches are used.

Although the Cleveland criteria utilize many of the same variables as are used by the Minnesota consolidated fund uniform criteria in making the level of care placement, the two systems differ in their specific cutoff points for each level and in their definitions of treatment settings and stages. As yet neither has been empirically validated. The lack of uniformity and of empirical validation are also characteristic of other sets of criteria currently in use and evoked concerns from the committee regarding their use—at least at present—as tools for decisions about level of care.

In addition to its consideration of existing sets of criteria, the committee also reviewed a list of criteria prepared by some of its members. These criteria were designed to provide guidance for the use of the most intensive and costly forms of care, namely, hospital and residential care. The guides for coverage would be as follows:

1. Detoxification and other forms of acute intervention should be carried out in the lowest cost setting of appropriate quality.
   a. Detoxification should be carried out in a residential setting if, and only if, one or more of the following conditions is present:
      1. potentially severe withdrawal symptoms or
      2. a nonsupportive psychosocial environment.
   b. Detoxification should be carried out in a medical or psychiatric inpatient hospital setting if, and only if, one or more of the following concomitant health conditions is present:
      1. withdrawal symptoms that require close medical monitoring and continuous nursing care;
      2. severe comorbid medical conditions; or
      3. severe comorbid mental illness.

2. Rehabilitation should occur in the lowest cost setting of appropriate quality.
   a. Rehabilitation should be carried out in a nonresidential (outpatient or day care) setting as the preferred treatment strategy.
   b. Rehabilitation should occur in a residential setting if, and only if, it is required by the disruption of the individual's psychosocial environment.
   c. Rehabilitation should take place in a medical or psychiatric inpatient hospital setting if, and only if, one or more of the following concomitant

health conditions is present in addition to the disruption of the individual's psychosocial environment:

1. severe comorbid mental illness or
2. severe comorbid medical conditions.

Although the Minnesota consolidated fund criteria allow for exceptions and some committee members endorsed the continuing use of clinical judgement, other committee members felt that allowing providers to waive coverage restrictions could, in select circumstances, lead to excessive use of the inpatient option. When the clinical judgment system is used, criteria such as the two sets presented above can form the basis for postadmission audits to determine whether clinicians who are allowed to use their clinical judgement are using each level of care appropriately. Of course, in the long run, outcome monitoring would determine the appropriateness of any set of placement criteria and any exceptions allowed. As was discussed in Chapter 11, placement at the proper level of care is essentially a problem in matching, and any set of criteria must be empirically tested against the criterion of most favorable outcome and lowest marginal cost.

Although the committee does not recommend a particular set of criteria for inpatient coverage in this report, it has concluded that, in general, a significant number of persons now cared for in inpatient facilities could receive appropriate care in less restrictive and less costly settings, if and when treatment in such settings were available. As discussed in Chapters 11 and 18, *the committee recommends that a consensus activity be carried out to develop a common set of definitions and criteria for determining appropriate type and level of care placement at each stage of treatment, and that the criteria that are adopted be based on available research as well as the broadest range of shared clinical experience.* Although a number of vehicles could be designed to conduct this activity, an expert committee convened on a regular basis to review what is known about matching would seem to be the most appropriate vehicle.

There was agreement within the committee that, if more alternative treatment approaches and guidelines for their use are to be placed in the existing system in order to achieve a redistribution of resource use, a transition period would be essential. Such a transition, while providing the mechanisms for redistribution (including restrictions and incentives), would take into account the overall effects of such a policy on patient care. In particular, it is imperative that the alternative forms of less intensive and less costly treatments (e.g., partial hospitalization, social setting detoxification, outpatient care) should be available before constraints are placed on more intensive treatments. The committee reflected on other experiences germane to this consideration—for instance, the problems that arose with the deinstitutionalization of patients from psychiatric hospitals (IOM, 1988) and the decriminalization of public intoxication (Finn, 1985; Wittman and Madden, 1988). In these situations less intensive or alternative services were specified but were not adequately provided in many communities. The committee wishes to emphasize that what it is recommending here is an expansion and redistribution of resource utilization and not an abrupt curtailment of existing services.

These recommendations avoid, on the one hand, the current problem of a lack of realistic coverage for more cost effective outpatient alternatives and, on the other hand, the problem of inpatient use expanding to the maximum number of days for which coverage is available. Specifying in insurance documents the conditions or disorders for which certain types of treatment are appropriately covered is bound to be imperfect; consequently efforts to match persons to sites or types of treatment will add benefits to this system. As proposed, coverage does, however, cover the spectrum of treatment alternatives so that any appropriate match should carry coverage along with it.

At one extreme end of the spectrum, coverage for inpatient treatment is unlimited in terms of days but is limited in terms of conditions. At the other extreme, it may not even be necessary to pay explicitly for brief interventions: the advice and information that constitute such "treatment" may already be included in a covered medical encounter or may be of such low cost that explicit coverage is unnecessary to encourage use. In both cases, there is considerable room for research to refine these indications. Moreover, these recommendations speak only to minimum desirable coverage. A buyer, especially a private buyer, who wants to provide more generous coverage would, of course, be free to do so if the cost were covered either through the premiums paid or the tax revenue available.

The ideal method would be to cover treatment for alcohol problems in the same manner that coverage is provided for effective treatment of medical problems, rather than under a separate benefit with the restrictions described above. Inappropriate use would then be controlled by the same mechanisms that are available for other medical conditions, and any restrictions would become part of the utilization review standards rather than a model benefit. *Therefore, the committee recommends that coverage for the treatment of alcohol problems should be subject to the same deductibles, coinsurance, limits, case management, and utilization review as are applied to coverage of treatment for other medical conditions.* Of course, as the coverage in conventional insurance changes—whether that change is a modification in cost sharing or in greater use of case management—the same sort of change would be appropriate for the coverage of treatment for alcohol problems. This "uniform coverage" recommendation is most easily applicable when the insurance policy is a so-called "comprehensive" policy, paying the same fraction of approved charges for all medical services after the deductible is covered. If the base plan provides different levels of coverage for different types of treatment (e.g., Medicare), coverage for treatment for alcohol problems would follow the same general rules as does coverage of treatment for physical problems.

Paying for the Current Treatment System

If these propositions about desirable, undesirable, and possibly desirable (or optional) insurance coverage are near the mark, how should they affect policy in private and public insurance, the two major methods of paying for treatment of alcohol problems? This question is considered in the discussion that follows.

Encouragement, Subsidization, or Mandation of Private Health Insurance There are several ways to affect private group health insurance purchases. One way is simply to provide information to buyers about which coverage makes the most sense, which coverage does not make sense, and why. Benefits managers, whether employed by the employer or by a union, do not want to waste money and do not want to deny benefits of high value (e.g., Tsai et al., 1988). Consequently, they may well pay attention to such encouragement, especially if the information and advice is embodied in a model policy that is carefully constructed.

A second method is subsidization. Group health insurance already receives substantial federal and state/local tax subsidies because of the exclusion of premiums and benefits from taxation. For many firms (as noted earlier), especially large firms with high-wage workers, this subsidy has been sufficient to stimulate coverage. Because the size of the tax subsidy rises with the marginal tax rate on wages, the subsidy, not surprisingly, is strongly related to an employee's likelihood of receiving coverage for treatment of alcohol problems (or any coverage). The notion that the current tax subsidy is not well designed to achieve efficiency, equity, and social objectives is not new (Pauly, 1986); the additional possibility here would be to limit tax deductibility to coverage that meets the appropriateness criterion the committee has outlined. If inpatient treatment of alcohol problems should be reserved for a restricted subset of persons with alcohol problems, there is no obvious reason to permit payments for such coverage for other individuals (should someone wish to offer them such coverage) to escape taxation. Any taxes collected on such payments could be used to enhance the tax subsidy to appropriate coverage, especially for low-wage workers.

The mandating of coverage by government is a third method of affecting private health insurance purchases. As discussed in Chapter 18, many state governments now mandate that treatment for alcohol problems be covered in any health insurance policy, or that its coverage be offered as an option. Frequently, the mandate specifically includes inpatient treatment and sometimes does not include outpatient treatments or treatment in nonmedical settings.

Therefore, the committee recommends that existing state mandates and public programs be modified to be consistent with its recommended strategy. Should new mandates and public programs be enacted, they should be designed to reflect these recommendations. Those national organizations which have been involved in the development of model benefit packages (e.g., the National Council on Alcoholism, the National Association of State Alcohol and Drug Abuse Program Directors, NIAAA, the Alcohol and Drug Problems Association, the National Association of Insurance Commissioners) should be encouraged to develop a model policy format that embodies these principles.

The committee, however, did not take a position on state mandates per se. On the one hand, encouraging coverage for effective treatment that provides substantial benefit is obviously desirable. On the other hand, the encouragement mandates may give to self-insurance and the possibility that other mandated benefits that push up premiums will accompany mandates for treatment for alcohol problems, possibly driving premiums out of reach of some purchasers, suggest that mandates are not always the best way to encourage coverage. In some circumstances providing persuasive information on the benefits of coverage for treatment of alcohol problems may well be preferable to new mandates. Conducting adequate research on the cost-effectiveness of alternative treatments is critical to providing such information to those who develop the specifics of financing policy; it is also necessary for any strong endorsement of mandates. The lack of research in this area is one of the causes of the continuing discomfort on the part of third-party payers with current treatment providers.

Recognizing the difficult and complex nature of mandated coverage of all types, the committee is not prepared to suggest either extension or contraction of this mechanism. The committee suggests that mandates be reviewed to determine whether they support the principles outlined in this chapter (i.e., the committee's interpretation of the current research findings). Judicious use of case management, described in the next section, may be an effective way to deal with existing mandated inpatient benefits under the current treatment system.

Case Managed Coverage As discussed in Chapter 18, case management has become a more prominent strategy for obtaining appropriate resource use and cost containment by both public and private third-party payers (e.g., Temkin-Geser and Clark, 1988; Tsai et al., 1988). The focus of case management has been primarily on reducing the cost of lengthy inpatient stays, and the treatment of alcohol problems within expensive hospital settings has been a major target of these efforts. If case management could be perfect, if case management could be costless, if case management could be the alter ego of ideal matching, recommending coverage policy would be simple: there should be complete coverage of a whole spectrum of services with case management determining what would actually be covered in each individual case. There is no rigorous evidence on the cost or the effects of case management, however; nor is it known how to bring about an approximation of perfection.

On the positive side, it certainly seems sensible to encourage work toward a system of case managed coverage for treatment of alcohol problems, the more so because case management fits so well with the matching approach the committee believes, in principle, to be most effective for delivering treatment. The development of model benefit packages and model case management procedures should be a high priority. Such an approach would permit the treatment of alcohol problems to be covered in the same nominal way as any other medical service, although case management for this type of care might lead to a quite different pattern of actual benefits.

The committee prefers to speak of the required function and role of case managers as "continuity assurance" (see Chapter 13). This distinction is critical in that case management has become identified (primarily by providers, although also by employers and persons seeking treatment) with the effort to cut costs by reducing the care provided, rather than by developing a plan for matching a person to the most appropriate treatment regimen at each treatment stage. The committee's stance is that the addition of assessment and reassessment, coupled with the emphasis on outcome monitoring in its proposed system, makes case management a legitimate clinical endeavor, one that has been severely lacking in the treatment of alcohol problems under a unitary model of problems and treatment.

The information-subsidization-mandation question also arises regarding case managed coverage. Such coverage should, if it fulfills its promise, virtually sell itself to most insurance buyers, public or private. Mandation, however, raises some additional issues. The employer or union that only adds benefits for treatment of alcohol problems only because of a mandate will presumably seek a case manager that is especially adept at limiting benefit payments. It may prove administratively difficult to deal with a mandated case-managed benefit, and the committee's previous cautions on mandation also apply here. One strategy to prevent reluctant employers or unions from limiting benefits through case management would be to set a minimum average or expected value for such benefits.

Supply Side or Reimbursement Limits   Reimbursement or payment policy can also be used to promote more cost-effective care. Payment on a prospective basis, payment of an amount sufficient on average to pay only for outpatient care, and other uses of reimbursement incentives that restrict access to certain settings may be worthwhile. Specific evidence of the impact of these strategies on the treatment of alcohol problems is lacking at this time. Therefore, it is premature to criticize these approaches or to suggest the adoption of one or more specific mechanisms.

Given the committee's recommendation that the coverage of treatment for alcohol problems be the same as that for all medical conditions, it sees no reason to exclude this treatment from the current experimentation with alternative reimbursement methods. It suggests only that there be very careful study of the specific effects of reimbursement methods on utilization and outcome. If a population of persons with alcohol problems could be identified, the payment of providers on a capitation basis would probably be desirable.

Public Financing and Public Insurance   Governments, especially state governments, currently play a major role in the financing and delivery of treatment for alcohol problems. Historically, the role has been undertaken as part of government's function of expressing the community's concern about the well-being of its less fortunate citizens. Beyond this, however, it is difficult to find a coherent articulation of the public sector's special role in financing treatment or in providing treatment for people with alcohol problems. The enormous variation across states in the extent of public involvement probably reflects this uncertainty. The committee views public provision of care (the source of care paid for through taxes) as largely an expression of the state's welfare function—a manifestation of the desire of all citizens that those who might injure themselves or others be helped if they do not have the resources to help themselves.

Governmental involvement in the treatment of alcohol problems takes a variety of forms. At one extreme, some people are eligible for various kinds of government insurance that pays for some treatment of alcohol problems. (For example, Medicare provides limited coverage and Medicaid provides a more extensive range of benefits for the categorically eligible poor and disabled, all available through providers of care who conform to the medical model of treatment.) Some states effectively administer their categorical program of treatment for alcohol problems as if it were a disease-specific insurance policy for the categorically eligible poor and disabled. State programs generally are available through a wide range of providers who use both the social and medical models. At the other extreme, some state and county systems are basically producers of treatment for alcohol problems, controlling production, volume, and cost directly by means of ownership or contracting, or both.

For historical reasons, states have been major funders and providers of public treatment for alcohol problems. The federal government's role has receded in recent years, while that of local governments seems to be growing. Since more than half of all specialty treatment for alcohol problems is paid for by state and local funds, and the states and local governmental units are major providers of treatment as well, practical and political considerations suggest that the main locus of governmental control should remain with the states. To the extent it is possible, this financial obligation should then be matched with the financial control embodied in a consolidated fund which would permit more rational spending of public funds. The Minnesota Consolidated Chemical Dependency Treatment Fund is an example of mechanisms for controlling access and cost which should be followed by other state alcoholism authorities and the federal government. The federal government, in particular, needs to consider such consolidation in both its contributions to community-based service provision through the block grant, Medicare, Medicaid, and the federal employees' health insurance program and its direct operations in the Department of Defense, the Department of Veterans Affairs, and the Indian Health Service.

The kind of "coverage" that would be provided by governmentally sponsored public health insurance would not differ in design from the coverage for appropriate care that was discussed earlier in this chapter. It seems to be well-established practice that such appropriate care need not be as extensive, as costly, or (often) as inefficient as what well-to-do citizens might choose to buy for themselves. The notion of appropriateness here seems quite consistent with that of the President's Commission for the Study of Ethical Problems in Medicine and Biomedical Behavioral Research (1983).

Practical and political considerations also imply that state spending for treatment will probably remain means tested through a sliding scale of charges or subsidies (e.g., eligibility and fee level determined by income and other expenses). At some sufficiently adequate income level, the state subsidy would be terminated altogether and the person expected to pay the full cost, either directly or through private insurance.

The same considerations that were applied to private insurance regarding case management and reimbursement limits are pertinent to public financing. Again, the committee asserts that the same general principles for determining optimum coverage and for controlling costs should govern both publicly and privately financed treatment for alcohol problems.

Financing the Ideal Treatment System

In considering methods for financing the treatment system proposed by the committee, the overall principle is that public and private insurance financing should cover a broad range of treatment alternatives so that care will be effective and worth the cost. The new method of screening for and treating alcohol problems described in Section III of this report is justified, the committee believes, on the grounds of producing large benefits relative to its cost. Moreover, intrinsic to the method is a set of devices for matching and monitoring the quality and cost of care that should limit care to that which is appropriate.

As a consequence, it should not be necessary to use out-of-pocket payments or benefit limitations as substitute methods for controlling costs.

The committee recognizes that broadening the base of the spectrum of intervention responses to include more individuals with mild and moderate alcohol problems and sharpening the apex to include more outpatient treatment capacity may raise concerns that it is recommending vast increases in the amount of funding needed for treatment. Although data on which to develop projections of any additional costs are not available, the committee believes that any additions can be largely paid for by the savings generated from matching persons to the most appropriate intervention strategies early in the course of development of their alcohol problems when treatment is likely to be more effective and less costly.

Yet sound estimates of any additional costs to be generated or any costs to be saved cannot be developed because there are few good data available. The committee attempted to develop such projections and rejected the approach because of the paucity of sound data of costs in each of the sectors that will be impacted by the change. Instead, the committee has chosen to illustrate how the new system would be financed and what its cost-benefit would be by continuing to elaborate on the vignettes introduced earlier (see Chapter 2). Consider, for instance, the case of Elizabeth who lives and works in the California wine country. Elizabeth was hospitalized after vomiting blood and passing out. Her high level of daily wine consumption, which was previously thought to be in conformity with the practices of her family, is now identified as a problem, and she is seen by her physician as requiring specialist treatment. She is employed and has health insurance that will cover up to 30 days of rehabilitation for alcohol problems in a general hospital; the policy has a $1,000 limit on outpatient treatment. She would probably be willing to seek treatment, and the prognosis would be good. Given the orientation of the majority of treatment programs under the current system, her presenting symptoms, and insurance coverage, referral would most likely be to a fixed-length 28-day medically supervised, hospital-based primary rehabilitation program at a cost of approximately $15,000 (based on the 1987 average cost per day of $537 for 28 days). In contrast, working from the alcohol problems perspective, as presented in Chapter 2 and Section III, Elizabeth would be seen as experiencing substantial alcohol problems and to be a good candidate for outpatient rehabilitation in a freestanding day care program with medical consultation (following her discharge from the hospital for treatment of her physical problems) at a cost of $3,900 ($130 per session for 30 sessions). There would also be the likelihood of a substantial cost offset, (that is, a reduction in future costs for treating the alcohol-involved physical illness); consequently, the net cost would be reduced for both treatments if she entered treatment immediately.

The prevalence of persons with substantial alcohol problems, like Elizabeth, is estimated at 6 percent of the adult population (18 years of age and above). The likelihood that she and others who are experiencing substantial problems will be identified and referred to treatment is unknown, but estimates range from 15 to 55 percent. Persons with problems similar to those of Elizabeth are estimated to account for approximately two-thirds of those who enter specialist treatment in hospital settings under the current system in which the full spectrum of intervention responses is not available. Assuming that a significant proportion of these individuals can be identified earlier and can be treated in lower cost residential and outpatient settings or in brief intervention settings involving no additional cost, there should be sufficient savings to pay for the cost of outcome monitoring and continuity assurance and to increase the proportion of persons who can be treated. The amount of savings depends on the proportion of current admissions that can be redirected. There is no set of studies available that can be used to develop projections. Such studies are sorely needed.

Consider Patrick, the foundry worker who enjoys drinking with his workmates in the evening and on weekends. Under the current system, Patrick's need for rehabilitation would probably not be identified despite his recent absenteeism and family history. In the proposed system, however, Patrick's moderate level of alcohol problems would be picked up through screening; the optimal referral would be to a brief intervention in the general health care system or, if available, in his company's employee assistance program. The additional cost for a brief intervention if done in the general health care system is estimated to be zero or, at most, $280 ($70 per session for 4 sessions), if done in the specialist system. These costs are in contrast to a zero explicit medical cost under the current system.

Under the current system, David, the star salesman whose drinking is injuring his health, is most likely to be referred by his physician to a specialist inpatient hospital program because of his health problems, his "denial" of the existence of excessive drinking, and his work environment, which is not considered to be supportive of recovery. In any event, David would probably refuse a referral to any treatment, particularly an inpatient program. More appropriate choices would be a brief intervention or a course of outpatient rehabilitation. If David's physician were trained in brief intervention and relapse prevention techniques, then this method would be appropriate and less likely to be resisted. For David, like Patrick, this brief intervention would add a cost where there had been none previously. Bringing additional persons with a moderate level of alcohol problems like David and Patrick into treatment suggests an aggregate cost increase. Estimates of the prevalence of this level of problems or of the number of such individuals now in treatment at each level of care are not available to serve as the basis for projecting aggregate costs and savings. Provided such persons can be successfully treated using brief interventions, however, any increase should be small. Yet any near term cost increase is likely to be much less than if either David or Patrick continued drinking and later needed more intensive and expensive medical, psychiatric, or alcohol problems treatment.

Let us assume that Sally, the young assistant receptionist with a speech impediment, has recognized spontaneously that her daily relief drinking has become a problem and seeks assistance. Her spontaneous recognition that she had moved from drinking to relieve her anxiety to drinking for enjoyment makes her a good candidate for treatment. Under the current system, Sally most likely would be referred for a course of outpatient treatment. Under the committee's proposed system, Sally would be an excellent candidate for a brief intervention. Here, the savings in the individual case could be approximately $1,800, the difference between the cost of an outpatient rehabilitation episode and a brief intervention. Once they have been identified and referred to formal specialist treatment, the proportion of persons with mild alcohol problems like Sally who are treated in outpatient settings is estimated to be about one-third under the current system in which the full spectrum of intervention responses recommended by the committee is not available. This proportion is projected to decrease by half under the proposed comprehensive system. Redirecting to brief interventions those persons with mild problems (e.g., Sally) who are now being treated in outpatient programs should also yield a net savings.

Consider the cases of Jimmy, who has chronic severe alcohol problems, and William, who has chronic but intermittent substantial alcohol problems. Jimmy has been through standard inpatient rehabilitation programs and Alcoholics Anonymous several times, relapsing after a period of several months on each occasion and continuing to deteriorate emotionally, physically, and socially. William has not received any formal treatment and manages to maintain a marginal work and social existence between drinking bouts. Both require extended formal treatment (maintenance and relapse prevention) of the type that does not now exist in most communities—Jimmy in a long-term alcohol-free living facility (categorized as custodial/domiciliary in the 1987 NDATUS) and William in an outpatient setting. There is likely to be no savings generated in either of these cases, because the activity required is not currently available. In Jimmy's case, a cost offset may occur as the lower cost supportive living environment reduces the need for repeated hospitalizations to treat DTs, pancreatitis, and other physical illnesses. Again, however, the prevalence of such cases and their costs under the current and proposed systems are only speculative at this time, given the lack of comparative data.

The committee has reviewed several schemes for moving beyond these vignettes to project changes in referral patterns and utilization levels but finds that none are adequate to provide policy guidance at this time. Its review does suggest that there could be a decrease of about one-third of the current admissions to inpatient programs if the proposed comprehensive system were put in place. Redirecting those persons to day care or outpatient programs or to brief interventions could yield a substantial net saving from current levels of spending. However, the committee recognizes that any savings to be achieved in this area of funding could be absorbed by the increase in services involved in broadening the base of treatment to include those with mild and moderate alcohol problems. It is the committee's hope that the creation of alternatives and the ability to match persons to the appropriate treatment will bring additional persons with severe and substantial problems who are not now being seen into both nonspecialist brief interventions and specialist treatment. Prompt early treatment can decrease the need for later, more expensive treatment.

Implementing the new treatment system described in Section III will require that benefit plans offered by all payers, both public and private, incorporate the principles outlined in these recommendations into a single strategy. Such an approach must include the use of empirically determined matching criteria that are continuously validated through outcome monitoring as the method of access to the appropriate setting and modality at each stage of treatment. Given the redirection aspect of the proposed system (i.e., providing prompt treatment in lower cost sites), the committee anticipates that the savings offered by the system would be sufficient to cover the costs of the expanded treatment options and the continuity assurance activities, as well as to attract more persons into treatment. Indeed, the committee would make the same recommendations even if there were short-term increases in costs because of the long-term reductions in social costs that can be anticipated.

Therefore, the committee recommends that sufficient insurance coverage be provided to facilitate adequate access to the continuum of services included in the new system: screening, assessment, treatment, reassessment, maintenance, and continuity assurance. Because the new system will use both matching and a type of case manager to provide continuity assurance, the use of inappropriately costly care should be less likely than under the old system. Accordingly, more generous coverage for the new system might be possible. The committee reiterates its support for and recommendation of the "uniform coverage rule" here as the minimum required coverage—that is, coverage for the treatment of alcohol problems should be governed by the same principles as coverage for physical problems.

Financing the Vision: Paying for Specialized Treatment Services for the Poor and the Uninsured

In the committee's view, it is clear that payment for the cost of specialized treatment services should ultimately be included in some system of comprehensive coverage for all citizens and for all conditions. For the poor, this premise means that, in an ideal setting, the payment system ought to combine the dollars available from all sources for covering treatment for alcohol problems and in turn combine those dollars with the resources available in the health care system for covering other kinds of treatments. In line with the principle of insuring treatment for alcohol problems on the same basis and in the same way as other treatment for illnesses is insured, no distinction in coverage should be made based on the condition requiring the treatment.

Yet moving the financing of alcohol problems treatment from its current state to what is ultimately recommended, even when the ideal treatment system comes into existence, is no small task. However logical the uniform payment approach, the current problem of paying for treatment for poor citizens is complicated by the fact that these citizens are either covered by Medicaid or a state or locally financed medical assistance plan or are uninsured. The problem in paying for other citizens is that some fraction of them is not insured privately or publicly as well. Minnesota's consolidated fund administered by the state alcoholism authority is one approach for fostering integration of the diverse sources of public funds that must be used to pay for the proposed comprehensive system. *The committee recommends that, in addition to monitoring the progress of this effort, demonstrations of other approaches also be undertaken and evaluated.*

For those low-income people covered by Medicaid, the situation is complicated because these services are covered in a variety of ways across states (Toff, 1984). Although there may be some scope for allowing states to vary the form of coverage in accord with their circumstances and to vary the extent of coverage with state taxpayer generosity, the committee believes that there should probably be more uniformity—and a higher basic level of coverage—than at present. In a few states, the service dollars earmarked for the treatment of alcohol problems are combined with Medicaid funds when the Medicaid recipient requires specialized alcohol treatment services. This integration fits well with the committee's concept of combining alcohol treatment financing generally with insurance for other medical conditions. Outcomes are ultimately constrained by the availability of resources, but using those resources for Medicaid beneficiaries in a more integrated way would probably be more efficient and more equitable.

Nevertheless there is still a long way to go. Most states have not integrated their Medicaid and their categorically funded programs for treatment of alcohol problems. In addition, many of the poor are not eligible for Medicaid. Their "default insurance" is frequently uncompensated care in a hospital's emergency room, a budgetary account which is difficult to combine with state treatment monies into a single fund in any case (Gage et al., 1988). For people who are not poor but are uninsured, neither Medicaid nor uncompensated care are viable options.

For the uninsured, both poor and nonpoor alike, the state-funded specialist treatment system is likely to be the real insurer for the treatment of alcohol problems. At least until the problem of the generally uninsured is solved, it may be best to try to make this system work. That commitment probably means more generous funding of treatment for alcohol problems so that all who need care can receive it. In addition, it probably means using a method of payment that makes use of the entire medical care treatment system, rather than relying only on specialist state-provided alcohol treatment services. It probably also means using a sliding scale of fees (low or zero for the poor but rising for others) so that a reasonable percentage of out-of-pocket revenues are generated in each state and the public treatment system does not become more attractive than private insurance coverage.

The ultimate objective is clear: everyone should have some insurance and that insurance should combine alcohol treatment funding into a single policy or plan, to be supplemented by out-of-pocket payment in instances when doing so will not discourage cost-effective treatment. While we wait for the emergence of a fully rational and complete system of health care financing, an interim solution would be to build on and improve Medicaid and the state categorical funding systems now in place. For Medicaid, this strategy would mean the combination of funds into a payment package that is appropriately generous in terms of coverage and payment to providers for appropriate treatments. For the other uninsured, it means a revision of the state financing system to produce one with better funding (i.e., funding that is more equitable across states and tied to need), more flexible "coverage" of alternative providers in different settings, and a sliding scale of fees tailored to the responsiveness of the demand for treatment.

States are featured prominently in this transitional system because they are of central importance in the current approach to paying for treatment of alcohol problems and because there does not seem to be a principle that would argue against this role. However, as discussed in Chapters 7 and 8, the states now vary substantially in their financing and administration of alcohol treatment services. Research tells us that state spending varies enormously (Institute for Health and Aging, 1986) (see Chapter 8). It also reveals that the availability of alternative forms of treatment varies tremendously across the states (see Chapter 7). What is not known is what such variation means for access to needed treatment; in part, the reason for this uncertainty arises from a lack of knowledge about the need for effective and economical treatment.

As one means to reduce that variability, the committee recommends that the state-funded specialist systems incorporate an income-related sliding scale of fees. A federal minimum standard could be developed and made part of the federal block grant requirements. Specific priority should be set to determine the allocation of funds to free care for the poor versus partially paid programs for the nonpoor who are not covered for specific treatment of alcohol problems.

One could well envision the formulation of a federal minimum standard requirement, for both Medicaid and state specialist programs (through the alcohol, drug abuse, and mental health services block grant) which ensures that benefits and eligibility do not sink below some minimal level. Above this level, states should try to choose the level of coverage and form of reimbursement that supports only the most effective programs in terms of treatment and costs.

As noted earlier, however, existing knowledge does not identify that minimum level or the most effective programs. As new information becomes available, states should be strongly encouraged to structure their "categorical benefit plans" toward what are known to be the most effective forms of treatment. Any federal minimum level of coverage should also be varied as new information becomes available on the effectiveness of alternative treatment forms. The proposed expert committee described above could provide independent, objective monitoring of the data.

What is known at present is that maximum effectiveness requires the matching of persons with alcohol problems to treatment methods at each stage of the treatment process. Currently, Medicaid and state categorical programs do not include the full range of effective treatment options and are not designed to encourage assessment and matching. The committee encourages greater cooperation between these programs at the federal and state levels of government to design "consolidated" trials of the vision of treatment offered in this report.

One further step, which is difficult to implement in the current era of cost containment and budget stringency but worth considering for the near future, would be to test a program that provides automatic access for a year to Medicaid coverage for anyone below a specified income level who is judged to need specialized services for the treatment of alcohol problems and who continues in a treatment program. In this sense, the presence of serious alcohol problems would become one of the categories for Medicaid eligibility, and continued eligibility for Medicaid would depend on remaining in treatment. The state-funded specialist treatment system would continue to treat people who are unable to continue in the Medicaid specialist program. The attractiveness of Medicaid coverage for treatment of other medical care needs would offer some incentive to comply with and stay in the alcohol treatment program.

These considerations are crucial in developing a mechanism for financing the proposed comprehensive system that integrates the specialist financing of treatment for alcohol problems with the other major vehicle of financing treatment of medical problems for the poor and uninsured. Their importance leads the committee to recommend that Medicaid and the state-funded specialist systems should be expanded to provide integrated coverage of treatment of alcohol problems for those eligible for Medicaid and for the uninsured. This treatment should be available in a variety of medical model and social model settings and should implement the principles of the "vision" as much as is possible.

As better results on the effectiveness and cost-effectiveness of alternative treatment modalities, settings, and insurance coverage become available, the committee recommends that they be incorporated into the design of these consolidated state systems. Including provisions for outcome monitoring is crucial for such feedback and refinement.

REFERENCES

Davis, K. 1987. The organization and financing of alcohol and drug abuse services. Presented to the Annual Meeting of the Institute of Medicine, Washington, D.C., October 21.

Finn, P. 1985. Decriminalization of public drunkenness: Response of the health care system. Journal of Studies on Alcohol 46:7-22.

Gage, L. S., D. P. Andrulis, and V. Beers. 1987. America's Health Safety Net: A Report on the Situation of Public Hospitals in our Nation's Metropolitan Areas. Washington, D.C.: National Association of Public Hospitals.

Gordis, E. 1987. Accessible and affordable health care for alcoholism and related problems: Strategy for cost containment. Journal of Studies on Alcohol 48:579-585.

Harwood, H. J., P. Kristiansen, and J. V. Rachal. 1985. Social and economic costs of alcohol abuse and alcoholism. Issue Report No. 2. Research Triangle Institute, Research Triangle Park, N.C.

Harwood, H. J. D. M. Napolitano, P. L. Kristiansen, and J. J. Collins. 1984. Economic Costs to Society of Alcohol and Drug Abuse and Mental Illness: 1980. Prepared for the Alcohol, Drug Abuse, and Mental Health Administration. Research Triangle Park, N. C.: Research Triangle Institute.

Hoffmann, N. G., J. A. Halikas, and D. Mee-Lee. 1987. The Cleveland Admission, Discharge and Transfer Criteria: Model for Chemical Dependency Treatment Programs. Prepared for the Northern Ohio Chemical Dependency Treatment Directors Association. Cleveland: Greater Cleveland Hospital Association.

Institute for Health and Aging. 1986. Review and Evaluation of Alcohol, Drug Abuse and Mental Health Services Block Grant Allotment Formulas: Final Report. Prepared for Alcohol, Drug Abuse, and Mental Health Administration. San Francisco, Calif.

Institute of Medicine. 1988. Homelessness, Health, and Human Needs. Washington, D.C.: National Academy Press.

Minnesota Chemical Dependency Program Division. 1987. Biennial Report to the Governor and the Minnesota Legislature. St. Paul: Minnesota Department of Human Services.

Minnesota Chemical Dependency Program Division. 1989. Report to the State Legislature on the Status of the Consolidated Chemical Dependency Treatment Fund. St. Paul: Minnesota Department of Human Services.

Minnesota Department of Human Services. 1987. Consolidated Chemical Dependency Treatment Fund: County and Reservation Training Manual. Saint Paul, Minn.: Minnesota Department of Human Services.

Pauly, M. 1986. Taxation, health insurance, and market failure in the medical economy. Journal of Economic Literature 24:629-675.

President's Commission for the Study of Ethical Problems in Medicine and Biomedical Behavioral Research. 1983. Securing Access to Health Care: The Ethical Implications in the Availability of Differences. Washington, D.C.: U.S. Government Printing Office.

Temkin-Geser, H., and K. T. Clark. 1988. Ethnicity, gender, and utilization of mental health services in a Medicaid population. Social Sciences in Medicine 26:989-996.

Toff, G. E. 1984. Mental Health Benefits under Medicaid: A Survey of the States. Washington, D.C.: Intergovernmental Health Project, George Washington University.

Tsai, S. P., S. M. Reedy, E. J. Bernacki, and E. S. Lee. 1988. Effect of curtailed insurance benefits on the use of mental health care: The Tenneco plan. Medical Care 26:430-440.

U.S. Department of Health and Human Services (USDHHS). 1986. Toward a National Plan to Combat Alcohol Abuse and Alcoholism. Report submitted to the United States Congress. Rockville, Md.: National Institute on Alcohol Abuse and Alcoholism.

U.S. Department of Health and Human Services (USDHHS). 1987. Sixth Special Report to the U.S. Congress on Alcohol and Health. Rockville, Md.: National Institute on Alcohol Abuse and Alcoholism.

Wittman, F. D., and P. A. Madden. 1988. Alcohol Recovery Programs for Homeless People: A Survey of Current Programs in the U.S. Rockville, Md.: National Institute on Alcohol Abuse and Alcoholism.

21 Leadership

Before discussing what needs to be done in the future to implement its recommendations and its vision, the committee wishes to acknowledge and to commend what has been accomplished in the past. The Cooperative Commission on the Study of Alcoholism was the first body that attempted to consider the treatment of alcohol problems from a national perspective; the commission was originally established in 1961 through the efforts of the North American Association of Alcoholism Programs, an organization of United States and Canadian government programs, with funding provided by the National Institute on Mental Health. In the slightly more than 20 years since the commission issued its report (Plaut, 1967), there has been a remarkable increase in the scope, quality and availability of treatment for alcohol problems. A review of some of the commission's conclusions and recommendations can be helpful in illustrating the progress that has been made in recent years. As noted in its report, the state of affairs when the commission began its work in 1967 was problematic:

> Public attitudes and feelings about drinking and about alcohol abuse have significantly influenced the way services for alcoholics have developed. The belief that the problem drinker cannot be helped—sometimes referred to as "therapeutic nihilism"—and the view that the condition is "self inflicted" result in the problem drinker's frequently being ignored by most helping agencies and by many professional workers.
>
> Hospitals, psychiatric agencies, public welfare departments and social agencies among others are often reluctant to provide care and treatment for problem drinkers; they tend to neglect or reject them. An understanding of the nature of problem drinking and its management is often limited in such helping agencies. Certain services generally available to patients with other disorders are frequently denied to problem drinkers by policy or practice. These include hospital insurance coverage, admission to general hospitals, assistance by public-welfare agencies, voluntary admission to mental hospitals and participation in most mental hospital after-care programs. (Plaut, 1967:53)

Surveys of the general U.S. population and of care givers indicate that alcohol problems are now seen as treatable. Some pessimism, however, remains among legislators, the general public, and professionals (e.g., Skinner, and Holt, 1987), and vestiges of the attitudes encountered by the commission are still present. Yet the questions raised today are less likely to be about whether treatment is effective or whether treatment should be provided than about the relative effectiveness and cost-effectiveness of different treatment approaches with specific subgroups. There has, in a word, been considerable growth in the level of overall sophistication about alcohol problems and their management. The common distinction between the pessimist and the optimist applies in determining where we stand today as a nation in regard to the effectiveness of treatment for alcohol problems: either the glass is half empty, or the glass is half full. Based on its deliberations, the committee is optimistic. We choose to regard the glass as half full and to emphasize that great progress has been achieved in making treatment more available and in increasing favorable treatment outcomes. Our goal is now to fill the glass beyond the halfway point.

Our Vision: The Committee's Recommendations

To continue the progress that has been made, the committee has engaged in a lengthy process of observation and consultation.   We have reviewed the literature, site-visited a number of treatment programs, and heard presentations from researchers, practitioners, and representatives of professional associations, trade associations, insurers, and citizens groups. We received written communications and copies of studies and reports from more than 200 researchers, practitioners, and administrators, many of whom provided summaries of the research and practice in a given area of alcohol problems treatment and specific recommendations. We have also drawn heavily on the experience, expertise, and creativity of the members of the committee and its task forces. During this process we have become increasingly aware of the uneasiness and deep concern that attend many of the changes that have taken place in the heath services arena. Yet we have also seen a readiness to change when a direction was identified. There is growing awareness that the structure and orientation of the service delivery system that was initiated some 20 years ago through the efforts of the Cooperative Commission and NIAAA must continue to evolve. Salutary as the historical development of treatment for alcohol problems has been, however, the committee has found reasons to recommend that further changes be made. In so complex an area as health care delivery, and even in so specialized a part of that area as the treatment of alcohol problems, it would be surprising if in the short space of a few years all that was required had already been accomplished. This report is only one of a long series of efforts, begun by the Cooperative Commission, to contribute to an incremental movement toward better treatment. There have been previous reports in recent years (e.g., Pattison, 1977; IOM, 1980; Saxe et al., 1983; IOM, 1989) and there will undoubtedly be others.

Two basic observations have informed the development of the committee's recommendations. One is that the range of alcohol problems and of the individuals who manifest them is very broad indeed. The other is that a multiplicity of treatments have evolved over time to deal with these problems and with those who are troubled by them. Because research on the outcomes of these treatments has indicated that none is universally effective but that many are highly effective with certain individuals and certain kinds of problems, the focus of the committee's attention has been on the interactions among persons, problems, and treatments.   Its recommendations have proposed how this interaction might more effectively be structured.

As discussed in Chapter 10, the committee views a comprehensive pretreatment assessment as the cornerstone of a sound therapeutic approach. With the knowledge this comprehensive assessment provides, explicit guidelines can subsequently be used to match individuals seeking treatment with what is likely to be the most effective treatment for them. To employ matching a broad range of well-specified treatment interventions must be made available if appropriate treatment is to be offered to all who seek it.   In each community, there must be an appropriate mix of services and settings that are available and financially accessible across the entire spectrum of problems. This mix must take into account the differing levels of severity and need for social supports. Moreover, matching must occur not only at the beginning of the process of treatment but throughout its course.

For this reason, as well as many others, it is vitally important to have ongoing knowledge of the outcome of treatment. One crucial use of such knowledge of outcome is to modify the treatment process so that it works more effectively and efficiently in the future. Guidelines for matching individuals to appropriate treatments should be continually modified in the light of outcome information so that matching becomes increasingly precise. If this is done, the treatment process becomes self-correcting. Thus, the evolution and development of the treatment system as a whole and of its component parts must be systematically monitored through the collection of uniform data on the persons entering treatment, the specific treatments that they receive, the costs of treatment, and the immediate and long-term outcomes. The cost-effectiveness of each treatment and its active ingredients must be carefully studied.

A way of summarizing these recommendations is to look toward the integration of presently existing treatment programs into a treatment system as described in Chapter 13. That system in essence is the cornerstone of our vision. Combining the resources of two or more treatment programs would enable a much more efficient conjoint implementation of such functions as assessment, matching, outcome determination, and continuity assurance. The resources required to implement these functions could arise from a broader base, and the functions themselves could be shared. Prototype examples are available in some jurisdictions in the public sector (e.g., Minnesota's consolidated fund, Ontario's independent assessment and referral centers) and in some organizations in the private sector (e.g., utilization management companies, employee assistance programs), although much is still required in the way of further development.

The committee has also strongly recommended that the base of treatment be broadened (see Chapter 9). Much evidence has accumulated that a majority of persons with alcohol problems seek various kinds of assistance from health, social service, and other agencies rather than from specialized treatment agencies. The detection of these problems has received more emphasis in recent years and the implementation of brief, low-cost interventions has been shown to be effective and should be implemented on a comprehensive basis. Although this action will not eliminate the need of some persons for specialized treatment, available information suggests it is likely to prove the most effective way of reducing the overall burden of alcohol problems on American society.

In addition to broadening the base of treatment, the treatment structure must be sharpened at the apex. The foregoing recommendations may need to be modified in order to deal with the needs of special populations (see Section IV). The unique social, cultural, psychological, and biological characteristics of large subgroups of American society would not be well served by a treatment system of the type we proposed if it did not take such differences into consideration. The committee believes the proposed system is capable of accommodating such a requirement, but it also believes that special effort must be exerted to see that it does. Specifically, additional research is needed on the effectiveness of proposed but untested culturally sensitive treatments advanced for each of the special populations.

Finally, there is the bottom line: all of this needs to be paid for. No pretense need be entertained that the burden of alcohol problems can be significantly eased without additional cost, and improvements in treatment could be costly. However, the current cost of treatment is, even by conservative estimates, a tiny fraction of the total monetary cost of alcohol problems (quite apart from their devastating toll of human misery and lost potential). If the improvement of treatment effectiveness results in a higher level of positive outcomes, the costs involved may be to a significant degree offset by a decrease in the cost of alcohol problems. Improved methods of financing treatment may contribute to this balance in an important way. The cost of increasing treatment availability and effectiveness through our vision could, indeed, come from the savings to be achieved by changing the emphasis on inpatient detoxification and rehabilitation to a focus on assessment, brief intervention, and outpatient treatment and by matching persons with the most effective form of treatment. There are no solid data on which to base estimates of either costs of current inappropriate use or projections of savings because of the lack of adequate surveys and cost-effectiveness studies (see Chapters 8, 19, and 20). There is a need for greatly expanded program of research on the cost-effectiveness of alternative treatments.

Such are the committee's vision and its specific recommendations, spelled out in much greater detail in the preceding chapters. One thing is certain: they will not implement themselves. Indeed, in many regards, a total reorientation in our thinking about "alcoholism" is required—a shift away from the conception that all alcohol problems involve a chronic progression that can only be deterred through a single treatment approach. Although there has been some movement in this direction, strong leadership will be required for any significant level of implementation. Who will provide the requisite leadership?

Opportunities for Leadership

It is tempting to think in terms of a single designated leader—an individual, an office, an organization—who would be assigned the task of providing for the future of the treatment of alcohol problems. In this way, responsibility is clearly delegated, and an accounting can readily be demanded. Despite its advantages, the committee rejects this strategy. The range of alcohol problems is too large and too complex to yield to unitary leadership. There is no one federal agency, no one advocacy group, no one sector that can manage the job. Leadership in the future development of diversified treatment for alcohol problems must be shared. In what follows, possible initiatives that might be taken by some of the principal actors on the scene will be mentioned for illustrative purposes.

The Leadership Opportunity for Congress

The federal government has been, through the initiatives of Congress starting with the Hughes Act and continuing with the recent reviews of services, a keystone in the development of treatment services for alcohol problems. In recent years, Congress has shown an increasing willingness to share this role with the states through the development of the block grant mechanism to fund categorical services for the uninsured and indigent. It is also sharing the role with the employers who are the major purchasers of private health insurance by its unwillingness to pass legislation mandating a specific benefit for the treatment of alcohol problems. Congressional concern has been expressed as an unwillingness to impose mandates on purchasers when the efficacy of various treatments is still unknown (e.g., Florio, 1988).

Although, the committee focuses these comments on Congress which commissioned this study, it recognizes that the administration and each of the agencies involved in the delivery, financing, and study of treatment for alcohol problems can also provide leadership by taking the initiative to implement those parts of the committee's vision which are relevant to their operations.

The federal government itself is both a major purchaser and a major provider of treatment services for alcohol problems (see Chapters 4, 8, and 18). In the aggregate, the treatment capability operated by federal agencies (i.e., the Indian Health Service hospitals and clinics, as well as its contracted treatment programs; the Department of Defense hospitals, clinics, and freestanding residential and outpatient units; and the Department of Veterans Affairs inpatient and outpatient units and contracted halfway houses) constitutes one of the largest pools of treatment resources in the country. None of these services is currently operating in the manner envisioned by the committee. Congressional initiatives to introduce the comprehensive system proposed in this report into each of the system operated by federal agencies would create an important model for other providers to emulate.

The federal government is also one of the major purchasers of all health care services. It pays (according to the best available data) more than 25% of the total cost of treatment for alcohol problems through its direct operations, grant programs, and public insurance programs. Congress has played a key role in the development of federal support for the nation's current system of treatment services for alcohol problems and retains oversight responsibility for it. The role of the federal government as a purchaser of health care has been described in terms that are quite applicable to the specific case of purchases of treatment for alcohol problems:

> In the federal government's role as a *primary* purchaser of health care, the Congress has, over time, developed a number of different programs. Each of these has been established to address the needs of a different beneficiary population, and each has viewed peer review in a different frame of reference. Although, in the abstract, and perhaps, in a public policy frame of reference, it would appear that the federal government should actively seek to develop a uniform benefit program (and a uniform cost-containment/quality assurance mechanism) for all its beneficiaries, and thus, at a minimum, use its considerable purchasing power (i.e., size) and experience to ensure the most cost-effective benefit package possible—in reality, this is not what has occurred. Each of these programs come under the jurisdiction of different congressional (sub) committees and as a result, each is considerably different in philosophical orientation and benefit structure. (DeLeon et al., 1988:287)

Obviously, the situation described here is not what the committee advocates. None of the federal purchase-of-care programs have mechanisms in place that require conformity to the elements of effective treatment as recommended in this report. Federal programs differentially support alternative treatment strategies without adequate, coordinated discussion and review. Medicare and Medicaid have narrow provider eligibility criteria that exclude providers who offer social model alternatives; they continue to support only a medical model of hospital-based detoxification and rehabilitation whereas the majority of states, using block grant funds, support a mixed medical and social model that also includes maintenance and extended care in nontraditional, nonhospital settings. While different oversight committees are involved for the different federal treatment programs, all could use similar or identical guidelines to review the current manner in which pretreatment assessment, referral and matching to treatment, treatment itself, and outcome monitoring are carried out. Alternatively, oversight responsibility could be restructured and perhaps consolidated so that a single committee reviews all treatment for alcohol problems paid for with federal funds.

Pursuant to its review, the committee suggests that all federally operated treatment systems as well as the grant and insurance programs, should include both medical model and social model residential, intermediate (day care), and outpatient assessment, detoxification and other forms of acute intervention, rehabilitation, and maintenance activities as options in their benefit packages so that each can be used when clinically appropriate. The implementation of brief, low-cost interventions should be initiated immediately through the training of generalist health care and social services staff as well as specialist staff. This recommendation is merely a restatement of the committee's advice to all purchasers of care as outlined in Chapter 20. *The committee recommends that Congress using these principles as a means of demonstrating its leadership initiate a total review of the programs for which it has oversight responsibility and create a uniform benefit structure.*

For example, programs offering inpatient hospital-based treatment in Minnesota are more expensive than a structured day program, but the intermediate care option has not been covered as fully as the hospital option by either public or private payers. After reviewing the research on the effectiveness of the two options, the Minnesota legislature adopted a consolidated approach that was designed to place persons needing treatment in the most appropriate setting. Medicaid and the alcohol, drug abuse, and mental health services block grant are part of the current effort by the Minnesota Chemical Dependency Program to determine whether there can be cost savings with a statewide system of preadmission screening and assessment using uniform level of care placement criteria that include provisions for intermediate care. Medicare is not participating in the system. Conversely, the alcohol, drug abuse, and mental health block grant and many of the state alcoholism authorities exclude hospital-level service from their funded options because of cost. Yet there are times when such services are clinically appropriate and should be available, through the appropriate matching procedures. The Minnesota consolidated fund approach, now undergoing evaluation, represents a naturalistic study of all these modalities and can provide data to supplement the HCFA-NIAAA demonstration (Lawrence Johnson and Associates, Inc., 1986). This effort should be closely monitored by Congress as it decides which path to follow.

In short, treatment should be determined by clinical need rather than by the design of benefits or by ideological constraints. Clinical need should be determined by careful pretreatment assessment and continued reassessment as described in Section III of this report. Leadership from the major purchasers of care, including Congress, will be required for such changes in clinical practice and financing policies to occur on a nationwide basis. The importance of the federal government as a provider and a purchaser of services suggests that its initiatives would be influential guides for all purchasers and providers.

Another area of alcohol problems treatment in which Congress might exercise some influence is through support for research on the organization and financing of effective treatment services. Data on the effectiveness of specific treatment approaches must be continuously available to encourage purchasers of care to include—or exclude—a given procedure or type of provider. *The committee strongly urges that Congress support an enhanced program of clinical and services research on the treatment of alcohol problems.* One unintended effect of the introduction in 1982 of the block grant system of funding treatment and prevention services appears to have been a reorientation of federally funded research in the direction of basic biomedical research accompanied by a relative deemphasis of clinical and services research and a cutback in monitoring the development of the treatment system and in conducting services research. (This effect will be discussed in more detail below in the section on leadership opportunities for the NIAAA.)

Only limited funding has been available for treatment evaluation and technology transfer. The result has been a slowing down in efforts devoted to the refinement of treatment strategies and practices through the comparative study of their cost effectiveness. Also lacking are mechanisms to transfer into practice the knowledge that has been gained about the effectiveness of specific treatments. What is needed are expanded training in the conduct of alternative approaches that have been shown to be effective (e.g., brief interventions) and funding support for programs that implement these more cost-effective approaches.

Several recent developments that have occurred during the course of this study are noteworthy. NIAAA placed a renewed emphasis on its treatment research function in establishing a Treatment Research Branch in its new Division of Clinical and Prevention Research and will be funding studies for evaluating effectiveness when persons are matched to specified treatment strategies (Noble, 1989). In addition, NIAAA received explicit authorization to fund services research projects as part of the Anti-Drug Act of 1988. Support for these activities, however, remains minimal; more substantive funding and staffing must be found and an expanded research agenda articulated if the needed studies are to be carried out using adequate experimental methods so that their findings are accepted and can lead to changes in practice.

The Leadership Opportunity for the States

Within the current legislative framework, the states have the primary responsibility for funding, planning, implementing, regulating, and monitoring the quality of treatment for alcohol problems (e.g., USDHHS, 1986). At present, each state now has an identifiable agency that is responsible for the development, maintenance, and evaluation of its service delivery system. The scope and authority of the agencies differ slightly from state to state, as do the components of the service delivery system. In states that have adopted the Uniform Act, the definitions of treatment and the continuum of care for alcohol problems are similar (see Chapters 3 and 4). Generally, state alcohol agencies do not operate facilities or treatment programs (although some states do).

Most state governments are the largest single purchasers of treatment for alcohol problems in their jurisdictions, either through the categorical agency which administers the federal block grant or through their Medicaid program, or using a combination of these funding sources. The beneficiaries on whose behalf these services are purchased tend to be low-income persons who do not have private health insurance coverage for treatment of alcohol problems. The elements in the continuum of care supported by the benefit package in each state program differ from those of other states, although there are certain common features. Increasingly, however, state alcohol agencies are accepting the research findings that have demonstrated the effectiveness of lower cost mixed medical and social model detoxification and rehabilitation carried out in outpatient and intermediate care settings.

The issue of consistency among the states in relation to treatment standards and the establishment of a continuum of care based on the best available research information continues to be of prime importance (see Chapters 3 and 7). The Minnesota and Oregon legislatures' recent efforts constitute an important model for state action. The Oregon legislature recognized that the treatment system that had been put in place over 20 years earlier had not had a major review. It established a special committee to review the need for services in the state, the existing local service delivery system, and the administrative relationships and operations of the various state and local agencies involved in treatment funding and provision. The result of the review was a significant body of recommendations that was submitted to the legislature for adoption (Special Committee on Alcohol and Drug Abuse Policy, 1984; J. Kushner, Oregon Office of Alcohol and Drug Abuse Programs, personal communication, 1988).

The recommendations formulated in this report could be used in a similar fashion by state legislatures and state alcoholism authorities to review program standards and policies utilized by the state in funding specialist treatment for alcohol problems. Whether such funding is part of the categorical program administered under the state alcoholism authority or supplied by Medicaid, the following questions are relevant:

- Do the standards and policies include a provision for comprehensive pretreatment assessment?

- Do the standards and policies require outcome monitoring and performance contracting?

- Do the standards and policies require a demonstration that particular services are either appropriate for heterogeneous groups or should be limited to those persons for which that specific level and type of care has been shown to be effective?

- Do the standards and policies allow alternative treatments to be offered to all persons seeking assistance?

- Do the standards and policies require matching of the person to the appropriate setting at each stage of treatment?

- Do the standards and policies provide for brief interventions with demonstrated effectiveness as part of the state-funded continuum of care?

- Does the state supported continuing education and credentialing program include training in brief intervention techniques, assessment strategies, and continuity assurance? Are there training opportunities for each of the key disciplines involved (physicians, psychologists, social workers, and nurses, as well as counselors)?

The findings and recommendations formulated in this report could also be used to review the continuum of care in those states that have in place legislation mandating particular insurance benefits. As discussed in Chapter 19, the committee makes no recommendation per se on whether there should or should not be mandates. The committee maintains, however, that the principles for determining appropriateness of coverage for a given approach should be applied to mandates as well as to individual benefit plans. For example, does the mandate include a provision for comprehensive pretreatment assessment? Does it include the variety of settings and alternative treatments needed by the heterogeneous subgroups that require treatment? Does the mandate call for matching to the appropriate setting and intensity of treatment at each treatment stage? Does it allow for reassessment and outcome monitoring? Does it include a predefined number of inpatient days or outpatient sessions? Does it call for outcome monitoring and continuity assurance?

If there are concerns about the cost of implementing the vision of treatment presented by the committee, the states can take the lead in evaluating the feasibility of the proposed comprehensive system by conducting their own naturalistic and experimental studies. One possibility for conducting such a feasibility study involves the extensive network of drinking-driver services that developed in each state out of the Alcohol Safety Action Program (see Chapters 4 and 16). Questions have been raised regarding the effectiveness of DWI intervention and treatment in comparison with other sanctions (Hagen, 1986). There have been few adequate studies of the potentially positive effects of matching persons in DWI clinics to the appropriate treatment modality; typical first-offender programs involve only the options of education or limited treatment for all individuals (Wells-Parker et al., 1986). Using the network of drinking-driver programs as test sites, some of the newer brief intervention strategies along with comprehensive pretreatment assessment and continuity assurance could be introduced and evaluated following a process outlined below.

State-administered and state-regulated drinking-driver programs already have in place a prototype version of the comprehensive assessment process discussed in Chapter 10, as well as a network of probation specialists responsible to the court for reports on offenders' progress and outcome. In addition, most states now have in place an outcome monitoring system for program evaluation. However, these systems have not been formalized with regard to such matters as assessment, matching decision rules, and continuity assurance procedures. Consequently, the committee proposes adding a more sophisticated assessment and outcome monitoring capability, as well as additional alternative interventions, to the DWI referral and case-monitoring programs already in place. The augmented system should be capable of matching the DWI offender to different brief interventions and to different conditions of continuing treatment. Rather than being introduced in all DWI programs in a state, such an approach could be given a trial to determine its feasibility and effectiveness in one or more of the state's jurisdictions and outcomes compared among jurisdictions.

A more elaborate, multisite study could be developed by the states working cooperatively with the NIAAA and the National Highway Traffic Safety Administration. There has been no comprehensive national study of these programs in recent years, despite their importance as one of the keystones of the nation's policy to decrease driving after drinking. Studies that have attempted to develop typologies of drinking-driver offenders through more extensive assessment suggest that treatment as a countermeasure can be made more effective in reducing both relapse and recidivism by the differential assignment of persons to brief or intensive interventions (e.g., Pisani, 1986; Scoles et al., 1986; Wells-Parker et al., 1986). Given the importance of the drinking-driver problem, such a national study merits serious consideration.

The Leadership Opportunity for Employers and Private Insurers

Insurers and employers are major purchasers of health care in general and of treatment for alcohol problems in particular. Similarly to the federal and state governments that also purchase these services, employers and insurers are seeking answers to questions about the effectiveness of treatment services to aid in cost containment and benefit design. Our vision provides the tools to obtain the data necessary to make informed choices among the alternative treatments which are presented to them by providers as "successful."

Increasingly, purchasers of care use a variety of mechanisms to contain costs; these include preadmission certification, required second opinions when a costly procedure is being considered, concurrent and retrospective reviews of medical necessity, and case management. Increasingly, purchasers are entering into managed care and preferred provider arrangements with practitioners and facilities that incorporate these mechanisms along with discounts and other forms of risk sharing that were pioneered in HMOs. Questions have been raised regarding the effectiveness of these techniques to accomplish the dual purposes of containing costs and maintaining the quality of care (e.g., Ellwood, 1988). A new "outcomes management" approach has been suggested; this approach is similar to the vision of a comprehensive system presented by the committee in this report.

Employers as purchasers of treatment for alcohol problems (either directly through self-insurance or through commercial insurance carriers) can respond to these concerns by using the committee's recommendations to evaluate their current benefits or any new benefit design they seek to adopt. The committee has chosen to provide the schematics for an idealized comprehensive treatment system that can be used as a template to evaluate the continuum of care supported by a particular purchaser of services. The purpose of presenting this system is not to suggest that each employer, insurer, or government agency adopt this particular framework; the committee is well aware that other approaches are possible. Rather, its goal is to provide purchasers with an example of how a model comptrehensive system can be used to assess their particular approach. To assist in this evaluation we have included examples of the assessment tools and placement criteria currently available.

In sum, we are suggesting that each and every government agency and business that purchases treatment services on behalf of its "beneficiaries" review the continuum of care supported by its "benefit package" to determine whether the plan enables a person to receive the appropriate match at each stage of treatment or whether its structural features (e.g., provider eligibility rules, "payment caps") serve as disincentives to proper matching. Leadership will require the asking of some difficult questions:

- Does the benefit pay for an objective assessment to determine the appropriate match to level of care (setting) and treatment modality at each stage of treatment?

- Are the requisite screening and assessment and outcome monitoring mechanisms in place to allow for matching?

- Are those medical model and social model venders that provide the most cost-effective treatment part of the continuum and eligible to participate in the plan?

- Are the participating venders capable of providing the alternative treatments (e.g., brief interventions, ambulatory detoxification, day care) that should be available? Have the venders' staff had training in brief intervention techniques, assessment strategies, and continuity assurance?

- Do the participating venders conduct outcome monitoring?

- Is there a detailed description of each treatment that is part of the continuum and that is covered under the plan? Is there a mechanism to monitor the adequacy of the treatment's implementation as well as its outcome?

- Does the benefit plan provide incentives that motivate individuals to choose the treatment that is most cost-effective for them?

- Does the benefit plan provide incentives for venders to offer the most cost-effective treatment determined through assessment and matching?

Employers and insurers can take the lead in the private sector in the development and testing of the vision through their already existing employee assistance programs (EAPs) and managed care activities. Like the drinking driver programs in the public sector, many of these employer-and insurer-sponsored plans have partially instituted key elements of the proposed comprehensive system; they can thus serve as testing grounds to evaluate the benefits to be gained by introducing our vision—or another variation that will allow employers and insurers to make data-based, empirically testable choices for their employees and customers, respectively, among the competing treatment strategies. Employers and insurers can carry out their own studies, introducing the comprehensive system in specific sites and not in others and then comparing outcomes. Again, like the states, employers and insurers can also design more elaborate experimental studies to test various combinations of practices; here, the participation of NIAAA and private foundations in funding multisite studies would be appropriate.

In some measure as a response to the recommendations of the Cooperative Commission (Plaut, 1967), there are now an estimated 10,000 EAPs covering approximately 25% of the work force (see Chapter 18 and Appendix D). A recent survey by the Bureau of Labor Statistics found that approximately 50 percent of businesses with more than 250 employees had an EAP. Many EAPs have become caught up in their sponsoring company's efforts to cut down escalating health insurance costs, and as a result some concern has been expressed for their future as programs. The committee shares this concern in the absence of any change in the basic pattern of operation of EAPs. Nevertheless, it sees this situation as a potential opportunity for leadership if the cost-containment efforts are combined with efforts to maintain and improve positive outcomes through the implementation of the committee's recommendations.

In some respects EAPs are similar in form and function to the kind of mechanism recommended in this report. (See, for example, the discussion in Chapter 13.) Like DWI programs, they have in place rudimentary assessment and continuity assurance mechanisms. EAP counselors even now have informal means for evaluating treatment agencies and for matching their referrals to them. The EAP counselor already functions in some respects as a case manager, although there is ongoing debate as to whether this is an appropriate function if the emphasis is on cost containment rather than cost-effectiveness. In general, it is important to prevent "financial case management" and "clinical case management" from working at cross purposes (see Chapters 13 and 20).

Thus an opportunity exists for EAPs, working in concert with their company's top management and benefit administrators, to implement the committee's vision and to achieve a balance between cost containment and treatment quality. Recently, several companies have introduced assessment and case management systems (e.g., that introduced by General Motors and the United Auto Workers working with Family Services of America and Connecticut General Corporation [Butler, 1987]) that are quite reminiscent of this report's recommendations of this report. However, assessment and structured outcome monitoring have not routinely been undertaken in these arrangements.

Employers and insurers can also provide leadership by requiring the implementation of the committee's recommendations in any managed care arrangement which they develop or with which they contract, be it an HMO or a preferred provider network. The HMO or preferred provider network should include an organized system for the treatment of alcohol problems that includes screening and the opportunity for brief intervention in the generalist system before referral to the specialist system (see Chapter 9). The managed care specialist system should include pretreatment assessment, matching at each stage of treatment, continuity assurance, and outcome monitoring.

Through such activities, the private sector, without waiting for federal or state initiatives, can take the lead in modeling changes in practice that are needed to make cost-effective treatment possible.

The Leadership Opportunity for Treatment Providers

According to the most recent survey, there are over 5,000 specialist treatment programs for alcohol problems (see Chapter 7). At the time of the report of the Cooperative Commission in 1967, there were fewer than 400. This remarkable growth, in its richness and variety, offers a major opportunity for implementing the recommendations of this report in various ways and under various circumstances.

As has been repeatedly noted, the majority of providers offer only a single approach to treatment. The continuation of such single-focus efforts was criticized in one recent state report, which recommended that such programs not be eligible for third party reimbursement (New Jersey Department of Insurance, 1988). In those instances, in which programs have the resources to offer alternative interventions within their own organization, but have not yet done so, the committee hopes that its recommendations will encourage them to proceed with such a strategy.

As an alternative, treatment programs could implement arrangements by which they cooperatively offer a broad panoply of interventions and jointly provide those functions (e.g., comprehensive assessment, matching, outcome determination, and continuity assurance or case management) that would be difficult for individual programs to implement.

Because providers have traditionally been creative in their approaches to treatment, there is reason for optimism regarding the creativity they may bring to the forging of cooperative arrangements. It is the committee's hope that the adoption of the broad perspective on alcohol problems that it endorses (see Chapter 1) may facilitate this process.

A worthy goal might be for the providers in a given area to work out cooperative arrangements in such a way that those seeking treatment in that area have a truly broad spectrum of alternatives on which to draw. Usually, large-scale arrangements of this kind are initiated by government agencies or other payers. If polycentric leadership is to become a reality, however, providers may also need to be initiators. In general, they can be expected to be much more aware of the service needs of their regions than a centralized governmental agency can be. Many communities already have in place a specialized information and referral agency that can serve as a hub for these activities (see Chapter 4). In addition there are many independent information and referral agencies are operated by local affiliates of the National Council on Alcoholism. These organizations can work to bring providers together in this effort and create for their community a comprehensive system with objective assessment, outcome monitoring, and continuity assurance.

Implementation of the committee's recommendations that there be an organized system of care in each community will require cooperation between treatment providers and third party purchasers of treatment services. Providers, individually or collectively through their associations, can approach the major sources of reimbursement in their community to support the effort to create a coordinated broad spectrum of treatments with a centralized objective assessment and continuity assurance function. Each community could work toward implementing the comprehensive spectrum of intervention responses that constitutes the vision of this committee—including the opportunity for brief intervention in the generalist system before referral to the specialist system, as well as pretreatment assessment, matching, continuity assurance, and outcome monitoring in the specialist system.

The Leadership Opportunity for the Professions and Training Programs

One of the focuses of the Cooperative Commission's recommendations in the late 1960s was development of enhanced services for problem drinkers within existing health, welfare, and community mental health agencies as well as on the development of a separate network of specialized services (Plaut, 1967). The Commission's recommendation for enhancing nonspecialist services within the nonspecialist sector has not yet been implemented. This report also includes suggestions (see Chapter 9) toward the achievement of this end. Yet what was not possible earlier may now be achievable because of the impressive gains in knowledge and experience over the past 20 years. Encouragement in this area may also be drawn from the experiences of other nations: screening and brief intervention in the nonspecialist sector has become a cornerstone of the approach to treatment for alcohol problems in developing countries (see Appendix C).

In its focus on enhanced generalist services for alcohol problems, the Cooperative Commission also emphasized the need for special clinical training programs. Until 1982, this recommendation was implemented through a number of training programs administered by NIAAA. Since 1982, it has been continued on a reduced level by NIAAA (primarily for physicians), by many state alcoholism authorities (primarily for counselors), and a variety of universities and professional schools (see Chapter 4).

However, as discussed earlier, the number and characteristics of the cadre of trained professionals (e.g., physicians, nurses, counselors, social workers, and clinical psychologists) who provide treatment for alcohol problems is unclear because there is a serious lack of accurate, timely work force data at the national level, and this lack of data compromises efforts to plan for future training and professional needs. A related issue is credentialing. While there is a growing consensus on the need for some external validation of the qualifications of a given individual to engage in clinical work, there is little movement toward organizing and coordinating such efforts within the various groups involved, let alone across different groups. As a result, diverse practices are now the rule. A uniform—or at least a coordinated—policy of training and certification should to be considered, in large part because the characteristics of treatment personnel are significant contributors to treatment outcome (see Chapter 5).

Such a policy is also critical to the implementation of the committee's new vision of alcohol problems and their treatment. For example, the certification of counselors who work as primary therapists in the majority of specialist programs using a mixed medical and social model is an ongoing concern of the public and private funding sources that play an ever-increasing role in determining the direction in which the field is going. The certification of treatment personnel is an important quality assurance issue for these payers.

The committee suggests that a national strategy for the training, continuing education, and certification of persons who provide treatment for alcohol problems be formulated and implemented. The current division of responsibility suggests that the lead should be shared by the federal agencies involved, by the state alcoholism authorities acting through their national organization, and by the broadest possible coalition of professional associations whose members are actively engaged in the treatment of alcohol problems. As discussed in Chapter 4, there has been renewed interest and activity in the development of curricula and training programs as well as in credentialing. However, there does not appear to be a viable mechanism for coordination and cooperation among the disciplines and agencies involved. There should be better integration of the efforts for the various disciplines.

There are several sorts of training that need to be addressed. The training of physicians, because of their influence in the health care system, is crucial and developments that have taken place within this profession can serve as a model for what is needed for the other disciplines involved (psychology, nursing, social work, counseling). Training efforts can be important tools for bringing about the changes in institutions that are necessary to broaden the base in which screening and brief interventions will need to take place Many of the settings in which screening and brief intervention would occur, once the comprehensive system proposed by the committee was in place, are not now particularly conducive to dealing directly with alcohol problems. There needs to be a special effort by each of the professions to create training opportunities in brief interventions.

If there is to be further evolution of treatment for alcohol problems, the overall training and certification issue cannot remain unaddressed at a national level. Because a broad scope is required to develop the requisite data and to address the policy issues, the task is beyond the capability of any existing single organization. These concerns need be addressed not only for physicians or for counsellors but for all the disciplines. Clearly, a broadly based consortium of the professions involved needs to be developed. One or more of the professional organizations can take the lead in bringing together all these groups to initiate such efforts.

The Leadership Opportunity for the National Institute on Alcohol Abuse and Alcoholism

That there needed to be strong federal leadership, and discrete federal and state administrative entities working in close partnership, was the theme of several of the Cooperative Commission's recommendations (Plaut, 1967). NIAAA and the state alcoholism authorities were subsequently established, and the goal of a strong federal presence was achieved for many years. The strong leadership previously exercised by the

National Institute on Alcohol Abuse and Alcoholism in the development and maintenance of treatment for alcohol problems has been described in previous chapters and is widely acknowledged (Lewis, 1982, 1988; Cahalan, 1987).

NIAAA's role altered profoundly, however, with the introduction in 1982 of the block grant system of funding treatment and prevention. The shift to block grants, which was intended to place major responsibility for services development and enhancement on the states, coincided with a focusing of the agency's mission on research. Currently, a substantial amount of NIAAA's funding is expended for basic biomedical research, reflecting a pattern that is uniform across the three institutes (NIAAA, NIDA, and NIMH) that constitute the Alcohol, Drug Abuse, and Mental Health Administration (ADAMHA). This policy rests on a belief that advances in knowledge regarding the basic biological processes underlying the three institutes' target problems is required for advances in treatment (Goodwin, 1988).

With this reorientation came a perception in the field that there had been a sharp cutback in staff and resources and that NIAAA was no longer able to carry out the leadership role it had originally assumed in monitoring service development, services demonstration, or clinical training (Cahalan, 1987; Lewis, 1988). The perception is that there has been minimal financial and staff support for cooperative studies of treatment effectiveness, minimal communication about developments and refinements in treatment methodology, and the dissolution of a clinical and services surveillance and research infrastructure necessary for policymaking. There has been recognition that these areas have not been fully attended to and suggestions made for an expanded clinical and services research effort (e.g., Wallen, 1988; IOM, 1989). Currently, only 14 percent of the intramural research budget and 12 percent of the extramural research budget are devoted specifically to treatment research (IOM, 1989). These allocations are relatively small amounts, considering the need for research on treatment effectiveness outlined here and in the 1989 IOM report, *Prevention and Treatment of Alcohol Problems: Research Opportunities*.

Yet recently, there have also been some heartening changes: the creation of the Treatment Research Branch within NIAAA's new Division of Clinical and Prevention Research; the reestablishment of a specific services demonstration authority for NIAAA in the Anti-Drug Act of 1988 (P.L. 100-690, Sec. 1922); and the development of initiatives to study matching and financing. The recent program announcement for a cooperative agreement to study matching strategies is a major step toward implementing what should become an ongoing program to test the cost-effectiveness of alternative treatment strategies (see Chapter 19). A similar positive initiative is the recent program announcement for research on economic and socioeconomic issues in prevention, treatment, and epidemiology. This program solicits investigator-initiated applications for studies of the existing system (e.g., examinations of the geographic distribution and availability of treatment, studies on the use and costs of various treatment services and settings). Both of these relatively small initiatives, however, are dwarfed by the need for better data.

NIAAA's enhanced clinical and services research program is an important first step toward developing the body of research knowledge needed to further refine the maturing treatment system. Much more needs to be done, however. Some of the Institute's own programs can serve as prototypes. For example, NIAAA has creatively used the services demonstration grant to provide a mechanism to evaluate its projects for services to the homeless (Lubran, 1987; NIAAA, 1987). The committee recommends expanding this type of research, which involves both a project process evaluation and a national multisite outcome evaluation across all grantees, to other special population groups to study the comparative effectiveness of culturally relevant treatment approaches (see Chapter 18). It could also be used generally for multisite trials of significant specific treatments that have not yet been subjected to testing. The cooperative agreement and contracting mechanisms constitute flexible vehicles for mounting studies that can supplement the traditional investigator-originated grant submissions. These mechanism are beginning to be used by the Treatment Research Branch (NIAAA, 1989), although, their effective use, which involves a much more active partnership of the sponsoring organization with the participating test sites, depends heavily on an adequate complement of staff.

The committee believes strongly in the need to affirm the visibility and priority of clinical and services research in NIAAA. Otherwise there is cause for concern regarding the adequacy with which the organization can carry out its portion of the shared leadership responsibility that the committee sees as necessary to implement the recommendations of this report. One must also think beyond the extensive but necessarily limited purview of the present study: there will be a readily foreseeable future need for the conduct of this kind of research as a basis for policy and practice. However, any future study will also be hampered by the lack of relevant data if the current deployment of resources is not enhanced.

There is currently only one NIAAA-funded research center, located at the University of Connecticut Health Center, that is devoted to treatment research. The Department of Veterans Affairs also funds one clinical research center at the San Diego VA Medical Center (IOM, 1989). These two centers constitute a significant but inadequate effort. The committee sees a need for additional clinical research centers and activities, particularly if its concerns about the cost-effectiveness of existing treatment and referral patterns are to be addressed. An additional treatment research center, with a major focus on studies of cost-effectiveness of alternative treatment methods, would be a logical next step.

In accord with its recommendations for enhancing matching in Chapter 11, the committee recommends that consideration be given to establishing a multisite network of researchers who could conduct treatment evaluation studies on an ongoing basis. This multisite network could complement the work of the more traditional research centers and carry out those activities that cannot be studied through the investigator-initiated research grant mechanism. Developing such a network with sites that can undertake cooperative studies of the effectiveness of specific treatment approaches with specific target groups and ensuring that these centers are dispersed around the country will significantly improve the timeliness and relevance of treatment research.

For example, each of the sites could participate in multisite clinical trials organized in a manner similar to the VA cooperative studies of the efficacy of disulfiram (Fuller et al., 1986). The protocols of the studies would be developed by the participating center or centers in cooperation with the NIAAA Division of Prevention and Treatment Research. The network would be able to use feedback designs within a multiprogram format and analyses of the treatment process within a uniform measurement framework to determine the effectiveness of various treatments and to identify their "active ingredients." The sites can also serve as "quick response" mechanisms to develop rapid information on treatments, procedures, assessment instruments, costs, characteristics of persons seeking treatment, and so forth. This type of timely information gathering could be of great value to NIAAA and other federal agencies (e.g., HCFA, the Department of Defense, the VA) in their efforts to respond to new developments in practice.

A recommendation more directly tied to the implementation of its vision is the committee's suggestion that NIAAA be given the additional resources to fund clinical research consortia in several communities around the country to test the feasibility of implementing its proposed comprehensive system. Such a plan would involve the development of sites designed to undertake cooperative studies of the effectiveness of specific treatment approaches with specific target groups when assessment and outcome monitoring, including detailed cost data, are in place. These studies will not only enhance treatment research but will provide models of the vision for other programs and practitioners to emulate.

Each of the sites would involve a consortium of treatment agencies and include as the center of its operations a comprehensive assessment capability fully staffed by an assessment, referral, and clinical case management team supported by a data collection and analysis staff. Because most providers currently offer only one or two treatment approaches, each consortium should be associated with as many treatment programs as possible. The criteria for association should include an agreement to participate fully in the pretreatment assessment of individual patients and the posttreatment monitoring of outcome and, whenever possible, in clinical trials of specific treatments. The number of treatment programs involved in any one consortium is not as critical as having a range of treatments that represent the entire continuum of care.

Beyond what can be achieved through the expansion of NIAAA's treatment research centers, investigator-initiated studies of treatment effectiveness, and specific studies to test the feasibility of the committee's vision, there is a great need for increased communication in and support of the field as a whole. At present in this country, treatment activities related to alcohol problems lack a central focus. Although much can be done by the states themselves and by other groups in cooperation with them in cooperation with them, the treatment of alcohol problems is a national effort and needs to be viewed as such. In previous chapters, there were suggestions and recommendations made that, for maximum usefulness, require the achievement of a national consensus on practices and procedures. NIAAA can play a crucial role in forging such a consensus. The attenuation of its services funding role through the block grant mechanism not only does not relieve it of responsibility for leadership in other areas but, in an important way, makes its leadership more credible (i.e., if funding is a state and local matter, NIAAA cannot be viewed as imposing its views on treatment programs under the guise of creating a consensus). NIAAA needs to expand its role as a disseminator of research findings through the development of a national technical assistance program.

Local treatment programs and state agencies are in great need of assistance to identify and implement the latest developments in treatment delivery. Such mechanisms as technical assistance conferences, onsite demonstrations by practitioners experienced in a particular methodology, and the dissemination of technical advice manuals and training materials could provide this assistance. Consultant visits and like activities provide exchanges of information that break down the isolation that seems to be increasing for many programs in the field. The federal government, through NIAAA, could provide leadership that would end this isolation by establishing a program of technical assistance, continuing education, technology transfer conferences, consensus conferences, and consultation on matters pertinent to treatment that would be directed toward state alcohol agencies and other funders and toward providers of treatment for alcohol problems.

The Leadership Opportunity for Voluntary and Community Organizations

There are many voluntary and community organizations that are concerned with the prevention and treatment of alcohol problems (Matheson, 1982; Lewis, 1988). These organizations also have a major role to play in bringing about the changes required in our current system to move away from the present emphasis on undifferentiated treatment of those individuals with the most severe alcohol problems. Creating a comprehensive system that provides cost-effective treatment for persons at all levels of alcohol problems requires action at both the local and national levels. Thus, community and voluntary organizations must be encouraged to work to work closely with governmental agencies, treatment providers, professional organizations, employers, and insurance companies to implement these recommendations.

Much of the progress documented by the committee in relation to the establishment of a nationwide network of specialist treatment has been due to the assistance and, often, leadership of voluntary organizations, citizens groups, unions, service organizations, trade associations, private foundations, and church and clergy groups in the implementation of the recommendations of the Cooperative Commission on Alcohol Problems. Key roles have been played by organizations such as the National Council on Alcoholism, the Junior Chamber of Commerce, the National Congress of Parents and Teachers, the AFL-CIO and the United Auto Workers (UAW), the Junior League, and the Alcohol and Drug Problems Association of North America. Over the past 20 years, these groups have frequently endorsed programs of prevention, treatment, and research; they have also helped obtain wider access to treatment for persons with alcohol problems. Similarly, recovering persons and their family members have used these local and national organizations to express their concerns about the accessibility and adequacy of treatment resources . The successful efforts of these groups can be seen in the passage of legislation at the national, state, and local levels of government, as well as in the initiation of and continuing support for individual treatment programs.

In particular, the role of local churches and national religious organizations of all denominations is critical. Individuals and families often share their alcohol-related difficulties first with clergy and are counseled or referred to self help organizations or specialist treatment. Clergy and church groups also provide ongoing support in preventing relapse after formal treatment. In many instances in which no treatment programs existed, churches were active in their initiation. There is now an opportunity for them to play a leadership role again in combination with schools, service organizations, and other voluntary associations. One particularly useful course of action would be for all these groups to come together in each community to review the committee's conclusions and recommendations and to work with the providers and funders to evaluate how closely the current treatment system and the efforts to implement them come to having a comprehensive system. Their various national associations can come together for a similar review.

Frequently, the positions on various alcohol-related issues held by voluntary associations and community organizations are at variance with government policies. This divergence comes from the unique perspective these groups bring to community needs and interests and as such represent a substantial force for change in both the public and private sectors. It is the committee's hope that these groups can adopt the broad perspective on alcohol problems presented in Chapter 1 and work with the relevant government agencies, treatment providers, third-party payers, and professional associations to develop a full response in both the generalist and specialist sectors to persons at each level of the spectrum.

Thus, it is not only the professionals and legislators who should be involved in the reevaluation of the nation's approach to the treatment of alcohol problems but also those community members who have an ongoing stake in the outcome of treatment. Clearly, a broadly based consortium of the relevant community organizations asking these same questions about the system of care in their community can help to provide the leadership needed to bring about the necessary changes.

The Challenge for the Future

In sum, much has been accomplished in the treatment of alcohol problems since the pioneering work of the Cooperative Commission more than 20 years ago. Nevertheless, it should surprise no one that much remains to be accomplished. Alcohol problems, like other so-called "lifestyle" problems (e.g., smoking, eating habits) have increasingly risen to national attention as further knowledge is gained regarding the attendant morbidity and mortality. Now is the time for a major increment in efforts to deal effectively and efficiently with individuals at risk of or already experiencing alcohol problems. The committee hopes its recommendations will contribute to this process.

Implementing the recommendations contained in this report will require shared leadership and cooperation among those groups and agencies that have been involved since the report of the Cooperative Commission in efforts to expand the availability of quality primary treatment for alcohol problems. We have entered a period of stabilization for those gains that were achieved by the acceptance of alcohol problems as a condition that could be effectively treated. Now, those gains can be maintained only if there is a shift toward concern with the differential effectiveness of each treatment for specific individuals. The current emphasis on cost containment in all areas of health care must engender a positive response from those who provide treatment for alcohol problems, a response that emphasizes careful assessment of clinical status and the matching of individuals to the appropriate setting, intensity, and modality at each stage of treatment.

Rather than viewing these concerns as threats to the future of the field, the committee sees them as challenges that may allow the field to take the next steps along its path to maturity as an important, vital specialty area within mainstream health services. Meeting those challenges will demand the joint efforts of a wide range of leaders who are ready to adopt a broader, yet more precise, framework for treating alcohol problems.

REFERENCES

Butler, J. 1987. GM's approach to substance abuse treatment. Business and Health 4(3): 12-13.

Cahalan, D. 1987. Understanding America's Drinking Problem: How to Combat the Hazards of Alcohol. San Francisco: Jossey-Bass.

DeLeon, P. H., J. G. Willens, J. J. Clinton, and G. VandenBos. The role of the federal govrnment in peer review. Pp. 285-453 in G. Stricker and A. R. Rodriguez, eds. Handbook of Quality Assurance in Mental Health. New York: Plenum Press, 1988.

Ellwood, P. M. 1988. Outcomes management: A technology of patient experience. New England Journal of Medicine 318: 1549-1556.

Florio, J. J. 1988. Opening statement. Presented at the U.S. House of Representatives, Subcommittee on Commerce, Consumer Protection and Competitiveness hearing regarding insurance coverage of drug and alcohol abuse treatment. Washington, D.C., September 8.

Fuller, R. K., L. Branchey, D. R. Brightwell, R. M. Derman, C. D. Emrick, F. L. Iber, K. E. James, R. B. Lacoursiere, K. K. Lee, I. Lowenstam, I. Maany, D. Neiderhiser, J. J. Nocks, and S. Shaw. 1986. Disulfiram treatment of alcoholism: A Veterans Administration cooperative study. Journal of the American Medical Association 256:1449-1445.

Goodwin, F. K. 1988. Alcoholism research: Delivering on the promise. Public Health Reports 103:569-574.

Hagen, R. E. 1986. Evaluation of the effectiveness of educational and rehabilitation efforts: Opportunities for research. Journal of Studies on Alcohol Suppl. 10:179-182.

Institute of Medicine. 1980. Alcoholism, Alcohol Abuse, and Related Problems: Opportunities for Research. Washington, D.C.: National Academy Press.

Institute of Medicine. 1989. Prevention and Treatment of Alcohol Problems: Research Opportunities. Washington, D.C.: National Academy Press.

Lawrence Johnson and Associates, Inc. 1986. Evaluation of the HCFA Alcoholism Services Demonstration: Final Second Analytic Report. Prepared for the Health Care Financing Administration. Washington, D.C.

Lewis, J. S. 1982. The federal role in alcoholism research, treatment, and prevention. Pp. 385-401 in Alcohol, Science, and Society Revisited, E. Gomberg, H. White, and J. Carpenter, eds. Ann Arbor, Mich. and New Brunswick, N.J.: University of Michigan Press and Center of Alcohol Studies, Rutgers University.

Lewis, J. S. 1988. Congressional rites of pasage for the rights of alcoholics. Alcohol Health and Research World 12:241-251.

Lubran, B. G. 1987. Alcohol-related problems among the homeless: NIAAA's response. Alcohol Health and Research World 11(3):4-6, 73.

Matheson, J. D. 1982. The private sector. Pp. 355-367 in Prevention, Intervention, and Treatment: Concerns and Models, J. de Luca, ed. Washington, D.C.: U.S. Government Printing Office.

National Institute on Alcohol Abuse and Alcoholism (NIAAA). 1987. Request for Applications: Community Demonstration Grant Projects for Alcohol and Drug Abuse Treatment of Homeless Individuals, RFA AA-87-04. Rockville, Md.: NIAAA.

National Institute on Alcohol Abuse and Alcoholism (NIAAA). 1989. Request for Cooperative Agreement Applications: Matching Patients to Alcoholism Treatments, RFA AA-89-02a, Coordinating Center. Rockville, Md.: NIAAA.

New Jersey Department of Insurance. 1988. Report of Governor's Cabinet Working Group's Ad Hoc Advisory Committee on Funding Sources for Treatment for Alcoholism and Drug Abuse. Trenton, N.J.: New Jersey Department of Insurance.

Noble, J. A. 1989. Status report on the Division of Clinical and Prevention Research for the National Advisory Council on Alcohol Abuse and Alcoholism. National Institute on Alcohol Abuse and Alcoholism, Rockville, Md. May.

Pisani, V. D. 1986. DUI recidivism: Implications for public policy and intervention. [no page nos.] in Zeroing-in on Repeat Offenders: A Summary of Conference Proceedings: Papers Presented at the Conference on Recidivism, September 16, 1986. Atlanta, Ga.: National Commission Against Drunk Driving.

Pattison, E. M. 1977. Ten years of change in alcoholism treatment and delivery systems. American Journal of Psychiatry 134:261-266.

Plaut, T. F. A ., ed. 1967. Alcohol Problems: A Report to the Nation. New York: Oxford University Press.

Scoles, P. E., E. W. Fine, and R. A. Steer. 1986. DUI offenders presenting with positive blood alcohol levels at presentencing evaluation. Journal of Studies on Alcohol 47:500-502.

Skinner, H. A., and S. Holt. 1987. The Alcohol Clinical Index: Strategies for Identifying Patients with Alcohol Problems. Toronto: Addiction Research Foundation.

Saxe, L., D. Dougherty, K. Esty, and M. Fine. 1983. The Effectiveness and Costs of Alcoholism Treatment. Washington: U.S. Congress, Office of Technology Assessment.

Special Committee on Alcohol and Drug Abuse Policy. 1984. Report on Oregon State Programs for Alcohol and Drug Abuse Services. Prepared for the Oregon State Legislature. Portland, Oregon.

U.S. Department of Health and Human Services (USDHHS). 1986. Toward a National Plan to Combat Alcohol Abuse and Alcoholism. Report submitted to the United States Congress. Rockville, Md.: National Institute on Alcohol Abuse and Alcoholism.

Wallen, J. Alcoholism treatment service systems: A health services research perspective. Public Health Reports 103:605-611.

Wells-Parker, E., P. J. Cosby, and J. W. Landrum. 1986. A typology for drinking driving offenders: methods for classification and policy implications. Accident Analysis and Prevention 18:443-453.

Acknowledgments

The committee wishes to acknowledge the thoughtful and timely contributions of the numerous individuals who made this report possible. While it assumes full responsibility for whatever the faults of the study may be, the committee acknowledge at the same time that many of its virtues come from the generous input of others. Regrettably, it is able to thank explicitly only a small number of those to whom thanks is due.

Susan Farrell, Director of the Office of Policy Analysis of the National Institute on Alcohol Abuse and Alcoholism (NIAAA), and our project officer throughout the study, provided sympathetic but trenchant criticism of our work, guided us through the thickets of legislative and institutional history, and provided us with informed access to the bountiful material and personal resources of her organization. Our thanks go also to NIAAA director Enoch Gordis, who provided detailed initial guidance and helpful continuing support. Many other members of the staff of NIAAA and related federal agencies were of great assistance, including John Allen, Loran Archer, Richard Fuller, James Kaple, Barry Montague, John Noble, Al Woodward, and Herbert Yahr.

There are too many debts to the staff of the Institute of Medicine (IOM) to acknowledge fully. Samuel O. Thier, IOM President, provided support throughout and contributed to the deliberations of the committee. Fredric Solomon made available to us his many years of experience both with the division and with the organization as a whole. Nancy Diener, Lou Cranford, and Janet Stoll handled the financial intricacies of the project. Bradford Gray shared with us his detailed knowledge of health care in the private sector. Sam Johnson and the IOM Library provided crucial bibliographic support, and the reference staff of the library of the Addiction Research Foundation in Toronto were extremely helpful. Leah Mazade, our editor, is largely responsible for the clarity and directness of expression in the manuscript. Our particular thanks for consistent and thoughtful guidance go to Marian Osterweis.

A particular acknowledgment of the deepest gratitude must go to our chairman, Robert D. Sparks, M.D. Our ability to achieve consensus and complete this report owes more to his helmsmanship than to any other factor. His consistent humanity, balanced judgment, openness and flexibility were crucial to our efforts.

At the same time that this study was being conducted, two other related studies, one on a research agenda for treatment and prevention of alcohol problems, and another on coverage for substance abuse treatment, were also being conducted. We are particularly grateful to those who kept us abreast of developments within these studies, including especially Roger Meyer, Robert Murray, Larry Lewin, Alice Fraenkel, Dean Gerstein, and Rick Harwood. Three members of our committee, Thomas Babor, Merwyn Greenlick, and Mark Pauly, provided overlapping membership with these related studies. But thanks must also go to all members of the project committees, whose interchanges were unfailingly stimulating and useful.

Kaye Fillmore and her colleagues Elizabeth Hartka, Bryan Johnstone, Richard Speiglman, and Mark Temple contributed a background paper on "spontaneous remission." Rick Harwood contributed another on aspects of financing. Harold Holder, Richard Longabaugh, William Miller, and Anthony Rubonis contributed another on cost effectiveness. Marcus Grant and Bruce Ritson contributed the analysis of treatment services in other countries, collating and summarizing responses from their colleagues in the World Health Organization study on the effectiveness of brief intervention. All were extremely useful in the preparation of the report. More than fifty colleagues contributed summaries of their experiences and viewpoints on the assessment process.

Leonard Saxe shared with the committee his experience in traversing the same territory. Norman Hoffmann and Dan Newman addressed some of the problems involved in obtaining and interpreting data on treatment populations. William Butynski facilitated our access to much important information on treatment services, Irvin (Sam) Muszynski provided valuable advice on financing, and Thomasina Borkman elucidated many aspects of social model programs. Lauri Greig's assistance was critical in the preparation of the section on special populations.

Well over one hundred colleagues responded to a general request for information, and many participated in our public hearings. Particular thanks are due to Helen Annis, Leclair Bissell, Floyd Bloom, Sheila Blume, Vincent Dole, John Ewing, Jack Mendelson, Stanton Peele, Marc Schuckit, and George Vaillant, who responded generously to detailed requests for particular information. Many colleagues in many settings welcomed our visits and incessant questions. Marc Schuckit also provided extensive direct consultation with staff and committee members in areas of his special competency.

The committee members extend their great gratitude to Fred Glaser and Herman Diesenhaus, who as staff members always and colleagues generally, made the difficult task of preparing the written report possible. Secretarial and administratives services were provided to the committee through the effective and cheerful activities of Barbara Kelley; we thank her effusively. Elaine Lawson continued these efforts, seeing the report through to publication.

Finally, we acknowledge most particularly the forbearance of our families and friends. They sustained with grace and good humor the irretrievable loss of the many hours of companionship that were required for the completion of this task. We hope that what has been accomplished is in some way worthy of that sacrifice.

APPENDIXES

A   Task Forces

TASK FORCE ON TREATMENT OUTCOME EVALUATION

David C. Lewis, M.D., *Chair*
Professor of Medicine and Community
 Health and Donald G. Millar Professor
 of Alcohol and Addiction Studies, and
 Director, Center for Alcohol and
  Addiction Studies
Brown University Medical School
Providence, Rhode Island

Chad D. Emrick, Ph.D.
Assistant Clinical Professor of Clinical
 Psychology in Psychiatry
University of Colorado Health Sciences
 Center
Denver, Colorado

Richard K. Fuller, M.D.
Assistant Chief of Gastroenterology
 Service
Ceveland Veterans Affairs Medical
 Center
Cleveland, Ohio

Edward Gottheil, M.D., Ph.D.
Professor of Psychiatry
Jefferson Medical College
Philadelphia, Pennsylvania

Richard Longabaugh, Ed.D.
Professor of Psychiatry and Human
 Behavior
Brown University, and
Director of Evaluation
Butler Hospital
Providence, Rhode Island

William R. Miller, Ph.D.
Professor of Psycholgy and Psychiatry,
 and Director of Clinical Training
Department of Psychology
University of New Mexico
Albuquerque, New Mexico

TASK FORCE ON ASSESSMENT AND TREATMENT ASSIGNMENT

Harvey A. Skinner, Ph.D., *Chair*
Professor and Chairman
 Department of Behavioural Science
 Faculty of Medicine
University of Toronto, and
 Senor Scientist
Addiction Research Center
Toronto, Ontario, Canada

Thomas F. Babor, Ph.D.
Professor of Psycholgy
Department of Psychiatry
University of Connecticut Health Center
Farmington, Connecticut

A. Thomas McLellan, Ph.D.
 Research Professor
Department of Psychiatry
Veterans Affairs Medical Center and
University of Pennsylvania
Philadelphia, Pennsylvania

Stephen Holt, M.D., FACP
Professor of Medicine, and
Chief, Division of Gastroenterology
Department of Medicine
Southern Illinois University School of
 Medicine
Springfield, Illinois

Philip O'Dwyer M.A., C.S.W., C.A.C.
President, Brookfield Clinics
Garden City, Michigan

Bruce J. Rounsaville, M.D.
Director of Research, Substance Abuse
 Treatment Unit, and
Associate Professor of Psychiatry
Yale University School of Medicine
New Haven, Connecticut

TASK FORCE ON SPECIAL POPULATIONS

Roger Dale Walker, M.D., *Chair*
Professor of Psychiatry and Behavioral
 Sciences
University of Washington School of
 Medicine, and Chief, Addictions
 Treatment Center
Veterans Affairs Medical Center
Seattle, Washington

Barbara Ross-Lee, D.O.
Professor and Chairman
Department of Family Medicine
College of Osteopathic Medicine
Michigan State University
East Lansing, Michigan

Jim Francek, M.S.W., C.E.A.P.
President
Jim Francek and Associates, Inc.
Norwalk, Connecticut

Marsha Vannicelli, Ph.D.
Associate Professor of Psychology
 Department of Psychiatry
Harvard Medical School, and
Director, Appleton Outpatient Clinic
McLean Hospital
Belmont, Massachusetts

Joseph J. Westermeyer, M.D., Ph.D.
Professor and Chairman
Department of Psychiatry and Behavioral
 Science
University of Oklahoma Health Science
 Center
Oklahoma City, Oklahoma

A. Thomas McLellan, Ph.D.
Research Professor
Department of Psychiatry
Veterans Affairs Medical Center and
 University of Pennsylvania
Philadelphia, Pennsylvania

G. Alan Marlatt, Ph.D.
Professor of Psychology
University of Washington
Seattle, Washington

Dennis Donovan, Ph.D.
Associate Professor of Psychiatry
 and Behavioral Sciences
University of Washington School of
 Medicine
Seattle, Washington

TASK FORCE ON FINANCING

Mark V. Pauly, Ph.D., *Chair*
Robert D. Eilers Professor of Health
 Care Management and Economics,
 Professor of Public Management
 and Economics, and
 Executive Director, Leonard Davis
 Institute of Health Economics
University of Pennsylvania
Philadelphia, Pennsylvania

Merwyn R. Greenlick, Ph.D.
Vice President (Research)
Kaiser Foundation and Hospitals and
Director, Center for Health Research,
Kaiser Permanente, Northwest Region
Portland, Oregon

Harold D. Holder, Ph.D.
Director
Prevention Research Center
Berkeley, California

Steven S. Sharfstein, M.D.
Vice President and Medical Director
The Sheppard and Enoch Pratt Hospital
Baltimore, Maryland

Barry Montague (Liaison)
Special Assistant to the Director
Office of Policy Analysis
National Institute on Alcohol Abuse
 and Alcoholism (NIAAA)
Rockville, Maryland

B Treatment Modalities: Process and Outcome[a]

Evaluation research represents a key to the advancement of therapeutic effectiveness in alcohol treatment. Since 1980, more than 250 new studies have been published reporting outcome data on various approaches to the treatment of alcohol problems. This body of research has provided important new knowledge regarding optimal approaches to alcohol treatment, in addition to clarifying areas in which further research is most needed.

A major continuing problem for the field is a gap between available knowledge and current practice. Much of what is presently done in alcohol treatment has not been evaluated; thus, the efficacy of standard components of many current treatment programs has not been established. Other approaches for which there is promising evidence of effectiveness remain largely unused in treatment.

In an effort to close this gap, the sections below survey research focusing on a number of topics of interest: specific treatment approaches, traditional treatment programs, the intensity and duration of treatment, aftercare, and the treatment process itself. In the final section, the committee presents its conclusions and summarizes the opportunities for further progress in treatment research.

OUTCOME RESEARCH ON SPECIFIC TREATMENT APPROACHES

Most of the studies conducted since 1980 have focused on the effectiveness of particular treatment approaches or programs. This research includes many uncontrolled studies but also more than 60 studies that use controlled designs and more methodologically sophisticated approaches. "Controlled" studies comprise those employing randomization or matching procedures to assign individuals to alternative treatment methods or to treatment versus control conditions. Uncontrolled studies typically report outcome data following a single intervention, or employ quasi-experimental designs (Cook and Campbell, 1979) to provide partial control of extraneous variables. Although both types of research can yield informative findings, controlled studies are less subject to confounding and tend to produce more reliable and interpretable results. In this review, therefore, greater emphasis will be placed on the findings of properly controlled evaluations.

Evaluations of interventions for alcohol problems can also be divided according to the point at which intervention occurs. Preventive interventions, generally administered prior to the onset of serious alcohol problems, are discussed in Part I of this report. Within formal **treatment**, three phases can be distinguished: (1) detoxification; (2) active treatment and rehabilitation; and (3) relapse prevention.

Intervention procedures during the first phase, detoxification, are designed to carry the individual safely through the process of alcohol withdrawal, minimizing the risks associ-

[a] Chapter 9 from the Institute of Medicine report, *Prevention and Treatment of Alcohol Problems: Research Opportunities*, prepared by the Committee to Identify Research Opportunities in the Prevention and Treatment of Alcohol-Related Problems. Preparation of the report supported by Contract No. ADM 281-87-003 with the National Institute on Alcohol Abuse and Alcoholism. Additional support for the study was provided by the Pew Charitable Trusts and the National Research Council Fund.

ated with the abstinence syndrome for those who are more severely dependent on alcohol. Detoxification typically yields little or no long-term change in alcohol consumption and related problems and is usually viewed as a prelude to active treatment.

Phase 2, active treatment, seeks to bring about change in the individual's use of alcohol and other drugs and to reduce problems associated with that use. Typically, the goal of treatment programs has been total abstention from alcohol and other drugs of abuse. A wide range of treatment strategies is available to achieve this goal, and research on these alternative modalities is discussed in the subsections below. After each discussion are questions that identify opportunities for research in these treatment areas.

During the 1980s, increased attention has been devoted to the importance of relapse prevention as a third phase of treatment. The goal of these efforts is to help the individual avoid a relapse to previous patterns of problematic drinking. When this phase follows inpatient treatment, it is sometimes called aftercare. In essence, relapse prevention is a logical extension of treatment efforts in that it attempts to sustain and stabilize the beneficial changes that have occurred during the initial phases of treatment. Relapse prevention strategies have been incorporated into treatment programs. Principles underlying some of these strategies are described in Chapter 3. In this section of the report, they are discussed among the alternative treatment modalities.

Pharmacotherapies

The use of medications in the treatment of alcohol problems can be divided into three major strategies. *Antidipsotropic* medications cause adverse results when alcohol is consumed. Their intended effect is to suppress drinking. *Effect-altering* medications likewise are intended to suppress alcohol consumption but through a different mechanism. Rather than precipitating aversive reactions to alcohol, these medications are designed to diminish the reinforcing or intoxicating properties of ethanol. *Psychotropic* medications, by contrast, are designed to treat such concomitant disorders as depression, psychosis, or anxiety. Their intended effect is to alleviate psychopathology that may accompany alcohol abuse, thereby diminishing the likelihood of relapse to drinking and improving the person's overall functioning.

Antidipsotropics

Within the United States, the principal antidipsotropic agent is disulfiram (Antabuse). Taken on a regular basis, disulfiram induces an adverse reaction of variable severity if the person consumes alcohol. New studies have provided mixed evidence regarding the usefulness of disulfiram in promoting improvement. Like earlier research, recent studies (e.g., Duckert and Johnsen, 1987; Thurston, Alfano, and Nerviano, 1987) have reported a relationship between voluntary compliance with disulfiram and favorable treatment outcome. In such investigations, however, medication effects were confounded with individual difference variables affecting motivation and compliance.

Several new controlled trials have failed to show benefits from disulfiram. Powell and colleagues (1985) found no differences in outcome over 12 months of follow-up among groups that were assigned at random to receive medication (disulfiram plus the option of chlordiazepoxide), medication plus supportive counseling, or a control group receiving only monitoring of medical problems. In studies of alcoholics who were being treated in Veterans Administration methadone clinics, Ling and coworkers (1983) observed no differences in abstinence, treatment compliance, or breath test results between groups that were randomly assigned to receive disulfiram and those assigned to receive a placebo.

Schuckit (1985) also reported no difference in the 12-month outcome between alcoholics who were prescribed and agreed to take disulfiram and those who refused to take it.

Recent research further suggests that most or all of the therapeutic impact of disulfiram prescription (at least without compliance assurance) may not be attributable to specific medication effects. Fuller and Williford (1980), in a urinalysis of a randomized clinical trial, reported that two groups of alcoholics who were given disulfiram showed significantly higher abstinence rates at 12 months, compared with those who were given no disulfiram. Only one of the two medicated groups received a therapeutic dose, however, whereas the other was given only 1 milligram (mg), an inert dose. Thus, both groups who believed they were receiving disulfiram showed higher abstinence rates.

In the largest and most carefully designed clinical trial of disulfiram to date, Fuller and coworkers (1986) replicated their earlier study in a nine-site collaborative research program. Outpatient alcoholics were again randomly assigned to receive 250 mg (therapeutic) doses, 1 mg (inert) doses of disulfiram, or a vitamin supplement and no disulfiram. Over 12 months of follow-up, the three groups did not differ on measures of total abstinence, employment, or social stability. Compliance with medication (even the inert dose or the vitamin supplement) was highly associated with abstinence. Within the subgroup of individuals who were highly compliant with research procedures and provided complete data, those given the therapeutic dose reported significantly fewer drinking days than their counterparts in the two control groups.

Other studies have employed the surgical implantation of disulfiram in an attempt to avoid problems with compliance. Wilson, Davidson, and Blanchard (1980) found a substantially higher rate of abstinence in two groups undergoing surgical operations—one for the implantation of disulfiram, the other for an inert implant—relative to a random control group that was given no operation. No difference in outcome was observed between the disulfiram and inert implant groups. Johnsen and colleagues (1987) similarly found no differences in a double-blind randomization study comparing disulfiram and inert implantation. The failure of disulfiram implants to show a specific medication effect, however, may be due to the low probability of a disulfiram-ethanol reaction, even when the person drinks (Wilson et al., 1984; Johnsen et al., 1987). Future research may discover more effective methods administering long-acting doses of disulfiram. A danger attached to long-acting parenteral administration, however, is the difficulty of reversing an acute disulfiram-ethanol reaction if the individual consumes alcohol.

Thus, at present, oral administration is the standard procedure for administering antidipsotropics in the United States, and compliance is a crucial issue in the effectiveness of oral disulfiram. Recent studies have found few or no differences between disulfiram accepters and refusers on the basis of personality and demographic variables (O'Neil et al., 1982; Schuckit, 1985), which suggests that contextual or attitudinal factors may be important determinants of compliance (Brubaker, Prue, and Rychtarik, 1987). Motivational strategies to promote medication compliance appear to increase the impact of disulfiram treatment. Azrin and coworkers (1982) tested a simple disulfiram assurance procedure whereby the alcoholic took the medication daily in the presence of a significant other who provided praise and support for compliance. At the six-month follow-up point, those in the disulfiram assurance group showed substantially better outcomes than randomly chosen controls for whom disulfiram was prescribed but who were given no compliance intervention. The difference was greatest for married persons, perhaps because of the spouse's availability to serve as the reinforcing partner.

In another study, Kofoed (1987) found that a chemical monitoring system to verify disulfiram intake increased medication compliance in a controlled trial but did not affect compliance with other aspects of treatment. Keane and colleagues (1984) reported favorable results with a home-based disulfiram compliance program that involved monitoring and contracting with the spouse. Determination of the effects of mandated monitoring of disulfiram compliance on long-term outcomes, either by chemical testing or by direct observation (e.g., Sereny et al., 1986), has not yet been evaluated in a properly controlled trial.

Calcium carbimide, an alternative antidipsotropic medication, has been tested in other countries but has not yet been approved for therapeutic use in the United States. A pharmacologic comparison of carbimide and disulfiram indicated similar adverse reactions when alcohol is consumed, with the carbimide-ethanol reaction being somewhat more severe (Peachey et al., 1983). However, the pharmacodynamics of carbimide differ significantly from those of disulfiram. The more rapid onset and increased intensity of aversive effect with carbimide may offer advantages for certain therapeutic applications. Peachey and Annis (1985) proposed its use as part of a relapse prevention procedure whereby an individual could take it acutely in anticipation of a high-risk situation. Furthermore, carbimide appears to be less toxic and to yield fewer side effects than disulfiram (Peachey and Annis, 1984). Well-controlled clinical trials of carbimide have not yet been reported. If future trials reflect positive outcomes, however, carbimide should be made available in the United States as an alternative pharmacotherapeutic agent for the treatment of alcohol problems.

The potential benefits of antidipsotropics must be weighed against their side effects and the potential hazards associated with their longer term use, particularly in light of studies reflecting no differences between medication and control groups. Recent reports suggest that antidipsotropic medication may increase sexual dysfunction (Snyder, Karacan, and Salis, 1981; Jensen, 1984) and a craving for alcohol (Nirenberg et al., 1983; Stockwell, Sutherland, and Edwards, 1984), in addition to other commonly reported side effects. However, at least one double-blind study found no differences in side effects between disulfiram and placebo groups (Christensen, Ronsted, and Vaag, 1984).

The following questions represent opportunities for research on antidipsotropic medications:

- What motivational procedures most effectively increase compliance with antidipsotropic medications?
- What are optimal combinations of antidipsotropic medication with other treatment strategies?
- What are the characteristics of individuals who accept and respond favorably to the various classes of antidipsotropic medications?
- What are the effects of mandatory monitoring of compliance with antidipsotropics? Does this procedure increase abstinence during and after the period of mandatory monitoring?
- What are the effects of various antidipsotropic medications on subjective desire and craving for alcohol?
- What methods of administration, if any, could be used safely to sustain effective and long-acting doses of antidipsotropic medications?

Effect-Altering Medications

Effect-altering medications reduce the reinforcing properties of ethanol without producing illness. Rockman and coworkers (1979) reported that zimelidine, a serotonin uptake inhibitor, diminished alcohol intake by animals in a free-choice drinking paradigm. Similar results have been reported in rodent studies of other serotonin uptake inhibitors including norzimelidine, citalopram, alaproclate, fluoxetine, indalpine, viqualine, and fluvoxamine. In studies with nondepressed, nondependent, heavy-drinking humans, zimelidine and citalopram have been found to reduce alcohol intake (Naranjo et al., 1984, 1987).

The principal effect of zimelidine was found to be an increase in the number of abstinent days for heavy drinkers. Moreover, zimelidine was effective within the first two weeks of treatment, before its antidepressant effects normally occur (Naranjo et al., 1984). Amit and colleagues (1985) found that drinkers given a single dose of zimelidine reported a reduced euphoriant effect from alcohol as well as a decreased desire to drink. These effects of zimelidine may be due to an effect on the reinforcing properties of ethanol or to a generalized suppressant effect on both food and alcohol consumption (Gill and Amit, 1987).

Because zimelidine produced flulike symptoms and neuropathy in a significant number of subjects who were being treated for depression, it has been withdrawn from human use. Other serotonin uptake inhibitors such as fluoxetine and fluvoxamine would appear to be reasonable candidates for therapeutic trial in alcoholic patients (Linnoila, et al., 1987) but thus far have been tested only in heavy drinkers. Fluoxetine does not act synergistically with alcohol on physiologic, psychometric, or psychomotor activity; it also does not increase blood alcohol levels (Lemberger et al., 1985). Recent work by E. M. Sellers of the Addiction Research Foundation of Ontario (personal communication, 1988) suggests that fluoxetine affects the initiation of drinking behavior as opposed to moderating drinking episodes. Fluvoxamine is approximately three times as selective in serotonin uptake inhibition (relative to norepinephrine reuptake) as zimelidine. At the time of this report, one serotonin uptake inhibitor (fluoxetine) has been approved for the treatment of depressive disorders in the United States.

Effect-altering medications could be used in the treatment of alcohol-dependent persons much as opiate antagonists have been used in treating opiate addiction. It may be useful to combine such pharmacotherapy with psychological interventions designed to enhance motivation and medication compliance.

The following questions represent opportunities for research on effect-altering medications:

- What is the impact of various effect-altering medications on subjective desires and cravings for alcohol and on the perceived reinforcing effects of alcohol consumption?
- What motivational procedures most effectively increase compliance with effect-altering medications?
- What are the side effects and long-term risks involved in the use of various effect-altering medications?
- Do effect-altering medications promote long-term sobriety?
- What is an optimal duration for treatment with effect-altering medications to maximize therapeutic effects while minimizing side effects and medication-related risks?
- What are the characteristics of individuals who accept and respond favorably to various classes of effect-altering medications?
- What are optimal combinations of effect-altering medications and other treatment strategies?

Psychotropics

Psychotropic medications have three potential uses in the treatment of alcohol problems. First, certain medications are of demonstrated utility during alcohol detoxification (Liskow and Goodwin, 1987). The usefulness of such medications during acute withdrawal is now generally accepted, although detoxification can often be accomplished without medication in nonhospital settings (Whitfield et al., 1978; Whitfield, 1980; Sparadeo et al., 1982).

Second, as indicated in the discussion of effect-altering drugs, it has been suggested that some psychotropic medications may decrease the desire for and use of alcohol (McMillan, 1981). In addition to the antidepressants and serotonin uptake inhibitors discussed earlier, lithium has been investigated in this regard. Fawcett and colleagues (1987) found no differences on drinking measures between alcoholics given lithium and alcoholics given a placebo. Compliance with either medication was highly associated with abstinence. Among compliant individuals, those sustaining high blood levels of lithium did show a higher rate of abstinence than those with low lithium levels or placebo doses. No differences were observed between depressed and nondepressed alcoholics. Other investigations, including a major Veterans Administration collaborative study, have found no therapeutic impact of lithium on the drinking outcomes of either depressed or nondepressed alcoholics (Peck et al., 1981; Pond et al., 1981; Powell et al., 1986; Dorus, 1988). A variety of other psychotropic medications have been tested for their effects on drinking behavior and the desire to drink (Liskow and Goodwin, 1987).

A third potential use of psychotropic medications is in the treatment of "dual diagnosis" individuals, who manifest both alcohol abuse and another significant form of psychopathology. Current evidence indicates that untreated concomitant psychopathology generally predicts a poor prognosis for alcoholics (Rounsaville et al., 1987) and is associated with a high rate of treatment dropout (Kofoed et al., 1986). It is logical (although not yet conclusively demonstrated) that alcoholics with major depression that persists into sobriety would be significantly more likely to remain sober if their depression could be treated effectively by antidepressant medication or other means. Similarly, it is quite plausible that individuals with concomitant alcohol abuse and schizophrenia would benefit from antipsychotic medication and that alcoholics with bipolar affective disorder would have an improved prognosis if given lithium.

It is important to note here that apparent psychopathology that coincides with active alcohol and drug abuse frequently remits during the early weeks of sobriety (Nakamura et al., 1983). Sufficient time should be allowed for full withdrawal from abused drugs, and the diagnosis should be firmly established before psychotropic medication is considered. Nonpharmacological alternatives should also be considered in treating concomitant psychopathology (e.g., depression or anxiety). Extreme caution is warranted in the prescription of psychiatric medications with a high potential for abuse and dependence. However, many medications of known therapeutic value for other conditions (e.g., lithium, antipsychotic and antidepressant agents) pose few risks of abuse or dependence. Given proper consideration and precautions, there is no persuasive reason to deny such medications to alcoholics who manifest concomitant psychopathology for which these drug treatments are known to be effective therapeutic agents.

Finally, it is worth noting that no medication currently constitutes a primary treatment for alcohol problems. Pharmacotherapy is only an adjunctive treatment that is best used in combination with other strategies. Medications are not regarded as a "cure" for alcohol problems, but when properly used, they may be valuable aids in the recovery process.

The following questions represents opportunities for research on psychotropic medications:

• For persons with dual diagnoses (e.g., major depression, bipolar disorder, schizophrenia), does appropriate psychotropic medication reduce the risk of relapse and improve other aspects of outcome?

- What is the relative effectiveness in reducing relapse potential of psychotropic medication versus alternative drug-free strategies of treatment (e.g., cognitive-behavioral therapy) for individuals with concomitant psychopathology?
- Are certain psychotropic medications of value in reducing drinking or the desire to drink among alcoholics without concomitant psychopathology?
- What therapeutic doses, verified by appropriate means (e.g., serum monitoring), are essential to produce improvement in treatment outcome?
- When are the optimal time (in the continuum of detoxification, active treatment, and relapse prevention) and duration for administering psychotropic medications as an aid to recovery?

Aversion Therapies

Aversion therapy for alcohol abuse is based on the principle of counterconditioning. Attraction to, and positive associations with, alcohol are replaced by conditioned aversive reactions. Unlike the antidipsotropic medications, aversion therapy is designed to produce an enduring adverse reaction to alcohol in the absence of medication. In aversion therapy, alcohol is associated with unpleasant experiences or images. The typical and intended effects are a loss of desire for alcohol and avoidance of drinking.

Various methods have been used to produce conditioned aversive responses to alcohol. Electrical and apneic aversion have fallen into justifiable disuse, and no new studies have appeared since 1980 (Miller and Hester, 1986a; Wilson, 1987). Chemical aversion pairs alcohol with nausea and vomiting induced by emetic drugs. Aversion therapy is a mainstay of alcohol treatment in the Soviet Union and continues to be used in some U.S. treatment centers.

In the 1980s, however, chemical aversion therapy has come under sharp attack (National Center for Health Care Technology, 1981; Wilson, 1987). Although uncontrolled studies have reported relatively high rates of abstinence (Miller and Hester, 1980; Neuberger et al., 1980, 1981, 1982), support from controlled studies has been weak, and the absolute impact of chemical aversion treatment beyond or in the absence of adjunctive therapeutic approaches is unclear. Cannon, Baker, and Wehl (1981) found no long-term differences between a group treated with chemical aversion and a control group receiving only standard hospital treatment, although both fared better than a group that received electrical aversion. Richard (1983) found no effects of an aversion procedure based on nausea induced by motion sickness. Thurber (1985) expressed cautious optimism based on a meta-analysis of controlled studies of chemical aversive counterconditioning. The Council on Scientific Affairs of the American Medical Association (1987) likewise found "positive results" from aversion therapies but called for further controlled trials. Wilson (1987), in contrast, concluded that the use of chemical aversion therapy for alcoholism is unwarranted, given its stressful and potentially hazardous nature and the absence of clear evidence for its efficacy.

One strength of the chemical aversion approach is its foundation in basic research and learning theory. Acquired and persistent taste aversion is a well-established phenomenon in mammals, including humans. Elkins (1984) demonstrated a strong relationship between the intensity of induced nausea and the persistence of taste aversion. Elkins and Hobbs (1982) likewise demonstrated a potent genetic influence on the susceptibility to taste aversion learning, perhaps mirroring human individual differences in response to this treatment modality. This inherited susceptibility factor appears to be quite specific to taste aversion and is not generalized to other learning paradigms such as electric shock aversion (Hobbs and Elkins, 1983; Elkins, 1986). Recent human research has demonstrated that chemical aversion therapy does produce a conditioned aversive response to alcohol and that the strength of conditioning is predictive of treatment outcome (Cannon and Baker, 1981; Cannon, Baker, and Wehl, 1981; Baker et al., 1984; Cannon et al., 1986). The robustness of these experimental findings and of the taste aversion conditioning phenomenon itself warrants further investigation of taste aversion therapy for alcohol problems.

Covert sensitization is an alternative aversive counterconditioning procedure employing only imagery. It requires no use of drugs or shock, is less physically stressful, and can be administered in outpatient treatment. Recent studies have demonstrated that conditioned aversion to alcohol can be produced by covert sensitization and that (as with chemical aversion) the strength of conditioning is predictive of treatment outcome (Elkins, 1980; Miller and Dougher, 1984). Olson and colleagues (1981) demonstrated greater suppression of drinking among alcoholics assigned at random to receive behavior therapy (including covert sensitization), relative to two groups receiving transactional analysis or milieu treatment alone. Covert sensitization administered in groups was found in two studies to be ineffective (Sanchez-Craig and Walker, 1982; Telch, Hannon, and Telch, 1984).

Finally, it should be noted that certain therapeutic procedures for alcohol problems (including some aversion therapies) require the administration of small amounts of alcohol to those undergoing treatment. Certain relapse prevention and cue exposure procedures may require exposure to the sight, smell, or taste of alcohol (see Chapter 12). Research on these procedures may thus require the presentation of alcohol to alcohol-dependent persons. Recent reports have specified clear ethical guidelines for the administration or exposure to alcohol of persons with alcohol problems, for research purposes (NIAAA, 1988). Available evidence indicates that when such guidelines are carefully followed, the administration of alcohol during research or treatment poses no significant risks to the individual's welfare.

The following questions represent opportunities for research on aversion therapies:

• Does the addition of chemical aversion therapy to an alcohol treatment program significantly improve long-term outcomes?
• Does covert sensitization suppress urges to drink and have beneficial effects on long-term outcomes?
• Do chemical aversion and covert sensitization differ in their relative impact on drinking behavior and on urges or the craving to drink?
• What individual factors predict the establishment of conditioned aversion and of favorable responses to aversion therapy?

Psychotherapy and Counseling

Controlled treatment outcome studies prior to 1980 failed to yield persuasive evidence for the effectiveness of psychodynamic psychotherapy with alcoholics (Miller and Hester, 1980). Recent controlled studies have not substantially altered this trend, although more promising results have been obtained in drug abuse populations (see Chapter 12). Olson and colleagues (1981) found that insight-oriented psychotherapy yielded no increase in effectiveness when added to a milieu treatment program and was less effective than behavioral approaches. Brandsma, Maultsby, and Welsh (1980) found somewhat fewer drinking days among mandated individuals assigned at random to either cognitive-behavioral or insight-oriented therapy, relative to untreated controls after one year. Braunstein et al. (1983) observed no differences in outcome between those assigned at random to aftercare that included individual counseling and group psychotherapy and two control groups that were given only medical monitoring. Annis and Chan (1983) similarly found no effect of confrontational group therapy in a random assignment design with incarcerated alcohol-related offenders.   Individuals low in self-esteem, however, showed detrimental effects from confrontational psychotherapy, whereas those higher in self-esteem evidenced some benefit.   In another randomized trial, Swenson and Clay (1980) observed no differences at an eight-month follow-up interval between drunk-driving offenders assigned to confrontational group therapy and those given only a home-study course.

There has been increased interest in and research on cognitive-behavioral therapy with alcoholics, although the results of outcome studies to date have been mixed. Oei and Jackson (1982) found significantly greater improvement among two groups of alcoholics that were randomly assigned to receive cognitive restructuring, relative to controls who received the same residential treatment without cognitive therapy. Modeling and reinforcement of positive self-statements appear to be important to the effectiveness of cognitive therapy with alcoholics (Oei and Jackson, 1984). Positive results have been reported from a prevention program based on cognitive-behavioral procedures (Botvin et al., 1984a). Other randomized clinical trials have reported no significant effect of cognitive therapies with drunk-driving offenders (Rosenberg and Brian, 1986) or halfway house residents (Sanchez-Craig and Walker, 1982; Walker, Sanchez-Craig, and Bornet, 1982).

Psychotherapy is also used in the treatment of concomitant psychopathology. For example, two types of psychotherapy (interpersonal and cognitive-behavioral) have been evaluated rigorously for their effectiveness in the treatment of outpatients with major depression; generally positive results have been reported (Elkin et al., 1989). For alcoholics with concomitant depression, then, psychotherapy may be effective not only in treating depression, but also in diminishing the likelihood of relapse to drinking. Such therapeutic effects with alcoholics, however, have not yet been demonstrated in properly controlled studies.

A common problem in research on psychotherapy and counseling is the definition and integrity of interventions. What constitutes the "psychotherapy" or "counseling" given? Evaluations should, as much as possible, specify and standardize the treatment being studied. Efforts should also be made to ensure the integrity and consistency of delivery of the specified psychotherapeutic procedures.

The following questions represent opportunities for research on psychotherapy and counseling:

• Are certain therapies (e.g., cognitive-behavioral therapy) differentially effective in preventing relapse to drinking for persons manifesting concomitant psychopathology (e.g., depression) for which the therapy is an effective treatment?

• In treating psychopathology concomitant to alcohol abuse, do psychotherapy and psychotropic medication differ in their impact on drinking?

• What are the components and processes of counseling as typically administered by alcohol counselors?

• What approaches to or components of alcohol counseling significantly improve treatment outcome?

• Are there additive effects of psychotherapy or counseling in combination with other therapeutic strategies (e.g., pharmacotherapy)?

• Within the continuum of detoxification, active treatment, and relapse prevention, when is the optimal time to initiate psychotherapeutic intervention?

• What individual difference variables (e.g., degree of residual cognitive impairment) are predictive of response to psychotherapy?

Didactic Approaches

Treatment programs frequently include educational lectures on alcohol and related problems. Interventions with drunk-driving offenders sometimes rely solely on educational strategies. Siegal (1985a,b) reported lower recidivism in two educational intervention groups than in a nonrandom control group whose members apparently were given jail sentences. Yet controlled research to date has failed to yield any persuasive evidence of the impact of such educational strategies on drinking behavior among problem drinkers or alcoholics (Uecker and Solberg, 1973; Swenson and Clay, 1980; Miller and Hester, 1986a). One concern here is whether cognitive impairment from excessive drinking may deter alcoholics from comprehending and retaining information presented in traditional educational approaches. Two studies reported very poor retention of treatment-relevant information by alcoholics (Sanchez-Craig and Walker, 1982; Becker and Jaffe, 1984).

The following questions represent opportunities for research on didactic approaches:

- What contributions to treatment outcome are made by educational lectures within the context of a multimodal treatment program?
- Does the level of cognitive impairment predict the response of alcoholics to educational interventions?
- What short-term changes, if any (e.g., information gain, attitude shifts, motivation increases) are predictive of long-term behavior change following educational interventions?
- What elements of newly developed educational technologies could be tested that might increase the effectiveness of traditional classes?

Mutual Help Groups

Although it has been in existence since 1935 and has been an important shaping force in alcohol treatment in the United States, Alcoholics Anonymous (AA) has been subjected to surprisingly little scientific study. In the 1980s, contributions to the literature on AA have continued to consist primarily of commentaries and summaries of available correlational data (Glaser and Ogborne, 1982; Kurtz, 1982; Emrick, 1987). Some progress has been made toward identifying the characteristics of individuals who are most likely to maintain affiliation with AA (Boscarino, 1980; Ogborne and Glaser, 1981), although favorable outcomes in AA are by no means limited to particular types of persons (Emrick, 1987). Correlational studies continue to support a relationship between abstinence and AA attendance (Alford, 1980; Polich, Armor and Braiker, 1980; Hoffman, Harrison, and Belille, 1983). Both correlational and controlled studies have suggested a relationship between AA attendance and greater severity of symptomatology if subsequent drinking does occur (Brandsma, Maultsby, and Welsh, 1980; Ogborne and Bornet, 1982; Walker, Sanchez-Craig and Bornet, 1982; Stimmel et al., 1983).

The findings of correlational investigations are difficult to interpret because differences (e.g., between AA attenders and nonattenders) may be attributable to a variety of factors that are confounded in such studies. Treatment-compliant individuals, for example, generally show better prognosis than those who are less compliant (Fuller et al., 1986; Fawcett et al., 1987). An observed relationship between treatment exposure and outcome, then, may be due not to specific characteristics of the treatment but to nonspecific individual difference factors that drive compliance.

Prior to 1980 only one controlled study had been conducted of outcomes of AA (Ditman et al., 1967). Only two controlled outcome studies of AA have appeared in the 1980s. Brandsma, Maultsby, and Welsh (1980) found no long-term differences between problem drinkers who were court-mandated to participate in AA and those who were assigned at random to a no-treatment condition. A second controlled evaluation (Stimmel et al., 1983) compared outcomes of alcohol-abusing methadone maintenance patients assigned at random to an AA-based therapy group, a controlled drinking training group, or a control group (no additional treatment beyond the methadone program). Among treatment completers (fewer than 20 percent), the controlled drinking and control groups showed decreased drinking on a measure of peak use, whereas the AA abstinence-focused group reported an increase on the same measure. (The relevance of this study for the principal target population of AA, namely alcoholics without other substance abuse problems, remains in doubt.)

Given its great importance in U.S. treatment programs, it is unfortunate that AA has not been the subject of more empirical research. The inherent anonymity of the treatment group presents special but not insurmountable challenges in studying its effectiveness. Advances in outcome assessment and in program evaluation methodology have increased the feasibility of conducting meaningful research on AA processes and effectiveness (Glaser and Ogborne, 1982). Alcoholics Anonymous is available in nearly every U.S. city, offering a free and highly accessible support system for recovering. alcoholics. Because it is free, on a cost-effectiveness basis AA is likely to compare favorably with alternative intervention approaches. Furthermore, the enduring success of this organization in attracting alcoholics to recovery is itself worthy of study. There is, therefore, a pressing need for high-quality research on the impact and mechanisms of AA.

In addition to AA, other U.S. mutual help movements currently include AlAnon, Women for Sobriety, and Adult Children of Alcoholics. The impact of affiliation on members of these groups and their families is unknown. Systematic outcome research on mutual help groups for alcoholics and their families represents a promising avenue for future study.

The following questions represent opportunities for research on mutual help groups:

- What are the long-term impact and cost-effectiveness of participation in mutual help groups, relative to alternative approaches? There is a particular need for outcome research employing a range of contemporary treatment assessment approaches.
- What role does mutual help group participation play in the context of multimodal treatment programs?
- What are the characteristics of individuals who maintain a stable affiliation with mutual help groups and experience favorable outcomes?
- What is the impact of mandated mutual help group attendance among offenders, relative to alternative interventions or legal sanctions alone?
- What are the key mechanisms of effective change for those who maintain successful affiliation with mutual help groups?
- What differentiates long-term affiliates from those who do not attend or who drop out after brief attendance?
- What common stages or processes of change may underlie (a) remission without formal treatment, (b) remission following formal treatment, and (c) remission associated with participation in mutual help groups?

Behavioral Self-Control Training

Behavioral self-control training (BSCT) as applied to the treatment of alcoholism consists of a set of self-management procedures that are intended to help problem drinkers reduce or stop alcohol consumption (Sanchez-Craig, 1984). Since 1980 there have been more studies on the effectiveness of BSCT than on any other single treatment modality for alcohol abuse.

A number of controlled studies compared alternative BSCT procedures or contrasted BSCT with other approaches. Brown (1980) found significantly greater reductions in drinking among driving-while-intoxicated (DWI) offenders who were given BSCT than among those receiving conventional alcohol education. Connors, Maisto, and Ersner-Hershfield (1986), who also worked with DWI offenders, reported that BSCT resulted in significantly reduced consumption, whereas two random control groups showed no change. Four controlled studies offering BSCT to outpatient problem drinkers and randomly assigning them to abstinence versus moderation goals found no long-term differences in outcome based on the assigned goal (Sanchez-Craig, 1980; Stimmel et al., 1983; Sanchez-Craig et al., 1984; Orford and Keddie, 1986; Graber and Miller, 1988)

Other research efforts have produced somewhat different results. Foy, Nunn, and Rychtarik (1984), working with inpatient alcoholics, assigned them at random to receive or not receive moderation-oriented BSCT training in addition to the abstinence-based award program. Those given the additional moderation training fared worse at short-term follow-up but showed no different long-term outcome from those receiving only abstinence-oriented treatment (Rychtarik et al., 1987). Other studies found comparable impacts from therapist-administered and self-administered BSCT (Miller and Taylor, 1980; Miller, Taylor, and West, 1980; Miller, Gribskov, and Mortell, 1981; Carpenter, Lyons, and Miller, 1985; Berg and Skutle, 1986; Skutle and Berg, 1987).

The outcomes of BSCT, even in controlled trials, have thus ranged from significant benefit (e.g., Brown, 1980) to a detrimental effect (Foy, Nunn, and Rychtarik, 1984). Comparisons with alternative treatment modalities have sometimes but not always yielded differences favoring BSCT. A plausible reason for this diversity of findings is the heterogeneity of populations included in these studies. Other causes of diversity include variations in content and in implementation effectiveness of the BSCT method. Treated populations have included inpatients on an alcohol unit (Foy, Nunn, and Rychtarik, 1984), heroin addicts on methadone maintenance (Stimmel et al., 1983), drunk-driving offenders (Brown, 1980), and self-referred problem drinkers from the community (Miller, Taylor, and West, 1980; Miller, Gribskov, and Mortell, 1981). Further study should be directed toward an examination of the characteristics of individuals and populations for whom BSCT procedures are optimally effective.

The following opportunities exist for research on behavioral self-control training:

• Studies are needed to address the following question: How effective is abstinence-oriented BSCT, relative to other approaches to abstinence?

Conjoint Therapies

Recent research supports a strong association between favorable family adjustment and sustained abstinence or problem-free drinking after treatment (Moos, Finney and Gamble, 1982; Billings and Moos, 1983; Moos and Moos, 1984). This association suggests that interventions to improve the relationship functioning of couples and families may enhance treatment outcome.

New data are available regarding conjoint couples therapy as an adjunct to alcohol treatment. One study found that, over six months of follow-up, alcoholics given behavioral marital therapy showed more rapid reductions in drinking and somewhat better maintenance of sobriety than two control groups (McCrady et al., 1987). Similarly, Stout and colleagues (1988) reported that alcoholics who undertook behavioral marital therapy showed superior outcomes at longer follow-up points, relative to those treated with only an alcohol problem focus.   However, a four-year follow-up study supported earlier findings that joint hospitalization of alcoholics and their spouses did not improve outcome relative to hospitalization of the alcoholics alone (McCrady et al., 1982).

Conjoint therapy has also been found to decrease the probability of treatment dropout (Noel et al., 1987; Weidman, 1987). O'Farrell, Cutter, and Floyd (1985) compared group behavioral marital therapy with an "interactional" couples group focusing on mutual support, discussion of feelings, and insights. Couples in behavioral marital therapy showed greater improvement in marital functioning than those in the interactional group, relative to controls who received no marital therapy. On a measure of alcohol-free days, all groups showed improvement, but individuals in behavioral marital therapy improved significantly more than those treated by interactional couples group therapy.

Interventions with spouses of alcoholics have also been tested. In one controlled study (Dittrich and Trapold, 1984), wives of alcoholics who were given eight weeks of treatment showed significantly greater reductions in anxiety and enabling behavior and significantly enhanced self-concepts relative to a random waiting list control group.

Although recent studies provide support for the effectiveness of behavioral marital therapy, current alcohol treatment programs include a much wider range of interventions for couples and families. These include confrontational family sessions, AlAnon and AlaTeen meetings, groups for young and adult children of alcoholics, and a variety of other conjoint and group approaches to marital and family counseling. The effectiveness of these approaches, however, is unknown. Reports of studies that compare alternative approaches have only recently begun to appear (e.g., Zweben, Pearlman and Li, 1988).

Current research has focused largely on couples in which both spouses were cooperative and willing to participate in treatment. Yet a common problem in treatment is the uncooperative partner. Unilateral interventions have been described for working with one spouse (Thomas and Santa, 1982; Thomas et al., in press). The effectiveness of such unilateral marital/family therapy interventions, with either the alcoholic or the alcoholic's spouse, is unclear at present.

Furthermore, only couples therapies have been systematically evaluated (most evaluations have focused on behavioral marital therapy), and the effectiveness of treating alcoholics within the context of the whole family is unknown. New research is needed to explore the effects of conjoint therapies, not only on the drinking of the alcoholics but also on the adjustment of spouses, children, and other family members.

The following questions represent opportunities for research on conjoint therapies:

• What couples and family therapy approaches contribute significantly to favorable outcomes for treated alcoholics and their families?

• What is the relative effectiveness of treating the individual alcoholic, the couple, or the entire family?

• In what ways and by what processes do conjoint therapies contribute to long-term favorable outcomes?

• What dimensions of adjustment should be assessed as prognostic and outcome measures in family members?

• For what subpopulations is conjoint therapy effective, ineffective, or contraindicated?

• In the continuum of detoxification, active treatment, and relapse prevention, at what point is it most effective to introduce conjoint therapy?

• When the spouse (without alcohol problems) is unwilling to enter treatment, what unilateral interventions are effective in improving relationship functioning for the couple or family and in decreasing the likelihood of relapse?

Broad-Spectrum Treatment Strategies

The term "broad spectrum" applies to treatment strategies that address not only alcohol consumption but other problem areas that may be functionally related to alcohol abuse. Broad-spectrum treatments have been generally (although not necessarily) derived from a social learning theory approach to alcohol problems. Evidence increasingly indicates that appropriately planned broad-spectrum treatment is associated with lower rates of relapse to alcohol abuse (Miller and Hester, 1986a). Broad-spectrum treatment strategies should not be seen as treating an "underlying cause" of alcohol problems. Rather, these strategies appear to be useful in relapse prevention after the stabilization of alcohol problems. This is consistent with other findings which suggest that posttreatment problems and experiences are major determinants of long-term outcomes (Cronkite and Moos, 1980; Finney, Moos, and Mewborn, 1980).

Social skills training appears to be an effective adjunct in promoting sobriety among alcoholics who are deficient in social skills. Oei and Jackson (1980) found significantly greater improvement on drinking and other measures among those assigned at random to receive social skills training, relative to those assigned to traditional supportive therapy. These findings were replicated in a later study that showed significant beneficial effects of both social skills training and cognitive restructuring, with an apparent additive effect of the two interventions (Oei and Jackson, 1982). Ferrell and Galassi (1981) reported substantially higher one-and two-year abstinence rates among alcoholics given assertiveness training in addition to standard treatment procedures.

A Norwegian study similarly found that inpatients given social skills training, relative to controls who received only standard hospital treatment, had twice as many days of sobriety and employment in the subsequent year, sustained abstinence for longer periods, and experienced fewer than one-fourth as many days of institutionalization (Eriksen, Bjornstad, and Gotestam, 1986). Jones, Kanfer, and Lanyon (1982) reported that both a social skills training program and a social coping discussion group significantly improved drinking outcomes for inpatient alcoholics, relative to controls who received only hospital treatment. Chick and his colleagues (1988) found that alcoholics who received "extended treatment" that included group social skills training showed significantly greater reductions in alcohol-related problems at the one-year follow-up point, relative to two control groups who received brief "advice" interventions. Skills training has also been found to be effective in substance abuse prevention (Botvin et al., 1984a,b; Gilchrest et al., 1987).

Stress management training likewise may be helpful to alcoholics in staying sober, particularly when anxiety is a significant concomitant problem (Miller and Hester, 1986a). Although three studies found no overall effect of relaxation training on drinking measures (Miller and Taylor, 1980; Miller, Taylor, and West, 1980; Sisson, 1981), Rosenberg (1979) found that biofeedback-assisted relaxation training did contribute to reductions in drinking, but only for individuals who were high in anxiety. Controlled studies with nonalcoholic drinkers have found modest short-term suppression of alcohol consumption through aerobic exercise but not through meditation (Murphy, Pagano, and Marlatt, 1986), although uncontrolled studies suggest a correlation between the long-term practice of meditation and a reduction in substance abuse (Aron and Aron, 1980, 1983). A general stress management training program has also produced promising results (Rohsenow, Smith, and Johnson, 1985).

The community-reinforcement approach (CRA) is a comprehensive broad-spectrum treatment strategy that addresses many life-style areas related to alcohol abuse, including unemployment, marital problems, isolation, use of leisure time, and social support. The CRA combines a variety of behavioral strategies in an attempt to make the person's nondrinking life-style more rewarding than drinking. It includes job-search training, behavioral marital therapy, monitored disulfiram, and counseling focused on alcohol-free social and recreational activities. Prior evaluations of the CRA (Hunt and Azrin, 1973; Azrin, 1976) indicated a large effect on treatment outcome. More recently, Azrin and coworkers (1982) randomly assigned alcoholics to a CRA group versus traditional outpatient treatment. At the six-month follow-up point, the CRA group showed nearly total abstinence and employment, whereas most controls had relapsed and showed high rates of drinking and unemployment. In another controlled experiment, Mallams and colleagues (1982) found that one specific component of the CRA, the encouragement to attend an alcohol-free social club, likewise led to greater sobriety.

The following questions represent opportunities for research on broad-spectrum treatment strategies:

• What broad-spectrum treatment strategies (social skills training, stress and mood management training, etc.) effectively decrease the likelihood of relapse following treatment?

• Is a high level of pretreatment distress, life problems, or skills deficits a differential predictor of favorable outcome for broad-spectrum interventions?

• At what point in the treatment and relapse prevention process is it optimal to undertake broad-spectrum treatment strategies?

Relapse Prevention

In the early 1980s Marlatt introduced a conceptual model and new treatment procedures that were broadly described as "relapse prevention." Marlatt suggested that relapse was best understood not as a sudden discrete event but rather as a developmental process. He described a sequence of cognitive and behavioral events that lead to relapse and a set of strategies that might be used to decrease its likelihood (Cummings, Marlatt, and Gordon, 1980; Marlatt and Gordon, 1985). Other cognitive-behavioral models for relapse prevention have been introduced more recently, including Annis's self-efficacy approach (1986b) and Litman's "survival" model (1986). As discussed in the writings of Gorski (e.g., Gorski and Miller, 1982), relapse prevention strategies have been popularized and integrated into the 12 step approach used by AA.

The approach's intended effect is that the addition of relapse prevention procedures to a treatment program will reduce the probability and rapidity of relapse. At present, only three controlled studies of cognitive-behavioral relapse prevention procedures with problem drinkers have been reported. Rosenberg and Brian (1986) reported no differences on drinking outcome measures between an "unstructured therapy" control group and two treatment groups for DWI offenders, one of which was based on Marlatt's relapse prevention model. Missing data from the control group, however, compromised the interpretability of this study. In a large, controlled evaluation, Annis and coworkers (1988) found a modest impact of cognitive relapse prevention procedures on treatment outcome. However, Ito, Donovan, and Hall (1988) found no differences in outcome between groups given a cognitive-behavioral relapse prevention program based on Marlatt's model and an interpersonal process aftercare program based on a more psychodynamic approach.

Reactivity to alcohol stimuli has been found to be predictive of relapse. A plausible but still experimental relapse prevention strategy is cue exposure, in which the goal is to diminish alcoholics' responsivity to cues that may precipitate the desire to drink or relapse to drinking (Rankin, 1986). Empirical support for the cue exposure approach is currently limited to case reports (Blakey and Baker, 1980) and evidence that cue exposure decreases the subjective desire to drink and reduces the perceived difficulty of resisting relapse (Rankin, Hodgson, and Stockwell, 1983).

The following questions represent opportunities for research on relapse prevention:

• What relapse prevention procedures—when added to alcohol treatment programs significantly reduce the frequency, severity, or duration of posttreatment relapses?

• Are cue exposure strategies effective in reducing the desire for and relapse to drinking after treatment?

• At what point in the treatment process are relapse prevention strategies best taught? Is it more effective to offer relapse prevention training during intensive treatment or after formal treatment as a follow-up strategy?

• What individual characteristics most strongly predict relapse and which traits predict a favorable response to relapse, prevention procedures?

• What change processes do individuals use successfully to avoid or cope with relapses?

• Do relapse prevention strategies constitute an effective treatment in themselves? What is the optimal combination of relapse prevention strategies with other procedures?

RESEARCH ON TRADITIONAL TREATMENT PROGRAMS

In practice, alcoholism treatment programs in the United States typically offer a combination of modalities that includes detoxification and health care, AA groups, lectures and films, group therapy, individual counseling, recreational and occupational therapy, medication, and aftercare group meetings. Claims of high success rates are sometimes made for such programs. For example, in testimony before the Senate Committee on Governmental Affairs, McElrath (1988) stated that the Hazelden approach (the Minnesota model) "is the most successful form of treatment for chemical dependency in recorded history."

Scientific evidence regarding traditional multicomponent programs thus far has been limited to uncontrolled studies, several of which have been reported since 1980. Gilmore, Jones, and Tamble (1986) reported the results of 6-and 12-month follow-up questionnaires completed by patients of Hazelden and two other treatment facilities. Excluded from the study were short-stay patients, those who were deceased or absent without leave, and those who refused to complete the questionnaire. In the remaining Hazelden sample, 70 percent of the 6-month follow-up questionnaires were completed, among which 73 percent (51 percent of the total sample) reported abstinence from alcohol. At 12 months (74 percent completed), 58 percent (43 percent of the total sample) reported continuing abstinence. Validity checks were made by interviewing significant others in an unspecified number of cases.

A similar uncontrolled study by CompCare (1988) reported a telephone follow-up survey of 1,002 patients discharged from 50 care units. Short-stay patients not receiving normal discharge were excluded from the study. At 12 to 15 months after discharge, with a 72 percent follow-up completion rate, 43 percent (31 percent of the total sample) reported continuous abstinence from alcohol and drugs, with an additional 18 percent (13 percent of the sample) having had one to four relapses. These two groups were combined to constitute a 61 percent "recovering" rate (44 percent of the total sample). No verification of the accuracy of the self-reports of the respondents was included in the report of the study. Compliance with treatment and aftercare recommendations was reported to be a strong predictor of favorable outcome.

A third recent study was an uncontrolled evaluation of patients treated at Edgehill Newport, a private for-profit hospital (Wallace, et al.). From a target treated sample of 380, an interviewer was able to screen 257 (68 percent) eligible respondents for the study.

Of these, 65 cases (25 percent) were excluded because they were unmarried, were living apart from their spouses, or failed to complete treatment; 11 others refused to participate. Of the remaining 181, 169 were interviewed by telephone during a follow-up survey six months later. This figure represents 93 percent of the attempted interviews, although only 44 percent of the original target sample. A collateral informant was interviewed in 98 percent of the found cases, and the less optimistic report of outcome was accepted as accurate. The reported rate of abstinence varied, depending on the criteria used, from 57 percent (continuous abstinence from alcohol and other drugs for six months) to 72 percent (current abstinence from alcohol only). Rate of abstinence was found to be correlated with the frequency of attendance at meetings of Alcoholics Anonymous or Narcotics Anonymous.

Two recent studies employed more conservative methodological standards. Alford (1980) reported two-year follow-up data for 56 patients who completed 5 to 11 weeks of inpatient treatment and received staff-approved discharges. Verification of self-reports was obtained from significant others, and evaluation focused on employment and social stability as well as drinking variables. At two years, 66 percent were reported to be either "essentially abstinent" (51 percent) or light to moderate drinkers (15 percent). When more stringent criteria were employed that required abstinence with few slips, employment, and good social adjustment, 41 percent were rated as successful at two years.

In the second study, Pettinati and coworkers (1982) accounted for 100 percent of 255 patients who were followed annually for four years after inpatient treatment at the Carrier Foundation. As in the Alford study, collateral verification was obtained, and evaluation included a broad range of outcome dimensions. Abstinence (allowing for a few slips) was reported in 40, 45, 51, and 55 percent of cases at one-, two-, three-, and four-year follow-ups, respectively. When cases that showed "drinking with good adjustment" were included, these figures rose to 48, 51, 56, and 60 percent. However, about half of the cases in the study showed fluctuation in outcome status over follow-up points, and only 22 percent evidenced continuous abstinence (29 percent were mostly abstinent with slips) over the four-year period. These studies exemplify how reported success rates are significantly influenced by the stringency of outcome criteria.

Reports of uncontrolled studies pose difficulties in interpretation. Because random assignment and control groups are absent (they are often regarded as unacceptable in traditional treatment settings), the absolute effectiveness of treatment cannot be inferred. Positive outcomes may be attributable, at least in part, to favorable pretreatment characteristics or posttreatment experiences of the clinical population (Finney, Moos, and Mewborn, 1980). Consequently, despite some very useful information that can be gleaned from uncontrolled program evaluations (e.g., predictors of outcome within a program), such studies cannot support causal inferences or yield reliable estimates of the absolute or relative magnitude of treatment effects. Furthermore, it is difficult to determine which elements of a multicomponent program may account for the positive outcomes that are observed.

Methodological shortcomings can also inflate the reported rates of favorable outcomes. For example, patients who cannot be located for follow-up generally have a poorer prognosis than those who participate in follow-up studies; thus, the exclusion of the cases that are lost to follow-up is likely to yield overestimates of success within the total population. The exclusion of short-stay and noncompliant cases, dropouts, and irregular discharges likewise biases a study sample toward inflated remission rates in that compliance with treatment recommendations is known to be a favorable prognostic indicator regardless of treatment modality. Some studies have also eliminated unmarried or less stable cases, again with the likely effect of inflating success rates (e.g., Wallace et al., in press). The reliability and validity of self-reports (e.g., questionnaires or telephone interviews) without objective verification are also questionable.

As a quasi-experimental alternative to a randomized design, Grenier (1985) contrasted AA-based residential treatment for adolescents with a waiting list group. For the treated group, a 65.5 percent abstinence rate was estimated, based on two multiple choice questions administered to parents by telephone. The report did not specify the duration of reported abstinence, the length of follow-up, the percentage of cases that were not interviewed, or whether lost cases were included among nonabstinent cases. The waiting list group consisted of parents who had contacted the treatment center expressing a "sincere interest in admitting an alcohol-or drug-abusing adolescent for treatment" (p. 383), but who for unstated reasons had not done so for 3 to 18 months after initial contact. The telephone follow-up completion rate for this group was reported to be 36 percent, although outcome data were reported for only 26 percent. Among the waiting list parents, 47 percent reported improvement, including 20 percent who reported total abstinence. Several abstinent cases were excluded because they had received alternative treatment, leaving a 14 percent abstinence rate among located, untreated cases.

Contrasting the study's 65.5 and 14 percent abstinence rates, Grenier (1985, p.389) concluded that residential treatment for adolescents "was a significant causal factor in the reduction of chemical use." Causal interpretations of such findings, however, cannot be made with confidence. Individuals who remain on a waiting list for 18 months do so for a wide variety of reasons, which introduces substantial selection differences between treated and "control" groups. In addition, the accuracy of unverified self-reports is impossible to ascertain—perhaps even more so when data are gathered by mailed questionnaires or by telephone rather than in personal interviews. A high rate of uncompleted interviews also introduces interpretation difficulties because unlocated cases are not likely to be representative of those interviewed.

Uncontrolled and quasi-experimental designs may yield useful information about treatment impact, particularly when controllable methodological problems are properly addressed. Important new knowledge may be obtained regarding predictors of outcome. In addition, special populations that are seen in private treatment programs may not be found in public programs in which controlled research is more commonly conducted. Yet uncontrolled studies cannot substitute for properly controlled, randomized designs in determining the absolute and relative effectiveness of treatment programs and modalities. *Increased attention should be devoted to the possibility of conducting controlled trials in a broader range of treatment facilities.* Even in cases in which conditions constrain randomization to untreated or alternative treatment groups, it may be feasible to conduct well-controlled evaluations by comparing the addition or deletion of specific treatment components designed to enhance motivation or prevent relapse (Miller, 1980, 1985). Such studies yield information of immediate clinical utility by indicating the value of adding specific components to ongoing treatment programs.

The following types of studies, which offer opportunities for research on traditional treatment programs, are particularly needed at this time:

- evaluations conducted in ongoing treatment settings, involving collaborations of research teams with traditional treatment personnel and programs;
- specification of the treatment methods and procedures that constitute typical and traditional alcohol treatment programs;
- evaluations of the effectiveness of generic, traditional treatment procedures as offered by typical U.S. programs;
- controlled additive designs evaluating the effectiveness of traditional treatment programs with and without additional innovative treatment strategies; and
- unpackaging designs to identify the "active ingredients" of traditional treatment programs.

RESEARCH ON THE INTENSITY AND DURATION OF TREATMENT

It is a commonsense assumption that if one kind of treatment is longer, more intensive, offered in a hospital, or more expensive than another, that treatment should also be more effective than the other. Reimbursement policies of health care insurers have often followed this maxim, paying preferentially for more intensive and expensive forms of alcohol treatment.

Uncontrolled studies have long reported a positive correlation between length of stay in treatment and favorable outcome, and studies since 1980 have continued this trend (e.g., Finney, Moos, and Chan, 1981; McLellan et al., 1982), although there are exceptions (e.g., Booth, 1981). As discussed earlier, however, such correlational findings confound treatments with important individual determinants of outcome (e.g., compliance) and thus are difficult to interpret.

Fortunately, more than two dozen controlled studies have addressed this issue. In the typical study, individuals eligible for either form of care (excluding those who urgently need intensive treatment) have been assigned at random to more versus less intensive treatments or settings or to longer versus shorter treatment. With great consistency, these controlled studies have found no differences in outcome based on the duration or intensity of treatment or the setting (e.g., inpatient versus outpatient) in which it is offered (for reviews, see U.S. Congress, Office of Technology Assessment, 1983; Annis, 1986a; Miller and Hester, 1986b). Recent studies continue to find no overall advantage of residential treatment over nonresidential alternatives (McLachlan and Stein, 1982; Longabaugh et al., 1983; Eriksen, 1986; Chapman and Huygens, 1988). Similarly, recent controlled studies have found that increasing the length of alcohol treatment does not result in improved outcomes relative to briefer interventions (Miller and Baca, 1983; Walker et al., 1983; Powell et al., 1985; Eriksen, 1986; Zweben, Pearlman, and Li, in press).

Treatment settings may differ importantly, however, in cost and cost-effectiveness. Treatment is often substantially more expensive in residential and longer treatment programs. Several studies have reported that individuals treated in residential settings show increased future use of hospital-based treatment with no offsetting advantage in long-term outcome, relative to those treated in nonresidential settings (Miller and Hester, 1986b). If these increased costs are not offset by superior outcomes, less expensive forms of treatment are preferable on a cost-effectiveness basis.

Even if there is no *overall* advantage in outcome from longer, more intensive, or hospital-based treatment programs, *there remains the question of whether certain subpopulations of alcoholics may benefit differentially from such approaches.* Currently available data are limited but suggest that intensive residential treatment may be warranted for socially unstable individuals (e.g., unemployed or homeless persons; drinkers with more severe psychopathology) and for individuals with more severe alcohol dependence. Socially stable and less severely dependent persons, by contrast, appear to do as well or better in less intensive treatment (Miller and Hester, 1986b). The interactions of severity and treatment approaches are complex, however (see McLellan et al., 1983), and require further investigation.

The following questions represent opportunities for research on the intensity and duration of treatment:

- For what types of individuals is residential treatment differentially effective or more cost-effective than nonresidential alternatives?
- For particular treatment approaches, what minimum length or intensity is sufficient to yield most of the benefits attendant to the treatment? What length and setting are optimal for maximum cost-effectiveness?

●   What is the relative cost-effectiveness of different treatment settings (e.g., residential, day hospital, social model, outpatient) when consistent content is offered?

RESEARCH ON AFTERCARE

Relapse prevention as more broadly conceived includes any intervention that is designed to diminish, forestall, or attenuate relapses following treatment. Program components that are referred to as "aftercare" have traditionally been designed to promote this same goal of maintaining gains following treatment. Aftercare is not itself a form of treatment but rather a phase of treatment—continued contact with, and services to, clients or patients following the termination of a formal phase of treatment. The term is typically used only in conjunction with residential treatment, in which discharge is a discrete event. Research on aftercare, then, is essentially research on the optimal timing of various treatment procedures. Most of the treatment strategies previously discussed in this section could, in this sense, be offered as "aftercare."

Progress has been made toward defining interventions that decrease relapse during the aftercare period. Correlational and quasi-experimental studies generally point to a strong relationship between aftercare attendance and sustained remission (Costello, 1980; Ornstein and Cherepon, 1985; Ito and Donovan, 1986) although there are exceptions (Gilbert, 1988). Experimental studies of aftercare procedures have begun to appear. In a randomized trial (Ahles et al., 1983), individuals who were given a behavioral contracting intervention and a calendar designating scheduled aftercare sessions were significantly more likely to attend, to be abstinent at 3-, 6-, and 12-month follow-ups, and to sustain continuous abstinence. In that study, this simple intervention doubled the treatment success rate during the first year (after residential treatment) from 39 to 78 percent. One placebo-controlled study reported that acupuncture significantly suppressed drinking episodes, readmissions, and urges to drink following treatment (Bullock et al., 1987). However, the effectiveness of specific alternative aftercare approaches may vary with the pretreatment characteristics of participants (e.g., McLachlan, 1972, 1974), which suggests a need for individualized matching of aftercare strategies.

Other studies have failed to support the impact of aftercare procedures. Fitzgerald and Mulford (1985), in a randomized trial, found no effect of biweekly telephone contacts over a year of follow-up after inpatient treatment. Another controlled study found no differences in outcome between inpatients assigned at random to medical monitoring only versus aftercare that consisted of biweekly group therapy, individual counseling, family therapy, and social service support (Braunstein et al., 1983). Ito, Donovan, and Hall (1988) found no differences in outcomes from two alternative aftercare programs based on cognitive-behavioral versus interpersonal process models.

Although controlled and correlational studies now indicate that participation in aftercare increases the effectiveness of residential treatment, it is unclear to what extent hospital treatment contributes to long-term prognosis above and beyond the effects of aftercare itself (Miller and Hester, 1986b).

The following questions offer opportunities for research on aftercare:

●   What variables predict and what interventions increase aftercare participation?
●   Do alternative aftercare procedures differ in their impact or cost-effectiveness?
●   Is there an optimal sequencing for specific treatment interventions? Are certain modalities best offered after a period of prior detoxification and treatment?
●   What characteristics of individuals predict differential response to alternative aftercare approaches?

- What are the relative contributions of residential treatment versus outpatient aftercare procedures to long-term outcome? Does a preceding period of inpatient treatment improve prognosis, given an effective "aftercare" program? If so, for what types of individuals are there differential benefits?

TREATMENT PROCESS RESEARCH

Whereas outcome research provides data regarding the overall impact of therapeutic interventions, process research yields information about the active ingredients of treatment efficacy. Process and outcome research are not wholly separable approaches and in fact are best conducted conjointly. The central concern of the former, however, is to investigate the underlying processes involved in treatment. Three emerging areas of treatment process research are considered here: (1) mechanisms of treatment efficacy; (2) therapist variables; and (3) motivation.

Mechanisms of Treatment Efficacy

Most therapeutic interventions include at least three kinds of components: (1) active ingredients that have specific and direct effects on outcome; (2) placebo or nonspecific elements that also contribute to outcome but are not unique to the particular treatment; and (3) inert components that have no impact on outcome. Treatment interventions may also inadvertently contain components that are detrimental to recovery. Such research strategies as dismantling or additive designs can be used to identify which elements of treatment are crucial to positive outcomes.

Research on brief-treatment strategies indicates that, for some individuals, sufficient conditions for change can be contained within relatively minimal interventions. Common elements within currently documented brief-treatment strategies appear to be: (1) motivational feedback to increase the perception of risk, (2) clear advice or guidelines for change; and (3) an empathic approach that fosters self-efficacy and perceived choice (Miller, 1985; Orford, 1986; Miller, Sovereign and Krege, in press).

Within particular treatment modalities, specific mechanisms of efficacy can be tested for consistency with the theoretical model underlying the treatment. A client-centered treatment perspective, for example, would posit a strong relationship between treatment outcome and the level of "critical conditions" (e.g., empathy) offered by the therapist during therapy. Empirical support exists for this position (Miller, Taylor and West, 1980; Valle, 1981; Miller and Sovereign, 1988). Oei and Jackson (1984) found that therapist self-disclosure and reinforcement of positive client self-statements are crucial components of cognitive therapy with alcoholics. The effectiveness of social skills training would presumably rely on the improvement of the individual's interpersonal skills (e.g., Greenwald et al., 1980). In treatment programs that subscribe to a traditional disease model, it would be predicted that certain processes (e.g., reduction of denial, acceptance of oneself as alcoholic, recognition of alcoholism as a disease, working the early steps of AA's "Twelve Steps" program) would be crucial prerequisites for recovery.

The Pavlovian learning theory basis of aversion therapies would require the establishment of a conditioned aversion response to alcohol as a precondition for successful outcome. Studies of both chemical aversion (Baker et al., 1984; Cannon et al., 1986) and covert sensitization (Elkins, 1980; Miller and Dougher, 1984) show a strong relationship between treatment outcome and the strength of the conditioning that is established during treatment. When administered in a manner that is unlikely to produce conditioned aversion, covert sensitization appears to be ineffective (Telch, Hannon and Telch, 1984).

This type of process research supports the integrity of a specific treatment approach and clarifies the critical elements that should be included when the treatment is replicated.

A limited but nonetheless potentially fruitful strategy for clarifying treatment process is to ask treated individuals which elements of the program they have found most useful or have continued to use during the follow-up period. Self-reports do not necessarily identify the true determinants of outcome, but such inquiries can provide useful leads for further exploration.

The following questions represent opportunities for research on the mechanisms of treatment efficacy:

- For a particular treatment approach (e.g., cognitive therapy, marital/family therapy, AA), what are predicted to be the necessary and sufficient conditions for recovery to occur? Do these process dimensions, when operationally defined and measured, prove to be strong predictors of treatment outcome?
- What do those who have been treated perceive to be the crucial elements of treatment that is, the elements that most account for their outcomes?

Therapist Variables

Although therapist skills and characteristics have long been regarded as important factors in treatment outcome, these variables have remained largely unexamined within the alcohol treatment field (Cartwright, 1981). A few studies prior to 1980 pointed to important relationships between therapist attributes and treatment motivation, dropout, or outcome (Miller, 1985).

Some studies have focused on client/patient perceptions of therapist empathy, a variable with a plausible but still unclear relationship to treatment outcome. Two studies (Lawson, 1982; Kirk, Best, and Irwin, 1986) reported that alcoholics' perceptions of counselor empathy were unaffected by whether the counselor was a recovering alcoholic, although other perceived therapist dimensions may be influenced by this factor (Lawson, 1982). Recent reports continue to reflect no significant difference in treatment outcomes between treatment by counselors who are themselves recovering substance abusers and treatment by those who are not (Aiken et al., 1984).

Other research has included direct measures of the interpersonal functioning of therapists. One therapist characteristic that appears to be related to favorable motivation and treatment outcomes is therapist empathy. "Empathy" in this context refers not to the ability to identify with others based on similar personal experiences but rather empathic understanding as operationally defined by Carl Rogers and his students (Truax and Carkhuff, 1967). A therapist attitude of empathic understanding has been a common element in brief interventions that have been reported to have substantial impact on alcohol problems (Chafetz, 1961; Chafetz et al., 1962; Edwards et al., 1977; Kristenson et al., 1983). In a study assigning alcoholics at random to different counselors, Valle (1981) found a significant relationship between therapist empathy skill and treatment outcomes at 6, 12, 18, and 24 months. Miller, Taylor, and West (1980) found that therapist empathy during behavioral treatment accounted for two-thirds of the variance in 6-month treatment outcome ($r = .82$) and that a strong relationship persisted in outcomes measured at 12 and 24 months (Miller and Baca, 1983). Analyzing tapes of therapeutic interventions, Miller and Sovereign (1988) found that confrontive and directive therapist behaviors (experimentally controlled) were associated with increased client/patient resistance and higher rates of drinking at the 12-month follow-up point, whereas therapist supportive and listening behaviors were associated with lower resistance and more positive outcomes.

Other therapist behaviors may be important determinants of outcome. As noted in the previous discussion on mechanisms of treatment efficacy, Oei and Jackson (1984), in an experimental study, found greater improvement among individuals whose therapists practiced self-disclosure and reinforced clients' positive self-statements. Cartwright (1980) reported a relationship between therapist self-esteem and positive attitudes toward alcoholics. McLachlan (1972, 1974) reported differential effects of therapist "conceptual level" (directiveness versus nondirectiveness), depending on a corresponding personality type among alcoholic patients. A variable found to be important in research on the treatment of other problems (e.g., depression) is the extent to which the therapist consistently adheres to specific treatment procedures. Still another dimension for exploration is the impact of the therapist's personal history of alcoholism.

The following questions represent opportunities for research on therapist characteristics:

- What role do therapist characteristics (e.g., empathy, self-disclosure, optimism, confrontiveness) play in influencing client/patient dropout, motivation for change, and treatment outcome?
- Do certain types of people respond better to therapists with particular characteristics or styles (e.g., empathic versus confrontational)?
- Is therapist effectiveness influenced by the consistency with which the therapist adheres to specific treatment strategies?
- How great are differences in therapist effectiveness within specific treatment strategies?
- What factors influence client/patient perceptions of therapist empathy, likability, and effectiveness? Are such perceptions predictive of long-term outcome?
- Do recovering persons differ from others in their effectiveness as therapists? If so, in what ways do they use their recovering status in the process of treatment?
- What forms of training or credentialing for treatment providers will improve the effectiveness of their services?

Motivation

Motivation has long been recognized as a key factor in recovery. Early writings conceptualized motivation in alcoholics as a trait or personal characteristic of the individual. Consistent with this perspective, many studies continue to focus on dispositional or demographic predictors of treatment noncompliance (e.g., Bander et al., 1983; Beck et al., 1983; Ornstein and Cherepon, 1985). Yet the dispositional markers of compliance identified in such studies have shown few consistencies, suggesting that individual pretreatment characteristics interact with attributes of the particular treatment setting (Fink et al., 1984).

Research has generally failed to support a trait view of alcoholics as poorly motivated, prone to particular defense mechanisms (e.g., denial), inherently resistive, or possessing a characteristic personality. Rather, motivation or resistance appears to be determined by a range of factors in the treatment situation, many of which are influenced by the therapist (Miller, 1985). Studies do, however, continue to find positive relationships between treatment compliance and outcome (Finney, Moos, and Chan, 1981; Westermeyer and Neider, 1984; Fuller et al., 1986; Fawcett et al., 1987). Consequently, the emphasis in research has shifted from alcoholic traits to a search for intervention procedures that increase compliance and the motivation for change.

Interventions that provide personal feedback about risk appear to have a particular impact on motivation and may be sufficient to induce change in many problem drinkers

(Kristenson et al., 1983; Miller, 1985). Two recent controlled evaluations of a "Drinker's Checkup" intervention indicate that problem drinkers significantly reduce their alcohol consumption after receiving feedback about personal harm and risks (Miller and Sovereign, 1988; Miller, Sovereign, and Krege, in press). Such interventions appear to interact with therapist style as well. Risk feedback that is given in a supportive, empathic style appears to induce more change than risk feedback presented in a confrontational and directive style (Miller, 1983; Miller and Sovereign, 1988).

Compliance

Relatively simple interventions have been demonstrated in controlled studies to have powerful effects on treatment entry, persistence, and compliance (Miller, 1985). Moreover, recent studies have added new tools to the armamentarium of motivation-boosting techniques. Pretreatment exposure to videotape role modeling (Craigie and Ross, 1980), participation in a prescreening group (Olkin and Lemle, 1984), and participation in an orientation group (Panepinto et al., 1980) have been found to increase the frequency of return for treatment. Zweben and Li (1981) found that a "role induction" preparation for treatment increased continuation in therapy. For white-collar workers, a role induction conducted by an ex-patient proved less effective than inductions administered by a therapist or by staff using videotape.

In another study, Ossip-Klein and colleagues (1984) provided a wall calendar marked with the dates of aftercare meetings and negotiated a behavioral contract for aftercare attendance. This simple intervention doubled the rate of aftercare compliance, relative to a random control group. Procedures adapted from Azrin's community reinforcement approach were found in three studies to increase treatment entry (Sisson and Azrin, 1986), attendance at AA and AlAnon meetings (Sisson and Mallams, 1981), and medication compliance with subsequent abstinence (Azrin et al., 1982). In another controlled study, a simple contingency contracting procedure substantially increased aftercare participation (Ahles et al., 1983). Correlational studies point to the potential importance of other variables in precipitating or preventing dropout: staff attitudes toward alcoholics (Velleman, 1984), the length of delay between appointments (Leigh, Ogborne and Cleland, 1984), spouse involvement in treatment (Zweben, Pearlman, and Li, 1983), and the availability of treatment groups that include peers of one's own gender or age (Duckert, 1987; Kofoed et al., 1987). Other studies have contributed to our knowledge of motivation by finding a surprising *lack* of beneficial impact from what would be expected to be an effective intervention. Rees (1985), for example, demonstrated that health beliefs predicted treatment compliance and outcome; in a subsequent experimental study, however, the same investigator found that an intervention which increased the relevant health beliefs had no impact on compliance (Rees, 1986).

Mandated Treatment

An increasingly common practice is the mandating of treatment interventions by requiring individuals to choose between accepting treatment or suffering adverse consequences (e.g., imprisonment, loss of employment). Despite their widespread current use, intervention strategies such as "constructive confrontation" (Trice and Beyer, 1984) and group confrontational intervention (Johnson, 1980) have not as yet been subjected to adequately controlled evaluations of their impact on outcome.

Uncontrolled studies reflect roughly comparable outcomes among mandated and voluntary participants in treatment (Freedberg and Johnston, 1980). Yet direct comparisons of mandated interventions with control groups have yielded inconsistent results. Salzberg and Klingberg (1983), replicating the findings of two previous studies, found that DWI offenders who were given deferred sentencing and then referred for alcohol treatment, showed significantly higher rates of recidivism relative to a comparison group that was given only legal sanctions. Swenson and colleagues (1981) found no differences between two treatment programs for DWI offenders and a home-study control group given a single 30-minute session and educational reading matter. With few exceptions (e.g., Brown, 1980), educational and treatment intervention have not been shown in properly controlled trials to improve long-term outcome and to suppress recidivism to a greater extent than such ordinary legal sanctions as monitored probation (cf. Brandsma et al., 1980; Ditman et al., 1967).

With increasing frequency, employee assistance programs (EAPs) refer employees to treatment when an alcohol or other drug problem is detected, often with the condition that continued employment depends on participation and improvement. Uncontrolled studies of EAPs (e.g., Spickard and Tucker, 1984) continue to report high rates of favorable outcomes in such programs. Several recent studies have focused in particular on the outcomes of impaired physicians who seek treatment in order to retain or regain their license to practice. Among those completing such programs, reported "success" rates near 80 percent are not uncommon (Shore, 1982, 1987; Gualtieri, Cosentino, and Becker, 1983; Morse et al., 1984). Such rates are sometimes inflated by the exclusion of lost, deceased, or uncooperative cases (e.g., Morse et al., 1984).

The contribution of particular intervention components is difficult to assess in this context. Improvement may be motivated simply by the crisis of being identified as having a problem or by the desire to maintain employment, license, or liberty. Morse and coworkers (1984) found that physicians who were closely monitored and in jeopardy of loss of license showed a higher improvement rate than a comparison group of nonphysicians in treatment for alcohol and drug dependence without such scrutiny and contingencies. As with court probation cases, formal treatment may make little or no contribution to outcome above the effects attributable to the threatened loss of liberty or livelihood. Another important factor to consider is the extent to which threatened penalties for noncompliance in "mandated" programs are actually enforced. Perceived stringency of enforcement may be an important determinant of the impact of mandatory treatment. Thus, the level of enforcement of participation should be documented, and perceived enforcement should be assessed.

The following questions represent opportunities for research on motivation, compliance, and mandated treatment:

• What interventions, therapist characteristics, or situational factors increase the probability that a problem drinker will enter, continue, and comply with treatment?

• What measures of motivation best predict a favorable response to treatment? What proportion of variance in outcome is accounted for by dispositional versus situational aspects of motivation and by compliance with specific components of treatment?

• What approaches will instill a motivation for change in individuals who display hazardous alcohol consumption patterns but do not regard themselves as problem drinkers or in need of treatment?

• What are the short-and long-term effects on outcome of coercive motivational strategies (e.g., court-mandated treatment, employee assistance programs, confrontational interventions), relative to less coercive or intrusive alternatives?

CONCLUSIONS

The foregoing discussion constitutes a comprehensive review, within the context of knowledge from earlier research, of what has been learned in treatment outcome studies since 1980. In this section, specific conclusions based on the preceding review will be drawn in order to summarize the opportunities for further progress in treatment research.

Does Treatment Work?

As an introduction to such conclusions, it is important to address what is an inevitable and broader question: Does treatment work? Although attention to this issue was not part of the committee's specific charge, this fundamental question necessarily underlies any consideration of research opportunities. Indeed, the answer to this question may be what many readers of this report most wish to obtain through an examination of well-designed research.

Clearly, clinicians believe sincerely in the efficacy of their interventions; otherwise they would probably not be involved in the treatment enterprise. The history of medicine, as well as recent psychological and medical research, however, abundantly shows that clinician confidence in a treatment is not a reliable indicator of its specific effectiveness. Judgments of whether treatment works must rely on more valid criteria than the certitude of treatment agents or the testimonials of clients or patients.

Given the hundreds of clinical studies now available, what meaningful answer can be given to this question? The answer depends, of course, on what is meant by the question. The first problem to be considered in seeking an answer is the great heterogeneity of treatments for alcohol problems. A very broad array of different treatment approaches has been evaluated in clinical research, and a still wider range has been implemented in practice. If the question, Does treatment work? is understood to mean, Do *all* of these treatments work?, the answer is plainly, no. Some methods (several of which remain in widespread use) have consistently failed to show a significant impact on alcohol problems. Other currently or previously used treatment methods remain unproved. More than half of controlled clinical trials of alcohol treatment approaches have yielded negative results; that is, no significant differences in outcome among groups. Clearly, no blanket blessing can be given to all or unspecified treatments as "effective."

If, on the other hand, the question is taken to mean, Are *any* of these treatments effective?, one can more confidently answer, Yes. Several different treatment modalities have been found in a number of clinical trials to produce significantly better outcomes than occur in the absence of the treatment or with alternative treatment. Thus, we are in the happy position of having at our disposal a variety of promising treatment strategies with a positive record of success in well-designed studies.

A third interpretation of the question might be: Is there a single treatment of choice that is superior to all other approaches? Here, the answer is an unambiguous no. No treatment method is universally effective. Few have been found to yield favorable outcomes in even a majority of cases over the long run. Some approaches have poor records of success, whereas others have demonstrated encouragingly consistent benefits, but no particular treatment can lay justifiable claim to superiority over all others. Instead of a single outstandingly effective strategy, there are a number of promising alternatives, each of which appears to be effective with different types of individuals. Behavioral self-control training, for example, appears to be most effective with individuals showing less severe alcohol-related problems and dependence, whereas AA tends to be more effective with individuals who have histories of more severe alcohol problems and dependence.

This picture is consistent with human therapeutics in other fields. In medicine, for example, no single medication is effective against all infections. Nevertheless, the judicious use of the entire range of available medications, effectively deployed on an individual case basis, produces an excellent record against infection. There is no one therapeutic method for dealing with cancer, but the combined use of surgery, chemotherapy, and radiation in differing degrees in individual cases has produced notable reductions in suffering and mortality. Likewise, there are now not one but multiple potentially effective ways to treat diabetes mellitus, depression, anxiety disorders, heart disease, and hypertension. All of these examples are no longer regarded as uniform or unitary problems; rather, each is properly regarded as a family of related disorders that are diverse in etiology as well as optimal treatment. Alcohol problems are fruitfully understood in this same light as heterogeneous disorders, admitting of variety in etiology and proper treatment.

Thus, depending on the meaning of the question, Does treatment work?, the answer can be gloomy or optimistic. The grounds for optimism are not to be found in the efficacy of all treatments or in the established superiority of any particular approach. Instead, this committee, in reviewing its charge, is optimistic about the encouraging array of promising treatment procedures that have been identified through research and about the opportunities for continued research to improve the effectiveness of treatment. The following conclusions should be read within this general context.

Specific Conclusions

Significant progress has been made in alcohol treatment research since 1980. Based on currently available empirical research, the nine following conclusions appear to be supported:

1. The provision of appropriate, specific treatment modalities can substantially improve outcome. A variety of specific alcohol treatment methods have been associated with increased improvement, relative to no treatment or alternative treatments, in controlled studies. Future research should continue to evaluate the effectiveness of alternative current and new treatment modalities.

2. There is no single superior treatment approach for all persons with alcohol problems. Although a number of different treatment methods show promise with particular groups, no single approach stands out as significantly more effective overall. Reason for optimism about alcohol treatment lies in the range of promising alternatives that are available, each of which may be optimal for different types of individuals. Rather than seeking to establish the superiority of a single approach by testing specific interventions in heterogeneous populations, treatment outcome studies should delineate the characteristics of the subpopulation for whom particular modalities are maximally effective.

3. Therapist characteristics have been underestimated as determinants of outcome. Treatment is not offered by neutral agents. Therapist skills and attributes appear to be important factors that influence treatment outcome. Interactions of therapist factors with treatment and client/patient variables, as well as the main effects of therapist characteristics, may account for a substantial amount of variance in client/patient motivation, dropout, compliance, and outcome. Future research should examine the impact of therapist attributes and behaviors on treatment outcome.

4. Alcoholics Anonymous, one of the most widely used approaches to recovery in the United States, remains one of the least rigorously evaluated. Given its widespread availability and potential cost-effectiveness, there is a need for well-designed studies to elucidate the impact and mechanisms of change within AA. There is a particular need for outcome research that employs a range of contemporary treatment assessment strategies.

5. Treatment of other life problems related to drinking can improve alcohol treatment outcome. Posttreatment problems and experiences have been shown to be important determinants of outcome. Social skills training, marital and family therapy, antidepressant medication, stress management training, and the community reinforcement approach all show promise for promoting and prolonging sobriety. Such broad-spectrum strategies appear to affect sobriety by helping to resolve other significant problems that, left untreated, could precipitate relapse. Future research should continue to explore the impacts of posttreatment adjustment and the treatment of other life problems on outcome.

6. Outcome may be predictable from treatment process factors. Individual difference variables that are nonspecific (e.g., resistance) or specific to particular approaches (e.g., the establishment of a conditioned aversion response) may predict treatment outcome. Future studies should seek to clarify treatment process factors that are key determinants of outcome within specific treatment modalities and to build stronger theoretical models of treatment efficacy.

7. The overall effectiveness of treatment with unselected patients appears to be no different in residential versus nonresidential programs or in longer versus shorter inpatient programs. Although health care reimbursement systems have emphasized more expensive forms of treatment, studies to date fail to show an offsetting increase in overall effectiveness relative to less expensive alternative forms of intervention. Residential care may be differentially effective for individuals who are socially unstable (e.g., homeless, unemployed) as well as those who have more severe levels of alcohol dependence and psychopathology. Socially stable individuals without severe alcohol dependence or psychopathology appear to be treatable by less intensive approaches without compromising effectiveness and at substantially less cost. The validation of differential criteria for admission to various treatment settings and for flexible movement between them during the course of an individual's treatment is an important task for future research.

8. Both experimental and quasi-experimental designs contribute important new knowledge regarding treatment outcome. Randomized, controlled trials yield data from which conclusions of specific effectiveness can be drawn more confidently than from uncontrolled demonstrations; moreover, such studies have tended to yield more consistent results. Experimental studies may be more expensive (although a number of published controlled trials have been conducted at relatively low cost), but given the incremental new knowledge they yield, well-designed controlled clinical trials remain a cost-effective investment of research funds. Contemporary quasi-experimental designs offer sound alternatives in instances in which controlled trials are not feasible. Properly designed nonexperimental studies likewise can yield useful incremental information regarding treatment outcome.

9. The implementation of any treatment procedure warrants careful consideration of the relative risks and benefits that are likely to be derived. A treatment is justifiable when the probable benefits demonstrably outweigh the risks and costs involved in the proposed treatment procedures. Probable benefits may be judged, in general or for specific subpopulations, from the weight of current evidence in treatment outcome research. Treatments with documented special risks merit particular consideration of the risk-benefit balance. Future research should address the relative benefits, risks, and costs attached to specific alternative treatment modalities.

REFERENCES

Ahles, T. A., D. G. Schlundt, D. M. Prue et al. Impact of aftercare arrangements on the maintenance of treatment success in abusive drinkers. Addict. Behav. 8:53-58, 1983.

Aiken, L. S., L. A. LoSciuto, M. A. Ausetts et al. Paraprofessional versus professional drug counselors: The progress of clients in treatment. Int. J. Addict. 19:383-401, 1984.

Alford, G. Alcoholics Anonymous: An empirical study. Addict. Behav. 5:359-370, 1980.

Amit, Z., Z. Brown, A. Sutherland et al. Reduction in alcohol intake in humans as a function of treatment with zimelidine: Implications for treatment. In C. A. Naranjo and E. A. Sellers, eds. Research Advances in New Psychopharmacological Treatments for Alcoholism. Amsterdam: Elsevier, 1985.

Annis, H. M. Is inpatient rehabilitation of the alcoholic cost effective? Con position. Advances in Alcohol and Substance Abuse 5:175-190, 1986a.

Annis, H. M. A relapse prevention model for treatment of alcoholics. Pp. 407-433 in W. R. Miller and N. Heather, eds. Treating Addictive Behaviors: Processes of Change. New York: Plenum, 1986b.

Annis, H. M., and D. Chan. The differential treatment model: Empirical evidence from a personality typology of adult offenders. Criminal Justice and Behav. 110:159-173, 1983.

Annis, H. M., C. S. Davis, M. Graham et al. A controlled trial of relapse prevention procedures based on self-efficacy theory. Unpublished manuscript. Toronto: Addiction Research Foundation, 1988.

Aron, A., and E. N. Aron. The transcendental meditation program's effect on addictive behavior. Addict. Behav. 5:3-12, 1980.

Aron, E. N., and A. Aron. The patterns of reduction of drug and alcohol use among transcendental meditation participants. Bull. Soc. Psychol. Addict. Behav. 2:8-33, 1983.

Azrin, N. H. Improvements in the community-reinforcement approach to alcoholism. Behav. Res. Ther. 14:339-348, 1976.

Azrin, N. H., R. W. Sisson, R. Meyers et al. Alcoholism treatment by disulfiram and community reinforcement therapy. J. Behav. Ther. Exp. Psychiatry 13:105-112, 1982.

Baker, T. B., D. S. Cannon, S. T. Tiffany et al. Cardiac response as an index of the effect of aversion therapy. Behav. Res. Ther. 22:403-411, 1984.

Bander, K. W., N. A. Stilwell, E. Fein et al. Relationship of patient characteristics to program attendance by women alcoholics. J. Stud. Alcohol 44:318-327, 1983.

Beck, N. C., W. Shekin, C. Fraps et al. Prediction of discharges against medical advice from an alcohol and drug misuse treatment program. J. Stud. Alcohol 44:171-180, 1983.

Becker, J. T., and J. H. Jaffe. Impaired memory for treatment-relevant information in inpatient men alcoholics. J. Stud. Alcohol 45:339-343, 1984.

Berg, G., and A. Skutle. Early intervention with problem drinkers. Pp. 205-220 in W. R. Miller and N. Heather, eds. Treating Addictive Behaviors: Processes of Change. New York: Plenum, 1986.

Billings, A. G., and R. H. Moos. Psychosocial processes of recovery among alcoholics and their families: Implications for clinicians and program evaluators. Addict. Behav. 8:205-218, 1983.

Blakey, R., and R. Baker. An exposure approach to alcohol abuse. Behav. Res. Ther. 18:319-326, 1980.

Booth, R. Alcohol halfway houses: Treatment length and treatment outcome. Int. J. Addict. 16:927-934, 1981.

Boscarino, J. Factors related to "stable" and "unstable" affiliation with Alcoholics Anonymous. Int. J. Addict. 15:839-848, 1980.

Botvin, G. J., E. Baker, N. L. Renick et al. A cognitive-behavioral approach to substance abuse prevention. Addict. Behav. 9:137-148, 1984a.

Botvin, G. J., E. Baker, E. M. Botvin et al. Prevention of alcohol misuse through the development of personal and social competence: A pilot study. J. Stud. Alcohol 45:550-552, 1984b.

Brandsma, J. M., M. C. Maultsby, and R. J. Welsh. The Outpatient Treatment of Alcoholism: A Review and Comparative Study. Baltimore, MD: University Park Press, 1980.

Braunstein, W. B., B. J. Powell, J. F. McGowan et al. Employment factors in outpatient recovery of alcoholics: A multivariate study. Addict. Behav. 8:345-351, 1983.

Brown, R. A. Conventional education and controlled drinking education courses with convicted drunken drivers. Behav. Ther. 11:632-642, 1980.

Brubaker, R. G., D. M. Prue, and R. G. Rychtarik. Determinants of disulfiram acceptance among alcohol patients: A test of the theory of reasoned action. Addict. Behav. 12:43-52, 1987.

Bullock, M. L., A. J. Umen, P. D. Culliton et al. Acupuncture treatment of alcoholic recidivism: A pilot study. Alcoholism Clin. Exp. Res. 11:292-295, 1987.

Cannon, D. S., and T. B. Baker. Emetic and electric shock alcohol aversion therapy: Assessment of conditioning. J. Consult. Clin. Psychol. 49:20-33, 1981.

Cannon, D. S., T. B. Baker, and C. K. Wehl. Emetic and electric shock alcohol aversion therapy: Six-and twelve-month follow-up. J. Consult. Clin. Psychol. 49:360-368, 1981.

Cannon, D. S., T. B. Baker, A. Gino et al. Alcohol-aversion therapy: Relation between strength of aversion and abstinence. J. Consult. Clin. Psychol. 54:825-830, 1986.

Carpenter, R. A., C. A. Lyons, and W. R. Miller. Peer-managed self-control program for prevention of alcohol abuse in American Indian high school students: A pilot evaluation study. Int. J. Addict. 20:299-310, 1985.

Cartwright, A. K. J. The attitudes of helping agents towards the alcoholic client: The influence of experience, support, training, and self-esteem. Br. J. Addict. 75:413-431, 1980.

Cartwright, A. K. J. Are different therapeutic perspectives important in the treatment of alcoholism? Br. J. Addict. 76:347-361, 1981.

Chafetz, M. E. A procedure for establishing therapeutic contact with the alcoholic. Q. J. Stud. Alcohol 22:325-328, 1961.

Chafetz, M. E., H. T. Blane, H. S. Abram et al. Establishing treatment relations with alcoholics. J. Nerv. Ment. Dis. 134:395-409, 1962.

Chapman, P. L. H., and I. Huygens. An evaluation of three treatment programmes for alcoholism: An experimental study with six and 18-month follow-ups. Br. J. Addict. 83:67-81, 1988.

Chick, J., B. Ritson, J. Connaughton et al. Advice versus extended treatment for alcoholism: A controlled study. Br. J. Addict. 83:159-170, 1988.

Christensen, J. K., P. Ronsted, and U. H. Vaag. Side effects after disulfiram: Comparison of disulfiram and placebo in a double-blind multicentre study. Acta Psychiatr. Scand. 69:265-273, 1984.

CompCare. Care Unit Evaluation of Treatment Outcome. Newport Beach, CA: Comprehensive Care Corporation, 1988.

Connors, G. J., S. A. Maisto, and S. M. Ersner-Hershfield. Behavioral treatment of drunk-drinking recidivists: Short-term and long-term effects. Behav. Psychotherapy 14:34-35, 1986.

Cook, T. D., and D. T. Campbell. Quasi-experimentation: Design and Analysis Issues for Field Settings. Boston: Houghton-Mifflin, 1979.

Costello, R. M. Alcoholism aftercare and outcome: Cross-lagged panel and path analyses. Br. J. Addict. 75:49-53, 1980.

Council on Scientific Affairs, American Medical Association. Aversion therapy. J. Am. Med. Assoc. 258:2562-2566, 1987.

Craigie, F. C., Jr., and S. M. Ross. The use of a videotape pre-therapy training program to encourage treatment-seeking among alcohol detoxification patients. Behav. Ther. 11:141-147, 1980.

Cronkite, R. C., and R. H. Moos. Determinants of the posttreatment functioning of alcoholic patients: A conceptual framework. J. Consult. Clin. Psychol. 48:305-316, 1980.

Cummings, C., G. A. Marlatt and J. R. Gordon. Relapse: Prevention and prediction. In W. R. Miller, ed. The Addictive Behaviors: Treatment of Alcoholism, Drug Abuse, Smoking, and Obesity. Oxford: Pergamon Press, 1980.

Ditman, K. S., G. G. Crawford, E. W. Forgy et al. A controlled experiment on the use of court probation for drunk arrests. Am. J. Psychiatry 124:160-163, 1967.

Dittrich, J. E., and M. A. Trapold. A treatment program for wives of alcoholics: An evaluation. Bull. Soc. Psychol. Addict. Behav. 3:91-102, 1984.

Dorus, W. Lithium carbonate treatment of depressed and non-depressed alcoholics in a double-blind, placebo-controlled study. Presented at the annual meeting of the Research Society on Alcoholism, June 3, 1988.

Duckert, F. Recruitment into treatment and effects of treatment for female problem drinkers. Addict. Behav. 12:137-150, 1987.

Duckert, F., and J. Johnsen. Behavioral use of disulfiram in the treatment of problem drinking. Int. J. Addict. 22:445-454, 1987.

Edwards, G., J. Orford, S. Egert et al. Alcoholism: A controlled trial of "treatment" and "advice." J. Stud. Alcohol 38:1004-1031, 1977.

Elkin, I., M. T. Shea, J. T. Watkins et al. National Instiute of Mental Health Treatment of Depression Collaborative Research Program: General Effectiveness of Treatments. Arch. Gen. Psychiatry 46:971-982, 1989.

Elkins, R. L. Covert sensitization treatment of alcoholism: Contributions of successful conditioning to subsequent abstinence maintenance. Addict. Behav. 5:67-89, 1980.

Elkins, R. L. Taste-aversion retention: An animal experiment with implications for consummatory-aversion alcoholism treatments. Behav. Res. Ther. 22:179-186, 1984.

Elkins, R. L. Separation of taste-aversion-prone and taste-aversion-resistant rats through selective breeding: Implications for individual differences in conditionability and aversion-therapy alcoholism treatment. Behav. Neuroscience 100:121-124, 1986.

Elkins, R. L., and S. H. Hobbs. Taste aversion proneness: A modulator of conditioned consummatory aversion in rats. Bull. Psychonomic Soc. 20:257-260, 1982.

Emrick, C. D. Alcoholics Anonymous: Affiliation processes and effectiveness as treatment. Alcoholism Clin. Exp. Res. 11:416-423, 1987.

Eriksen, L. The effect of waiting for inpatient treatment after detoxification: An experimental comparison between inpatient treatment and advice only. Addict. Behav. 10:235-248, 1986.

Eriksen, L., S. Bjornstad, and K. G. Gotestam. Social skills training in groups for alcoholics: One-year treatment outcome for groups and individuals. Addict. Behav. 11:309-330, 1986.

Fawcett, J., D. C. Clark, C. A. Aagesen et al. A double-blind, placebo-controlled trial of lithium carbonate therapy for alcoholism. Arch. Gen. Psychiatry 44:248-256, 1987.

Ferrell, W. L., and J. P. Galassi. Assertion training and human relations training in the treatment of chronic alcoholics. Int. J. Addict. 16:959-968, 1981.

Fink, E. B., S. Rudden, R. Longabaugh et al. Adherence in a behavioral alcohol treatment program. Int. J. Addict. 19:709-719, 1984.

Finney, J. W., R. H. Moos, and D. A. Chan. Length of stay and program component effects in the treatment of alcoholism: A comparison of two techniques for process analyses. J. Consult. Clin. Psychol. 49:120-131, 1981.

Finney, J. W., R. H. Moos, and C. R. Mewborn. Posttreatment experiences and treatment outcome of alcoholic patients six months and two years after hospitalization. J. Consult. Clin. Psychol. 48:17-29, 1980.

Fitzgerald, J. L., and H. A. Mulford. An experimental test of telephone aftercare contacts with alcoholics. J. Stud. Alcohol 46:418-424, 1985.

Foy, D. W., B. L. Nunn, and R. G. Rychtarik. Broad-spectrum behavioral treatment for chronic alcoholics: Effects of training in controlled drinking skills. J. Consult. Clin. Psychol. 52:218-230, 1984.

Freedberg, E. J., and W. E. Johnston. Outcome with alcoholics seeking treatment voluntarily or after confrontation by their employer. J. Occup. Med. 22:83-86, 1980.

Fuller, R. K., and W. O. Williford. Life-table analysis of abstinence in a study evaluating the efficacy of disulfiram. Alcoholism Clin. Exp. Res. 4:298-301, 1980.

Fuller, R. K., L. Branchey, D. R. Brightwell et al. Disulfiram treatment of alcoholism: A Veterans Administration cooperative study. J. Am. Med. Assoc. 256:1449-1455, 1986.

Gilbert, F. S. The effect of type of aftercare follow-up on treatment outcome among alcoholics. J. Stud. Alcohol 49:149-159, 1988.

Gilchrest, L. D., S. P. Schinke, J. E. Trimble et al. Skills enhancement to prevent substance abuse among American Indian adolescents. Int. J. Addict. 22:869-879, 1987.

Gill, K., and Z. Amit. Effects on serotonin uptake blockade on food water and ethanol consumption in rats. Alcoholism Clin. Exp. Res. 11(5):444-449, 1987.

Gilmore, K., D. Jones, and L. Tamble. Treatment Benchmarks. Center City, MN: Hazelden, 1986.

Glaser, F. B., and A. C. Ogborne. Does A.A. really work? Br. J. Addict. 77:123-129, 1982.

Gorski, T. T., and M. Miller. Counseling for Relapse Prevention. Independence, MO: Herald House-Independence Press, 1982.

Graber, R. A., and W. R. Miller. Abstinence and controlled drinking goals in behavioral self-control training of problem drinkers: A randomized clinical trial. Psychol. Addict. Behav. 2:20-33, 1988.

Greenwald, M. A., J. D. Kloss, M. E. Kovaleski et al. Drink refusal and social skills training with hospitalized alcoholics. Addict. Behav. 5:227-228, 1980.

Grenier, C. Treatment effectiveness in an adolescent chemical dependence treatment program: A quasi-experimental design. Int. J. Addict. 20:381-391, 1985.

Gualtieri, A. C., J. P. Cosentino, and J. S. Becker. The California experience with a diversion program for impaired physicians. J. Am. Med. Assoc. 249:226-229, 1983.

Hobbs, S. H., and R. L. Elkins. Operant performance of rats selectively bred for strong or weak acquisition of conditioned taste aversions. Bull. Psychonomic Soc. 21:303-306, 1983.

Hoffman, N. B., P. A. Harrison, and C. A. Belille. Alcoholics Anonymous after treatment: Attendance and abstinence. Int. J. Addict. 18:311-318, 1983.

Hunt, N. H., and N. H. Azrin. A community-reinforcement approach to alcoholism. Behav. Res. Ther. 11:91-104, 1973.

Ito, J. R., and D. M. Donovan. Aftercare in alcoholism treatment: A review. Pp.435-456 in W. R. Miller and N. Heather, eds. Treating Addictive Behaviors: Processes of Change. New York: Plenum, 1986.

Ito, J. R., D. M. Donovan, and J. J. Hall. Relapse prevention and alcohol aftercare: Effects on drinking outcome, change process, and aftercare attendance. Br. J. Addict. 83:171-181, 1988.

Jensen, S. B. Sexual function and dysfunction in younger married alcoholics. Acta Psychiatr. Scand. 69:543-549, 1984.

Johnsen, J., A. Stowell, J. Bache-Wiig et al. A double-blind placebo controlled study of male alcoholics given a subcutaneous disulfiram implantation. Br. J. Addict. 82:607-613, 1987.

Johnson, V. I'll Quit Tomorrow. New York: Harper and Row, 1980.

Jones, S. L., R. Kanfer, and R. I. Lanyon. Skill training with alcoholics: A clinical extension. Addict. Behav. 7:285-290, 1982.

Keane, T. M., D. W. Foy, B. Nunn et al. Spouse contracting to increase Antabuse compliance in alcoholic veterans. J. Clin. Psychol. 40:340-344, 1984.

Kirk, W. G., J. B. Best, and P. Irwin. The perception of empathy in alcoholism counselors. J. Stud. Alcohol 47:834-838, 1986.

Kofoed, L. L. Chemical monitoring of disulfiram compliance: A study of alcoholic outpatients. Alcoholism Clin. Exp. Res. 11:481-485, 1987.

Kofoed, L. L., J. Kania, T. Walsh, and R. Atkinson. Outpatient treatment of patients with substance abuse and coexisting psychiatric disorders. Am. J. Psych. 143:867-872, 1986.

Kofoed, L. L., R. L. Tolson, R. M. Atkinson et al. Treatment compliance of older alcoholics: An elder-specific approach is superior to "mainstreaming." J. Stud. Alcohol 48:47-51, 1987.

Kristenson, H., H. Ohlin, M. B. Hulten-Nosslin et al. Identification and intervention of heavy drinking in middle-aged men: Results and follow-up of 24-60 months of long-term study with randomized controls. Alcoholism Clin. Exp. Res. 7:203-209, 1983.

Kurtz, E. Why A.A. works: The intellectual significance of Alcoholics Anonymous. J. Stud. Alcohol 43:38-80, 1982.

Lawson, G. Relation of counselor traits to evaluation of the counseling relationship by alcoholics. J. Stud. Alcohol 43:834-838, 1982.

Leigh, G., A. C. Ogborne, and P. Cleland. Factors associated with patient dropout from an outpatient alcoholism treatment service. J. Stud. Alcohol 45:359-362, 1984.

Lemberger, L., H. Rowe, R. F. Bergstrom et al. The effect of fluoxetine on psychomotor performance, physiologic response, and kinetics of ethanol. Clin. Pharmacol. Ther. 37:658-64, 1985.

Ling, W., D. G. Weiss, V. C. Charuvastra et al. Use of disulfiram for alcoholics in methadone maintenance programs: A Veterans Administration cooperative study. Arch. Gen. Psychiatry 40:851-861, 1983.

Linnoila, M., M. Eckardt, M. Durcan et al. Interactions of serotonin with ethanol: Clinical and animal studies. Psychopharm. Bull. 23:452-457, 1987.

Liskow, B. I., and D. W. Goodwin. Pharmacological treatment of alcohol intoxication, withdrawal and dependence: A critical review. J. Stud. Alcohol 48:356-370, 1987.

Litman, G. Alcoholism survival: The prevention of relapse. Pp. 391-405 in W. R. Miller and N. Heather, eds. Treating Addictive Behaviors: Processes of Change. New York: Plenum, 1986.

Longabaugh, R., B. McCrady, E. Fink et al. Cost-effectiveness of alcoholism treatment in partial vs. inpatient settings: Six-month outcomes. J. Stud. Alcohol 44:1049-1071, 1983.

Mallams, J. H., M. D. Godley, G. M. Hall et al. A social-systems approach to resocializing alcoholics in the community. J. Stud. Alcohol 43:1115-1123, 1982.

Marlatt, G. A., and Gordon, J. Relapse prevention: Maintenance strategies in the treatment of addictive behaviors. New York: Guilford Press, 1985.

McCrady, B. S., J. Moreau, T. J. Paolino, Jr., et al. Joint hospitalization and couples therapy for alcoholism: A four-year follow-up. J. Stud. Alcohol 43:1244-1250, 1982.

McCrady, B. S., N. E. Noel, D. B. Abrams et al. Comparative effectiveness of three types of spouse involvement in outpatient behavioral alcoholism treatment. J. Stud. Alcohol 47:459-467, 1986.

McElrath, D. The Hazelden treatment model. Testimony before the U.S. Senate Committee on Governmental Affairs, Washington DC, June 16, 1988.

McLachlan, J. F. C. Benefit from group therapy as a function of patient-therapist match on conceptual level. Psychother. 9:317-323, 1972.

McLachlan, J. F. C. Therapy strategies, personality orientation, and recovery from alcoholism. Can. Psychiatr. Assoc. J. 19:25-30, 1974.

McLachlan, J. F. C., and R. L. Stein. Evaluation of a day clinic for alcoholics. J. Stud. Alcohol 43:261-272, 1982.

McLellan, A. T., L. Luborsky, C. O'Brien et al. Is treatment for substance abuse effective? J. Am. Med. Assoc. 247:1423-1428, 1982.

McLellan, A. T., G. E. Woody, L. Luborsky et al. Increased effectiveness of substance abuse treatment: A prospective study of patient-treatment "matching." J. Nerv. Ment. Dis. 171:597-605, 1983.

McMillan, T. M. Lithium and the treatment of alcoholism: A critical review. Br. J. Addict. 76:245-258, 1981.

Miller, W. R. Maintenance of therapeutic change: A usable evaluation design. Prof. Psychol. 41:773-775, 1980.

Miller, W. R. Motivational interviewing with problem drinkers. Behavioral Psychotherapy 11:147-172, 1983.

Miller, W. R. Motivation for treatment: A review with special emphasis on alcoholism. Psychol. Bull. 98:84-107, 1985.

Miller, W. R., and L. M. Baca. Two-year follow-up of bibliotherapy and therapist-directed controlled drinking training for problem drinkers. Behav. Ther. 14:441-448, 1983.

Miller, W. R., and M. J. Dougher. Covert sensitization: Alternative treatment approaches for alcoholics. Paper presented at the Second Congress of the International Society for Biomedical Research on Alcoholism, Santa Fe, 1984.

Miller, W. R., and R. K. Hester. Treating the problem drinker: Modern approaches. In W. R. Miller, ed. The Addictive Behaviors: Treatment of Alcoholism, Drug Abuse, Smoking, and Obesity. Oxford: Pergamon Press, 1980.

Miller, W. R., and R. K. Hester. The effectiveness of alcoholism treatment: What research reveals. Pp. 121-174 in W. R. Miller and N. Heather, eds. Treating Addictive Behaviors: Processes of Change. New York: Plenum, 1986a.

Miller, W. R., and R. K. Hester Inpatient alcoholism treatment: Who benefits? American Psychologist 41(7):794-805, 1986b.

Miller, W. R., and R. G. Sovereign. A comparison of two styles of therapeutic confrontation. Unpublished manuscript, University of New Mexico, 1988.

Miller, W. R., and C. A. Taylor. Relative effectiveness of bibliotherapy, individual and group self-control training in the treatment of problem drinkers. Addict. Behav. 5:13-24, 1980.

Miller, W. R., C. J. Gribskov, and R. L. Mortell. Effectiveness of a self-control manual for problem drinkers with and without therapist contact. Int. J. Addict. 16:1247-1254, 1981.

Miller, W. R., K. A. Hedrick, and C. A. Taylor. Addictive behaviors and life problems before and after behavioral treatment of problem drinkers. Addict. Behav. 8:403-412, 1983.

Miller, W. R., A. L. Leckman, and M. Tinkcom. Long-term follow-up of controlled drinking therapies, unpublished, 1988.

Miller, W. R., R. G. Sovereign, and B. Krege. Motivational interviewing with problem drinkers. II. The drinker's check-up as a preventive intervention. Behav. Psychother, in press.

Miller, W. R., C. A. Taylor, and J. C. West. Focused versus broad-spectrum therapy for problem drinkers. J. Consult. Clin. Psychol. 48:590-601, 1980.

Moos, R. H., and B. S. Moos. The process of recovery from alcoholism. III. Comparing functioning in families of alcoholics and matched control families. J. Stud. Alcohol 45:111-118, 1984.

Moos, R. H., J. W. Finney, and W. Gamble. The process of recovery from alcoholism. II. Comparing spouses of alcoholic patients and matched community controls. J. Stud. Alcohol 43:888-909, 1982.

Morse, R. M., M. A. Martin, W. M. Swenson et al. Prognosis of physicians treated for alcoholism and drug dependence. J. Am. Med. Assoc. 251:743-746, 1984.

Murphy, T. J., R. R. Pagano, and G. A. Marlatt. Lifestyle modification with heavy alcohol drinkers: Effects of aerobic exercise and meditation. Addict. Behav. 11:175-186, 1986.

Nakamura, M., J. E. Overall, L. E. Hollister et al. Factors affecting outcome of depressive symptoms in alcoholics. Alcoholism Clin. Exp. Res. 7:188-193, 1983.

Naranjo, C. A., E. A. Sellers, C. A. Roach et al. Zimelidine-induced variations in alcohol intake by non-depressed heavy drinkers. Clin. Pharm. Ther. 35:374-381, 1984.

Naranjo, C. A., E. A. Sellers, J. T. Sullivan et al. The serotonin uptake inhibitor citalopram attenuates ethanol intake. Clin. Pharmaco. Ther. 41:266-274, 1987.

National Center for Health Care Technology. Assessment of Chemical Aversion Therapy for Alcoholism. Washington DC: National Center for Health Care Technology, 1981.

National Institute on Alcohol Abuse and Alcoholism. Draft recommended council guidelines on ethyl alcohol administration in human experimentation. Washington, DC: NIAAA, November 1988.

Neuberger, O. W., J. D. Matarazzo, R. E. Schmitz et al. One-year follow-up of total abstinence in chronic alcoholic patients following emetic counterconditioning. Alcoholism Clin. Exp. Res. 4:306-312, 1980.

Neuberger, O. W., N. Hasha, J. D. Matarazzo et al. Behavioral-chemical treatment of alcoholism: An outcome replication. J. Stud. Alcohol 42:806-810, 1981.

Neuberger, O. W., S. I. Miller, R. E. Schmitz et al. Replicable abstinence rates in an alcoholism treatment program. J. Am. Med. Assoc. 248:960-963, 1982.

Nirenberg, T. D., L. C. Sobell, S. Ersner-Hershfield et al. Can disulfiram use precipitate urges to drink alcohol? Addict. Behav. 8:311-313, 1983.

Noel, N. E., B. S. McCrady, R. L. Stout et al. Predictors of attrition from an outpatient alcoholism treatment program for couples. J. Stud. Alcohol 48:229-235, 1987.

Oei, T. P. S., and P. R. Jackson. Long-term effects of group and individual social skills training with alcoholics. Addict. Behav. 5:129-136, 1980.

Oei, T. P. S., and P. R. Jackson. Social skills and cognitive behavioral approaches to the treatment of problem drinking. J. Stud. Alcohol 43:532-547, 1982.

Oei, T. P. S., and P. R. Jackson. Some effective therapeutic factors in group cognitive-behavioral therapy with problem drinkers. J. Stud. Alcohol 45:119-123, 1984.

O'Farrell, T. J., H. S. G. Cutter, and F. J. Floyd. Evaluating behavioral marital therapy for male alcoholics: Effects on marital adjustment and communication before and after treatment. Behav. Ther. 16:147-167, 1985.

Ogborne, A. C., and A. Bornet. Abstinence and abusive drinking among affiliates of Alcoholics Anonymous: Are these the only alternatives? Addict. Behav. 7:199-202, 1982.

Ogborne, A. C., and F. B. Glaser. Characteristics of affiliates of Alcoholics Anonymous: A review of the literature. J. Stud. Alcohol 42:661-675, 1981.

Olkin, R., and R. Lemle. Increasing attendance in an outpatient alcoholism clinic: A comparison of two intake procedures. J. Stud. Alcohol 45:465-468, 1984.

Olson, R. P., R. Ganley, V. T. Devine et al. Long-term effects of behavioral versus insight-oriented therapy with inpatient alcoholics. J. Consult. Clin. Psychol. 49:866-877, 1981.

O'Neil, P. M., J. C. Roitzsch, J. P. Glacinto et al. Disulfiram acceptors and refusers: Do they differ? Addict. Behav. 7:207-210, 1982.

Orford, J. Critical conditions for change in the addictive behaviors. Pp. 91-108 in W. R. Miller and N. Heather, eds. Treating Addictive Behaviors: Processes of Change. New York: Plenum, 1986.

Orford, J., and A. Keddie. Abstinence or controlled drinking in clinical practice: A test of the dependence and persuasion hypotheses. Br. J. Addict. 81:495-504, 1986.

Ornstein, P., and J. A. Cherepon. Demographic variables as predictors of alcoholism treatment outcome. J. Stud. Alcohol 46:425-432, 1985.

Ossip-Klein, D. J., W. VanLandingham, D. M. Prue et al. Increasing attendance at alcohol aftercare using calendar prompts and home based contracting. Addict. Behav. 9:85-90, 1984.

Panepinto, W., M. Galanter, M. Bender et al. Alcoholics' transition from ward to clinic: Group orientation improves retention. J. Stud. Alcohol 41:940-944, 1980.

Peachey, J. E., and H. M. Annis. Pharmacologic treatment of chronic alcoholism. Psych. Clin. N. Am. 7:745-756, 1984.

Peachey, J. E., and H. M. Annis. New strategies for using the alcohol-sensitizing drugs. Pp. 199-216 in C. A. Naranjo and E. M. Sellers, eds. Research Advances in New Psychopharmacological Treatments for Alcoholism. Amsterdam: Excerpta Medica, 1985.

Peachey, J. E., D. H. Zilm, G. M. Robinson et al. A placebo-controlled double-blind comparative clinical study of the disulfiram-and calcium carbimide-acetaldehyde mediated ethanol reactions in social drinkers. Alcoholism Clin. Exp. Res. 7:180-187, 1983.

Peck, C. C., S. M. Pond, C. E. Becker et al. An evaluation of the effects of lithium in the treatment of chronic alcoholism. II. Alcoholism Clin. Exp. Res. 5:252-255, 1981.

Pettinati, H. M., A. A. Sugerman, N. DiDonato et al. The natural history of alcoholism over four years after treatment. J. Stud. Alcohol 43:201-215, 1982.

Polich, J. M., D. J. Armor, and H. B. Braiker. Patterns of alcoholism over four years. J. Stud. Alcohol 41:397-416, 1980.

Pond, S. M., C. E. Becker, R. Vandervoort et al. An evaluation of the effects of lithium in the treatment of chronic alcoholism: I. Clinical results. Alcoholism Clin. Exp. Res. 5:247-251, 1981.

Powell, B. J., E. C. Penick, M. R. Read et al. Comparison of three outpatient treatment interventions: A twelve-month follow-up of men alcoholics. J. Stud. Alcohol 46:309-312, 1985.

Powell, B. J., E. C. Penick, S. Rahaim et al. The dropout in alcoholism research: A brief report. Int. J. Addict. 22:283-287, 1986.

Rankin, H. Dependence and compulsion: Experimental models of change. Pp. 361-374 in W. R. Miller and N. Heather, eds. Treating Addictive Behaviors: Processes of Change. New York: Plenum, 1986.
Rankin, H., R. Hodgson, and T. Stockwell. Cue exposure and response prevention with alcoholics: A controlled trial. Behav. Res. Ther. 21:435-446, 1983.

Rees, D. W. Health beliefs and compliance with alcoholism treatment. J. Stud. Alcohol 46:517-524, 1985.

Rees, D. W. Changing patients' health beliefs to improve compliance with alcoholism treatment: A controlled trial. J. Stud. Alcohol 47:436-439, 1986.

Richard, G. P. Behavioral treatment of excessive drinking. Unpublished dissertation, University of New South Wales, 1983.

Rockman, G. E., Z. Amit, G. Carr et al. Attenuation of ethanol intake by 5-hydroxytryptamine uptake blockade in laboratory rats. I. Involvement of brain 5-hydroxytryptamine in the mediation of the positive reinforcing properties of ethanol. Arch. Int. Pharmacodyn. Ther. 241:245-259, 1979.

Rohsenow, D. J., R. E. Smith, and S. Johnson. Stress management training as a prevention program for heavy social drinkers: Cognitive, affect, drinking, and individual differences. Addict. Behav. 10:45-54, 1985.

Rosenberg, H., and T. Brian. Cognitive-behavioral group therapy for multiple-DUI offenders. Alcoholism Treat. Q. 3:47-65, 1986.

Rosenberg, S. D. Relaxation training and a differential assessment of alcoholism. Unpublished doctoral dissertation (University Microfilms No. 8004362), California School of Professional Psychology, San Diego, 1979.

Rounsaville, B. J., Z. S. Dolinsky, T. Babor et al. Psychopathology as a predictor of treatment outcome in alcoholics. Arch. Gen. Psychiatry 44:505-513, 1987.

Rychtarik, R. G., D. W. Foy, T. Scott et al. Five-year follow-up of broad-spectrum behavioral treatment for alcoholism: Effects of training controlled drinking skills. J. Consult. Clin. Psychol. 55:106-108, 1987.

Salzberg, P. M., and C. L. Klingberg. The effectiveness of deferred prosecution for driving while intoxicated. J. Stud. Alcohol 44:299-306, 1983.

Sanchez-Craig, M. Random assignment to abstinence or controlled drinking in a cognitive-behavioral program: Short-term effects on drinking behavior. Addict. Behav. 5:35-39, 1980.

Sanchez-Craig, M. Therapist's Manual for Secondary Prevention of Alcohol Problems: Procedures for Teaching Moderate Drinking and Abstinence. Toronto: Addiction Research Foundation, 1984.

Sanchez-Craig, M., and K. Walker. Teaching coping skills to chronic alcoholics in a coeducational halfway house. I. Assessment of programme effects. Br. J. Addict. 77:35-50, 1982.

Sanchez-Craig, M., H. M. Annis, A. R. Bornet et al. Random assignment to abstinence and controlled drinking: Evaluation of a cognitive-behavioral treatment program for problem drinkers. J. Consult. Clin. Psychol. 52:390-403, 1984.

Schuckit, M. A. A one-year follow-up of men alcoholics given disulfiram. J. Stud. Alcohol 46:191-195, 1985.

Sereny, G., V. Sharma, J. Holt et al. Mandatory supervised antabuse therapy in an outpatient alcoholism program: A pilot study. Alcoholism Clin. Exp. Res. 10:290-292, 1986.

Shore, J. H. The impaired physician: Four years after probation. J. Am. Med. Assoc. 248:3127-3130, 1982.

Shore, J. H. The Oregon experience with impaired physicians on probation: An eight-year follow-up. J. Am. Med. Assoc. 257:2931-2934, 1987.

Siegal, H. A. The intervention approach to drunk driver rehabilitation. I. Evolution, operations, and impact. Int. J. Addict. 20:661-673, 1985a.

Siegal, H. A. The intervention approach to drunk driver rehabilitation. II. Evaluation. Int. J. Addict. 20:675-689, 1985b.

Sisson, R. W. The effect of three relaxation procedures on tension reduction and subsequent drinking of inpatient alcoholics. Unpublished doctoral dissertation (University Microfilms No. 8122668), Southern Illinois University at Carbondale, 1981.

Sisson, R. W., and N. H. Azrin. Family-member involvement to initiate and promote treatment of problem drinkers. J. Behav. Ther. Exp. Psychiatry 17:15-21, 1986.

Sisson, R. W., and J. H. Mallams. The use of systematic encouragement and community access procedures to increase attendance at Alcoholics Anonymous and Al-Anon meetings. Am. J. Drug Alcohol Abuse 8:371-376, 1981.

Skutle, A., and G. Berg. Training in controlled drinking for early-stage problem drinkers. Br. J. Addict. 82:493-501, 1987.

Snyder, S., I. Karacan, and P. J. Salis. Disulfiram and nocturnal penile tumescence in the chronic alcoholic. Biol. Psychiatry 16:399-406, 1981.

Sparadeo, F. R., W. R. Zwick, S. D. Ruggiero et al. Evaluation of a social-setting detoxification program. J. Stud. Alcohol 43:1124-1136, 1982.

Spickard, W. A., and P. J. Tucker. An approach to alcoholism in a university medical center complex. J. Am. Med. Assoc. 252:1894-1897, 1984.

Stimmel, B., M. Cohen, V. Sturiano et al. Is treatment of alcoholism effective in persons on methadone maintenance? Am. J. Psychiatry 140:862-866, 1983.

Stockwell, T., G. Sutherland, and G. Edwards. The impact of a new alcohol sensitized agent (nitrefazole) on craving in severely dependent alcoholics. Br. J. Addict. 79:403-409, 1984.

Stout, R. L., B. S. McCrady, R. Longabaugh et al. Marital therapy helps enhance the long-term effectiveness of alcohol treatment. (Abstract) Alcoholism: Clin. and Exper. Res. 11:213,1987.

Swenson, P. R., and T. R. Clay. Effects of short-term rehabilitation on alcohol consumption and drinking-related behaviors: An eight-month follow-up study of drunken drivers. Int. J. Addict. 15:821-838, 1980.

Swenson, P. R., D. L. Struckman-Johnson, V. Ellingstad et al. Results of a longitudinal evaluation of court-mandated DWI treatment programs in Phoenix, Arizona. J. Stud. Alcohol 42:642-653, 1981.

Telch, M. J., R. Hannon, and C. F. Telch. A comparison of cessation strategies for outpatient alcoholism. Addict. Behav. 9:103-109, 1984.

Thomas, E. J., and C. A. Santa. Unilateral family therapy for alcohol abuse: A working conception. Am. J. Fam. Ther. 10:49-60, 1982.

Thomas, E. J., C. A. Santa, D. Bronson et al. Unilateral family therapy with spouses of alcoholics. J. Soc. Serv. Res., in press.

Thurber, S. Effect size estimates in chemical aversion treatments of alcoholism. J. Clin Psychol. 41:285-287, 1985.

Thurston, A. H., A. M. Alfano, and V. J. Nerviano. The efficacy of A.A. attendance for aftercare of inpatient alcoholics: Some follow-up data. Int. J. Addict. 22:1083-1090, 1987.

Trice, H. M., and J. M. Beyer. Work-related outcomes of the constructive-confrontation strategy in a job-based alcoholism program. J. Stud. Alcohol 45:251-259, 1984.

Traux, C. B., and R. R. Carkhuff. Toward Effective Counseling and Psychotherapy. Chicago: Aldine, 1967.

Uecker, A. E., and K. B. Solberg. Alcoholics' knowledge about alcohol problems: Its relationship to significant attitudes. Q. J. Stud. Alcohol 34:509-513, 1973.

U.S. Congress, Office of Technology Assessment (OTA). The Effectiveness and Costs of Alcoholism Treatment. Washington, D.C.: OTA, 1983.

Valle, S. K. Interpersonal functioning of alcoholism counselors and treatment outcome. J. Stud. Alcohol 42:783-790, 1981.
Velleman, R. The engagement of new residents: A missing dimension in the evaluation of halfway houses for problem drinkers. J. Stud. Alcohol 45:251-259, 1984.

Walker, K., M. Sanchez-Craig, and A. Bornet. Teaching coping skills to chronic alcoholics in a coeducational halfway house. II. Assessment of outcome and identification of outcome predictors. Br. J. Addict. 77:185-196, 1982.

Walker, R. D., D. M. Donovan, D. R. Kivlahan et al. Length of stay, neuropsychological performance, and aftercare: Influences on alcohol treatment outcome. J. Consult. Clin. Psychol. 51:900-911, 1983.

Wallace, J., D. McNeill, D. Gilfillan et al. Six-month treatment outcomes in socially stable alcoholics: Abstinence rates. J. Substance Abuse Treatment, in press.

Weidman, A. Family therapy and reductions in treatment dropout in a residential therapeutic community for chemically dependent adolescents. J. Substance Abuse Treat. 4:21-28, 1987.

Westermeyer, J., and J. Neider. Predicting treatment outcome after ten years among American Indian alcoholics. Alcoholism Clin. Exp. Res. 8:179-184, 1984.

Whitfield, C. L. Non-drug treatment of alcohol withdrawal. Curr. Psychiatr. Ther. 19:101-119, 1980.

Whitfield, C. L., G. Thompson, A. Lamb et al. Detoxification of 1,024 alcoholic patients without psychoactive drugs. J. Am. Med. Assoc. 239:1409-1410, 1978.

Wilson, A., W. J. Davidson, and R. Blanchard. Disulfiram implantation: A trial using placebo implants and two types of controls. J. Stud. Alcohol 41:429-436, 1980.

Wilson, A., R. Blanchard, W. J. Davidson et al. Disulfiram implantation: A dose response trial. J. Clin. Psychiatry 45:242-247, 1984.

Wilson, G. T. Chemical aversion conditioning as a treatment for alcoholism: A re-analysis. Behav. Res. Ther. 25:503-516, 1987.

Zweben, A., and S. Li. The efficacy of role induction in preventing early dropout from outpatient treatment of drug dependency. Am. J. Drug Alcohol Abuse 8:171-183, 1981.

Zweben, A., S. Pearlman, and S. Li. Reducing attrition from conjoint therapy with alcoholic couples. Drug Alcohol Depend. 11:321-331, 1983.

Zweben, A., S. Pearlman, and S. Li. A comparison of brief advice and conjoint therapy in the treatment of alcohol abuse: The results of the marital systems study. Br. J. Addict., 83(8):899-916, 1988.

C International Review of Treatment and Rehabilitation Services for Alcoholism and Alcohol Abuse

M. Grant and E. B. Ritson

This review is concerned with trends in treatment policy for alcohol problems from an international perspective. It reflects opinions and data from a range of different cultures and states of socioeconomic development. However, it makes no claim to be a comprehensive account of all worldwide experiences or a statement of World Health Organization (WHO) policy. Much of the evidence discussed below was obtained from investigators in nine countries who were participants in a WHO multicenter cross-national study on the effectiveness of brief interventions. Each center was asked to prepare a short report on its current national policy and future plans concerning the treatment of alcohol problems. They were asked to address this topic under the following headings: (1) What types of alcohol problems are most common in your country? (2) What types of treatment responses are offered to these problems? (3) What are the criteria for admission to these different types of treatment? (4) Are some treatment services also offered for special population groups (e.g., adolescents, women) and if so on what basis? (5) What information is available regarding the outcome of treatment for alcohol problems in your country? (6) How are treatment services financed, and how does the cost structure impact on patients, private institutions (e.g., insurance companies), and the public purse? (7) What important issues are currently being discussed in your country with respect to the future of alcohol treatment services?

The countries involved were Australia, Bulgaria, Costa Rica, Kenya, Mexico, Norway, the United Kingdom, the USSR and Zimbabwe. The United States also participated in the study but for obvious reasons was not concerned in this particular enquiry. The opinions expressed therefore come from a reasonable geographic spread of countries with a diversity of political systems and economies.

There have been a number of cross-national studies of alcohol policies during the past decade, and WHO has played a major role in promoting or participating in many of them. The value of cross-national research was the subject of a publication in the annals of the New York Academy of Sciences (Babor, 1986). This report reviewed the findings of a large number of cross-national studies and international initiatives.

A major WHO study entitled *The Community Response to Alcohol-Related Problems* (Rootman and Moser, 1984; Ritson, 1985) was concerned with the need to provide services that were more responsive to the pattern of alcohol-related problems existing in the population. Communities within three countries (Mexico, the United Kingdom, and Zambia) were studied. The investigation consisted of a general population survey on drink-

An edited version of the report submitted to the IOM Committee for the Study of Treatment and Rehabilitation Services for Alcoholism and Alcohol Abuse, August, 1988. Marcus Grant is a Senior Scientist with the Division of Mental Health, World Health Organization (WHO), Geneva, Switzerland. E. Bruce Ritson is a Consultant Psychiatrist with the Department of Psychiatry, University of Edinborough, Scotland and serves as a consultant to the WHO Collaborative Study on the Identification and Treatment of Persons with Harmful Alcohol Consumption. Investigators who contributed to this review are S. W. Acuda, Nairobi, Kenya; M. Boyadjieva, Pleven, Bulgaria; C. Campillo-Serrano, Mexico City, Mexico; R. Hodgson, Cardiff, UK; N. N. Ivanets, Moscow, USSR; M. Machona, Harare, Zimbabwe; S. Montero, San Jose, Costa Rica; J. B. Saunders, Camperdown, Australia; and A. Skutle, Bergen, Norway.

ing patterns and the problems arising from alcohol. Enquiries were also made of a wide range of different agencies who were concerned with care giving or social control. They were asked about their experience of alcohol problems among their clients and their views about the management of alcohol problems in the community. When these views were considered alongside the opinions of specialist service providers, it was clear that the majority of alcohol problems never reaches specialist attention. This finding has been shown on many previous occasions and seems to be true even in the presence of an elaborate network of treatment agencies. The WHO project also showed that many different first-echelon services devote a great deal of time to working with the consequences of intoxication or habitual excessive drinking and yet rarely attempt to focus on their clients' drinking behavior in a constructive way. These generalists, whether social workers, primary health care workers, casualty staff, or law enforcement officers, were often reluctant to become involved in this work either because they did not see it as part of their job or more often because they felt that they lacked skills in working with "problem drinkers" and regarded this as a task for "specialists."

Thus, primary-level workers are encountering clients with alcohol problems often at an early stage in their drinking careers. Such workers seem to be ideally situated to intervene in a simple and nonstigmatizing way, and yet in many countries there is an obvious reluctance to take on this task. In some countries, quite elaborate specialist services exist for the more severely damaged problem drinkers, whereas in others there is no possibility of developing these services even if it were seen as desirable. The WHO European Regional Office (WHO EURO) organized a series of meetings concerned with the merits of intervention at the primary level and with the relationship between primary level and specialist treatment (WHO, 1986, 1987). Participants came from a wide range of European countries, and among the conclusions reached was the view that,

> ... in addition to major efforts aimed at the prevention of alcohol-related problems, there is an outstanding need for the recognition of incipient alcohol problems and for intervention starting at an early stage. Such tasks can be undertaken only with the collaboration of personnel in PHC [primary health care] services. Their willingness and ability to assume such functions, however, is generally impeded by their lack of training for such work and by the inadequacy of the available assessment and intervention techniques for use within the PHC setting. (WHO, 1986)

Mobilizing PHC services toward the early recognition and management of alcohol problems is a widely agreed upon goal in many countries, but there are also many barriers to achieving it. The community response project referred to above is being continued in modified form within the European section of WHO. It is too early to comment on its findings, but there is good evidence of the feasibility of innovative community action that is extremely cost-effective and that removes the necessity for transfering many problem drinkers to treatment facilities that are remote and of unproven value. It is also clear that there are very evident barriers to change the reluctance of PHC workers to be involved in a task they regard as difficult and of limited effectiveness. The evidence in favor of simple intervention is accumulating, and techniques are being developed (Babor et al., 1986). The WHO project concerned with the evaluation of simple interventions, whose participants provided much of the data that follow, has been employing an instrument that seems effective in detecting alcohol problems at an early stage and in a wide range of different cultures (Saunders and Aasland, 1987). The project has moved on to examine in a variety of settings the potential of simple interventions for modifying damaging drinking habits.

In summary, there are clear trends toward a new perspective in responding to alcohol problems, which can be found in a number of international reports and collaborative studies. It should be pointed out that almost all of these reports make it clear that primary prevention should be given greatest priority. This report focuses on treatment, but this narrow focus must not obscure the fact that developments in this area must be seen as part of a broader national alcohol policy.

What follows is a short review of the extent of alcohol problems in the nine countries that participated in the enquiry. This will be followed by a review of their treatment policies. Unless otherwise stated, throughout this text, quotations ascribed to particular countries have been derived from the country reports.

Types of Alcohol Problems Experienced

Before reviewing the extent of the problems reported, it is important to remember that these data are very susceptible to cultural variation. The following brief overviews of the most common alcohol problems encountered in five rather different countries illustrate both similarities and differences.

Kenya

The whole range of alcohol problems occurs in Kenya, and these problems can be classified as physical, psychological, and social problems. The physical problems that are frequently seen can be acute, subacute or chronic. The acute problems that normally present in emergency rooms include gastritis, intoxication, hypoglycemic coma, injuries and pancreatitis. The subacute and chronic problems include malnutrition, gastric ulcers and liver disease, and dementia.

The psychological complications of prolonged heavy alcohol abuse generally present in mental hospitals and psychiatric clinics, and also at the casualty departments of general hospitals and police stations. By far the commonest is alcohol psychosis. This condition may include delirium tremens, alcoholic paranoia, hallucinosis, blackouts, and "mania apotu." A recent study has shown that 21 percent of consecutive admissions into a mental hospital in Nairobi had alcohol psychosis. The other psychological presentations, which are more often detected among outpatients, are depression (occasionally with a suicide attempt), anxiety, chronic insomnia, and other nonspecific physical complaints (e.g., poor general health, weakness). Infrequently, patients may present with one or more features of the alcohol dependence syndrome such as inability to abstain despite awareness that harm is being done and uncontrollable intoxication lasting several days.

The social problems attendant upon chronic alcohol abuse are equally common though only a few come to the attention of psychiatrists. These range from domestic problems, including violence, to problems at work and economic hardships. A recent investigation into the drinking history of factory workers in Nairobi who had retired prematurely on medical grounds showed that chronic alcohol abuse seemed to be the commonest cause of retirement. A systematic study of such employees initiated by the Ministry of Labour is now in progress.

Mexico

Alcohol consumption has a strong impact on the health of the population in Mexico. For the last two decades, mortality rate from hepatic cirrhosis has varied from 20 to 23 per 100,000 inhabitants. These rates are among the highest in Latin America. Hepatic cirrhosis is one of the first ten causes of mortality in the population over 20 years of age in both sexes. Among males from 25 to 44 years of age, it ranks first. It has been estimated by Jellinek's formula that the rate of alcoholism in the population over 20 years of age is 5.37 per 1,000 inhabitants. Thus, the total number of alcoholics in the country is 1.7 million.

Alcohol-related problems are reflected in various aspects of everyday life. The biggest proportion of these problems is of a psychosocial nature and is associated with acute intoxication. For example, 5 percent of suicides in Mexico are committed under the effects of alcohol. (In a sample of 80 autopsies, alcohol was present in the blood of 28 percent of the people that died by suicide.) It has also been calculated that on the highways in Mexico, 4 percent of the drivers are drunk. In Mexico City this rate increases to 15 percent.

With relative frequency, the medical services cover problems of the acute type. Eleven percent of all the cases that were seen in the emergency services in five hospitals in Mexico City were identified as being intoxicated with alcohol, and 22 percent of the cases in similar services had positive alcohol levels. It is estimated that 28 percent of the patients in general hospitals suffer from alcohol-related pathology. During surveys for minor psychiatric disorders with self-evaluation questionnaires, it was estimated that 8 percent of the patients in family medicine services also have drinking problems.

Alcohol-related problems in the legal, family, and labor areas are also prevalent. Alcohol has been associated with 19 percent of the nation's cases of child abuse. The percentage of jail sentences resulting from the effects of alcohol was 18 percent and 24 percent, in 1975 and 1981, respectively. It is calculated that alcohol is involved in most cases of work absence.

Gender is the sociodemographic variable that shows the greatest differences. In Mexico, males drink much more than females. Different studies have shown that the rates of abstinence vary between 15 percent and 20 percent in men. Ten percent of men drink heavily and have problems with their consumption. The period when heavy drinking is most common is between 30 and 50 years of age; younger or older people drink less. Young drinkers, however, have many more problems than do older drinkers. Social class differences are not crucial, and in rural areas rates of drinking are higher.

The rates of abstinence among females vary from 50 to 60 percent. Three percent of women consume alcohol in a problematic way. There are almost no differences among age groups or among the social classes. Females in rural areas drink slightly more than females elsewhere.

The typical consumption pattern is infrequent drinking circumscribed to special occasions such as parties, celebrations, or weekends. On each occasion, however, large quantities are often ingested, and drinking may last for several hours with high degrees of resulting intoxication. Quite often, drinking takes place at the drinker's home, and females are usually excluded. Yet, in spite of the fact that drinking is not frequent, that the rate of consumption per capita is low, and that a high proportion of the population is nondrinkers, alcohol-related problems are numerous because of the way alcohol is consumed.

England and Wales

The average health district in England and Wales serves about 250,000 adults, and, using 1984 government data, it has been estimated that the prevalence of alcohol-related problems in such a district will be as follows:

Drinking heavily: 22,000
Based on a rate of 90 adults per 1,000 drinking more than 35 units a
week (men) or 20 units a week (women)

Admit to problems: 7,500
30 adults per 1,000 admitting to problems in a household survey

Known to agencies: 1,250
5 adults per 1,000 known to at least one agency to have problems
associated with drinking

Admitted to psychiatric hospitals: 125
0.5 adults per 1,000 admitted to psychiatric hospital units with an alcohol-
related diagnosis

The majority of these problem drinkers will be male. A recent survey showed that
more than 90 percent of women drink less than 15 units a week, and 70 percent drink less
than 5 units. However, indices of harm are rising faster among women than among men.
Between 1979 and 1984 in the United Kingdom, women's deaths from liver disease and
cirrhosis rose by 9 percent compared with a 1 percent fall for men. There has also been
a large increase in the number of women seeking alcohol counseling services.

The 18-24 age group has the highest proportion of heavy drinkers (i.e., 37 percent,
compared with 22 percent among the 25-35 age group). In addition, there has been a
marked rise in official figures for teenage drunkenness, from 1,852 in 1964 to 4,805 in
1976. Between 1950 and 1978 deaths from alcoholic cirrhosis of the liver in England and
Wales increased by 61 percent. United Kingdom studies have shown that alcohol
intoxication is involved in 60 percent of parasuicides, 54 percent of fire fatalities, 50
percent of homicides, 42 percent of patients admitted with serious head injuries, 30 percent
of deaths through drowning, and 30 percent of all domestic accidents.

It has also been estimated that, in England and Wales, alcohol intoxication is
implicated in the deaths of more than 500 young people each year, which is about 10
percent of all deaths in persons under 15. It is salutary to compare the absence of media
coverage of these tragedies with the extensive coverage of deaths of young people from
solvent abuse (about 25 per annum).

Between 1950 and 1977 the number of proven offenses of drunkenness in England
and Wales increased by 100 percent. In one recent investigation it was found that alcohol
usage was associated with assaults in 78 percent of cases; it was linked with breaches of the
peace in 80 percent of cases and with criminal damage arrests in 88 percent of cases.
Furthermore, 93 percent of people arrested between the hours of 10:00 p.m. and 2:00 a.m.
were intoxicated. In the United Kingdom, a 1974 study carried out by the Transport and
Road Research Laboratory showed that one in three drivers killed in road accidents had
blood alcohol levels above the statutory limit. On Saturday night, this figure rose to 71
percent.

Australia

The comparative prevalence of various alcohol problems may be gauged from
mortality data, morbidity data as judged by hospital admissions, and surveys of the general
population and specific target groups. The two most common causes of alcohol-related
deaths are trauma as a result of road accidents (approximately 1,600 deaths per annum)
and chronic liver disease (approximately 1,000 deaths per annum). Dependence and
withdrawal syndromes are common reasons for hospitalization; in New South Wales they
account for 150 to 200 admissions per 100,000 population per year, compared with 20 to
30 per 100,000 for chronic liver diseases. Between 10 and 30 percent of patients admitted
to general or psychiatric hospitals have an alcohol-related problem. In general, Australia

experiences the whole gamut of alcohol-related disorders including trauma and other acute sequelae, chronic physical and neuropsychiatric complications, dependence and withdrawal, and psychosocial problems, including industrial losses. The cost to the national economy has been estimated to exceed a A$2,500 million per annum.

Union of Soviet Socialist Republics (USSR)

The following brief comment from the USSR not only shows the overall extent of alcoholism but points out the enormous regional variation in patterns of problems that must be taken into account in most countries.

> Epidemiological research reveals that levels of alcoholism prevalence in different regions of the country differ considerably. The highest level is registered in the Russian, Ukrainian, Byelorussian, Latvian and Moldavian Soviet Socialist Republics. The lowest ones—both in the past and nowadays —are registered in the Georgian, Azerbeijan and Armenian SSRs: 7-16 times lower as compared to the average country level. But in general the contingent of alcoholics who are on the books is rather large and at present it accounts for more than 4.5 million persons and treatment of alcoholism is still one of the most urgent problems.

The five descriptions given above inevitably reflect the different resources, attitudes, and preoccupations of the countries concerned, but they also reveal many similarities. The problems may be broken down into those that are medical, social, or psychological. They may be consequences of intoxication or injudicious drinking, which result, for instance, in accidents, assaults, criminal damage, or overdose, or they may be those that are the end stage of many years of habitual drinking such as alcoholic cirrhosis, delirium tremens, or "alcoholism."

Treatment Responses

Most of the countries had some form of specialist treatment for alcohol problems, although in some cases it was almost exclusively embedded within the general wards of a psychiatric hospital. For example, in Kenya, recognition of the extent of the problem has been coupled with the realization that, apart from a few overburdened psychiatrists, no other profession is "offering treatment seriously" and that "treatment is currently being carried out mainly either in psychiatric hospitals or general medical hospitals on either an inpatient or outpatient basis depending on the mode and severity of presentation. In either setting, treatment unfortunately stops with detoxification, usually Benzodiazepine cover, vitamin supplement and treatment of any coexisting physical illness."

Typically, these institutional services are augmented by various community-based, often voluntary groups. Again quoting from the Kenya experience:

> Various voluntary and religious groups have also started some forms of counselling services. But their efforts have been curtailed by lack of knowledge and skills in counselling alcoholics or drug dependent persons. On many occasions they have requested psychiatrists to assist in training their personnel in this respect. Of all these voluntary groups, it is the Alcoholics Anonymous group which is most active in Kenya, especially in the Nairobi city. Both psychiatrists and other counsellors frequently refer

clients to the group.   The AA meetings are announced daily in both
national newspapers. It seems they have two daily meetings: one for the
upper socio-economic group (in English) and the other for the working
class (in Swahili).   Finally there are various traditional healers and
herbalists who claim that they cure all psychiatric illnesses including alcohol
problems. Their claims however cannot be verified as they do not permit
other therapists to witness or even to know their clients.

The way in which services have developed in a variety of countries is probably best
illustrated by the following series of discussions from the reports received.

Australia

A range of hospital, community-based, and private-sector treatments is available.
Hospital treatment is provided for persons with trauma and acute physical sequelae, chronic
physical complications (e.g., cirrhosis), and chronic neuropsychiatric disorders (e.g.,
Wernicke-Korsakoff syndrome). There is a shortage of long-stay facilities in some states.
There have also been moves to place such patients in community hostels. Increasingly,
patients who are intoxicated or in withdrawal are admitted to specially built detoxification
units for alcohol dependence.   Inpatient treatment is currently less favored.   Many
outpatient drug and alcohol services are now located in general hospitals, a development
which has taken place over the past 5-7 years.

Community or health clinics tend to cater to problem drinkers who have minor or
major psychosocial problems. There is an emphasis on assessment and referral to drug and
alcohol agencies.   Many of these agencies are community based and offer counseling,
behavior modification, or psychotherapy.   Self-help groups are well established.   They
include Alcoholics Anonymous, which was introduced into Australia in 1955, Al-Anon, Al-
Ateen, and Adult Children of Alcoholics.

Private medical practitioners may also undertake the management of alcohol
problems, although probably to a lesser extent than in other Western countries.
Involvement by psychiatrists, general physicians, and others varies considerably from state
to state. There is considerable interest in early intervention programs, but there are few
service units offering early intervention.

Norway

Traditionally, the treatment of alcohol and drug problems in Norway has been
organized independently from ordinary health care services. Special institutions for people
with alcohol problems have existed since the beginning of the century, and specific laws
regulate these activities. Originally, only alcohol problems were considered, but during the
1950s the legislation was amended to include problems related to the use of drugs.

Since 1969 the Directorate for the Prevention of Alcohol and Drug Problems has
been responsible for the development of treatment services for persons with alcohol
problems, as well as for primary prevention efforts. The directorate reports to the Ministry
of Health and Social Affairs.   There has been a gradual increase in the number of
institutions, and today, there are more than 70 treatment facilities. There is at least one
institution for each of the 19 counties, and the total number of beds is approximately 3,000.

The treatment centers vary with regard to which groups of patients they serve and
which programs they offer. The treatment system is based on idea that the various groups
of problem drinkers have different service needs that may range from intensive inpatient

treatment programs to sheltered homes.   Yet the relatively broad differentiation of institutions that has existed in the past seems to be gradually disappearing, yielding a new financial structure distinguishing between emergency institutions (e.g., detoxification centers), institutions for treatment and rehabilitation, and institutions for permanent residence.   In addition, Norway appears to have an increasing number of outpatient facilities for people with alcohol and drug problems.   They are usually linked to one of the inpatient treatment services and offer outpatient treatment to the general population as well as offering follow-up to some treated inpatients.

England and Wales

The principle of community-based, multidisciplinary teams has now been embraced by Health and Social Services within mental health generally and within alcohol services in particular.   During the last 10 years there has been a steep rise in the number of community alcohol teams because they appear to be the most cost-effective way of providing the type of service outlined in the previous section.   There are now 14 community alcohol teams throughout England and Wales with others being planned and negotiated.   These teams are usually based in a building away from the hospital environment; most teams include community psychiatric nurses, a psychologist, a social worker, counselors, and an administrator/clerk.   Some teams also have the support of a psychiatrist, usually on a consultant basis.   The team is involved in consultation, education, and prevention (e.g., drinking and driving), as well as counseling and skills training.

There are 64 services that fall into the category of advisory and counseling services, 20 of which are within Greater London.   They are often called either councils on alcoholism or alcohol advisory services.   The size of these projects varies.   For example, the North East Council on Addictions employs 46 staff, but most councils employ from 2 to 6 staff.   Local councils are accountable to an executive committee that usually includes representatives from Health, Social Services, and Probation.

Recently, a number of councils established formal links with community alcohol teams.   Another recent trend is to combine an alcohol and drug service.   Local councils on alcoholism carry out a range of tasks that, to some extent, overlap with the functions of an alcohol team.   The most important functions are (a) providing advice and counseling to people with drinking problems; (b) informing the public and the media about alcohol misuse; (c) providing education and training, particularly to primary care workers; (d) acting as a coordinating body on alcohol misuse within their areas; and (e) initiating and developing strategies to prevent alcohol misuse locally.

There are 256 day centers that provide services primarily for people with drinking problems.   They make up 10.5 percent of alcohol services and employ 340 people (12 percent of the alcohol problems work force).   Of these, 141 (41.5 percent) are full-time, 127 (34 percent) are part-time and 72 (21.1 percent) are volunteers.   Day services are offered mostly in inner cities and tend to fall into two types.   Most are nonstatutory and provide food, shelter, and low-level support on request, dealing mainly with welfare rights, claims and accommodation problems.   A few offer individual counseling, group psychotherapy, drama therapy, and relaxation groups.

There are 248 alcohol agencies in England and Wales, and, of these, 81 (32.7 percent) are residential hostel projects.   They provide a total of 1,487 beds and employ 499 staff (a quarter of whom are part-time) with 129 volunteers.   Seventeen of these projects provide day support for a further 293 people.   More than half of the projects provide 12 or fewer beds.   Most projects are registered with their local authorities, 28 percent are registered housing associations, and a further 24 percent are linked with a housing association.

Residential projects allow people to spend time in an alcohol-free environment in which they can learn to break their dependence on drinking and develop alternative ways of living. The length of stay ranges from three months to a year or more. The projects have tended to attract problem drinkers who are homeless (or without a secure home base), single, unemployed, and male. This pattern is beginning to change in some areas, however, and home-based people are coming in for shorter periods.

Most residential projects are in the inner cities, although there are some in small towns. Some are linked closely to an existing community-based service; for instance, the Hastings hostel in Leicester receives its referrals through the local community alcohol team.

Ideally, residential projects should be part of an integrated network of services so they can be used more flexibly. Including them in such a network, however, would entail a reexamination of their objectives, as well as a less rigid form of funding. In particular, it would involve determining whether residential alcohol services were primarily aimed at helping homeless people who have a drinking problem or helping drinkers who need a temporary home away from their normal environment.

Alcohol treatment units (ATUs) are the major National Health Services treatment institutions for people with drinking problems. Set up in the 1960s, there are now 30 such units, and they provide varying services. Initially, they were supposed to provide services to an entire region, but it soon became clear that this expectation was unrealistic, and many now restrict their services to the surrounding community. Most ATUs require total abstinence from inpatients. Some use group work exclusively; others employ individual counseling. A few emphasize occupational therapy, and many encourage the involvement of Alcoholics Anonymous.

ATUs are now shifting their focus from institutional psychiatry to community psychiatry and are developing many links with community agencies. Many areas plan to close their ATUs that operate as separate units within hospitals and move them into the community.

Help for coping with withdrawal symptoms and the other immediate physical consequences of giving up alcohol may be provided either in a general or in a psychiatric hospital ward. Detoxification may also be linked to a period in an alcohol treatment unit. One recent development has been the growth of home detoxification in which the individual is helped to cope with withdrawal at home under the supervision of a general practitioner and a community psychiatric nurse. This procedure is best carried out with support from a close relative or friend. Many alcohol agencies find it difficult to persuade hospitals to accept individuals for detoxification, especially since the closure of many psychiatric and other types of hospitals.

The largest and best known UK self-help group is Alcoholics Anonymous (AA), which has approximately 1,350 groups throughout England and Wales and 25 regional contact points. Each group is self-supporting and autonomous, although they all subscribe to the basic philosophy of AA and follow the 12 steps laid down in the AA "Big Book." AA sees itself as a "fellowship of men and women who share their experiences, strength and hope with each other so that they may solve their common problem and help others to recover from alcoholism." The primary goals of AA members are "to stay sober and help the alcoholics to achieve sobriety". One of the basic tenets of belief in AA is that alcoholism is a disease, for which the only cure is total abstinence.

A recent innovation in the alcohol field is the development of Drinkwatchers groups. These groups are intended for people who have not yet developed serious problems of alcohol dependence but who want to do something about their present level and pattern of drinking before it gets too serious. Some people may attend only one meeting of the group. However, at that meeting, they will receive a copy of the Drinkwatchers manual, which suggests ways of cutting down, and for some people this may be all the help they need to resolve their problem.

The number of private clinics that cater to people with alcohol problems has grown from 6 in 1982 to at least 15, with more on the way. Private clinics usually operate on a residential basis and offer programs lasting two or three months. Most subscribe to the "disease" model of alcoholism and have close links with Alcoholics Anonymous. Some of the recently established clinics subscribe to the Minnesota model of treatment, and several cater to people with both drug and alcohol problems.

Norway and a number of other countries have emphasized the importance of a national plan and of government initiative in stimulating fresh thinking about the organization of services. Mexico, the USSR, and Zimbabwe provide further examples.

Mexico

Before 1982 there were a number of different institutions that dealt with health policies, and there was little coordination of their efforts. There was a lack of appropriate distribution of responsibility among the agencies, and there was also strong centralization: most of the responsibility for health measures belonged to the federal government.

Since 1982 the Ministry of Health has assumed greater responsibility and has established the rules for health policies at a national level. As a result, the total population receives more legal protection owing to that fact that the right to such services has been raised to a constitutional level. The roles of each health institution are specified, and actions are now regulated by a legal framework. The general policy is harmonized and unified by the General Health Law and also by the introduction of the National Health System. One of the intents of the new system is for each state to share the responsibility of arranging policies and administrating funds.

Alcohol treatment in Mexico has benefited from the above-mentioned changes. The Health Ministry considers alcohol problems to be a priority. A National Antialcoholic Council was installed in 1985 and is coordinated by the Health Ministry. It includes representatives of social, governmental, and private sectors, and its purpose is to develop preventive actions at legal, educational, and assistance levels. The National Antialocoholic Council has elaborated a national program that contemplates treatment measures as a priority issue. Unit now, only a few programs in this field are being undertaken. The changes that have occurred in the alcohol field in Mexico now permit coordination of the different institutions, as well as the sharing of responsibilities at various governmental levels: federal, state, and district.

There are three basic systems of care for a population of about 75 million people. The first system assists individuals in the lower socioeconomic levels (about 24 million people), offering virtually free services. It is administered by the Ministry of Health (SSA), the National and State Family Integration System (DIF), the municipal services, state boards, the Mexican Institute of Social Security (IMSS) and city hospitals. The second system which assists a population of a higher socioeconomic level (approximately 32.8 million people), is a social security program financed by employers and employees with regular jobs. It includes the Institute of Social Security and Services for Government Employees (ISSSTE) and the IMSS for the rest of the working class. The third system embraces private institutions and practitioners and covers the higher socioeconomic levels (approximately 7 million people). It is also important to point out that, for various reasons, approximately 14 million Mexicans do not have access to health facilities.

As can be seen, the Mexican government provides most of the available medical assistance programs, but in general they are crowded and insufficient to assist the whole population. As a result, there are few (specialty) treatment programs for alcolhol problems. Rather, such services are integrated with other treatment programs, most often in the form of acute detoxification centers.

Despite the small number of programs in this area, Mexican government health authorities and the professionals related to this field are conscious of the need to establish others because they recognize the magnitude and extention of the problems created by high rates of alcohol consumption. Alcohol problems already represent a substantial burden for the country's health services, and it is evident that, in the future, this burden will increase, mainly as a result of the pyramidal structure of the population, which is wider at the base. As was mentioned earlier, the group of greatest morbidity is between 35 to 50 years of age. In the near future, however, the larger younger population will be in this age range, and, consequently, there will be a larger number of drinkers who will require medical assistance.

It is generally accepted in Mexico that alcohol-related problems should be treated by medical personnel, even though drinkers are ashamed to recognize the problem and ask for help. Priests are among the agents who are trusted by drinkers and who are often sought out for help. The personnel who work in agencies that handle alcohol-related problems (policemen, doctors, nurses), clearly understand that these problems are frequent, but they consider themselves untrained in handling alcohol problems and lack the time to deal with them. Nonetheless, they report that they would like to have more knowledge on this topic and that they would be willing to undertake special training.

USSR

The impact of a recent national campaign in the USSR related to alcohol problems has been substantial, not only for preventive strategies but also for treatment services. For the past two and a half years since the start of this campaign, the number of specialist doctors/narcologists has increased by 45 percent, and the number of beds in narcological departments has risen by 25 percent. In addition, while outpatient facilities have more than doubled.

The following extract outlines the current organizational structure of alcohol treatment services in the USSR:

In the USSR there are different organizational forms of treatment of alcoholics: outpatient, inpatient, one-halfway settings. Treatment may be voluntary and involuntary. To choose the most adequate form one should consider a number of clinico-social characteristics: severity of patient's clinical state, whether there is a desire for treatment, social behaviours, etc.

A specialized narcological service organized in the USSR in 1976 is just the organizational structure in charge of treatment of alcoholics. Its basic unit is [the] narcological dispensary assigned to some definite area (city district, city, province). A dispensary structure usually includes [facilities] of divisional psychiatrist-narcologists, narcological [facilities] for young people, narcological consulting rooms and medical attendants' narcological posts at industrial and other enterprises, room of alcohol dizziness detection by experts, anonymous treatment rooms, rooms of anti-alcohol propaganda and preventive medical aid, specialized rooms of neuropathologist, psychologists, physicians, inpatient departments (including those organized at industrial and other enterprises); organizational-methodical advisory departments, medical offices and auxiliary subunits (clinicodiagnostic laboratory, room of functional diagnosis and others). Inpatient departments may exist as a separate narcological hospital. In the departments of this type treatment is free of charge. Alongside with these establishments, self-financing (requiring payment) narcological departments and specialized consulting rooms of self-financing and budget polyclinics [have] become more and more popular. As a rule they are staffed with highly qualified specialists who treat patients anonymously (without registration) for some moderate payment. Not so long ago, there appeared one more form of outpatient treatment of alcoholics requiring payment: cooperative establishments, which include doctors, psychologists and other specialists.

In addition to voluntary treatment there is a forced [treatment], which is organized in specialized establishments—treatment-and-labour camps run by the USSR Ministry of Internal Affairs. Alcoholics leading an antisocial way of life and giving no consent to undergo treatment voluntarily are placed there at court [discretion]. The terms of forced treatment [vary] from 6 months up to 2 years. Additionally in public health establishments there are specialized departments for forced treatment at a court [discretion] of alcoholics with antisocial behaviour or disabled by severe somatic diseases, who cannot be sent to the treatment-and-labour camps of the USSR Ministry of Internal Affairs.

The system of treatment of alcoholics in the USSR is based on the following principles: anti-alcohol therapy is continuous and long; it should be maximum; maximum differentiation of the therapy depending on patient's individual features; treatment is complex; direction of patient toward complete abstinence from alcohol; treatment should be conducted through consecutive stages, in successive order. As a rule treatment schemes for alcoholics consist of three stages. At the first stage alcohol abuse of a patient is interrupted, the state of alcohol intoxication is removed; pathologic bent for alcohol and severe abstinent syndromes are treated. Patient is examined, psychotherapeutic contact with him and his closely surrounding people is established. At the second stage an active anti-alcohol therapy is carried out. At the third stage supporting and anti-relapsing care together with rehabilitation measures [are] conducted.

Zimbabwe

In a very different setting the Zimbabwan government responded to various alcohol-related problems by creating a mental health department within the Ministry of Health and forming an intersectoral committee with a broad [portfolio] for mental health including alcohol problems. The government created the post of an officer for alcohol and drug abuse to coordinate its policy, which is summarized here in some detail because it ably illustrates the interplay of prevention and treatment strategies and the need for an intersectoral approach. It also shows the responsibilities assigned to different sectors within a country that has very limited resources. The role of each sector is described as follows:

The Ministry of Health provides preventive measures through the Department of Health Education. At the moment these comprise publication and distribution of posters on health dangers of alcohol and drug abuse. Formal lectures on alcohol and drug abuse have been incorporated into various levels of nurses training programmes. The

Ministry of Health provides curative services by providing outpatient and inpatient treatment in general and psychiatric hospitals for patients who have alcohol and drug related problems. Rehabilitative and Counselling services are offered by the occupational therapy staff, social workers and clinical psychologists in hospitals, psychiatric units and half-way houses. The Community Psychiatric Services provide counselling and support to patients with alcohol and drug abuse problems in the community and those discharged from Central, Provincial and District hospitals.

The Zimbabwe Council for Alcohol and Drug Abuse (ZIMCADA) is a voluntary organization that provides counselling for clients that have alcohol and drug abuse related problems. It liaises with health workers, social workers, clinical psychologists, GPs and medical consultants on issues related to alcohol and drug abuse. It provides public lectures on alcohol and drug abuse, whenever requested, to primary and secondary schools.

Alcoholics Anonymous (AA) is a fellowship of alcoholics and ex-alcoholics which provides psychological and moral support through the medium of group processes. The fellowship is guided by the famous "twelve traditions" of AA worldwide. The fellowship liaises with other agencies that counsel clients with alcohol and drug abuse related problems.

Al-Anon and Al-Ateen Family Groups are family and teenage children's groups where one member or members of the family suffer from alcohol related and drug abuse problems. The group helps members by providing moral support through group processes. Like AA, the groups are guided by the "twelve steps" and "twelve traditions" of AA worldwide.

Pharmacists Against Drug Abuse (PADA) is a recently launched association of pharmacists in Zimbabwe, supported by a local pharmaceutical company, that is attempting to provide public awareness of drug abuse by supplying pertinent information on drug abuse signs, damage to health and availability of drugs to parents, teachers, schools and other interested agencies countrywide.

The social workers in the Department of Social Welfare of the Ministry of Labour, Manpower Planning and Social Welfare provide counselling and support to clients with alcohol related and drug abuse problems. The department liaises with health workers, medical consultants and other agencies involved in problems of alcohol and drug abuse.

The Ministry of Justice, Legal and Parliamentary Affairs administers the legislation that permits and controls the sale and consumption of alcohol and drugs as contained in the Liquor Act, the Harmful Liquids Act, the Traditional Beer Act, and the Drugs and Allied Substances Control Act, in collaboration with the Ministry of Home Affairs and Ministry of Local Government. Recently, the Ministry introduced lectures on alcohol and drug abuse in the training of prison wardens and other prison staff. The Ministry of Home Affairs has recently stepped up policing for illicit brewing, selling and consumption of illicit beers [and] liquids and [for] any breaches of the alcohol and drug legislation. The Ministry has also provided training for police officers in the detection and management of drunk driving offenders.

Bulgaria

Bulgaria has a network of specialist (narcology) services and, as can be seen from its report, is moving toward an increasingly community-based approach. Nevertheless, its report acknowledges enormous difficulties that need to be overcome if primary-level workers are to become more enthusiastic about managing alcohol-related problems.

The country is divided into 28 districts, and in every district there is a psychiatric dispensary with a narcological outpatient clinic. The main functions of this service are registration, follow-up, monitoring and assistance for alcoholic patients and drug addicts. When these clinics are active (i.e., with sufficient and well-educated staff), they offer in antialcohol education and organize clubs for self-help, as well as providing some forms of prevention. These clinics are also in contact with the various narcological hospitals and regularly exchange information about patients in the area: their present state, hospitalizations, treatment, accidents, family problems, and so forth. One of the most important tasks of the outpatient clinics is to discover and register new cases of harmful alcohol consumption and dependence. Usually, this task is accomplished with the aid of the primary health care service in the given district. The organization of these activities needs improvement, however, because of population mobility and other demographic processes, as well as (among other reasons) the lack of trained staff.

There are four specialized narcological hospitals Bulgaria, two of which are located at the medical faculties, in Sofia and Pleven. The total number of all in narcological hospital beds is 470. In addition, six of the large psychiatric hospitals in the districts contain specialized alcohol wards, which have approximately 250 beds. Thus, in all there are around 720 beds for the whole country. Bulgaria plans to create more outpatient services for alcoholics, as well as hospitals and rehabilitation centers, as a way to help people continue functioning (instead of building new hospitals and increasing the number of beds). In this respect, Bulgarian medical authorities appear to be embracing the current tendency to diminish the number of hospital beds for alcohol problems treatment and to increase the number of outpatient clinics.

Costa Rica

Most of the treatment services for alcohol problems within Costa Rica are the responsibility of the National Institute of Alcoholism and Drug Dependence. This agency provides detoxification within a general hospital and, for more deteriorated patients, an inpatient rehabilitation unit in which they may remain for one or two months. During this time, patients receive group, occupational, and behavioral therapy, as well as social and family rehabilitation. Costa Rica also has a network of outpatient clinics, which have links with the innovative *promotore* development. *Promotores* are workers based in local communities in which they are often already known, who are trained at the National Institute in detecting alcohol problems and in providing prevention measures and techniques. They can either deal with the problems themselves or refer those who are seeking help to the nearest outpatient clinic.

The report from Costa Rica also describes a universal scenario of many problem drinkers who experience various medical emergencies and yet whose underlying alcohol problem remains largely ignored. Conventional inpatient services can attend only to the most damaged alcoholics:

In cases of other medical emergencies or other symptoms, people can also go to the out-patient clinics or emergency rooms of the general hospitals, belonging to the Social Security System. Usually they will receive ambulatory treatment, medical assistance. In these cases the alcoholism is usually hidden. Patients are only hospitalized in case of severe medical complications, or for study.

In case of neuropsychiatric complications, or withdrawal symptoms with mental compromise (psychosis, hallucination, delirium tremens), they are referred to the neuropsychiatric hospital, both of them belonging to the Social Security System.

Summary

The country reports extracted or described above may seem repetitious. To the extent to which this is true, it provides a crude measure of the commonalities in treatment strategies around the world. Most of the countries involved provide a mix of institutional and community-based responses. Some (like the USSR) have a highly developed specialist narcology service; others (like Norway) appear to be dismantling much of their specialist institutional base and are moving toward services located within the community that will liaise with and support primary health care workers. The development of community alcohol teams in England and Wales is evidence of a similar trend. The rationale for these developments was ably summarized in the Australian National Health Policy on Alcohol:

> There is recognition that resources for specialist services will never be adequate to meet the needs as has been emphasized by the WHO Expert Committee reporting in 1980. It is accepted that generalists have an important role in treatment provision and that specialist units should operate within a consultation-liaison model as well as providing direct services. Among the principles that are endorsed are early detection and intervention, comprehensive assessment and matching of services to needs, the availability of services to all, irrespective of their socio economic or cultural background, and the availability of range of services including detoxification facilities, assessment, medical and psychiatric care, telephone counselling and residential and rehabilitation programmes. It is emphasized that the planning of services should take account of the prevalence of alcohol-related problems in the catchment population.

Levels of Intervention

In most countries, there are different levels of interventions as one moves from nonspecific toward increasingly specialized services. Most alcohol-related problems bear most heavily on the family and those closest to the drinker, as shown in Table C-1. At the first level is the drinker who may decide to change a damaging drinking habit because of past experience or pressure from workmates and friends and most often from family. This level is the essence of the informal community response that is the focus of much health promotion. The potential of the family as change agents in the life of the problem drinker deserves much more formal study and recognition. The WHO community response project

TABLE C-1 Levels of Increasing Specialized Intervention

Level	Types of Intervention	Examples
1	Informal Community Response	Drinker Family Friends
2	Formal Community Response	Workplace Traditional healers Police Social welfare agencies Pharmacists
3	Generalist Health and Social Services	Primary health care Casualty Social work Outpatient clinic
4	Specialist Services	Rehabilitation hostel Detoxification Center Day Program Outpatient clinic Work program Inpatient unit Self-help group

concluded that, "in each area, the family was the battle ground on which most alcohol-related problems were fought out." The high level of concern, for instance, among Mexican women about their husband's drinking is a reminder that alcohol-related problems are not confined to the drinker but affect many of those nearby. Very little work has been done (except within marital therapy) on helping family members channel their concern into a more effective response. A promising informal approach in this area may be found in the activities of the *promotores* in Costa Rica, an innovation that merits careful evaluation.

Moving from the domestic setting to a more public arena (Level 2 in Table C-1) alcohol problems frequently come to the attention of authorities because of impaired performance, drunkenness, or hazardous behaviour. The workplace is an important location for detecting problem drinking. Alcohol-in-employment programs are quite developed in the United States, and similar trends are evident although less pronounced elsewhere (e.g., England and Wales, Australia, Bulgaria, Costa Rica). In many Eastern European countries the worksite also plays an important part in rehabilitation and aftercare through the provision of support groups and supervision. The controls and motivation that such programs can impose appear to reinforce abstinence and cooperation; however, no adequate evaluation studies were reported in this enquiry.

In many countries a great deal of police time is devoted to dealing with alcohol problems. Police obviously are well placed to detect alcohol problems and encourage rehabilitation. In some countries (e.g., the USSR, Norway), the police are empowered to take drunken people to detoxification centers for treatment. However, many countries find the dual activities of law enforcement and care giving too dissonant to combine within a single role (Ritson, 1986).

Potential change agents may also be found in many other informal settings (e.g., pharmacies as in Zimbabwe, religious groups, lay counsellors). In some areas traditional healers play an important part in offering help to the problem drinker. The benefits of efforts by such change agents have not been fully examined.

The next level (Level 3 in Table C-1) comprises primary-echelon health and social services that have a responsibility to provide care or treatment. Many of their clients and patients have been shown to have alcohol problems, and it is at this level that many countries wish to pitch their initiatives in early detection and simple intervention. The philosophy has many attractions. Primary health care (PHC) is usually accessible and widespread within most countries, patients feel less stigma within the PHC network than is commonly felt in seeking specialist services. If PHC workers could be appropriately trained, they would become an enormous resource for simple intervention. In some countries such as the United Kingdom, Australia, and Norway, there have been promising initiatives in this direction, but the experiences of Bulgaria, Mexico, Zimbabwe, and the Netherlands have shown clearly that front-line medical staff often feel pessimistic about being able to help and are reluctant to take on an extra burden.

Many of the country reports showed that the treatment of alcohol-related problems ought to begin and be performed most effectively at the level of the primary health care services. But in fact, the general practitioners (GPs) have no special qualifications and knowledge in alcohol-related problems. They are not prepared to deal with them. The main causes are: (1) the traditional thinking that alcoholism and alcohol-related problems need specialized psychiatric care; (2) lack of general concept and competence about the origin and nature and the specificity of these problems; and (3) general practitioners are not obliged officially to treat and to be interested in alcohol problems they send directly to the specialized institutions.

Many of the reporting centers took part in a study of the management of alcohol problems in general practice (WHO, 1985). The study revealed that: (1) the involvement of the GPs in the treatment of alcoholics is occasional and superficial; (2) the participation of GPs in alcohol education is unsatisfactory; (3) the involvement of GPs in management of alcohol services in control and regulation on the development of alcohol policy and in alcohol research practically does not exist; and (4) GPs need competent knowledge and special qualifications concerning treatment and management of alcohol-related problems.

Enlisting the PHC clinician in work of this kind will require careful retraining and continuous support (WHO, 1987). The reluctance to be involved in this task is even stronger among casualty staff who see themselves as too busy with emergencies to be actively concerned with work of this kind (e.g., reported by Kenya, Mexico, and Australia). The relationship between specialist and nonspecialist services was the topic of a 1987 WHO EURO meeting. In some countries (e.g., USSR, Bulgaria) specialist services are located at the PHC level. Other countries have moved some of their experts into the community where they provide a facilitative and consultative function (e.g., community alcohol teams in England and Wales). This new outreach perspective of specialist services seems to be welcome in all countries, but its development will be inhibited unless some consideration is given to the appropriate retraining of existing specialists who have become accustomed to working in an institution. After an initial period of resistance, this process of change seems to be working well in Norway. The WHO EURO project commented on the problem of resources transformation:

> In the longer term it also seems likely that specialist services will be taking on a different role. If this is the case then they will require help in making the necessary transition to a more consultative and educational activity. For this new function to be effectively developed, specialist personnel will need to be less identified with the institutional setting. Personnel will require help and support in making this transition, otherwise there will be a tendency to feel under threat and [to] cling to established

patterns of working. Health administrators can do much to either help or hinder this change. For instance, in some circumstances, funding for specialist services for problem drinkers are still assessed on calculations based on bed occupancy and resources within the institution, rather than on a more service and activity orientated approach.

Redistribution of resources also requires a community and political will that such changes should occur. Such commitment can only be expected to arise in the context of a population which has been enlightened about the nature of alcohol-related problems. This implies a necessary investment in health education which will create a background of information from which responsible attitudes towards health and health promotion can develop.

Redistribution of resources is always a difficult and stressful time for those involved in the changes. Careful preparation and liaison is an essential first step in formulating such plans. The encouragement of health ministries and governments is needed to provide the necessary impetus and support to changes of this kind. These changes will have implications and will need to be discussed at regional, district and local levels if they are to prove effective. The aim should be to create a personal service which truly reflects the nature of alcohol-related problems and the way in which they present in the community.

The detail of the specialist services provided was described, albeit briefly, in most of the country reports. In most cases there has been an evident trend toward a greater investment in outpatient services and a reduction in lengths of stay among existing inpatient programs. However, there is also the possibility of a contrary trend among some private health treatment programs in England and Wales, Australia, and Costa Rica. It is interesting that the most expensive and exclusive treatment programs often provide a predominantly inpatient experience.

The only other area in which longer stay treatment appears to be the norm is in the rehabilitation of the severely damaged, cognitively impaired, and socially deteriorated drinker. Here, long-stay institutions, often with a work or occupational therapy component, are common (e.g., Australia, Norway, Costa Rica, the USSR).

Self-help groups (see Table C-1) also provide a specialist service and because of their low-cost and personal commitment represent one of the most attractive additions to any portfolio of services. Alcoholics Anonymous is, of course, the most widely known self-help group and has a prominent place in most countries (notably Australia and England and Wales, but also in Zimbabwe, Kenya, and Mexico). Other self-help support groups or clubs have also been promoted in several countries (e.g., Bulgaria, Yugoslavia, Costa Rica). Membership in these groups often follows an initial contact with a treatment agency, but the groups take responsibility for the continuance of sobriety and the development of alternative interests and forms of recreation. As noted earlier, in England and Wales, Drinkwatchers is a self-help group whose aim is to help individuals reduce their alcohol consumption when they feel they have been drinking too much without becoming dependent. All of these services merit more careful evaluation.

Criteria for Admission to Different Types of Treatment

The criteria for enrollment into a particular treatment program often depend on the mode of presentation and the state of the patient. Physical state is the main criterion for admission to general or psychiatric hospitals in Kenya and Mexico. In some circumstances, the ability to pay or the possession of health insurance is an important consideration, as revealed in the following examples from Zimbabwe:

> In Zimbabwe everybody has the right for treatment provided the person is seen to be ill and in need of such treatment. While this is mostly so with Government institutions, it may not be so for private ones, where one gets treatment on payment. Although governmental institutions also require able patients to pay for their treatment, those without money receive free treatment.

> There is a further criterion for rural clinics, where feeding of patients is a problem. If such patients are to be inpatients, then somebody must accompany them, who would cook and feed them.

> Violent patients with alcohol related problems who are a danger to themselves or to others are ordered by law to get treatment, whether they like it or not. Such patients may be kept in secluded institutions until their situation has improved.

The reply from Costa Rica illustrates the way in which criteria are deduced from physical state, degree of dependence, and social need as well as more subjective concerns such as motivation:

> In the case of the Unit of Detoxification which IAFA offers, the main condition is that they are not chronic nor deteriorated patients—mental patients [who] are hospitalized for the first time there and who are under intoxication levels and are not [capable] of stopping.

> In general hospitals, where alcoholic patients who are intoxicated are hospitalized, it is because they present medical emergencies or physical complications which can not be treated ambulatory.

> In case of withdrawal symptoms and mental compromise they are hospitalized at the neuropsychiatric hospital.

> In other community private services, the main criteria is that the patient wants to stop drinking—further on they will receive rehabilitation programs.

> The rehabilitation centre for alcoholics where patients remain for 2-3 months is mainly for chronic alcoholics. They are first disintoxicated and later on they are submitted to the centre's program of rehabilitation through occupational therapy and a multi-disciplinary approach.

In Norway the degree of dependence and damage experienced by the person is taken as a guide to the kind of treatment he or she is offered:

> The treatment programme usually offered to alcohol clients [is] a combination of a medical and psychological examination followed by an individually tailored treatment and/or group therapy. The majority of treatment centres allow the clients to choose [their] treatment goal—abstinence [or] controlled drinking.

During the last couple of years some new treatment programmes have developed in order to meet uncovered client needs. These have for instance been secondary prevention programmes recruiting people with a stable living situation revealing mild to moderate dependence symptoms. At first these programmes were part of research programmes, but were later integrated into the services of some of the out-patient units.

These secondary prevention studies have revealed relatively positive outcomes, and have to some extent contributed to a more positive attitude among health and social professionals towards persons with alcohol problems.

Where they exist, the community alcohol teams described in England and Wales take responsibility for placing clients appropriately among the agencies available in the area.

Considering the multiplicity of treatment approaches available in some communities, it is surprising that so little progress has been made in tailoring the programs that are offered to the needs of the patients. Some centers appear to use motivation and social stability as criteria for particular types of treatment; in a few centers, the degree of dependence (based on symptom measures and questionnaire assessment) is used as a guide to allocate clients to controlled drinking programs. In general, attempts at matching continue to be based on very subjective or crude assessments.

Treatment Services for Special Populations

Most countries recognize the special needs of certain groups, particularly women, but very few are in a position to provide differentiated services of that kind. Norway is an exception:

There are special programmes for women and families. The traditional treatment programmes have primarily been a service for the men not paying enough attention to the needs of the women. Many women developed alcohol problems due to a heavy burden, having a job and being [mainly] responsible for raising children. The stigmatizing effect is much larger for female problem drinkers than it is for males. As a result women feel more guilt about their drinking and prefer less stigmatizing strategies to "cope" with their drinking problem. Extensive use of psychopharmaca and psychiatric treatment [has] been a more common treatment approach among female problem drinkers compared to men drinkers. The special treatment programmes for women within some of the Norwegian treatment centres are efforts at meeting their particular needs.

Some centers stress their growing concern about alcohol problems among adolescents and the way in which such problems are often linked to other forms of drug abuse. The Australian comment is particularly apposite:

Treatment services specifically for adolescents barely exist and there is considerable debate about the most effective type of service. Formal detoxification is infrequently required for persons under 18 years. A more important requirement is accommodation for adolescents who have become estranged from their families. Polydrug and alcohol use is the predominant pattern, rather than abuse of alcohol exclusively. There is considerable emphasis on presentation of alcohol intoxication among adolescents in national media campaigns and community drug education campaigns.

In their reports, Costa Rica and Australia both describe several facilities designed specifically for women. Costa Rica also provides a counseling service for the children of alcoholics and in common with some other countries organizes support groups for the relatives of problem drinkers. This function is also provided in many areas by self-help from Al-Anon and Al-Ateen. A voluntary organization in England and Wales recently prepared a report on treatment services and their consideration of treatment provision for specialist groups is summarized below.

Women   All the advisory and counselling agencies offer their services equally to women and men, but most residential services are for men only. Only three agencies offer a specific service for women problem drinkers; one of these is privately run; two of the three are residential. 67 agencies (23 percent of the total) advertise women-only groups. Women often prefer female counsellors and groups.

Younger People   109 agencies (38 percent) operate a minimum age criterion. 61 of these are residential. 85 (29 percent) set minimum age of 18 or above. 56 percent of all residential agencies exclude people under 18. 19 agencies (6.5 percent) advertise young drinkers' groups. There are a small but growing number of projects aimed at young people and seeking to influence their drinking behaviour through non-alcohol cocktail clubs, temperance youth clubs, programmes for young drunken drivers and some group work by probation officers.

Black and Ethnic Minorities   The 6.6 percent of the population of England and Wales who belong to black and minority ethnic communities have two (0.7 percent of the total) agencies advertising a specifically appropriate response, both of them in London. The common experience is that referrals (including self referrals) from black and ethnic minority communities are rare, as are alcohol agencies which have any links with services which help those communities. It is possible that most people from black and minority ethnic communities experiencing alcohol-related problems are being received into general and acute mental health care as a result of disturbed behaviour and the relevance of the alcohol relationship is ignored.

Lesbian and Gay People   There is no specialist provision for lesbian and gay problem drinkers outside London. In London there are three AA groups which, although open, welcome lesbian and gay people: The Women's Alcohol Centre runs a group for lesbian and gay people with London Friend, Accept and the Alcohol Counselling Service based at Brixton. Services for lesbian and gay communities appear to depend on the presence of openly lesbian and gay workers.

Homeless   The overwhelming majority of agencies, including residential, offer a service to homeless people, three of these are Alcohol Advisory

Services. There is a range of specialist services for single homeless people, some operated within the alcohol field, and many run by a variety of statutory and voluntary agencies. They include day centres, drop-in services and various housing projects. Many residential projects within the alcohol sector cater for single homeless people with drinking problems.

Relatives, Friends and Children of People with Drinking Problems The only organization specifically set up for relatives and friends of people with drinking problems is Al-Anon. It has around 750 groups in the UK and Eire. It aims to bring partners and relatives together to provide mutual support and to share their common problems. However, it does not purport to teach any particular skills for coping with their drinking partners. Most counselling services encourage relatives and friends to attend either on their own or with the person who has the drink problem. However, their statistics would suggest that not many of the former attend. Al-Ateen is the only organization specifically for children. Al-Ateen has around 150 groups in the UK and Eire. Most other services have little, if any, contact with children.

Many studies have suggested that the treatment of problem drinking is more effective if family members can be involved. However, most services in England and Wales are organized in a way that concentrates on the drinker and not on families. Contacting the children of problem drinkers is difficult. One strategy is to develop links with the childcare organization.

Information Regarding the Outcome of Treatment Services

Very few countries reported outcome evaluation studies, although several had changed their treatment priorities in response to research conducted elsewhere (e.g., the evaluation reviews of Emrick [1974] and Miller and Hester [1986]). The work of Edwards and his team (1977) seems to have been a particularly influential approach. In addition, Norway has recently completed studies on the benefits of early intervention. Few reports of systematic monitoring were received, however. Costa Rica quoted a follow-up of 3,000 men treated in a rehabilitation center: the researcher found that relapse was particularly common among younger patients (Miguez, 1983).

Indeed, the move toward simpler interventions for alcohol problems, given at an early stage and often located in primary-level agencies, has been supported by a number of reports (Kristenson [1983] in Sweden; Chick et al. [1985] and Heather et al. [1987] both from Scotland; and Elvy et al. [1988] from New Zealand).

Thus, relatively few countries have conducted evaluation studies and, as the review by Miller and Hester (1986) points out, even fewer have been sufficiently well designed to draw reliable conclusions. Nonetheless, those with convincing methodologies do seem to have had some effect on decisions about the patterns of services in many countries and are quoted in support of the move toward simpler and more accessible intervention. The current WHO project studying the effectiveness of simple intervention should soon add a significant new dimension to this evidence.

How Are Treatment Services Financed?

Very little appears to be known in the various countries about the costs of treatment for alcohol problems. Kenya described a typical dilemma:

> Virtually nothing is known about the cost of treatment for alcohol problems in the country. Many patients are admitted, treated and discharged without the doctors being aware that the cause of the illness was alcohol. But even in cases where an accurate diagnosis is made, the clinicians are reluctant to enter a diagnosis of alcohol dependence because of stigma and the implication of such diagnosis on the patient's employment and future.

> The Kenya Government continues to provide free medical services to all its citizens including in-patient treatment in government institutions. Consequently all government health facilities are chronically congested and usually short of essential supplies such as drugs and laboratory materials. Health personnel at government hospitals or health centres usually have no more than five minutes per patient. Consequently disorders that usually require a bit more probing into for an accurate diagnosis, such as alcohol dependence are largely missed.

> For people who want to avoid the over-crowding in government hospitals or clinics and employees in the private sector, there are numerous private hospitals. Usually their health insurance policies cover all medical treatment including alcohol dependence, but the diagnosis of "alcoholism" is hardly ever entered in the case notes or on the sick sheet. Even in these settings the cost of treatment for alcohol problems remain unknown.

Many countries have a balance between services that are free to the user, those that must be paid for, and it is often difficult to cost these services. Fee-for-service and insurance-based services are costed with more clarity, but very few useful data were forthcoming. Two estimates of the cost to society of alcohol problems were received from England and Wales and Australia, but they do not address the issue of the cost-effectiveness or cost-benefit of special treatments. Consequently, the question of treatment costs of alcohol problems appears to be a much underresearched area. The paragraphs below briefly discuss the England/Wales and Australia estimates.

England and Wales

A recent attempt to quantify the cost to society of alcohol problems in the United Kingdom concluded that a low estimate of the social cost of alcohol use (using 1983 prices) is 1,614 million pounds. This figure includes costs to industry, costs to the National Health Service, and the social costs of drink-related offenses. It excludes the cost to society of family stress and the burden placed on probation and social services. Days lost from work because of alcohol-induced sickness are estimated at 8 million to 15 million days per year in the United Kingdom and 20 percent of male admissions to a general medical ward are also estimated to be related to alcohol use.

Australia

The costs of excessive alcohol consumption to the individual, his or her family members, the local community, and society as a whole are extremely difficult to quantify, either in human or financial terms. An econometric analysis undertaken by federal government economists concluded that the financial cost in 1980 was at least $2,500 million, constituting $454 million from health care, $501 million from welfare payments, $454 million from the costs of emergency services because of road accidents, and $898 million in losses to industry because of absenteeism, accidents, and reduced efficiency.

The Future of Alcohol Treatment Services

Almost all of the countries had or were about to formulate plans for the future of their treatment services. As already described, some countries (e.g., Mexico, the USSR) found that a central plan had proved a help to the development and status of treatment services. Prevention of alcohol problems through reduction in per capita consumption by controlling availability has been a major theme in recent national resolutions in Bulgaria and the USSR.

Australia has a national health policy on alcohol. The overall objective of the policy is "minimization of the harm associated with the use of alcohol." The policy comprises six components that are regarded as interdependent: (1) controls; (2) education; (3) treatment; (4) the non-governmental sector; (5) research; and (6) administrative arrangements. Essential to that policy is a clearly defined structure for communication and administrative purposes that would encompass national, state, regional and local government areas as well as the voluntary sector. The policy also calls for the formation of a specific subcommittee on alcohol to report to the Ministerial Council on Drug Strategy. In England and Wales a ministerial group, the Wakeham Committee, has been created to promote preventive and treatment policies. As already mentioned in relation to Zimbabwe, several countries now recognize the importance of an intersectoral approach to planning alcohol policies. It is also important that such policies are given ministerial backing and can establish a proper means of monitoring developments including costing and effectiveness.

Turning to more detailed plans regarding future trends in service delivery, there is an evident preference among the countries for the development of community-based projects and, as mentioned, the promotion of interventions at the primary level. In some countries this policy stems from the realization that very little treatment exists at present and that the creation of a costly specialized service would be totally inappropriate. The development will require new training initiatives, as explained in the following report from Kenya:

> It is important to reiterate that the existence of alcohol problems in the country has been recognized although accurate or actual figures are still lacking. The question now being asked more often is what should be done to curtail the problem. Two main approaches are being debated. There are those advocating preventive measures and those demanding the creation of treatment facilities and the production of manpower to man the facilities.
>
> Recent attempts at prevention by suppression of production, distribution and consumption of traditional alcoholic beverages have not made any impact on consumption of illicit alcoholic beverages. Consequently there have been repeated calls for the training not only of health personnel but other professionals as well to enable them to recognize and deal with al-

cohol problems wherever they may present. Most training curricula and syllabus for health personnel now include something on alcohol and other drugs.

Kenya has recently initiated pilot primary health care projects in at least three districts in the country. The future plan is to integrate alcohol and drug problems into the system so that alcohol problems can be treated as a primary health care problem. The curriculum for the training of primary health care workers is being finalized and it has a strong section on alcohol problems.

Costa Rica envisages a greater emphasis on community workers (*promotores*) facilitating the development of alternative activities, providing education, and possibly acting as change agents to help those who are beginning to drink in a damaging way. Costa Rica is also planning to study the prevalence of alcohol problems in casualty departments and to use the data obtained as a stimulus to more widespread recognition and treatment of alcohol problems in general hospitals.

The USSR regards its research into classification as leading to better matching of patients with treatment approaches:

> A rise of efficacy of alcoholic therapy in the near future can be achieved on the basis of deep knowledge of the disease pathogenesis and ever growing differentiation of therapeutic activities with consideration of the disease clinical picture peculiarities, premorbid structure of [the] patient's character and [the] influence of [the] micro-environment.

> Thus, it is possible to mark out several peculiarities of treatment of alcoholics in the USSR. In the first place, alcohol patients are treated by special narcological services, organized according to territorial principles. Secondly therapy is conducted in accordance with results of the alcoholism pathogenesis study. Thirdly psychotropic agents, applied differentially, depending on clinical peculiarities of the disease play an important role in the therapy of alcohol patients.

The USSR is unusual among the countries considered, in that it gives a great deal of attention to pharmacological and physical treatments, which received little mention by other countries except with respect to medical detoxification.

Some countries (e.g., Australia, England and Wales, Norway) are making a conscious effort to shift their existing services toward briefer community-based treatment. For example, in Norway it seems that this process is quite advanced:

> The county responsibility for the planning and administration of the treatment services will probably lead to a reduction of the number of inpatient treatment services, and a corresponding increase in the outpatient treatment capacity. Hopefully, the new "trend" within the alcohol treatment area will continue, characterized by a more differentiated treatment system, meeting various client needs. The ultimate goal must be to integrate some of the public responsibilities for these problems as fully as possible with the general health and social services. Only then will it be possible to undertake realistic secondary preventive measures and interventions. There have been relatively few treatment evaluation studies or prospective studies in Norway. It will be valuable to reinforce the efforts at doing treatment evaluation studies, and to reduce the gap

between research and clinical practice: how to implement our new knowledge about treatment programmes in the most cost-effective way. There are many challenges to be met in the future. The increased competence and level of knowledge among the health and social professionals in Norway have created a new optimism and positive attitudes towards clients with alcohol problems. This new optimism is a good basis for carrying on with the positive development we have seen the last couple of years.

In England and Wales changes of this kind are also occurring. The following issues and problems were preoccupying those concerned with alcohol services:

1. Joint working and joint planning: Most services involve health, social services and voluntary organizations. There is a great deal of debate about how to work together and plan together. Joint planning groups are usually given responsibility for both mental health and alcohol services and these groups are being given more power. A survey carried out in 1985 showed that only 18 percent of District Health Authorities had specific planning teams on alcohol and/or drug abuse.

2. Social services: Most social services departments give very low priority to alcohol-related problems in spite of the evidence that many of their clients experience such problems.

3. Probation: The response from the probation service depends upon the enthusiasm of local teams rather than central policy but there is an increasing interest within the National Association of Probation Officers.

4. Changes in the management of the National Health Service are placing much more emphasis on information and service evaluation.

5. There is a trend towards minimal interventions especially within District General Hospitals.

6. Services for drug abusers have been developing at quite a pace as a result of government commitment. No official government backing has yet been given to the development of alcohol services.

7. Should alcohol treatment units be closed and the resources used to develop or consolidate community services?

8. Should the alcohol treatment service be managed by a particular profession?

Conclusion

This selective review of treatment trends points to the following conclusions and comments:

- In most countries, alcohol-related disabilities are viewed as a major and costly problem with diverse manifestations.

- Alcohol problems are now seen as a much broader concept than "alcoholism" or alcohol dependence, although this changed perspective is not always reflected in the organization of treatment services.

- There is a trend toward the early recognition of hazardous drinking patterns and toward responding with simple interventions at this early stage.

- Low-cost interventions delivered at the primary level seem to be as beneficial as many more intensive treatments, but additional properly designed evaluation studies are required for treatments of all kinds including self-help groups.

- Very few programs have been properly evaluated from a cost-effective or cost-benefit viewpoint.

- Effective categorization of patients' needs and the matching of patients with programs remain underdeveloped and underresearched.

- The balance between specialist and nonspecialist services needs careful consideration as do the needs of both during a time of transition toward more community-based services.

- Some countries are examining the potential role of new kinds of change agents, such as *promotores,* pharmacists, or even the drinker's own family.

- Detoxification in the community or in the patient's own home is commonplace in some areas.

- The trend toward community management is placing new demands on primary-level workers who often feel ill equipped for this task. Their training needs require urgent consideration.

- National alcohol policies do seem to have provided a stimulus to new developments in many countries.

- The treatment component of such plans needs to be integrated within a broader preventive strategy and entails ministerial support and intersectoral collaboration.

- In several countries all forms of substance abuse are considered together, both in terms of planning and of service delivery.

- The enquiry produced disappointingly little information about the various strategies for funding services and their implications for cost and quality. This area needs further research.

- In some countries there is a tendency to continue with established programs in an uncritical way and refuse to be influenced by research findings from other centers.

- Improved communication between and within countries would facilitate innovation, but it is also important to recognize the barriers to change and to provide support to services while they are experiencing the change process.

REFERENCES

Babor, T. F., ed. 1986. Alcohol and culture. Annals of the New York Academy of Sciences 472:1-239.

Babor, T. F., E. B. Ritson, and R. J. Hodgson. 1986. Alcohol-related problems in the primary health care setting: A review of early intervention strategies. British Journal of Addiction 81:23-46.

Chick, J., G. Lloyd, and E. Crombie. 1985. Counselling problem drinkers in medical wards: A controlled study. British Medical Journal 290:965-967.

Edwards, G., J. Orford, S. Egert, S. Guthrie, A. Hawker, C. Hensman, M. Micheson, E. Oppenheimer, and C. Taylor. 1977. Alcoholism: A controlled trial of "treatment" and advice. Journal of Studies on Alcohol 38:1004-1031.

Elvy, G. A., J. E. Wells, and K. A. Baud. 1988. Attempted referral as intervention for problem drinking in the general hospital. British Journal of Addiction 83:83-89.

Emrick, C. D. 1974. A review of psychologically oriented treatments of alcoholism. Quarterly Journal of Studies on Alcohol 35:523-549.

Heather, N., P. D. Campion, R. G. Neville, and D. McCabe. 1987. Evaluation of a controlled drinking minimal intervention for problem drinkers in general practice. Journal of the Royal College of General Practitioners 37:358-363.

Kristenson, H. 1983. Studies on Alcohol-related Disabilities in Medical Intervention Programmes in Middle-aged Males. Skurup, Sweden: Lindbergs Blankett.

Miller, W. R., and R. K. Hester. 1986. The effectiveness of alcoholism treatment: What research reveals. Pp.121-174 in Treating Addictive Behaviours: Processes of Change, W. R. Miller and N. Heather, eds. New York: Plenum Press.

Miguez, L. 1983. El paciente aloholico en Costa Rica: Caracteristicas y resultados. Acta Psiquiat. Psicoliga America Latina 29:7-20.

Ritson, E. B. 1985. Community Response to Alcohol-Related Problems. Geneva: World Health Organization.

Rootman, I., and J. Moser. 1984. Community Response to Alcohol-related Problems. Washington, D.C.: U.S. Department of Health and Human Services.

Saunders, J., and O. G. Aasland. 1987. WHO Collaborative Project on Identification and Treatment of Persons with Harmful Alcohol Consumption. Report on Phase I: Development of Screening Instrument. Geneva: World Health Organization.

World Health Organization (WHO). 1984. Management of Alcohol-related Problems in General Practice. Geneva: World Health Organization.

World Health Organization (WHO). 1986. Treatment and Rehabilitation Programs in Alcohol Abuse: Report of a Meeting in Helsinki, November 1985. Copenhagen: WHO, Regional Office for Europe.

World Health Organization (WHO). 1987. The Respective Roles of Primary Health Care and Specialized Services: The Development and Implementation of Programs for Problem Drinkers. Report of a Meeting in Oslo, August 1986. Copenhagen: WHO, Regional Office for Europe.

D   COERCION IN ALCOHOL TREATMENT

Constance M. Weisner

At present, a wide range of measures representing varying degrees of coercion is an established component of entry to both public and private alcohol treatment. Although this development has occurred relatively recently within the context of the modern alcohol treatment system, the use of coercion is not an entirely new topic of debate. Involuntary treatment was an issue that received much discussion in English-speaking countries at the turn of the century, and the inebriate legislation that was passed to provide for coerced treatment still exists in many places.

Coercion is defined in this paper as a form of institutionalized pressure (with negative consequences as an alternative) that results in an individual entering treatment. In the cases in which it refers to pressure by the family, coercion means those procedures in which there is an organized strategy involving some institutional contact. The types of coercion that are found in alcohol treatment today and that are discussed here are civil commitments, referrals to alcohol treatment from the criminal justice system, workplace referrals, and family and early intervention programs. These categories form a rough continuum of coercion, ranging from those that are legally mandated to those that are less explicit. In addition, there is variation within each category in the level of coerciveness and the range of practices used.

Major shifts have occurred in all types of coercion within the past 20 years, and these rapid changes, along with its greater use, have gone largely unresearched. Many questions remain unanswered. Included among them but not addressed here is whether the treatment system is expanding to include these new groups of individuals or whether the new groups are replacing those who have traditionally been served.

In the sociological literature, issues related to the interface between the medical and treatment systems and the criminal justice and other coercive systems are usually discussed in terms of the "medicalization of deviance" (Conrad and Schneider, 1980). American society in recent decades has seen a shift from frank punishment to the therapeutic treatment of deviance, although countertrends are also present (e.g., for opiates in the 1920s, and more generally in the decline in "therapeutic corrections" ideals in criminology in recent decades). The "medicalization of deviance" literature reminds us that there are losses as well as gains in the shift from punishment to treatment—especially when one considers that frank punishment is often replaced by punishment cloaked as treatment—but minus the civil liberties protection that accompanies punishment (Christie and Bruun, 1969).

Although different issues relating to coercion may surface depending on the type of treatment involved, some issues are common. For example, proponents of employee assistance programs as well as those who favor the use of the criminal justice system describe their client groups similarly as having a health problem and as "deviants" (Trice and Beyer, 1984). It remains to be seen whether there will be long-term effects from rede-

The author is a senior scientist with the Alcohol Research Group, Institute of Epidemiology and Behavioral Medicine, Medical Research Institute of San Francisco. Preparation of this paper was supported by a National Alcohol Research Center grant (AA05595) from the National Institute on Alcohol Abuse and Alcoholism to the Alcohol Research Group. The author wishes to thank Thomas Babor, Herman Diesenhaus, Frederick Glaser, Robin Room, and Laura Schmidt for their consultation on earlier drafts of this paper.

fining the treatment population using a focus on deviant behavior rather than on illness.

The objective of this paper is to describe the patterns of coercion in public and private alcohol treatment programs today. More specifically, it describes (a) the nature and prevalence of coercive referrals to alcohol treatment; (b) the distribution of criminal justice and workplace referrals in public and in private programs; (c) the epidemiology of alcohol problems within these clinical populations; (d) treatment outcome related to these programs and populations; and (e) the general impact of the presence of a largely coerced population in the alcohol treatment system.

Before beginning the paper's main discussion, it should be noted that there are large gaps in the data related to these patterns and even in the vocabulary available for exploring these issues. First, definitions are problematic. In the literature, what is meant by coercion is often unclear; alternatively, varying terms and conceptions may be used. Second, data are lacking on the number and outcomes of coercive referrals to treatment. In a discussion of treatment outcome, examining the relationship between coercion and outcome seems crucial. This literature is not well developed, but related research suggests that coercion must affect motivation and readiness for treatment, the process of treatment, and the outcome of treatment. Wherever possible in this report, national data sets are used. Otherwise, state- and county-level data are presented to illustrate prevalent patterns across the United States. It should always be kept in mind, however, that there is often great diversity from state to state.

Types of Coercion

As noted earlier, there is a range of types of coerced treatment for people with alcohol problems forming a continuum from mandatory to less explicit coercion. These treatment types are discussed below.

Involuntary Treatment: Civil Commitments

Civil commitments lie at the most severe end of the coercion continuum. Commitments have long characterized mental health referrals; in fact, early psychiatric hospitalization was entirely involuntary. (It was not until the enactment of an 1881 Massachusetts law that voluntary admission to psychiatric hospitals was officially acknowledged and permitted.) By the 1870s, however, reform movements were under way to establish specific procedures for involuntary treatment, in part as a result of alleged misuse of the mechanism by the medical profession and because of cases of "railroading" by the families of some of those committed (Fox, 1978). By the end of the nineteenth century, these reforms had led to requirements for independent examinations and trial by jury in many states (Appelbaum, 1985).

In addition to psychiatric hospitals, in some states, inebriate asylums provided treatment for alcoholism. These large, publicly run institutions for the involuntary treatment of alcoholics were founded during the 1870s, 1880s, and 1890s (Baumohl, 1986; Baumohl and Room, 1987). They developed alongside community-based "inebriate homes" that had only voluntary admissions. Although only a few inebriate asylums were ever actually funded and established, the agitation to build them was a mark of therapeutic and public opinion regarding the historical place of involuntary treatment for alcohol problems. Influential doctors in the inebriate asylums movement spoke out strongly against voluntarism: "any concern about the liberty of drunkards was just so much `sentimental nonsense´." (quoted in Bauhmohl, 1986). There was a general feeling that voluntary inebriate homes were "wasting philanthropic dollars" and not adequately protecting families or society.   The temperance physician and author of the mid-1800s, Henry Gibbons, recommended that asylums be "placed on a proper footing to consist of a rural asylum operated under medical direction with patients committed by the courts."   Proponents of temperance also recommended that they become state institutions in order to have "powers to restrain patients" (quoted in Baumohl and Room, 1987).   In an 1874 statute, Connecticut passed legislation allowing the involuntary commitment of inebriates to private institutions; other states soon followed its example.

From the early 1900s until the late 1960s the predominant criterion for involuntary commitment, whether under mental health or inebriate laws, was "need for treatment." Most commitments of inebriates were to mental hospitals under mental health law for "alcoholic psychosis."   Under the Lanterman-Petris-Short Act, however, California in 1969 changed its criterion for mental health commitment to require evidence of dangerousness to self or others or evidence of "grave disability." That landmark legislation influenced the enactment of statutes in most other states (Hoge et al., 1989).   Consequently, in recent years, the focus of civil commitment in most states has been on mental illness resulting in imminent danger to the self or others (Dunham, 1985).

There are several issues relevant to a discussion of involuntary commitment today and its application in the field of alcohol problems. The issues discussed here are (a) the alcohol specificity of statutes (as well as specifications for procedures and the length of commitment); (b) the frequency of alcohol-related commitments; (c) changes in the criteria of dangerousness or of need for treatment used in statutes; (d) the philosophy of the least restrictive alternative, including outpatient commitments; and (e) distinctions between voluntary and involuntary admissions, including the official and unofficial functions served by commitments. Related to each of these issues is the question of alcohol's specificity—do alcohol-related commitments generally fit the pattern of commitments for mental illness?

Statutory Specifications for Alcohol-related Commitments States vary as to whether they have alcohol-specific commitment statutes, whether alcohol problems are included as a criterion within more general mental illness commitment laws, or whether alcohol problems are excluded as a criterion for commitment. There are also differences from state to state in the number and characteristics of different commitment sections in the various statutes. Within the general framework of commitment, there are many subsidiary issues (e.g., commitment for primary rehabilitation and extended care versus emergency commitment).[1] The states also differ in which departments are designated as responsible for commitment proceedings.   Grad and colleagues (1971) reported that 35 states had involuntary commitment procedures for alcoholism, whereas 32 states had some organizational division or commission on alcoholism that was listed as having programmatic responsibility for commitments.   The Grad team's compilation was a by-product of discussions in the late 1960s on decriminalizing public drunkenness arrests. There has not been a similar compilation since that time.

More recently, Beis (1983) reviewed involuntary mental health commitment legislation across the 50 states, although not with a focus on alcohol problems. His brief descriptions of commitment criteria include only six states in which alcoholism, chemical dependence, addiction, or substance abuse are named in the criteria. Three states explicitly exclude alcoholism. The picture is actually more complicated than this, however, and a reading of the broader literature reveals examples of states that have alcohol statutes but that are not listed in Beis's review (e.g., see Gilboy and Schmidt, 1979; Mestrovic, 1983; Carlyle, 1988). It is perhaps indicative of the low profile of alcohol problems in recent years in studies of mental health commitments that there has been no overall compilation of state laws focusing on involuntary commitment for alcohol problems since the early 1970s.

Across state statutes, the provisions for commitment often vary for mental health and alcohol problems in terms of the length of commitment and the specific commitment

Across state statutes, the provisions for commitment often vary for mental health and alcohol problems in terms of the length of commitment and the specific commitment procedures. For example, Texas does not require a medical certificate for an alcoholism commitment unless the court orders an examination; for a mental health commitment, however, two certificates are required (Carlyle, 1988). Because of the variation across states and the lack of comprehensive reviews on the subject, it is difficult to gauge the place of alcohol in the overall civil commitment framework.

Frequency of Alcohol-related Involuntary Commitments Little is known about the frequency of such commitments, although some figures are available on the total number of admissions for alcohol problems. Room (1980) reported that, for the United States, there were about 15,000 state and private mental hospital admissions for alcoholism in 1942 and about 128,000 in 1976 (from population bases of 133 million and 214 million persons, respectively). The proportion of involuntary admissions is unknown. Cameron (1983) reported that the rate of involuntary alcohol-related commitments to state hospitals in California per 100,000 persons in the civilian population aged 20 and older was 37.3 in 1950 and 0.2 in 1970. The peak was 45.6 in 1961, after which the rate gradually began to decline. It seems significant that a dramatic drop in the rate took place between 1969 and 1970 (18.7 to 0.2) after the commitment criteria were tightened (Cameron, 1983).

Recently, there have been a few state-level studies that include prevalence rates for alcohol-related commitments. It is not possible to generalize from the conclusions of these studies, however, because they include different alcohol-related categories (e.g., polysubstance abuse, substance abuse, alcoholism) and use different criteria (dangerousness, need for treatment, or both). One of these studies gives an indication of how prevalence rates for commitments might be affected by the use of different criteria. The Hoge team's (1989) study in Massachusetts found that substance abuse disorders were responsible for 15 percent of the primary diagnoses of all patients coming to emergency mental health services. Of those who met the criteria for commitment under the Massachusetts law (which uses the dangerousness and gravely disabled criteria), 9.5 percent had a primary diagnosis of substance abuse. Of those who met the criteria but did not voluntarily accept treatment, 12.3 percent had a primary diagnosis of substance abuse. Of those who met the Stone criteria,[2] 8.6 percent had a primary diagnosis of substance abuse. Thus, regardless of the criteria used, the proportion of cases with a substance abuse primary diagnosis remained about the same.

There are also some data available from other states. Mestrovic (1983) reported that 17.7 percent of a sample from a New York State psychiatric hospital had symptoms of alcoholism (18.2 percent had symptoms of drug use). (New York's state statutes do not include dangerousness as a necessary part of the commitment criteria; two-physician certificate is sufficient for establishing the need for treatment [Mestrovic, 1983].) Faulkner and colleagues (1989) reported that in a sample from an Oregon county, about half of the emergency commitment group and half of those in a temporary police holding group had a secondary diagnosis of either substance abuse or personality disorder. Cohen's (1987) study of civil commitments in Colorado found that polysubstance abuse was the fifth highest disability (14.9 percent) among commitments.

Finally, an Illinois study by Gilboy and Schmidt stresses the importance of examining the role of alcohol in commitment as seen by the courts even when alcohol problems are not reported as the primary diagnosis. They describe a commitment case in which the doctor gave a diagnosis of mental illness, and the judge asked outright, "Is the basis of this, alcohol?" The doctor responded: "There is underlying mental illness, but alcohol is a contributing cause" (Gilboy and Schmidt, 1979:447).

Trends in Statutory Criteria of Dangerousness or of Need for Treatment Whether existing criteria should be relaxed is perhaps the most widely debated issue involving mental health commitments today. This discussion is not related specifically to alcohol commitments, however, and there is no extant body of research to inform a discussion of how alcohol-related cases would be affected by changes in commitment policy.

Many of the writers who discuss suggested changes in criteria point out that there has always been dissatisfaction with the approach of any era. This viewpoint is summed up by Lidz and coworkers (1989:176):

> The routine use of civil commitment distinguishes psychiatric care from other medical specialties, and the proper restrictions that should be placed on this professional practice have been the source of continuing controversy. In general, the history of civil commitment in the U.S. has been a series of swings between rigorous, rule-bound standards and looser, more discretion-based procedures. Strict procedural systems have usually led to objections that people needing treatment were not receiving it. Looser standards have usually produced an outcry against the infringements of civil liberties accompanying the application of broad clinical discretion. The 1960s and 1970s saw the most recent swing in this continuing cycle, with the growth of more rigid standards of commitment focused around the notion of dangerousness to self or others.[3]

Appelbaum describes the move at the end of the 1960s to increase civil liberties by providing extensive legal safeguards and focusing on dangerousness as a "criminalization" of the commitment process and the mental health system (Appelbaum, 1985). He also makes the case that these changes, in their departure from the notion of a need for treatment, were intrinsically different from criteria that had been considered basic throughout the nineteenth and twentieth centuries (Appelbaum, 1985). In fact, the controversy over the boundaries of civil commitment may simply reflect the ongoing tensions among disciplines over the mental health domain. Psychiatrists and other mental health professionals have traditionally argued for greater discretionary power over commitment decisions; the legal profession, on the other hand, has favored enhanced legal and judicial checks on the commitment process and assurances of the protection of patient civil rights (Fox, 1978).

The changes during the past 20 years that have precipitated the move toward a criterion based on dangerousness have resulted in a different set of criticisms from mental health professionals and patients' family groups. Many of these criticisms center around dissatisfaction regarding access to care and "right to treatment" issues (Dunham, 1985; Stone, 1985). Currently, there is a move to broaden the criteria again. In 1983, for example, the American Psychiatric Association (APA) published its contribution to the debate, the Model State Law on Civil Commitment of the Mentally Ill (Stromberg and Stone, 1983). Essentially, the APA model law argues for a "seriously deteriorating" criterion to be appended to the existing dangerousness criteria upheld by most states. It has been greeted with varying responses from the psychiatric, patients' rights, and legal communities, as evidenced by the broad range of literature on the subject. Some states (e.g., California) have proposed legislation that would implement a seriously deteriorating criterion; the presentation of the model law in 1983 reflects a general trend, supported by psychiatrists, to relax involuntary commitment criteria.

There are good arguments on both sides of these issues. Civil rights proponents claim that relaxing the criteria would remove legal safeguards, and this significant change would occur without knowing whether inpatient hospitalization were effective (Rubenstein, 1985). Wexler (1985) claims that the process would not ensure fair, independent, and multiple evaluations. There are also concerns regarding the financial impact of relaxed commitment laws. On the other side, Dunham (1985) argues that such a statute change would make it possible to get help earlier for people with problems.

examined the impact of such legislation. In one of the early efforts of this group of studies, Durham (1985) in Washington State, reported that, after statutes were relaxed (in 1979), involuntary commitments increased by 91 percent the year after passage of the legislation. The "grave disability" criterion embraced three-quarters of the cases. One of the repercussions of the changes in criteria was that there were not enough facilities or resources available; as a result, involuntary commitments were given priority over voluntary admissions.[4] As might be expected, such findings have intensified the concerns of those who felt that the broadening of commitment criteria would result in undesirable net-widening.

Yet at least one other study had different results. The Hoge team (1989) conducted a study in Massachusetts that compared the number of applicable commitments under the Stone commitment criteria and under the dangerousness criterion. The study found that fewer people were committed under the dangerousness criterion. The sample for this and other similar studies, however, constituted those who were already there—that is, those who had been referred under the more stringent criteria. Thus, the change was likely to be in referrals to treatment, and the available pool of patients was likely to be larger if the criteria were relaxed. Interestingly, it was thought that the requirement of the Stone model that "efficacious treatment" for the subject's condition be available would be a sufficiently restrictive criterion to keep commitments down. Instead, the study found that this particular criterion was not restrictive, as 87 percent of patients were rated by psychiatrists as being able to be effectively treated. The authors attributed this sizable proportion to the availability and current popularity of pharmacological treatments. Of course, for alcohol-related commitments, this finding may not apply because the field cannot rely on such treatments to the same extent as in mental health.

Minnesota followed a course different from most of the other states by tightening its commitment laws in 1982. The criteria it uses include recent and overt dangerous behavior, a determination that the person has received full protection under prevailing due process guarantees, routing to the least physically restrictive treatment alternative, and screening by independent agencies of all applications. However, given such changes, no significant differences were found in numbers of commitments (Greeman and McClellan, 1985).

There is little research on the characteristics of persons admitted to institutions under the different types of criteria, but there is some suggestion the criteria may make a difference. In his review of civil commitment standards in three countries, Segal (1989) found that the criteria across the three nations could be divided into two categories: need for treatment and degree of dangerousness. His study showed that the different criteria brought different categories of individuals into treatment.

Thus, although the field of alcohol problems is at an important juncture regarding shifts in civil commitment criteria, research to date does not give any clear direction regarding the effects of different legislation. In the absence of extensive and replicated research, professional and other interests appear to have dominated the literature in this area with rhetorical arguments for and against their positions. The historical tension between the individual's right to treatment and his or her civil rights remains visible and central to discussions of civil commitment criteria.

Two institutional strains characterize the debate over commitment decisions. First is the strain between the legislature and the judiciary. The judiciary tends to hand down "unimplementable" civil rights decisions. For example, decisions made in the "right-to-treatment" cases of the late 1970s required treatment of an intensity that many facilities cannot manage. The judiciary has clearly found "need-for-treatment" statutes unconstitutional, yet under the pressure of psychiatrists (e.g., the APA model law dictum) states still try to legislate such statutes. The second strain is the tension between civil rights lawyers on one side and psychiatrists and patients' family groups (i.e., the National states still try to legislate such statutes. The second strain is the tension between civil rights lawyers on one side and psychiatrists and patients' family groups (i.e., the National Association for the Mentally Ill) on the other. This tension is the result in part of an old debate over professional boundaries (Schmidt, 1986). Although this debate takes place in the mental health arena, the issues relevant to alcohol commitments are carried along with it without being separately examined.

Commitment to the "Least Restrictive Alternative" This concept came out of the same movement that produced deinstitutionalization, patients' rights, and mainstreaming. It recognizes the existence of a continuum within the larger involuntary commitment spectrum, referring both to issues of setting (inpatient versus outpatient) and to type of treatment (e.g., electro-shock, psychotropic medications) (Keilitz et al., 1985). It can affect precommitment screening and evaluation, involuntary civil detention procedures, and the continuity of community-based services, as well as release, transfer and diversion, and guardianship. Keilitz and coworkers (1985) argue that although the concept is difficult to apply in real-world practice and does not deal with the issue of quality of care, it remains an important principle in guiding procedures at every level.

"Involuntary outpatient civil commitment (IOC)—the legal and psychosocial process whereby an allegedly mentally disordered and dangerous person is forced to undergo mental health treatment or care in an outpatient setting" is the most common implementation of this concept today (Keilitz and Hall, 1985:378). In their review of state laws regarding compulsory outpatient treatment, Keilitz and Hall define IOC as "the dispositional options (lying between inpatient hospitalization and outright release) available to a civil court after an `adjudication´ of involuntary civil commitment" (1985:378). Most states insist that the same criteria be applied to IOCs as apply to involuntary hospitalization, although four states use different criteria for the two types of commitment, and at least one of them appears explicitly to attempt to increase the potential of commitment with its use of the IOC mechanism. Almost all states now allow for the use of IOCs, whereas 26 states and the District of Columbia have explicit provisions for it; nevertheless, there are also many differences in procedures and approaches across jurisdictions.

The Distinction Between Involuntary and Voluntary Commitment[5] This distinction is another important factor in an understanding of commitment. In fact, the issue of civil commitment cannot be understood without examining the underlying reasons for involuntary treatment. Although they are seldom addressed in the literature, the so-called "latent" or "unofficial" functions of treatment are central to understanding why patients are involuntarily treated. For example, Baumohl and Room (1987) describe the latent functions being served by involuntary commitment in the late nineteenth century:

> What inebriety doctors sought from the state, at least in English-speaking countries, pointed in two directions—toward fee-paying, private patients, and toward poor, urban drunkards. For private, fee-paying patients, doctors sought procedures to complement treatment. At a minimum, doctors wanted to be able to enforce the completion of treatment where patients had voluntarily entered into it. Beyond that, they wanted provisions to compel private patients into treatment. Essentially, this meant putting a tool in the hands not only of the doctor but also of the drinker's family. (p. 45)

Sixty years after the period of the "inebriety doctors," Selzer (1958) reported that state boards of alcoholism and private psychiatrists were beginning to change their opinions about the motivational problems of involuntary commitments and to favor such commitments (because too many people left before treatment really began).

Some of the literature discusses the complicated question of the extent to which voluntary commitments are really voluntary. For instance, the appendix to the task panel reports of the President's Commission on Mental Health (1978) discussed three studies (with mixed results) that investigated whether voluntary or involuntary commitment was longer in duration and whether individuals who were voluntarily admitted really wanted to be there. Voluntary commitments may serve specific "latent functions"; for example, Gilboy and Schmidt (1979) reported on the practice of persuading people to sign a "voluntary" admission form to avoid a police custody form. The complexity and contradictoriness of the commitment process may also affect voluntary and involuntary commitments. For example, Mestrovic (1983) examined the intake process in a state hospital and reported on how the actual intake decisions were made. Some commitments were "overturned" by staff at different levels of the institution, and some intakes became "involuntary" when patients refused to sign voluntary forms. His study is especially rich in exploring the arbitrariness of the process of admission and commitment.

The commitment process is further complicated by a kind of plea bargaining that may occur when the patient waives due process rights in order to negotiate sanctions. Describing the process of deciding between voluntary and involuntary commitment, Cohen (1987) suggests the analogy to criminal plea bargaining. She summarizes the arguments on both sides of the issue, pointing out that the existence of involuntary commitment has had the overall effect of criminalizing the mental health system, whereas voluntary commitment uses fewer financial resources and often results in fewer sanctions for the individual.

The motives of the person facing a commitment are an additional factor. Lidz and colleagues (1989) point out that for some the hospital is a place to receive "safe and timely" housing. Mestrovic (1983) also describes this room and board function, pointing out that admission is often sufficiently important to people that they fake suicide attempts to gain admission. The existence of social support to the persons facing commitment has been reported as an important variable in hospitalization (Schmidt, 1986).

At the institutional level (as in Baumohl and Room's description of an earlier period), involuntary commitment is a way to avoid the early termination of treatment (Lidz et al., 1989). Lidz and coworkers also claim that the current treatment reimbursement structure often makes it financially imperative that a person be committed rather than admitted voluntarily. Another related issue involves determining for whom the commitment is being made. Is it for the sake of the person, the family, or the community (President's Commission on Mental Health, 1978)? Mäkelä (1980) discusses the functions of commitment in solving family and community problems and argues: "It should not be up to the medical profession to take care of public order and the safety of the drunkard's family" (p. 229).

It is important to examine the area of civil commitment because, although alcohol treatment commitments are rare in comparison with alcohol treatment generally, the coercion issues raised by the commitment process are more clear-cut and easier to discern.

Diversion from the Criminal Justice System

Referrals from the criminal justice system to alcohol treatment are the next level on a continuum of coercion.[6] Diversion programs came originally from a focus on drug abuse. Programs in several of the states influenced the federal interest—for example, California's Civil Addict Program of 1961 (Anglin, 1988), which allowed for a seven-year commitment, and New York's 1966 civil commitment program of the Narcotic Addiction Control Commission (Inciardi, 1988). This interest resulted in the passage in 1966 of the Narcotic Addict Rehabilitation Act (P.L. 89-793), which developed relationships between criminal justice and treatment agencies. It also allocated demonstration treatment funds and influenced the establishment of drug programs throughout the United States (Leukefeld and Tims, 1988). In 1972 the Treatment Alternatives to Street Crime (TASC) program set in motion a series of community-based diversion programs (Cook and Weinman, 1988). Such projects were often funded by the U.S. Law Enforcement Assistance Administration (LEAA) and focused on crimes associated with drugs (Mecca, 1975). They commonly included panels of criminal justice representatives, treatment officials, and citizens who assessed cases for diversion from the criminal justice system to community alcohol treatment programs.[7] Although federal funding of most such projects has ended, in some areas they were followed by state or locally funded formal diversion schemes. Even in areas in which no subsequent programs were developed the effects of the projects may still be felt. Their most important achievements were that they set a precedent and left behind an informal system of contact among the courts, probation officers, public defenders and other attorneys, and individual treatment agencies for referring people who commit a wide variety of criminal offenses.

Today, these offenses include public drunkenness, alcohol-specific crimes, and non-alcohol-specific crimes in which alcohol is nevertheless considered to be a factor in the offense. Diversion technically indicates the transferring of the individual from the criminal justice system to a treatment program before sentencing and the removal of criminal sanctions from the case on the successful completion of treatment. In common practice, however, it has evolved to more loosely designate referral to treatment at any point in the adjudication process; such treatment then becomes either part or most of the sanctions imposed. Using this definition, diversion may occur both formally and informally.[8] In some instances, a case is made by a probation officer, a public defender, a private attorney, or the defendant that the defendant has a serious problem with alcohol, that the alcohol problem is responsible for or related to the committing of the offense, and that alcohol treatment is more appropriate than the sanctions of the criminal justice system (Mosher, 1983). Cases in this category are sometimes referred to treatment after sentencing, and treatment is considered to be part of the sanctions. On the whole, courts first convict an individual and then take alcohol into account (Mosher, 1983). The offense is considered a crime, but the handling of it takes place in the alcohol treatment sector rather than solely within the criminal justice system. Sometimes the individual enters treatment through the suggestion of a police officer or through the encouragement of (or even a referral by) a public defender, attorney, or probation officer. The person may also enter treatment on his or her own initiative before the adjudication process is completed, a move that often affects later sentencing.

The literature on diversion for drug abuse is helpful in understanding the alcohol case because drug-related diversion policy has been more clearly specified and there are many commonalities between it and alcohol-related diversion categories. The report of a joint German-American commission studying coercion in drug treatment (Brown et al., 1987) details the points in the criminal justice process at which diversion can take place. Diversion can be pre- and postadjudicatory. Preadjudicatory diversion can take place in lieu of arrest—for instance, when a policeman gives someone an opportunity to go to a treatment facility rather than be arrested. (This particular category may be even more common on the alcohol side for public drunkenness, alcohol-related domestic violence offenses, and other such "crimes".) There is also postarrest but preadjudicatory diversion, which can take place after arrest but prior to filing charges, at the district attorney's discretion, or after filing charges. Preadjudicatory diversion can also involve conditional release (often with the treatment program having some or all responsibility for the diverted person); treatment referral with disposition to be decided later, depending in part on treatment outcome (case responsibility is placed with the district attorney, the judge, or some other party); or a plea of guilty prior to adjudication for a negotiated treatment option. Postadjudicatory diversion can occur before sentencing, at which point a referral can be made before the verdict is given or in lieu of a different sentence. Diversion can also occur after sentencing; in this case, sentencing is deferred while the individual is in treatment, or alternately, treatment may be a condition of release. These alternatives usually involve probation supervision as well (Brown et al., 1987). All of these points at which diversion may occur represent different levels of judicial review, different levels of potential alternative sanctions, and different levels of interaction between the criminal justice and treatment systems. All of these points are defined for drug-related diversion; however, the categories and processes are similar to those for diversion to alcohol treatment.

Historically, diversion for public drunkenness has received the most official attention. In 1971 the National Conference of Commissioners on Uniform State Laws recommended that all states enact the Uniform Alcoholism and Intoxication Treatment Act. This act was the culmination of a long history of attempts by various medical and legal interests to provide more humane treatment of the public inebriate (Kurtz and Regier, 1975). Its objective was to handle this population within a medical rather than a criminal justice framework. It suggested a policy stating that "alcoholics and intoxicated persons may not be subjected to criminal prosecution because of their consumption of alcoholic beverages" (Hart, 1977:674). As of 1985, 34 states had fully implemented the Uniform Act (Finn, 1985). To be in compliance, states were required to have a plan in place that provided for continuity of care. This requirement was instituted to avoid the fragmentation of services and to ensure entry into the full range of services an individual might need. To be in compliance, states were also required to have appropriate commitment legislation and judicial safeguards. This legislation could be part of the mental health civil commitment statute, or it could be a specifically alcohol-related commitment statute. Each state considered meeting the Uniform Act criteria, but there were many factors that deterred across-the-board compliance, including the mandate to provide a full range of services.

Because its purpose was to decriminalize an offense, the Uniform Act made diversion for public drunkenness significantly different from other types of criminal justice diversion. Yet its success is less than clear. Finn (1985) found mixed results in relation to how far responsibility for the public inebriate had moved from criminal justice to treatment. Overall arrest statistics indicated fewer arrests, but they had not always decreased as much as might be expected from the intent of the legislation. In addition, several states reported increases in other types of arrests, which suggested a possible legislative transfer function. Finn also reviewed the literature on the effectiveness of these programs and concluded that "the health care system has not improved the physical, emotional, or social condition of most public inebriates" (1985:16). It is interesting to note that this is one area of criminal justice-treatment interaction that was fully and officially sanctioned by law; yet it has not been fully implemented, either legally or practically.

Aside from public drunkenness, in which decriminalization is the issue, there are two types of cases that are diverted. First there are alcohol-specific criminal offenses, such as driving while intoxicated (DWI). Although there had been a history of traffic safety schools in many U.S. communities, the national attention given to a treatment approach for DWI individuals through the Alcohol Safety Action Projects has been important in establishing such interventions. Today alcohol treatment is an established sanction for DWI offenses, and in fact, many states have transferred much of the handling of DWI offenses to alcohol treatment programs. In some jurisdictions, many DWI drivers are given their choice of alcohol treatment or criminal justice sanctions; in other jurisdictions, they are automatically referred to alcohol treatment (U.S. Department of Transportation, 1976; Weisner, 1986; Stewart et al., 1987). Whether sanctions involve alcohol treatment alone or a combination of treatment and criminal justice generally depends on the policy of a particular state and on the number of DWI offenses a person has committed. The social movement (e.g., Mothers Against Drunk Driving) toward more stringent sanctions for drinking drivers has been quite influential in promoting these changes and has resulted in a strong criminal justice function for alcohol treatment in the context of this treatment population (Reinarman, 1988).

The second diversion category includes offenders who are diverted because of their history of alcohol abuse or the involvement of alcohol in a non-alcohol-specific crime. The distinction here is that the individual is not referred to treatment because of an intrinsic condition as much as for a legal problem related to alcohol. The types of offenses range from burglary to domestic violence. These cases fall under the various diversion categories described earlier. In many criminal justice diversion cases, there are other coercion-related issues involving the type of treatment setting and the type of treatment modality. For example, in some programs, the individual is required (either by the court or by the program) to take disulfiram (Antabuse) (U.S. Department of Transportation, 1976; Bloom et al., 1988). This requirement is a subtle form of coercion; an individual is not involuntarily given disulfiram but simply referred "back to the legal authority" if he or she refuses it (see, for example, Bloom et al., 1988). Another related issue is that an individual may not be given a choice between inpatient versus outpatient treatment settings. In fact, there is some indication that the treatment setting decision between residential and outpatient treatment is made on the basis of the seriousness of the crime rather than on the seriousness of the alcohol problem (Weisner and Room, 1984).

Raising issues on the other side, however, are recent moves toward evaluation and screening of individuals for referral into different types of treatment based on the seriousness of the alcohol problem (especially multiple-offender DWIs) (Klein, 1983). This practice raises difficult legal questions concerning punishment that fits the crime rather than the condition of the offender. These questions will need to be resolved if the trend toward diagnostic-based referral continues.

The Prevalence of Criminal Justice Referrals

Referrals to alcohol treatment from the criminal justice system are numerous (Boscarino, 1980; Furst et al.,1981; Speiglman, 1984; Weisner, 1987a,b; Connecticut State Drug and Alcohol Abuse Criminal Justice Commission, 1988;), a state of affairs that seems to prevail at the international level as well. (A World Health Organization study found that 20 of the 43 countries researched had some type of diversion legislation [Curran et al., 1987].)

There are two data systems that provide statistics on the prevalence of criminal justice referrals in treatment. NIAAA and NIDA collect data through the National Drug and Alcohol Treatment Unit Survey (NDATUS), a point prevalence survey of alcohol and drug treatment programs throughout the United States that has been carried out intermittently since 1979. Although it collects data on categories of individuals treated, the NDATUS does not collect individual-level data. Data are also compiled by the National Association of State Alcohol and Drug Abuse Directors, under contract with NIAAA and NIDA, and presented in the State Alcohol and Drug Abuse Profile (SADAP). The profile reports data from individual programs by state and is limited to those programs that are receiving some portion of their funds from the state. Because states do not organize services in the same way, the proportion of programs receiving funds from them varies dramatically. For some states the SADAP primarily excludes private for-profit and some nonprofit agencies. It has sociodemographic data on individuals in treatment, but the data are aggregated by agency for each program, which precludes individual-level data analysis. Thus, as will be discussed later, neither data system offers enlightenment us about the epidemiology of specific treatment populations because neither provides adequate client-level data. Also, neither provides data on the "unduplicated" client count.

Therefore, there is no accurate way to determine the overlap of clients from one alcohol program to another, although it is thought such an overlap occurs.

In sum, there are no data sources for obtaining an accurate count of the criminal justice referrals in the United States as a whole. The NDATUS collects information on the number of programs providing DWI services within its public and private sample but not on the number of individuals within those programs (except for the DWI programs that do not include any other client groups). The SADAP data base does have data on the number of DWI clients served by programs under state agency auspices. SADAP data for 1984 showed that for the Nation as a whole, there were 2,551 programs serving 864,000 individuals (Butynski, 1985). According to the same data, in California there were 118 programs with 288,222 individuals registered. It is likely that data from 1985 on will show much higher numbers of DWI clients in treatment. California was among the first of the states to adopt first-offender DWI treatment legislation (M.W. Perrine, 1984). Since that time, many other states have followed with similar statutes.

The DWI impact on treatment has been quite substantial. When state agencies were asked to identify the most significant changes during fiscal year 1980-1981, 25 named the "development or enhancement of DWI programs" (Butynski et al., 1987:66). In the 1985 SADAP report, an even larger impact was noted. To give just one example, Connecticut has had a 400 percent increase in DWI intakes in the past two years (Connecticut State Drug and Alcohol Abuse Criminal Justice Commission, 1988).

Using the 1987 NDATUS, Diesenhaus (1989) calculated the proportion of each state's overall total treatment units that provide DWI treatment. The variation and range were extensive. At the low end of the range were Alabama (12 percent), Texas (15 percent), Nevada (20 percent), California (21 percent), Georgia (21 percent), Tennessee (22 percent), Connecticut (23 percent), and Massachusetts (25 percent). At the high end were South Carolina (69 percent), Idaho (64 percent), Wyoming (61 percent), New Hampshire (56 percent), and Iowa (55 percent). The mean was 39 percent. These statistics seem to indicate that some states concede a large proportion of their overall treatment agenda to DWIs.

The examination of DWI statistics raises issues regarding the coerced population in relation to the self-referred. Gilbert and Cervantes (1987) reviewed a number of studies and reported that Mexican American clients had higher utilization rates for alcohol treatment than the general population. Their alcohol treatment utilization rates were also higher than their rates for general health services and mental health treatment utilization. The authors suggest that these statistics are a result of high arrest rates for Mexican Americans for offenses that the criminal justice system refers to alcohol treatment. Their review of admission data from states that together cover 78 percent of the Mexican American population in the United States found much higher proportions of that population than of the white population in categories of involuntary admissions. These nonvoluntary admissions included DWIs and other court referrals. Although studies have shown mixed results as to whether this higher proportion is due to discriminatory police or court practices or oversurveillance, the main interest here is to raise the issue of whether coercion is related to class or ethnicity. Consequently, although minorities may be found in treatment in larger numbers than before, this enlarged presence may only reflect their overrepresentation in criminal justice arrests, especially for drunk driving.

The number of DWI referrals in the public treatment system is so large that it overshadows other types of criminal justice referrals. Neither the NDATUS nor the SADAP collects data on the prevalence of these other criminal justice clients, a data gap that makes it impossible to calculate their presence in treatment. However, a few isolated state and local studies have provided some information. New York State reported that, in 1972, 35 percent of male and 42 percent of female new prison commitments were alcoholic. In addition, 46 percent of parolees were in need of alcohol problems treatment. Such sizable numbers of potential clients would obviously swamp the state's treatment system (New York State Governor's Task Force on Alcoholism Treatment in Criminal Justice 1986).

Connecticut is another state that was able to provide some data on referrals. A study conducted by the Connecticut State Drug and Alcohol Abuse Criminal Justice Commission (1988) found that 11,133 (25 percent) of the probation supervision cases are under court order to enter some form of alcohol or drug treatment. Alcohol residential programs receive 19 percent of their referrals from the criminal justice system, and outpatient programs receive 41 percent. The study also found that persons referred by the courts were often sent to detoxification programs when rehabilitation beds were not available. However, if all referrals were accepted by alcohol programs, court-referred individuals would use 64 percent of the rehabilitation beds available in the state.

Workplace Referrals

Referrals from the workplace are another form of coerced entry into alcohol treatment, although they usually involve less explicit coercion than that attached to criminal justice referrals. This treatment sector has evolved partly through its own impetus but also through the direct and indirect encouragement of NIAAA (Roman, 1988). The number of such programs and the weight they carry in the alcohol treatment and policy field regarding financing issues are unmistakably great. This prominence is all the more striking in that it has happened in less than 20 years (Lewis, 1987; Roman 1988). Over time, many of the major workplace programs and referrals have been subsumed under the employee assistance program (EAP) rubric. These programs include: (1) work organizations that have an employee who refers individuals to community resources, (2) work organizations that have formal contracts with external agencies, (3) programs run by unions within labor organizations, and (4) assistance programs for members of specific professions (Roman, 1988).

Within and across these four models there is a wide range of levels of coercion, ranging from voluntary referrals to job-jeopardy referrals. The range of types of referrals include at a minimum the following: self-referral; a coworker or supervisor unofficially suggesting referral; a coworker or supervisor arranging an intervention; a supervisor doing an informal performance evaluation and "suggesting" that the employee seek help from the EAP, which initiates the screening and referral process through "clinical evaluation" and "recommendation"; and the supervisor making referral to treatment through the EAP a formal condition of a performance evaluation, with a clear stipulation that termination will follow if performance does not improve with or without treatment (Diesenhaus, 1989). "The true voluntary EAP referral would be where the individual seeks out the EAP on his or her own because of a self-generated perception of a problem. Each of the others reflect extrinsic pressures, and they vary in the explicitness of the threat of sanction, the nature of sanction, and duration of threat" (Diesenhaus, 1989:2).

Many modifications in practice have occurred throughout the history of each model, as well as within the field in general. Semantically, the concept has evolved from "constructive coercion" to "constructive confrontation" as sensitivity to the term *coercion* has grown in the field (Trice and Beyer, 1982). There have also been many attempts to define the intrinsic characteristics of the programs. The most common defining principle is one of job performance or "job oriented diagnosis"; that is, the problem is diagnosed and the individual referred to treatment on the basis of job performance rather than on the basis of a diagnosis of alcohol problems (Roman, 1988).

Articles describing the workplace referral model and its implementation in various types of organizations and across different levels of employees are commonly found in journals today. In fact, to describe EAP's as one model is inaccurate because of the extensive differences across programs (Shain and Groeneveld, 1980). However, most descriptions point to a delicate balance between advice and coercion. There is some sentiment that the idealized model is a complicated one that is not easily applied by the variety of supervisors and managers who are currently implementing their version of it. What should also be noted is that the constructive confrontation approach is clearly different from other models of treatment (Roman, 1988), and it can claim to have brought many individuals, as well as new groups of individuals, to treatment.

The Prevalence of Workplace Referrals

There are no accurate data on the numbers of individuals who have entered treatment through EAPs or other workplace programs. The NDATUS collects information on the number of programs that provide EAP services; however, it does not provide statistics on the number of EAP- or other workplace-referred clients. NASADAD (i.e., the SADAP) does not collect these data either; indeed, its sample of public agencies would not be appropriate for such work. At present, then, it is not possible to assess the number of individuals in treatment as a result of workplace referrals.

There are, however, some estimates regarding the number of EAPs. Roman, for example, claims that there are more than 10,000 workplace programs in the United States today (1988:137). The National Survey of Worksite Health Promotion Activities, in its survey of worksites with 50 or more employees, found that, overall, 24 percent of the sites had EAPs. As the size of the organization increased, so did the proportion that had EAPs (14.8 percent of those with 50-99 employees and 51.7 percent of those with 750 or more employees). Although there has been no information collected on how many of these EAPs provided alcohol-related services, researchers in the field claim that the majority of EAPs has a visible emphasis on alcohol programs (Roman, 1988).

It is interesting to note the tremendous variation across states in the proportion of overall treatment units that offer EAP services. Diesenhaus (1989) used the 1987 NDATUS to calculate the overall proportion of each state's public and private units that reported offering EAP services. At the low end of the range were Puerto Rico (4 percent), Hawaii (17 percent), Colorado (20 percent), Arizona (23 percent), Massachusetts (23 percent), Connecticut (26 percent), California (28 percent), Texas (28 percent), and Oregon (29 percent). At the high end of the range were South Carolina (69 percent), Idaho (64 percent), Wyoming (61 percent), New Hampshire (56 percent), Iowa (55 percent), Maine (54 percent), North Carolina (54 percent), Montana (53 percent), South Dakota (52 percent), and Vermont (50 percent). The mean was 35 percent. Thus, states differ greatly in the proportion of units that specialize in or at least include work-initiated referrals.

Early Intervention Programs

At the end of the coercion continuum are early intervention or family intervention programs. This approach was begun and first documented by V. E. Johnson (1980, 1986), but it has become an increasingly popular and formalized method throughout the United States (Logan, 1983). Early or family intervention programs are a sophisticated development in institutionalizing and perhaps accelerating the natural process that has often occurred within families to persuade a family member who is having a problem to enter treatment. The approach is defined in terms of a process, and it typically begins with the identification of a "concerned person." It then involves other relatives and friends of the "chemically dependent person" in a structured, well-rehearsed process that the Johnson Institute (1987) describes as follows:

1) Gather together people who are very meaningful to the chemically dependent person and who are concerned about his alcohol/drug use. These people can be spouses, children, other relatives, close friends, ministers, doctors, or employers.

2) Have those people make written lists of specific data about the person's alcohol/drug use and its effects as well as their feeling responses.

3) Have the concerned persons decide upon a specific treatment plan that they expect the chemically dependent person to accept.

4) Have the concerned persons decide beforehand what they will do if the chemically dependent person rejects all forms of help.

5) Meet as a group with the chemically dependent person and present the data and recommendations in an objective, caring, nonjudgmental manner.

Workshops that teach this kind of intervention are numerous (see, for example, Faulkner Training Institute, 1983; Johnson Institute, 1983; Scripps Memorial Hospital, 1984). The approach is unique in that the "concerned person" rather than the person with alcoholic problems remains the client. Advocates of these programs claim that the process is helpful to the concerned persons, as well as to the alcoholic, in that they are educated and empowered by it. Most of the literature suggests that the interventions are conducted by staff within specific treatment programs; if the individual enters treatment it is most often in that particular program (rather than being referred to another program). These programs are most often found in the private sector. There are no statistics to indicate the number of individuals who have entered treatment as a result of these methods and no data on treatment outcome.

The Distribution of Criminal Justice and Employee Assistance Program Referrals: Public Versus Private Programs

There is some agreement that criminal justice referrals are more commonly found in public alcohol treatment programs whereas workplace referrals are more common in private treatment programs. Using the NDATUS data, Yahr (1988) reported that EAP referrals were predominantly located in private for-profit agencies (and in federal programs). They were seldom found in nonprofit and state or local alcohol treatment agencies. Programs for public inebriates were almost always placed in public-sector agencies. Jacob (1985) found some indication that publicly funded treatment agencies were not able to compete with those in the private sector for EAP referrals and that most of the competition was within the private sector rather than between it and the public sector.[9]

In her interviews with state and federal treatment officials, Jacob found that, on the whole, public programs had increased the amount of their revenue from third-party payments. This increase may indicate, at least to some extent, a rise in the number of workplace referrals to the system, although at least in California the increase in third-party revenue mainly reflects drinking-and-driving revenue (Weisner, 1986). However, there may be more competition in the future between public and private programs for DWI clients.

For example, Dalen (1987) reported that because of the evaluation and screening done for the courts by private programs, those programs ended up with the majority of drinking drivers and the resulting profits. California counties generally contract with publicly run or private nonprofit programs, but in some cases they also use private for-profit agencies to run their certified DWI programs. Mosse's (1989) comparison of 1982 and 1987 NDATUS data found increases in the number of DWI programs across all sectors. The increases of DWI programs during the five-year period expressed as percentages of total programs were as follows: private for-profit (26 to 43 percent); private nonprofit (30 to 35 percent); state funded (46 to 50 percent); and federally funded (23 to 33 percent). Yahr's (1988) analysis did not include DWI programs.

Coercion Versus Self-Referral

A discussion of coercive practices often raises questions about the concept of self-referral. The health belief models related to treatment entry, on which treatment programs base their education and outreach efforts, describe a process of increasing problems or, using Alcoholics Anonymous parlance, of "hitting bottom" as a basis for seeking help. Concomitantly, however, there has been a realization that most people enter treatment because of some family, health, or job-related pressure. Perhaps as the field has become more self-conscious about its coercion orientation, there has been a tendency to question whether self-referral is or has ever been a concept applicable to the process by which individuals seek treatment.

Yet there is a difference between family pressure on an individual to enter treatment and institutionalized coercion. Although the EAP literature uses the argument that coercion is always involved in treatment entry, it also claims that EAPs increase the number of self-referrals, thus acknowledging a distinction between coercion and self-referral. In fact, the EAP literature uses the concept of self-referral in claiming that, over time, the existence of EAPs has led to information about alcohol problems and resources for treatment and thus to an increasing number of individuals within work organizations who seek help on their own initiative (Roman, 1988). There is some question, however, as to the legitimacy of using the claim of self-referral within any coercive context (Trice and Sonnenstuhl, 1988). Some studies have found that individuals involved in processing with the criminal justice system may present themselves to alcohol treatment agencies as self-referred in a strong effort to gain admittance and avoid harsh criminal justice sanctions (Speiglman and Weisner, 1982). Researchers in the EAP field have also questioned whether informal or subtle coercion may exist in the workplace even for those whose intakes are recorded as self-referred (Heyman, 1976; Roman, 1988; Trice and Sonnenstuhl, 1988). Trice and Sonnenstuhl (1988) label self-referral a "cultural category." That label may be appropriate for this concept, which has been used to advantage by both sides of the coercion debate.

Alcoholics Anonymous and Coercion

Alcoholics Anonymous (AA) has become a frequent referral organization for various departments within the criminal justice system. In some jurisdictions, referrals to AA occur in ways similar to referrals to formal treatment programs (described above). This phenomenon is noteworthy in light of the barriers to this policy, both from criminal justice and within AA. From the perspective of the criminal justice system's usual criteria for diversion, AA is not a treatment program and traditionally has not had the same types of accountability as those programs. Probation officers and other criminal justice representatives have a long history of indirect encouragement to individuals to attend AA. In the past, however, such attendance was most often voluntary and did not affect criminal justice sanctions. In the case of AA, the self-help group has long been an organization that insists on anonymity, on independence from treatment, and on attendance "motivated by a sincere desire"—that is, on a voluntary basis (although it is recognized that many members are initially pressured by someone to attend). In spite of these barriers, however, a shift in policy has occurred. Now, observers in many localities report that courts refer to and expect evidence of attendance at AA as part of an offender's sentence for a variety of crimes, and AA group secretaries sign attendance cards for such individuals (Kramer, 1983; Phillips, 1989; R. Room, Alcohol Research Group, personal communication, 1989). This large criminal justice presence and the issue of monitoring attendance have resulted in substantial debate within the organization (AA, 1987). AA itself has formally commented on the positive and negative aspects of this relationship with criminal justice and suggested guidelines for cooperating with the courts, especially regarding "proof of attendance at AA meetings" (AA, 1987). Increasingly, articles on AA's role in working with criminal justice agencies are found in the literature (Young and Lawson, 1984; Read, 1987). Referrals to AA are made for such groups as drinking drivers, who are often hostile to such referrals and sometimes disruptive in AA meetings (Kramer, 1983; Phillips, 1989).

Unfortunately, data are not available on the number of individuals who attend AA as a result of court referrals. AA's policy of confidentiality includes not keeping records of the number of individuals attending meetings who are required to do so by the courts. Moreover, criminal justice systems do not collect statistics on the number of individuals they refer to AA.

The Epidemiology Of Individuals In Different Diversion Programs

The Criminal Justice-Referred Population

There is a long tradition of epidemiological research on individuals with DWI problems (see Vingilis, 1983 and Donovan et al., 1983 for reviews of earlier research; see Wilson and Jonah, 1985; Hoffmann et al., 1987; and B. Perrine, 1986, for later studies). Overall, the findings have been mixed as to the alcohol diagnosis of this population. Some studies have found the population to be different demographically and diagnostically from the general population, and some have found it to be different from clinical populations. There have been few studies that used comparable questions or even comparable geographic sample frames across the different populations to assess their alcohol problem status. Most often, epidemiological studies of persons with DWI problems have been compared with other clinical studies without the comparison being intrinsic to the overall design of the study. In general, these studies have found the DWI population to be a mixed group that lies somewhere between the clinical and the general population on most drinking pattern and drinking problem measures.

Epidemiological descriptions of DWI populations are especially important as first offenders with DWI problems increasingly enter alcohol treatment, but this new treatment group has only begun to be investigated epidemiologically (Ryan and Segars, 1983; Weisner, 1984; Reis and Davis, 1979; Hoffmann et al., 1987; Stewart et al., 1987). In addition, there has been no significant investigation of the alcohol problem characteristics of other criminal justice referrals. Most studies have taken place within the criminal justice system and are limited to describing the prevalence of individuals with alcohol problems within the various crime categories rather than counting those who go to treatment (Roizen, 1982;

R. Ross and Lightfoot, 1985). The Hubbard team's (1988) analysis of data from the Treatment Outcome Prospective Study (TOPS) found that, in the case of drug treatment, individuals diverted from criminal justice were often referred earlier than were voluntary clients as a result of their drug use and drug-related problems; similar study is needed of individuals diverted as a result of their alcohol problems.

The Employee Assistance Program Population

Despite the large number of individuals who come to alcohol treatment through workplace referrals, there is very little epidemiological information on these persons. There are studies that provide information on the types of occupations reported by individuals in clinical studies (see Fillmore and Caetano, 1982, for a review of these studies). There are also estimates of the prevalence of alcohol problems within some workplaces and studies of employed individuals in some localities (Parker and Farmer, 1988). Yet there are few data on the demographic characteristics and the drinking problems and practices of individuals referred to alcohol treatment through the workplace, especially as they compare with more traditional referrals.

One study claims that the main differences across public and private programs are socioeconomic and that because the private, for-profit programs seem to be intervening with individuals earlier, "those served by private-for-profit and successful non-profit programs may be younger and less dysfunctional than those served by the public-funded programs" (Jacob, 1985:9-10). Other studies have found the employed treatment population to be younger and to have fewer psychosocial problems (Chopra et al., 1979). In his review of the development of the EAP field and his discussion of EAP-initiated self-referrals, Roman raises the question, "To what extent are EAPs generating alcohol-troubled people with few if any signs of addiction, but who desire assistance in altering their life styles?" (1988:156). In sum, the typical EAP referral is younger and, on measures such as employment and education, quite different from the traditional referral.

Treatment Outcome in Coerced Populations

Given the presence of a considerable number of coerced clients in treatment, one would expect to find a substantial body of literature examining the relationship between coercion and outcome. In fact, little is known about that relationship. The existing literature on outcome for coerced clients focuses primarily on samples of drinking drivers and of workplace referrals. As noted earlier, the more general outcome literature indicates that certain sociodemographic characteristics (e.g., age, income, educational levels) influence outcome.[10] In this regard EAPs see the type of referrals who do best in outcome studies as compared with more traditional referrals (Trice, 1983; Roman, 1988). In fact, much of the argument in favor of workplace programs is based on the notion that this group does well in treatment because of its demographic characteristics and lower levels of alcohol problems. These characteristics are in general similar for individuals with DWI problems, especially first offenders (Armor et al., 1978; Weisner, 1984; Stewart et al., 1987).

Studies using samples of coerced individuals vary greatly in regard to the nature of comparison groups and outcome measures, and results have been mixed. For example, DWI studies tend to evaluate the effectiveness of different treatment strategies, or they may compare treatment with criminal sanctions (U.S. Department of Transportation, 1976; Cameron, 1979; Reis, 1981a,b; Stewart et al., 1987). On the whole, these studies have not shown significant differences across different treatment strategies.

Studies with other coerced samples may also lack design consistency. Studies often compare, within a workplace or criminal justice system, coerced and voluntary entrants into treatment; alternatively, results may be compared with other more general outcome studies that have different designs. Chopra and colleagues (1979) found that coerced individuals did better in treatment than others; however, because these individuals were also younger and had fewer psychosocial problems than the comparison group, the results are inconclusive. Smart (1974), on the other hand, reported that individuals who entered treatment voluntarily had higher recovery rates. Freedberg and Johnston (1978) found no outcome differences between employer-coerced and voluntary entrants. These findings are in contrast, however, to the strong positive results claimed by EAPs (see Trice, 1983; Roman, 1988). The review by Kurtz and coworkers (1984) considers the methodological problems in this area of research to be serious enough to discount most existing results. Several reviews of studies of court-referred individuals have found no substantiation to the claim that they do better than individuals who enter treatment voluntarily (Ward, 1979; Fagan and Fagan, 1982). Yet in comparing treated and nontreated criminal justice inmates, the New York State Governor's Task Force on Alcoholism Treatment in Criminal Justice (1986) reported lower recidivism rates for the treated group.

Outcome measures across studies and programs also vary greatly.[11] First, studies of criminal justice- and EAP-referred individuals often measure compliance rather than outcome (Rosenberg and Liftik, 1976; Gurnack, 1986; Peachey and Kapur, 1986; Stitzer and McCaul, 1987). Stitzer and McCaul (1987) reviewed studies on legal contingencies and compliance (i.e., program attendance) and reported that most studies found a relationship; they did not find evidence for a relationship between those findings and outcome.[12] Second, the political and economic realities that shape the structure of treatment and referral paths also result in different outcome goals for programs. For example, agencies that treat individuals with DWI problems are evaluated in the eyes of the public on the recidivism rates of their clients rather than on client drinking levels. Criminal justice studies often use recidivism rates as the outcome measure (New York State Governor's Task Force on Alcoholism Treatment in Criminal Justice, 1986; Colorado State Alcohol and Drug Abuse Division, 1988). Individuals who come to treatment through workplace referrals are technically in treatment because of "work performance" problems rather than levels of drinking. Thus, the factors that contribute to employer satisfaction with an EAP have more to do with job performance than with levels of drinking after treatment. One of the significant EAP studies explicitly states the intended outcomes of these programs: "1) to induce employees to admit their drinking problem and to accept treatment aimed at their rehabilitation, and 2) to improve deficiencies in work performance" (Trice and Beyer, 1984:393). Finally, both criminal justice and EAP referrals have been justified and considered to be successful on the basis of their increasing the number of individuals who receive treatment for alcohol problems, regardless of the outcome of that experience.[13]

Thus, these studies indicate that there are relevant issues to consider in future research. First, what is the appropriate comparison group? Should it consist of those individuals with alcohol problems who are not referred from the criminal justice system or from the worksite? Or should it be alcohol treatment clients who are not coerced to enter treatment? Second, what outcome measures should be used? Should they be based on traditional alcohol treatment measures, including drinking patterns? Or should they be based on treatment goals related to the referral (e.g., improved job performance, lack of DWI recidivism, reduced criminal behavior)? Perhaps compliance alone is an acceptable outcome measure, although more information is needed about the relationship between compliance measures and outcome. As noted in the earlier discussion on the civil commitments, a primary reason for commitment is compliance—to keep the patient in treatment until treatment is finished.

These issues regarding comparison groups and outcome measures reflect the underlying question of which process (therapeutic or social control) is primary. The social control definition might emphasize the nonreferred criminal justice client as the comparison group and include criminal justice-related outcome measures; the therapeutic definition might emphasize the noncoerced treatment client as the comparison group and include traditional alcohol treatment outcome measures. It can be argued that social control is the prevailing process in the case of DWI because studies have shown nontreatment strategies (e.g., drivers' license suspensions) to be more successful than treatment strategies in reducing recidivism rates (H. L. Ross, 1984).

An important next step in such research is the development of theoretical frameworks from which to begin to ask research questions. Some of the behavioral research on contingencies may be useful. Contingency contracting (or contingency management) is based on principles from operant conditioning. Its original form involves a contract between the therapist and the client, with rewards for progress and the removal of rewards or privileges for "slips." Traditionally, this strategy has been used almost exclusively with those who enter treatment voluntarily. Although there are problems with generalizing the method to coerced individuals, coercion can be broadly interpreted to be externally applied contingencies. At present, some of these principles are being used with nonvoluntary substance abuse clients (mainly drug abusers). In addition, some contingency management work with impaired physicians is alcohol related. The community reinforcement model (Hunt and Azrin, 1973; Azrin, 1976; Azrin et al., 1982) is an approach that applies some of the contingency principles to broad areas of the individual's life. It involves developing reinforcements related to drinking in such areas as work, family and other social support networks, and recreation.

Some of the drug research on legal contingencies may be relevant to alcohol, although the results from such studies have been mixed. Stitzer and McCaul (1987) describe drug treatment intervention approaches that include "intensive community supervision with relapse-contingent return to incarceration" and "methadone maintenance treatment either with or without additional criminal justice supervision" (p. 345). They claim, however, that research does not show whether criminal justice contingencies are related to successful outcome or even to compliance and that the generalization of results from parole and probation drug abusers would not indicate optimism. It may well be that such findings reflect different definitions of compliance and contingencies. The Hubbard team's (1988) analysis of TOPS data found compliance (defined as treatment duration) to be important in outcome. They also found that criminal justice-referred clients stayed in treatment longer.

Many contingencies operate in alcohol treatment. As noted earlier, large numbers of people are "pushed" through the treatment door in one way or another. The meaning and measure of that push should be part of assessment and outcome research. The lack of successful treatment for an individual may mean the loss of family, the loss of a job, or a jail sentence. The push through the treatment door frequently also comes without institutional leverage, and it bears consideration as an important variable then as well. For example, in looking at national survey data of individuals who had entered treatment for alcohol problems, Room (1987) found that few people came to treatment without having been pressured by family or friends about their drinking. In their Boston survey, Hingson and colleagues (1982) also found that the pressure exerted by family and friends was important in treatment entry for those who went.

An EAP-referred individual whose supervisor has suggested treatment without any job sanctions is obviously not experiencing the same degree of coercion as a criminal justice referral who has entered treatment as a condition of probation. Thus, the measurement of contingencies would vary greatly. There are also individual differences in the way people respond to contingencies. The types of contingencies relating to coerced clients that have been discussed in this paper include social, economic, career, and legal contingencies. They affect many areas of an individual's life and have a range of import. Depending on the arrangements made between an individual and a program (which are usually common across types of programs), contingencies may vary in length. For some types of problems, they end as soon as treatment begins; for others, they end after the successful termination of treatment; and for still others, they do not end until sometime in the future. The lack of consistent findings across outcome studies may be a function of differences in contingencies or coercion patterns governing entry and discharge from treatment in different programs and populations.

Although these differences are seldom documented when outcome studies are performed, it could be hypothesized that there is a differential effect based on the length of the contingencies. There is some evidence that behavior change does not always last after contingencies are removed (Stitzer and McCaul, 1987). Reis (1981b) conducted one of the few studies of persons with DWI problems using both an untreated control group and different treatment methods, including "contingent deferral of legal sanctions." He found that there were some effects for the latter group but that they were not sustained after sanctions were removed.

Stitzer and McCaul (1987) hypothesize that much of the strength of legal contingencies is related to how quickly and how strongly they are reinforced. In their EAP outcome study, Trice and Beyer (1984) speak of "progressive discipline" as an important part of the process and of the importance of "predictability." There is reason to question whether contingencies can be generally enforced. Individuals in treatment for alcohol problems may be told to attend AA meetings; they may be required to submit to random breathalyzer tests and so on. Yet although there are often certain consequences to their noncompliance, the contingencies have not always been delineated or enforced. For example, a commonly used contingency in DWI programs is referral back to court when program rules are broken. Because the number of these clients is very large, however, the courts have seen alcohol treatment referral as a way of reducing the court load, and they often respond by summarily referring the individual back again to treatment. Gallant (1968) found this to be the case also for individuals charged with public drunkenness whose jail sentence contingencies were not carried out. Another important consideration is whether contingencies are related to positive or negative reinforcement (incentives versus disincentives) (Cox and Klinger, 1988). In applying this notion to coercion, the relevant concept might be that punishment imposes an aversive consequence (e.g., jail, job loss) if a certain condition is not fulfilled (e.g., sobriety, improved work performance). Negative reinforcement removes a positive consequence (e.g., spouse's attention or praise, employer's paycheck) if the condition is not fulfilled.

The factors relevant to treatment entry are an additional area in which contingencies or pressures are an important consideration relative to outcome. Research in this area has predominantly focused on individual psychological factors, but recent work has begun to consider factors that relate to outside pressures as well (Hingson et al., 1982; Weisner, 1988). Assessments of the relationship to outcome of "readiness for treatment" and "treatment motivation" would gain from adding measures of the pressures or contingencies attached to treatment entry. This area of motivational analysis and counseling is expanding (Miller, 1985; Cox and Klinger, 1988). Some of the most recent research builds on the literature from other fields (e.g., smoking cessation) and examines motivational and readiness factors in terms of stages (McConnaughy et al., 1983; Prochaska and DiClemente, 1986). Yet although current research often focuses on factors intrinsic to the individual, it seems important to include extrinsic factors as well.

Many of the assessment inventories and scales—for example, the Alcohol Use Inventory (Wanberg et al., 1977; Wanberg and Horn, 1983)—include adverse consequence items (e.g., "Does your spouse get angry over your drinking?") (Lettieri et al., 1985:104). In addition, some of the clinical intake assessments (e.g., the Addiction Research Foundation's Cross-Study Shared Data Base Intake Interview, McCrady's Project for Alcoholic Couples Treatment Baseline Interview, the Polich team's Alcohol Treatment Center [ATC] Four-Year Follow-up Study] have a number of items relating to legal, job, and family adverse consequences from drinking (Lettieri et al., 1985). These measures, however, seem to focus on these consequences in terms of motivation to do well in treatment or remain sober and assessments of these factors. They do not obtain information on the importance or role of the adverse consequences in encouraging the individual to enter treatment; they also do not assess whether the negative consequences were contingencies to enter treatment or whether they were connected with treatment entry at all. Simply put, what is missing are such items as, "Did your spouse/the court, etc., insist that you come here?" or "Are you glad to be here?" Although the appropriate clinical approach takes the client pool as a given and assesses the motivational factors that affect staying sober, the appropriate policy approach would be to assess the effects of the various types of contingencies on the motivational measures.

Thus, an understanding of the contingencies that affect entrance into treatment, the treatment process, and treatment outcome is important. Rather than understanding coercion as a dichotomous variable of coerced versus noncoerced, there is reason to examine it as a multifaceted concept. The degree of coercion and the types of contingencies vary greatly. The crucial ingredients may include the immediacy, strength, enforceability, duration, and consistency of contingencies. In addition, the relationship of contingencies to treatment readiness, motivation, and other individual factors warrants consideration.

Implications for Alcohol Treatment

As the discussion has shown, in the past 20 years there have been many changes that affect the entry into and the conditions of alcohol treatment, and those changes have not been well documented. As a result, any attempt to understand the effects of those changes is more likely to raise questions than to provide answers.

First, although the data are persuasive that a significant shift has occurred in the manner of entering both public and private treatment, even basic statistics on the size of that change are lacking. The first task is to document the number of individuals who come to treatment by means of the various types of institutionalized coercion. This is not an easy assignment, given the nature of the health care system in the United States and the lack of overall and systematic data collection. Epidemiological data (e.g., sociodemographic characteristics, drinking patterns and problems, other drug use) for the various coerced populations should also be collected. If, for example, individuals in alcohol treatment increasingly have polydrug problems, the nature and prevalence of coercion are likely to be affected because coercion and diversion programs have much more of a footing in the drug treatment field.

A second issue relates to overall access to treatment. Is the treatment system expanding to include these new groups, or are they replacing those traditionally served? National data seem to indicate that the public system has not grown in proportion to the number of new referrals discussed here. The growth in the private sector also does not appear to offer a solution because the private sector provides many of its services to different groups of people (Jacob, 1985; Yahr, 1988). In those instances in which treatment services have expanded to accommodate these new client groups, are the numbers still so large that they overwhelm the alcohol treatment agenda? There appear to be tremendous differences across states in the proportion of services directed toward some of these new treatment groups (Diesenhaus, 1989), but there has been no consideration of the consequences of these differences for access and of the characteristics of treatment populations.

Third, does treatment work for these new groups? Treatment outcome studies are lacking. It is difficult to understand how such a systemwide transformation in treatment could take place without a solid research base. As has been pointed out, the outcome research is sparse and has methodological problems. Behind some of these problems (e.g., interchangeable comparison groups, mixed outcome measures) is the lack of conceptual framing—to the point that there may be no theoretical base even for the existence of these coercive programs. Is the purpose to provide access to new treatment populations so as to intervene in alcohol problems early on? Is it to treat those individuals for whom drinking is related to legal problems? Is it to be more humane, more effective, or even simply more efficient than other sanctions? Is it to solve overcrowding within the criminal justice system? For work referrals, is the primary motivation to treat individuals whose drinking is causing job problems, or is it to fill empty treatment slots? It is simplistic to answer that all of these purposes can be served, because these functions do not easily coexist. Indeed, the conflicts in purpose among the programs can be seen in looking at outcome measures in the research. To some extent, the alcohol treatment system, through these new programs, has taken on broad responsibility for major social problems.

Some of the larger questions relate directly to the functions of treatment (Speiglman, 1984). How far is the alcohol treatment field willing to go in taking on a social control function? Are there contradictions in combining social control and medical functions? For example, is it consistent to define alcohol problems in treatment as health problems, even as disease, and at the same time as deviant behavior? The EAP as well as the criminal justice literature uses both conceptions. Perhaps this inconsistency is the result of treatment referrals based more on individuals' unacceptable behavior than on their health problems.

There are also complex ethical issues regarding coercion that must be addressed by the alcohol field. One concerns the ethics of coercing someone to enter treatment when the effectiveness of that treatment is unknown. This issue is especially important in situations in which assessment for referral to appropriate treatment does not take place. This concern speaks to the lack of outcome research on coerced populations in general, as well as to the lack of outcome measures related more specifically to the different types and levels of coercion. As discussed earlier, individuals who enter treatment under pressure from one institution or another should not lose their rights; they should have alternatives to choose from, including an alternative to treatment itself. A second ethical issue relates to informed consent and the importance of providing the person with a full understanding of the proposed treatment program, as well as what is known about its efficacy. For both of these issues, it seems reasonable to extend the same protections as are granted individuals involved in research projects to persons entering treatment, especially when a person is entering treatment for reasons other than his or her own choosing.

Finally, what will be the long-term effects of the public image of the alcoholic or problem drinker—or the image of who belongs in treatment? Although one hears about celebrities who enter treatment, the mainstream treatment client whose presence is felt in communities across the United States is increasingly seen as deviant. Will the long-term effect of coerced treatment, whether through criminal justice or the workplace, be to erode the hard-won nonstigmatized public perceptions of this problem as a health issue?

This paper has attempted to point out that there are some strong, basic similarities related to coercion in treatment that cut across public and private institutions and across criminal justice and work-related referrals. It has also noted that there are new populations entering treatment, populations that are often entering treatment earlier in their experience of problems than in the past and whose diversity is invigorating the alcohol field and broadening its horizons. These populations also bring with them dilemmas and important overarching questions whose solutions must be vigorously sought if the field is to serve them effectively.

NOTES

1. Gostin (1987) provides an interesting description of the types of powers available for compulsory treatment of drug abusers in the context of testing for the human immunodeficiency virus (HIV) considered to be the cause of AIDS. In so doing he also provides a framework for looking at parallel issues for alcohol. Gostin describes three types of powers: (1) civil commitment, (2) referrals to treatment from the criminal justice system, and (3) public health powers (community health orders).

2. The Stone commitment criteria were developed by Dr. Alan Stone, who became one of the authors of the American Psychiatric Association's model act. His criteria are similar to the provisions of the model act, with two main exceptions: (1) the act does not have a criterion for dangerousness and (2) does not require a determination of incompetence to make a treatment decision (Hoge et al., 1989).

3. The judiciary took action in a number of states during the 1970s, striking down need-for-treatment legislation on the basis of due process and equal protection rights. The following discussions are relevant: Alabama—*Lynch v. Baxley*, 386 F. Supp. 387 (1974); Michigan—*Bell v. Wayne County General Hospital at Eloise*, 384 F. Supp. 1093 (1974); Kentucky—*Kendall v. Truc*, 391 F.Supp. 419 (1975); and Nebraska—*Doremus v. Farrell*, 407 F. Supp. 514 (1975) (Schmidt, 1986).

4. Zusman (1985) also speaks to this issue, saying that the changing of criteria has no practical implication in the real world if the system is not designed to handle the changes.

5. Appelbaum and colleagues (1987) elaborate a further question they consider pertinent to the overall discussion of voluntariness: Is the important issue involuntary versus voluntary treatment, or is it really which type of treatment should a person receive? Should a person who is being committed have the right to decide what type of treatment he or she will receive?

6. Treatment programs within the jails are the oldest interface of criminal justice and treatment. Modern examples date back to the 1940s, but programs in jails can be identified as far back as the early 1900s (Baumohl and Room, 1987).

7. Unlike the alcohol treatment sector, the drug treatment sector has a tradition of compulsory programs. Perhaps as a result of that history, as well as the fact that the drug sector is concerned with drugs as illegal commodities, coercion in treatment entry has not raised the same issues for that field as has been the case for alcohol treatment.

8. The fact of diversion outside of formal diversion programs cannot be overlooked. Informal diversion is found even in the drug treatment system, in which official diversion programs are more the case than in treatment for alcohol problems. For example, Hubbard and colleagues (1988) found that data from five cities involved in the Treatment Outcome Prospective Study (a long-term longitudinal study of drug users who receive treatment from publicly funded programs) indicated more criminal justice-referred clients who were non-TASC clients than TASC clients. They also found that TASC clients were referred earlier in the legal process than non-TASC criminal justice-referred clients.

9. In both of these studies (Yahr, 1988; Jacob, 1985), the distinction between public and private is not always clear because there are some nonprofit agencies in the public and some in the private sector. There are also agencies with mixed funding. It is assumed that "public" includes nonprofit agencies with some public funding to the agency, as opposed to agencies operating solely on a fee-for-service basis.

10. There is a body of outcome research on the treatment of the public inebriate, the group that, in general, lacks the characteristics discussed as most related to successful outcome. Finn (1985) reviewed this literature as part of an assessment of the Uniform Act and pointed out that outcome measures are most often based on recidivism rates in detoxification centers. Although the results are not usually favorable, it also bears mention that these treatments are often brief and custodial (see Chapter 16).

11. Much of the evaluation literature on referrals stemming from the workplace is related to cost-effectiveness. Some short-term studies of employed clients have found that health care costs decrease after they receive treatment (Holder and Hallen, 1981; Holder and Schachtman, 1987) (see Chapter 19).

12. Recently, there have been studies that examine outcome in terms of compliance (treatment completion). For example, the Colorado State Alcohol and Drug Abuse Division (1988) found significantly higher success rates (i.e., lower rearrest rates) among those who completed treatment. In all of these studies, results may

be biased by the characteristics of those who complete treatment and by the types and effect of the different contingencies that are applied.

13. The Walsh team's study (1988) currently in progress is significant in its design and should address some of the issues of concern here. It has three comparison groups: the first is an inpatient program with intensive follow-up and supervision; the second is similar except that those in this group receive outpatient rather than inpatient services initially; and the third involves client participation in selecting one of the two programs.

REFERENCES

Alcoholics Anonymous World Services, Inc. (AA). 1987. A.A. Guidelines: Cooperating with Court, A.S.A.P., and Similar Programs. New York: Alcoholics Anonymous World Services, Inc.

Anglin, M. 1988. The efficacy of civil commitment in treating narcotic addiction. Pp. 8-34 in Compulsory Treatment of Drug Abuse: Research and Clinical Practice, C. G. Leukefeld and F. M. Tims, eds. Rockville, Md.: National Institute on Drug Abuse.

Appelbaum, P. S. 1985. Special section on APA's model commitment law: An introduction. Hospital and Community Psychiatry 36:966-968.

Appelbaum, P. S., C. Lidz, and A. Meisel. 1987. Informed Consent: Legal Theory and Clinical Practice. New York: Oxford University Press.

Armor, D., J. M. Polich, and H. B. Stambul. 1978. Alcoholism and Treatment. New York: John Wiley and Sons.

Atkinson, R. 1985. Persuading alcoholic patients to seek treatment. Comprehensive Therapy 11(11):16-24.

Azrin, N. H. 1976. Improvements in the community-reinforcement approach to alcoholism. Journal of Behavioral Research and Therapy 14:339-348.

Azrin, N. H., R. W. Sisson, R. Meyers, and M. Godley. 1982. Alcoholism treatment by disulfiram and community reinforcement therapy. Journal of Behavioral Research and Therapy 13:105-112.

Baumohl, J. 1986. On asylums, homes, and moral treatment: The case of the San Francisco home for the care of the inebriate, 1859-1870. Contemporary Drug Problems 13:395-445.

Baumohl, J., and R. Room. 1987. Inebriety, doctors, and the state: Alcoholism treatment institutions before 1940. Pp. 135-175 in Recent Developments in Alcoholism, vol. 5, M. Galanter, ed. New York: Plenum Press.

Beis, E. 1983. State involuntary commitment statutes. Maryland Law Review 7(4):358-369.

Bloom, J., J. Bradford, and L. Kofoed. 1988. An overview of psychiatric treatment approaches to three offender groups. Hospital and Community Psychiatry 39:151-158.

Boscarino, J. 1980. A national survey of alcoholism centers in the United States: A preliminary report. American Journal of Drug and Alcohol Abuse 7:403-413.

Brown, B. S., G. Buhringer, C. D. Kaplan, and J. J. Platt. 1987. German/American report on the effective use of pressure in the treatment of drug addiction. Psychology of Addictive Behaviors 1:38-54.

Butynski, W. 1985. State Resources and Services for Alcohol and Drug Abuse Problems: An Analysis of State Alcohol and Drug Abuse Profile Data, Fiscal Year 1984. Washington, D.C.: National Association of State Alcohol and Drug Abuse Directors, Inc.

Butynski, W., N. Record, P. Bruhn, and D. Canova. 1987. State Resources and Services for Alcohol and Drug Abuse Problems, Fiscal Year 1986: An Analysis of State Alcohol and Drug Abuse Profile Data. Washington, D.C.: National Association of State Alcohol and Drug Abuse Directors, Inc.

Cameron, T. 1979. The impact of drinking-driving countermeasures: A review and evaluation. Contemporary Drug Problems 8(4):495-565.

Cameron, T. 1983. Trends in alcohol problems in California, 1950-1979. Pp. 124-145 in Consequences of Drinking: Trends in Alcohol Problem Statistics in Seven Countries, N. Griesbracht, M. Cahannes, J. Moskalewicz, E. Osterberg, and R. Room, eds. Toronto: Addiction Research Foundation.

Carlyle, E. U. 1988. Hospitalization for mental disorders and substance abuse. Texas Bar Journal 51(6):568-574.

Chopra, K., D. Preston, and L. Gerson. 1979. The effect of constructive coercion on the rehabilitative process. Journal of Occupational Medicine 21:749-761.

Christie, N., and K. Brunn. 1969. Alcohol problems: The conceptual framework. Pp. 65-73 in Lectures in Plenary Sessions. Vol. 2 of the Proceedings of the 28th International Congress on Alcohol and Alcoholism. Highland Park, N.J.: Hillhouse Press.

Cohen, I. 1987. Civil commitment: A study of legal intervention. Working paper, Colorado Alcohol and Drug Abuse Division, Colorado Department of Health, Denver, Col.

Colorado Alcohol and Drug Abuse Division, 1988. The effectiveness of education and treatment in reducing recidivism among convicted drinking drivers. Office of Planning and Evaluation, Colorado State Alcohol and Drug Abuse Division, Colorado Department of Health, Denver, Col.

Connecticut State Drug and Alcohol Abuse Criminal Justice Commission. 1988. The drug and alcohol abuse crisis within the Connecticut Criminal justice system. Connecticut State Drug and Alcohol Abuse Criminal Justice Commission, Hartfort, Conn.

Conrad, P., and J. W. Schneider, 1980. Deviance and Medicalization: From Badness to Sickness. St. Louis, Mo.: Moseby.

Cook, L. F., and B. A. Weinman. 1988. Treatment alternatives to street crime. Pp. 99-105 in Compulsory Treatment of Drug Abuse: Research and Clinical Practice, C. G. Leukefeld and F. M. Tims, eds. Rockville, Md.: National Institute on Drug Abuse.

Cox, W. M., and E. Klinger. 1988. A motivational model of alcohol use. Journal of Abnormal Psychology 97:168-180.

Curran, W. J., A. E. Arif, and D. C. Jayasuriya. 1987. Guidelines for Assessing and Revising National Legislation on Treatment of Drug and Alcohol-Dependent Persons. Geneva: World Health Organization.

Dalen, M. 1987. Ethical Considerations in Evaluation and Treatment of Court-Referred Clients. Mission, Kan.: Alcohol and Drug Services, Inc.

Diesenhaus, H. I. 1989. Memo and worksheets on coercion. Prepared for the IOM Committee for the Study of Treatment and Rehabilitation Services for Alcoholism and Alcohol Abuse, April.

Donovan, D., G. A. Marlatt, and P. Salzberg. 1983. Drinking behavior, personality factors, and high-risk driving. Journal of Studies on Alcohol 44:395-428.

Dunham, A. 1985. APA's model law: Protecting the patient's ultimate interests. Hospital and Community Psychiatry 36:973-975.

Durham, M. 1985. Implications of need-for-treatment laws: A study of Washington state's involuntary treatment act. Hospital and Community Psychiatry 36:975-977.

Fagan, R., and N. Fagan. 1982. The impact of legal coercion in the treatment of alcoholism. Journal of Drug Issues 12:103-114.

Faulkner, L. R., H. M. Bentson, and J. D. Bloom. 1989. An empirical study of emergency commitment. American Journal of Psychiatry 146:182-186.

Faulkner Training Institute. 1983. Intervention Workshop. (brochure for a training workshop for alcohol treatment professionals). Austin, Tex.: Faulkner Training Institute.

Fillmore, K., and R. Caetano. 1982. Epidemiology of alcohol abuse and alcoholism in occupations. Pp. 21-88 in Occupational Alcoholism: A Review of Research Issues. NIAAA Research Monograph No. 8. Washington, D.C.: U.S. Government Printing Office.

Finn, P. 1985. Decriminalization of public drunkenness: Response of the health care system. Journal of Studies on Alcohol 46:7-23.

Fox, R. W. 1978. So Far Disordered in Mind: Insanity in California, 1870-1930. Berkeley, Calif.: University of California Press.

Freedberg, E. J., and W. E. Johnston. 1978. Effects of various sources of coercion on outcome of treatment of alcoholism. Psychological Reports 43:1271-1278.

Furst, C., L. Beckman, C. Nakamura, and M. Weiss. 1981. Utilization of Alcohol Treatment Services in California. Los Angeles: Alcohol Research Center, Neuropsychiatric Institute, University of California, Los Angeles.

Gallant, D. M. 1968. A comparative evaluation of compulsory and voluntary treatment of the chronic alcoholic municipal offender. Psychosomatics 9:306-310.

Gilbert, M. J., and R. C. Cervantes. 1987. Alcohol services for Mexican Americans: A review of utilization patterns, treatment considerations and prevention activities. Pp. 61-95 in Mexican Americans and Alcohol, M. J. Gilbert and R. C. Cervantes, ed. Los Angeles: Spanish Speaking Mental Health Research Center, University of California, Los Angeles.

Gilboy, J. A., and J. R. Schmidt. 1979. "Voluntary" hospitalization of the mentally ill. Northwestern University Law Review 66(4):429-453.

Gostin, L. 1987. Public health and police powers available to government to impede the spread of HIV. Working paper. National Institute on Drug Abuse, Rockville, Md.

Grad, F., A. Goldberg, and B. Shapiro. 1971. Alcoholism and The Law. Dobbs Ferry, N.Y.: Oceana Publications, Inc.

Greeman, M., and T. A. McClellan. 1985. The impact of a more stringent commitment code for Minnesota. Hospital and Community Psychiatry 36:990-991.

Gurnack, A. M. 1986. Factors related to compliance to Wisconsin's mandatory assessment policy for alcohol-impaired drivers. International Journal of the Addictions 21:807-812.

Hart, L. 1977. A review of treatment and rehabilitation legislation regarding alcohol abusers and alcoholics in the United States: 1920-1971. International Journal of the Addictions 12:667-678.

Heyman, M. M. 1976. Referral to alcoholism programs in industry: Coercion, confrontation, and choice. Journal of Studies on Alcohol 37:900-907.

Hingson, R., T. Mangione, A. Meyers, and N. Scotch. 1982. Seeking help for drinking problems: A study in the Boston metropolitan area. Journal of Studies on Alcohol 43:271-288.

Hoffmann, N., F. Ninonueve, J. Mozey, and M. Luxenberg. 1987. Comparison of court-referred DWI arrestees with other outpatients in substance abuse treatment. Journal of Studies on Alcohol 48:591-594.

Hoge, S. K., P. S. Appelbaum, and A. Greer. 1989. An empirical comparison of the Stone and dangerousness criteria for civil commitment. American Journal of Psychiatry 146:170-175.

Holder, H., and J. Hallen. 1981. Medical Care and Alcoholism Treatment Costs and Utilization: A Five-Year Analysis of the California Pilot Project to Provide Health Insurance Coverage for Alcoholism. Prepared for the National Institute on Alcohol Abuse and Alcoholism. Chapel Hill, N.C.: H-2, Inc.

Holder, H., and R. Shachtman. 1987. Estimating health care savings associated with alcoholism treatment. Alcoholism: Clinical and Experimental Research 11:66-73.

Hubbard, R. L., J. J. Collins, J. V. Rachal, and E. R. Cavanaugh. 1988. The criminal justice client in drug abuse treatment. Pp. 57-81 in Compulsory Treatment of Drug Abuse: Research and Clinical Practice, C. G. Leukefeld and F. M. Tims, eds. Rockville, Md.: National Institute on Drug Abuse.

Hunt, G. M., and N. H. Azrin. 1973. A community-reinforcement approach to alcoholism. Behavioral Research and Therapy 11:91-104.

Inciardi J. A. 1988. Some considerations on the clinical efficacy of compulsory treatment: Reviewing the New York experience. Pp. 126-139 in Compulsory Treatment of Drug Abuse: Research and Clinical Practice, C. G. Leukefeld and F. M. Tims, eds. Rockville, Md.: National Institute on Drug Abuse.

Jacob, O. 1985. Public and Private Sector Issues on Alcohol and Other Drug Abuse: A Special Report with Recommendations. Rockville, Md.: Alcohol, Drug Abuse, and Mental Health Administration. October.

Johnson, V.E. 1980. I'll Quit Tomorrow. New York: Harper and Row.

Johnson, V. E. 1986. Intervention: How to Help Someone Who Doesn't Want Help. Minneapolis, Minn.: Johnson Institute Books.

Johnson Institute. 1983. Intervention Skill Development Seminar (brochure for a training workshop for alcohol treatment professionals). Minneapolis, Minn.: Johnson Institute.

Johnson Institute. 1987. How to Use Intervention in Your Professional Practice. Minneapolis, Minn.: Johnson Institute Books, Professional Series.

Keilitz, I., and T. Hall. 1985. Some statutes governing involuntary outpatient civil commitment. Maryland Law Review 9(5):378-397.

Keilitz, I., D. Conn, and A. Giampetro. 1985. Least restrictive treatment of involuntary patients: Translating concepts into practice. St. Louis University Law Journal 29:691-745.

Klein, A. 1983. Alcohol, the lubricant of crime. The Judges' Journal 22(4):4-7,55-57.

Kramer, A. 1983. The drunk driver: Where is he heading? The courts need a new sentencing policy to get the alcoholic offender on the right road to recovery. The Judges' Journal 22(4):8-11,63-64.

Kurtz, N., and M. Regier 1975. The Uniform Alcoholism and Intoxication Treatment Act: The compromising process of social policy formulation. Journal of Studies on Alcohol 36:1421-1440.

Kurtz, N., W. Googins, and W. Howard. 1984. Measuring the success of occupational alcohol programs. Journal of Studies on Alcohol 45:33-45.

Lettieri, D. J., J. E. Nelson, and M. A. Sayers, eds. 1985. Alcoholism Treatment Assessment Research Instruments. NIAAA Treatment Handbook Series No. 2. Rockville, Md.: National Institute on Alcohol Abuse and Alcoholism.

Leukefeld, C. G., and F. M. Tims, eds. 1988. Compulsory Treatment of Drug Abuse: Research and Clinical Practice. Rockville, Md.: National Institute on Drug Abuse.

Lewis, J. S. 1987. Fifteen years of alcoholism coverage--1972-1987: The thick and the thin. 16(2)1-8.

Lidz, C. W., E. P. Mulvey, P. S. Appelbaum, and S. Cleveland. 1989. Commitment: The consistency of clinicians and the use of legal standards. American Journal of Psychiatry 146:176-181.

Logan, D. 1983. Getting alcoholics to treatment by social network intervention. Hospital and Community Psychiatry 34:360-361.

Mäkelä, K. 1980. What can medicine properly take on? Pp. 225-223 in Alcohol Treatment in Transition, M. Grant, ed. London: Croom Helm.

McConnaughy, E. A., C. C. DiClemente, J. O. Prochaska, and W. F. Velicer. 1983. Stages of change in psychotherapy: Measurement and sample profiles. Psychotherapy: Theory, Research, and Practice 20:368-375.

Mecca, A. 1975. A state of the art assessment of the treatment alternatives to street crime programs. Doctoral dissertation, School of Public Health, University of California, Berkeley, Calif.

Mestrovic, S. 1983. Need for treatment and New York's revised commitment laws: An empirical assessment. International Journal of Law and Psychiatry 6:75-88.

Miller, W. R. 1985. Motivation for treatment: A review with special emphasis on alcoholism. Psychological Bulletin 98:84-107.

Mosher, J. 1983. Alcohol: Both blame and excuse for criminal behavior. Pp. 437-460 in Alcohol and Disinhibition: Nature and Meaning of the Link, R. Room and G. Collins, eds. Washington, D.C.: U.S. Government Printing Office.

Mosse, P. R. 1989. Growth and Development of the Alcohol Treatment System in the U.S. Prepared for the National Institute on Alcohol Abuse and Alcoholism. Alcohol Research Group, Berkeley, Calif.

New York State Governor's Task Force on Alcoholism Treatment in Criminal Justice. 1986. Alcoholism Treatment in Criminal Justice: Task Force Report to the Governor. Albany, N.Y.: New York State Governor's Task Force on Alcoholism Treatment in Criminal Justice. October.

Parker, D., and G. Farmer. 1988. The epidemiology of alcohol abuse among employed men and women. Pp. 113-129 in Recent Developments in Alcoholism, vol. 6, M. Galanter, ed. New York: Plenum Press.

Peachey, J. E., and B. M. Kapur. 1986. Monitoring drinking behavior with the alcohol dipstick during treatment. Alcoholism 10:663-666.

Perrine, B. 1986. Varieties of drunken and of drinking drivers: A review, a research program, and a model. Alcohol, Drugs, and Traffic Safety—T86, Proceedings of the 10th Annual International Conference on Alcohol, Drugs, and Traffic Safety, Amsterdam, September 9-12.

Perrine, M. W. 1984. Analysis of DUI processing from arrest through post-conviction countermeasures. Vol 1 of An Evaluation of the California Drunk Driving Countermeasures System. Sacramento, Calif.: Research and Development Office, Department of Motor Vehicles.

Phillips, M. 1989. The American criminal justice system and mandates to alcohol treatment: The role of Alcoholics Anonymous. Alcohol Research Group, Berkeley, Calif.

President's Commission on Mental Health. 1978. Appendix. Vol. 4 of the Task Panel Reports Submitted to the President's Commission on Mental Health. Washington, D.C.: U.S. Government Printing Office.

Prochaska, J. O., and C. C. DiClemente. 1986. Toward a comprehensive model of change. Pp. 3-27 in Treating Addictive Behaviors, W. R. Miller and N. Heather, eds. New York: Plenum Press.

Read, E. 1987. The alcoholic, the probation officer, and AA: A viable team approach to supervision. Federal Probation 50(1):11-15.

Reinarman, C. 1988. The social construction of an alcohol problem: The case of Mothers Against Drunk Driving and social control in the 1980s. Theory and Society 17:91-120.

Reis, R. E. 1981a. Analysis of the Court Referral and Random Assignment Process: Internal Validity of the Research Designs—1980 Annual Report, vol. 30. Final Report, DOT HS-806-553. Washington, D.C.: U.S. Department of Transportation, National Highway Traffic Safety Administration.

Reis, R. E. 1981b. Analysis of the Traffic Safety Impact of Educational Counseling Programs for Multiple Offense Drunk Drivers—1980 Annual Report, vol. 5. Comprehensive Driving Under the Influence of Alcohol Offender Treatment Demonstration Project (CDUI). Interim Report, DOT HS-806-555. Springfield, Va.: National Technical Information Service.

Reis, R., and L. A. Davis. 1979. DUI client characteristics: An interim analysis of the random assignment process. Comprehensive driving under the influence of alcohol offender treatment demonstration project, DOT HS-805-587. County of Sacramento Health Department, Sacramento, Calif.

Roizen, J. 1982. Estimating alcohol involvement in serious events. Pp. 179-219 in Alcohol Consumption and Related Problems. Alcohol and Health Monograph No. 1. Washington, D.C.: U.S. Government Printing Office.

Roman, P. 1988. Growth and transformation in workplace alcoholism programming. Pp. 131-158 in Recent Developments in Alcoholism, vol. 6, M. Galanter, ed. New York: Plenum Press.

Room, R. 1980. Treatment-seeking populations and larger realities. Pp. 205-224 in Alcoholism Treatment in Transition, G. Edwards and H. Grant, eds. London: Croom Helm.

Room, R. 1987. The U.S. general population's experiences with responses to alcohol problems. Presented at the Alcohol Epidemiology Section of the International Congress on Alcohol and Addictions, Aix-en-Provence, France, June 7-12.

Rosenberg, C. M., and J. Liftik. 1976. Use of coercion in the outpatient treatment of alcoholism. Journal of Studies on Alcohol 37:58-65.

Ross, H. L. 1984. Deterring the Drinking Driver: Legal Policy and Social Control. Lexington, Mass.: Lexington Books.

Ross, R., and L. Lightfoot. 1985. Treatment of the Alcohol-Abusing Offender. Springfield, Ill.: Charles C. Thomas.

Rubenstein, L. S. 1985. APA's model law: Hurting the people it seeks to help. Hospital and Community Psychiatry 36:968-977.

Ryan, L., and B. Segars. 1983. San Diego County first conviction program population description. Alcohol Program, San Diego County Department of Health Services, San Diego, Calif. January.

Schmidt, L. 1986. The proposed "seriously-deteriorating" commitment standard: Some concerns for California mental health. Working paper, Alcohol Research Group, Berkeley, Calif.

Scripps Memorial Hospital. 1984. Intervention (brochure for a training workshop for alcohol treatment professionals). La Jolla, Calif.: Scripps Memorial Hospital.

Segal, S. P. 1989. Civil commitment standards and patient mix in England/Wales, Italy, and the United States. American Journal of Psychiatry 146:187-193.

Selzer, M. 1958. On involuntary hospitalization for alcoholics. Quarterly Journal of Studies on Alcohol 19:660-667.

Shain, M., and J. Groeneveld. 1980. Employee Assistance Programs: Philosophy, Theory and Practice. Lexington, Mass.: Lexington Books.

Smart, R. 1974. Employed alcoholics treated voluntarily and under constructive coercion: A follow-up study. Quarterly Journal of Studies on Alcohol 35:196-209.

Speiglman, R. 1984. Alcohol treatment and social control: Contradictions in strategies for California's skid rows. Presented at a meeting of the International Group for Comparative Alcohol Studies, Stockholm, October 23-27.

Speiglman, R., and C. Weisner. 1982. Accommodation to coercion: Changes in alcoholism treatment paradigms. Presented at the Annual Meeting of the Society for the Study of Social Problems, San Francisco, September 3-6.

Stewart, K., L. G. Epstein, P. Gruenewald, S. Laurence, and T. Roth. 1987. The California first DUI offender evaluation project: Final report. Prepared for the California Office of Traffic Safety. Pacific Institute for Research and Evaluation, Berkeley, Calif. February.

Stitzer, M. L., and M. E. McCaul. 1987. Criminal justice interventions with drug and alcohol abusers: The role of compulsory treatment. Pp. 331-360 in Behavioral Approaches to Crime and Delinquency, E. K. Morris and C. J. Braukmann, eds. New York: Plenum Press.

Stone, A. A. 1985. A response to comments on APA's model commitment law. Hospital and Community Psychiatry 36:984-989.

Stromberg, C. D., and A. A. Stone. 1983. A model state law on civil commitment of the mentally ill. Harvard Journal on Legislation 20:275-396.

Trice, H. 1983. Treatment and rehabilitation. Pp. 53-58 in The Encyclopedia of Crime and Justice. New York: The Free Press.

Trice, H., and J. Beyer. 1982. Social control in worksettings: Using the constructive confrontation strategy with problem-drinking employees. Journal of Drug Issues 12:21-49.

Trice, H., and J. Beyer. 1984. Work-related outcomes of the constructive-confrontation strategy in a job-based alcoholism program. Journal of Studies on Alcohol 45:393-404.

Trice, H., and W. Sonnenstuhl. 1988. Constructive confrontation and other referral processes. Pp. 159-170 in Recent Developments in Alcoholism, vol. 6, M. Galanter, ed. New York: Plenum Press.

U.S. Department of Transportation. 1976. Vol. 1, Description of ASAP Diagnosis, Referral and Rehabilitation Functions. Vol. 1 of Program Level Evaluation of ASAP Diagnosis, Referral and Rehabilitation Efforts. Final Report, Contract No. DOT-HS-191-3-759. Washington, D.C.: National Highway Traffic Safety Administration.

Vingilis, E. 1983. Drinking drivers and alcoholics: Are they from the same population? Pp. 299-342 in Research Advances in Alcohol and Drug Problems, vol. 7, R. Smart, F. Glaser, Y. Israel, H. Kalant, R. Popham, and W. Schmidt, eds. Toronto: Plenum Press.

Walsh, D. C., R. W. Hingson, and D. M. Merrigan. 1988. A randomized trial comparing inpatient and outpatient alcoholism treatments in industry—a first report. Presented at the Annual Meeting of the Alcohol Epidemiology Section of the International Council on Alcohol and Addictions, Dubrovnik, Yugoslavia, June 9-13, 1986. (updated, January 1988).

Wanberg, K. W., and J. L. Horn. 1983. Assessment of alcohol use with multidimensional concepts and measures. American Psychologist 38:1055-1070.

Wanberg, K. W., J. L. Horn, and F. M. Foster. 1977. A differential assessment model for alcoholism. Journal of Studies on Alcohol 38:512-543.

Ward, D. A. 1979. The use of coercion in the treatment of alcoholism: A methodological review. Journal of Drug Issues 9:387-398.

Weisner, C. 1984. The changing alcohol treatment system: A profile of clients. Presented at a meeting of the International Group for Comparative Alcohol Studies, Stockholm, October 23-27.

Weisner, C. 1986. The transformation of alcohol treatment: Access to care and the response to drinking-driving. Journal of Public Health Policy 7:78-92.

Weisner, C. 1987a. The social ecology of alcohol treatment in the United States. Pp. 203-243 in Recent Developments in Alcoholism, vol. 5, M. Galanter, ed. New York: Plenum Press.

Weisner, C. 1987b. Studying alcohol treatment as a system: Research issues and data sources. Presented at the Alcohol Treatment Service Systems Research panel at the Alcohol and Drug Problems Association National Conference, St. Louis, Missouri, September.

Weisner, C. 1988. The alcohol treatment seeking process from a problem perspective: Responses to events. Presented at the 14th Annual Alcohol Epidemiology Symposium, Kettil Bruun Society, Berkely, Calif., June 5-11.

Weisner, C., and R. Room. 1984. Financing and ideology in alcohol treatment. Social Problems 32:167-188.

Wexler, J. D. 1985. APA's model law: A commitment code by and for psychiatrists. Hospital and Community Psychiatry 36:981-983.

Wilson, J., and B. Jonah. 1985. Identifying impaired drivers among the general driving population. Journal of Studies on Alcohol 46:531-536.

Yahr, H. T. 1988. A national comparison of public- and private-sector alcoholism treatment delivery system characteristics. Journal of Studies on Alcohol 49:233-239.

Young, T., and G. Lawson. 1984. AA referrals for alcohol related crimes: The advantages and limitations. International Journal of Offender Therapy and Comparative Criminology 28:131-139.

Zusman, M. D. 1985. APA's model commitment law and the need for better mental health services. Hospital and Community Psychiatry 36:978-980.

INDEX

D

Data bases. *See also* National Drug and
   Alcoholism Treatment Unit Survey; State
   Alcohol and Drug Abuse Profile
   assessment information, 248-249
   computerization of, 248
   on funding and costs of treatment, 441-444
   outcome information, 316
   on special populations, 350-351
Data-driven treatment selection, 293-294
Day treatment, 104, 123, 133. *See also*
   Intermediate care
   cost-effectiveness of, 460
   mandated insurance and, 430
Delirium tremens, 74
Demographic variables, 256-257, 281, 282, 345
Denoix, P. F., 253
Depression
   and alcohol problems, 385-386
   and matching, 282
   treatment for, 76, 358, 516, 519
   women and, 357
Detoxification, 49, 59, 61, 64, 65, 313, 511-512,
   555
   costs of, 204
   health maintenance organizations and, 434
   insurance coverage for, 71, 464, 468
   managed care and, 436
   Minnesota programs, 114-115
   NDATUS classification, 122-123, 169
   Oregon programs, 418-419
   pharmacotherapies, 73, 74, 515-516
   placement criteria, 472
   prospective payment system and, 421
   setting for, 72
   social model and, 52, 56
   treatment capacity, 170-172
Detoxification centers, 48, 387, 408
Diagnosis, 303. *See also* Assessment,
   pretreatment
   and matching, 281, 282
   psychiatric 251, 358
Diagnosis-related groups (DRG), 61, 204, 420-
   421
Diagnostic Interview Schedule (DIS), 229, 251,
   255, 256
Diagnostic programs, 105
*Diagnostic and Statistical Manual of the American
   Psychiatric Association* (DSM-III-R), 27,
   29-30, 244, 255
Directory of Chemical Dependency Programs
   (Minnesota), 116
DIS. *See* Diagnostic Interview Schedule
Discharge and transfer criteria, 309-310
Discrimination
   against persons with alcohol problems, 413,
   426, 428
   and treatment utilization, 371
Disease, alcoholism as, 51, 385, 408, 559
Disease Concept of Alcoholism (Jellinek), 27-28
Disease and illness, 20, 152
District of Columbia, 415

Disulfiram (Antabuse), 14, 51, 52, 58, 75-76, 589
   matching and, 282
   outcome information, 333
   studies of, 512-514
Disulfiram-ethanol reaction (DER), 75, 76
Domiciliary care, 63, 66, 122, 169, 170
Donwood Institute (Toronto), 331
Dopamine, 77
Doxepin, 76
Drinking drivers, 232, 381-385, 399
   coerced treatment, 156, 534-535, 588-589,
      590, 593-594, 595, 596, 599
   in Mexico, 553
   programs for, 47, 111, 114, 492-493, 522
   as special population, 345, 346, 348, 349
   youth, 388, 389
"Drink-related disabilities," 29
Drinkwatchers groups, 108, 558-559, 567
Drug problems, 3, 102, 257, 348, 587
   in Alcoholics Anonymous membership, 109
   treatment programs, 118, 198
Drug therapy. *See* Pharmacotherapies
DSM-III. *See Diagnostic and Statistical Manual of
   the American Psychiatric Association*
"Dual-diagnosis" patients, 385-386, 387, 516
Duke University Medical Center, 145
DWI. *See* Drinking drivers

E

Early intervention, 45-46, 213, 592-593 *See also*
   Brief intervention
Economic Opportunity Amendments (1968 and
   1969), 410
Edinburgh study, 222, 233
Educational programs, 46, 82, 291
   for college students, 390, 391
   for drinking drivers, 382, 383, 384, 520
Educational settings for intervention, 231-232
Edwards, Griffith, 33
Edwards, Justin, 14
Edwards and Orford study, 221
Effect-altering medications, 512, 514-515
Effectiveness and Costs of Alcoholism Treatment
   (OTA), 1
Elderly
   Medicare and, 419
   as special population, 345, 348, 349, 350, 351,
      352, 364-365
Electrical aversion therapy, 78
Emergency treatment, 65, 66. *See also*
   Detoxification
   health maintenance organizations, 434
   hospital, 229, 406, 481
   for poor, 481
   Uniform Act guidelines, 48, 49
Employee assistance programs (EAP), 68, 111-
   112, 114, 232, 363, 411
   coerced referrals to treatment, 579, 591-592,
      593, 594, 596, 597, 598
   cost offset and, 456
   federal employees, 350

N

O

P